Therapeutic Modalities

Fourth Edition

Chad Starkey, PhD, AT, FNATA
Professor
Coordinator, Division of Athletic Training
Ohio University
Athens, Ohio

F.A. **Davis Company** • Philadelphia

F. A. Davis Company
1915 Arch Street
Philadelphia, PA 19103
www.fadavis.com

Copyright © 2013 by F. A. Davis Company

Printed in the United States of America

Last digit indicates print number: 10 9 8 7 6 5 4 3 2 1

Senior Acquisitions Editor: Quincy McDonald
Developmental Editor: Richard Morel
Manager of Content Development: George Lang
Art and Design Manager: Carolyn O'Brien

As new scientific information becomes available through basic and clinical research, recommended treatments and drug therapies undergo changes. The author(s) and publisher have done everything possible to make this book accurate, up to date, and in accord with accepted standards at the time of publication. The author(s), editors, and publisher are not responsible for errors or omissions or for consequences from application of the book, and make no warranty, expressed or implied, in regard to the contents of the book. Any practice described in this book should be applied by the reader in accordance with professional standards of care used in regard to the unique circumstances that may apply in each situation. The reader is advised always to check product information (package inserts) for changes and new information regarding dose and contraindications before administering any drug. Caution is especially urged when using new or infrequently ordered drugs.

Library of Congress Cataloging-in-Publication Data

Starkey, Chad, 1959-
  Therapeutic modalities / Chad Starkey.—4th ed.
      p. ; cm.
  Includes bibliographical references and index.
  ISBN 978-0-8036-2593-8 (hardcover : alk. paper)
  I. Title.
  [DNLM: 1. Athletic Injuries—therapy. QT 261]

  617.1'027—dc23

                                        2012023681

Preface to the Fourth Edition

Now in its Fourth Edition and 20th year of publication, *Therapeutic Modalities* has evolved to reflect the current status of health-care principles—specifically, its emphasis on therapeutic modalities as primarily an adjunct to active exercise. Concurrent with these changes are deletions and additions to the devices described. As in the prior editions, the text is organized into five sections.

The first two chapters of Section One describe the body's response to injury: the injury response and pain—to provide the context of the therapeutic modalities presented in subsequent sections and the basis for the Development and Delivery of Intervention Strategies (Chapter 3) and the Administrative Considerations (Chapter 4) pertinent to the use of these devices. Chapter 3, authored by Sara Brown, has been updated to include sections on the World Health Organization's International Classification of Functioning, Disability, and Health; developing patient-based clinical questions and outcomes, and searching for and incorporating evidence into patient care.

Section Two consists of two chapters. Chapter 5 addresses the physiological effects of cold and superficial heat. The clinical applications of these techniques are described in Chapter 6. The biophysical effects and clinical application of deep-heating agents—therapeutic ultrasound and shortwave diathermy—are presented in Section Three.

Electrical stimulation is covered in Section Four. The basic principles of electricity and therapeutic electrical currents are presented in Chapter 11, followed by the biophysical effects and the electrical stimulation goals covered in Chapter 12. Chapter 13, Clinical Application of Electrical Agents, describes how to deliver electrical current to the body based on the current's parameters.

Many mechanical agents are described in individual chapters in Section Five: intermittent compression (14), continuous passive motion (15), cervical and lumbar traction (16), massage (17), electromyographic feedback (18), and laser (19). Several long-standing therapeutic techniques, such as infrared and ultraviolet lamps, have been removed. Several techniques that do not demonstrate physiological or clinical efficacy are still included but with the rationale as to why they may be ineffective treatment devices.

This edition continues to build on its tradition of incorporating current research (evidence) into the discussion and limitations of the devices' effects. When relevant, chapters include a discussion of the overview of the evidence supporting or refuting a device's effects. As noted in Chapter 3, reviewing and applying the evidence of therapeutic interventions are less straightforward than diagnostic techniques. My hope is that the information presented here will help students and clinicians in making informed treatment decisions. Likewise, I attempt to instill in the reader the personal responsibility to remain up-to-date in research.

This edition carries over most of the existing features of its predecessor, such as the At a Glance, Treatment Strategies, Practical Evidence, and Clinical Techniques boxes. Examination of Orthopedic and Athletic Injuries have been adapted for use with therapeutic modalities. These helpful bits of evidence have a clinical slant and will, I hope, be easy for students to understand and apply. Schematics of the effect(s) that each type of modality has on physiology and healing response should help remove some of the mystery of how the energy affects healing. New to this edition is a series of Animated Learning Modules, available to students on the text's DavisPlus Web site (at http://davisplus.fadavis.com). These Animated Learning Modules work hand-in-glove with the text to provide a strong visual understanding of key concepts in *Therapeutic Modalities*.

As always, I encourage reader feedback, and I am always willing to respond to questions or help clarify any of this information for instructors or students (but I will not do your homework for you!). Feel free to contact me at scalenes@gmail.com.

Preface to the First Edition

This is an introductory text designed to fill the void between the baseline knowledge of undergraduate student athletic trainers and the information presented in existing therapeutic modality texts. Its scope and content are written in a style that will accommodate a wide range of students with varying educational backgrounds. The presentation of these modalities has a strong slant toward their application but not at the expense of theory and research. Traditional application techniques are supported or refuted based on current literature.

The aim was to write this text to the students in a manner that facilitates their comprehension of the material. The information in this text is presented in a sequential manner. Each chapter begins with the "basics" and progresses to higher levels of information. Terms that may be new to the student are defined on the same page for quick reference, and the text also includes a complete glossary. Chapters conclude with a short quiz to measure the student's learning.

The focal point of this text is Chapter 1, which presents the body's physiological and psychological response to trauma. Each subsequent chapter relates how individual modalities affect the injury response process. Chapter 2 discusses the basic physics involved in the transfer of energy.

Specific modalities are categorized by the manner in which they deliver their energy to the body. Chapter 3 presents thermal agents and the diathermies. Chapter 4 covers the principles, effects, and application of electricity. Chapter 5 deals with mechanical agents. Each modality is prefaced by an introductory section that is followed by the specific effects that the energy has on the injury response process. The unit then progresses to the modalities' instrumentation, set-up, and application and concludes with the indications, contraindications, and precautions of its use.

Chapter 6 introduces clinical decision making through the use of the problem solving approach and is supplemented through the use of case studies. The text concludes with a chapter addressing organizational and administrative concerns in the use of therapeutic modalities.

Contributors

Sara D. Brown, MS, ATC
Clinical Associate Professor
Boston University
Boston, Massachusetts

Kerry Gordon, MS, ATC, CSCS
Las Vegas, Nevada

Brian G. Ragan, PhD, AT
Assistant Professor
School of Applied Health Sciences and
    Wellness
Division of Athletic Training
Ohio University
Athens, Ohio

Reviewers

Amanda A. Benson, PhD, ATC
Department Chair, Program Director
Athletic Training
Troy University
Troy, Alabama

Steve Cernohous, EdD, ATC, LAT
Assistant Professor, Clinical Coordinator
Physical Therapy & Athletic Training
Northern Arizona University
Flagstaff, Arizona

Shawn D. Felton, MEd, ATC, LAT
Athletic Training Clinical Education
    Coordinator/Instructor
Physical Therapy & Human Performance
Florida Gulf Coast University
Fort Myers, Florida

Joseph A. Gallo, DSc, ATC, PT
Director, Associate Professor
Sport & Movement Science Department
Salem State University
Salem, Massachusetts

Peter M. Koehneke, MS, ATC
Professor, Director
Sports Medicine, Health & Human
    Performance
Canisius College
Buffalo, New York

Michele D. Pruett, MS, ATC
Clinical Coordinator
College of Physical Activity & Sport Sciences
West Virginia University
Morgantown, West Virginia

Jennifer Volberding, MS, ATC
Instructor
Health, Sport & Exercise Science
University of Kansas
Lawrence, Kansas

Scot A. Ward, MS, ATC
Coordinator of Clinical Education
Physical Education
Keene State College
Keene, New Hampshire

Delaine Young, ATC, LAT
Associate Professor, Assistant Athletic Trainer
Health & Fitness Sciences
Lindenwood University
St. Charles, Missouri

Acknowledgments

The Acknowledgments of the Third Edition concluded with the question whether there would be a Fourth Edition. The cliffhanger is over. This edition is the result of countless hours of work by many people. I thank the staff at F.A. Davis: Senior Acquisitions Editor Quincy McDonald, Developmental Editor Richard Morel, Head of Development George Lang, Associate Development Editor Stephanie Rukowicz, and Marketing Manager Julia Carp. This manuscript would not have been possible without their support and input.

Additional thanks go to Kerry Gordon, Brian Ragan, and Sara D. Brown for their contributions. They worked tirelessly to help improve the quality of the information provided within this text. They certainly accomplished this goal.

Contents

Section THREE

Deep-Heating Agents 167

Chapter 7

Chapter 8

Clinical Application of Therapeutic Ultrasound 189

Chapter 9

Shortwave Diathermy 200

Section FIVE

Mechanical and Light Modalities   303

Chapter 14

Intermittent Compression

Chapter 15

Continuous Passive Motion

Chapter 16

Cervical and Lumbar Traction

Injury Response and Treatment Planning

This section describes the body's physiological and psychological responses

to injury and their subsequent influence on treatment planning. Administrative

factors in the planning and delivery of therapy are also discussed.

Chapter 1

The Injury Response Process

This chapter provides an overview of the body's physical and psychological reactions to stress and injury. It also introduces many of the terms and concepts used throughout the text. The physiological response to trauma and the subsequent healing process are affected by the therapeutic modalities described later in this book. Pain, a major factor limiting function, is presented in Chapter 2.

● Why does a text dealing with therapeutic modalities focus its initial attention on the cell? To understand the purpose and effects of therapeutic modalities, we must first gain a basic knowledge of the body's response to injury. We will see that when therapeutic modalities are applied to living tissue, we are not just treating an ankle or a knee. We are applying **stress** • to the cells that will influence their metabolic function and assist healing.

Few, if any, modalities actually *speed* the healing of an injury. The body heals the injury at its own rate. However, by treating an injury with thermal, electrical, mechanical, or light energy, we attempt to provide the optimal environment for healing to occur. But what is a therapeutic modality? For the purposes of this text, a modality is a form of stress applied to the body for the purpose of eliciting an involuntary physiological response.

Defining the term "therapeutic" is needed to understand the principles behind the application of energy to the body. To be deemed therapeutic, the stress applied to the body must be conducive to the healing process of the injury in its current healing state. The optimum conditions for healing require a balance between protecting the area from further distresses and restoring tissue function at the earliest possible time.[1] The application of a modality at an improper point in its recovery may hinder, if not set back, the healing process. To complete this definition, therapeutic modalities involve the application of the correct form of energy, based on stage of inflammation, that best promotes healing.

To illustrate this concept, consider a lacerated finger. If dirt and grime are allowed to enter the cut, an infection occurs and delays the healing process by hindering the normal physiological healing response. If the area is

---

Stress: A force that disrupts the normal homeostasis of a system.

cleaned, an antibiotic ointment applied, and the wound covered with a dressing, the healing progresses relatively unhindered. Modalities function similarly; we use these devices to influence the body's physiological functions to provide the traumatized tissue with the best healing environment.

■ Stresses Placed on Tissues

Any type of mechanical, chemical, thermal, or emotional force placed on the body can be regarded as stress. Although we often think of stress as only being negative, many of the "stresses" in life are positive. Indeed, to be without stress is to be without life.

Consider the various types of stressors encountered by an athlete: the cardiovascular benefits associated with conditioning, the physical contact associated with sports such as football, the repeated pounding of the feet when running, the emotional elation or anguish related to the outcome of a game, and the damaged ligament tissue associated with an ankle sprain. If stress, regardless of its nature, is applied at a sufficient magnitude, the body undergoes several physiological changes at the cellular (tissue) and **systemic** ● levels.

The Physical Stress Theory describes how tissues react relative to the amount of stress they receive relative to normal[2]:

Physical Stress Level	Tissue Response
None to low	Cell death
Low	Decreased tolerance (e.g., atrophy)
Normal	Maintenance
Moderate (positive overload)	Increased tolerance (e.g., hypertrophy)
High	Injury
Extreme	Cell death

Extremes of physical stress—too low or too high—are detrimental to the body. The primary difference between the two extremes is the amount of time required to result in tissue changes. Too much stress causes a more rapid onset of negative consequences; the effects of too little stress accumulate over time. With a sprain cell death occurs in an instant, while tendinopathy and atrophy occur over time. The Physical Stress Theory explains this relationship as the exposure, calculated as the magnitude (force per unit area), time (duration, frequency, etc.), and direction (increased or decreased stress levels).[2]

While serving as a good theoretical basis for describing a cell's reaction to positive and negative stress, the Physical Stress Theory does not address the effect of injury on the patient's level of function. The outcome—improvement—of the care rendered is the yardstick by which therapeutic interventions are measured. Chapter 3 describes the process of developing and measuring the effectiveness of patient intervention plans.

The General Adaptation Syndrome

In the early 1900s, researchers observed that hospitalized patients shared a common set of symptoms regardless of their **pathology** ●. These symptoms included diffuse aches and pains in the joints, loss of strength, loss of appetite, and an elevated body temperature. These striking similarities led to the conclusion that the body's systems have a common mechanism for coping with stress. This phenomenon, the General Adaptation Syndrome, described three stages of stress response[3]:

1. Alarm stage
2. Resistance stage
3. Exhaustion stage

The **alarm stage,** best exemplified by the "flight-or-fight response," is the body's initial sudden reaction to a change in **homeostasis** ●. The body's systems spring to life, mobilizing its resources to respond to the effects of the stressor by readying its defensive systems. Increased blood supplies are routed to areas needing the resources by elevating the heart rate, cardiac stroke volume, and the force of myocardial contractions. The blood supply to nonessential areas is decreased by **vasoconstriction** ● of the superficial and abdominal arteries. **Cortisol** ● is released into the bloodstream to regulate inflammation, stimulate cellular level energy production, and otherwise help to prepare the body to deal with trauma. Some proteins are broken down into **amino acids** ● in preparation for long fasting periods to provide a potential energy source in the event that injury does occur.

After the alarm stage, there is a plateau in the body's adaptation to the stress: the **resistance stage.** The body continues to adapt to the stressor by using homeostatic resources to maintain its integrity. This is the longest phase of the general adaptation syndrome, lasting many days, months, or years. During this stage of stress response, the individual achieves physiological resistance or, as it is commonly referred to in exercise, "physical fitness."

Systemic: Affecting the body as a whole.

Pathology: Changes in structure and/or function caused by disease or trauma.

Homeostasis: State of dynamic equilibrium in the body and its systems that provides a stable internal environment.

Vasoconstriction: Reduction in a blood vessel's diameter. This results in a decrease in blood flow.

Cortisol: A cortisone-like substance produced in the body.

Amino acids: Building blocks of protein.

When the body can no longer withstand the applied stresses, it reaches the **exhaustion stage.** At this point, one or more of the body's systems cannot tolerate the stress and therefore fails. This stage may also be referred to as the point of distress, the point where the stressors produce a negative effect. Clinically, the exhaustion stage may show itself in the form of traumatic or overuse injuries.

Physical Stress' Relationship to Trauma

People experience beneficial or harmful stresses as a part of everyday life. Harmful stresses may take the form of an **acute** • injury such as a **sprain** •, **strain** •, or fracture. In these types of injuries, the body is overwhelmed by too much force in too short a time (macrotrauma).[4] Distresses may also result from repeated, relatively low-intensity forces, as exemplified by stress fractures, **chronic** • inflammatory conditions, and muscle soreness (microtrauma). Periods of immobilization or inactivity will result in decreased muscle mass and cardiorespiratory function.

The amount of stress applied to the body must be of a proper intensity and duration for the body to develop physiological resistance. If the stimulus is too intense or of too long a duration, the body reacts negatively to the stress, potentially causing injury. In the context of exercise, little (if any) physiological benefit occurs if a person trains at an insufficient intensity and duration. Conversely, if the intensity of the workout is too great, the body is placed in the stage of exhaustion, and injury can occur.

The body has certain mechanisms to balance the effects of positive and negative stressors. According to Wolff's law, bone adapts to the forces placed on it (Box 1-1). This remodeling may be exemplified by the

---

Box 1-1. WOLFF'S LAW

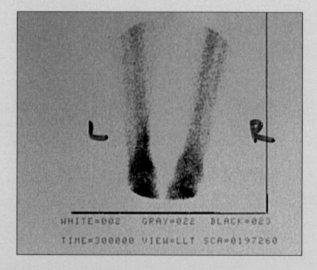

WHITE=002   GRAY=022   BLACK=023
TIME=300000 VIEW=LLT SCA=0197260

Bone scan showing stress fractures of the left foot (dark area).

Bones remodel and adapt to the forces placed on them by increasing their strength along the lines of mechanical stress. Based on fluctuations in the intrinsic electrical current of bones, the osteoblastic and osteoclastic activity changes in response to the presence or absence of functional stress. Bone is removed from sites of little or no stress and is formed along the sites of new stress.

Most commonly, these stresses are caused by compressive, distractive, or shear forces associated with running, throwing, and so on. However, the removal of these stresses can also result in the bone's remodeling itself. If a limb is immobilized, the daily stresses placed on its bones are removed. As a result, the body adapts to the lack of stress by decreasing bone density.

Acute: Of recent onset. The period after an injury when the local inflammatory response is still active.
Sprain: A stretching or tearing of ligaments.
Strain: A stretching or tearing of tendons or muscles.
Chronic: Continuing for a long period; with injury, extending past the primary hemorrhage and inflammation cycle.

deposition of **collagen** • fibers and inorganic salts in response to prolonged presence of stressors. This adaptation is based on the balance between the activities of **osteoblasts,** cells that build bone, and **osteoclasts,** cells that absorb and remove unwanted bone. For example, the repeated physical stresses associated with running increase the rate of osteoblastic activity along the lines of stress. This increased osteoblastic remodeling results in new areas of structural strength and increased bone density. If this stress is applied without time for the body to adapt, osteoclastic activity is greater than osteoblastic activity, resulting in a stress fracture. In contrast, a femur immobilized for 20 days can lose up to 30% of its mineral deposits, causing it to become porous and fragile.[5]

Physical Stress and Its Relationship to Treatment

The principles described by the Physical Stress Theory, the General Adaptation Syndrome, and Wolff's Law also apply to the use of therapeutic modalities. If the intensity of the modality application is too low or the treatment duration is too short, little or no benefit is gained. A 60-degree "cold" pack applied for 5 minutes would not penetrate deeply enough into the tissues to effect change. If the magnitude of the modality is too great, such as a moist heat pack with no covering or if it is applied at the wrong point in the healing process (e.g., during the acute state) further injury occurs.

✳ Practical Evidence

> For any form of therapeutic intervention to be successful it must be applied at the proper intensity for the proper duration to evoke the needed physiological response. These concepts are described by the Arndth-Schultz Principle (see Appendix A).

■ Types of Soft Tissue Found in the Body

This text focuses on epithelial, adipose, muscular, nervous, and connective tissue. This is also the order through which different forms of therapeutic energy must pass to affect the tissues that are the focus of the treatment, the **target tissues.** Based on its cellular structure, each tissue type has unique properties that allow it to reproduce after trauma (Table 1-1). When an injury occurs, the scope and severity of the trauma are generally in direct proportion to the number and type of cells that have been damaged.

TABLE 1-1 Types of Cells Found in the Body

Type	Tissues Where Found	Ability to Regenerate
Labile cells	Skin, intestinal tract, blood	Good
Stable cells	Bone	Some
Permanent cells	Muscle	Some
	Peripheral nervous system	Some
	Central nervous system	None

The regenerative potential and the ability of each of these types of tissues to transmit or absorb various forms of energy must be considered when selecting therapeutic modalities.

Epithelial Tissues

Epithelial tissues line the skin (stratified squamous epithelium), heart and blood vessels (simple squamous epithelium), hollow organs (transitional epithelium), glands, and external openings. This type of tissue is able to secrete and absorb various substances and has the distinction of being devoid of blood vessels. Epithelial tissue has excellent potential to regenerate, a fortunate trait because it is the tissue most commonly injured. Imagine how our bodies would appear if our skin failed to regenerate each time we suffered a minor cut.

The skin's outer layer is formed by the stratum corneum, a layer of flat, densely packed dead cells (Fig. 1-1). Unlike living cells, which are filled with cytoplasm, the stratum corneum cells are filled with keratin, a dry, fibrous protein. This structure forms a barrier that prevents many external substances, such as germs, from entering the body and helps keep the body's fluids inside.

Most forms of energy produced by the therapeutic modalities must pass through the stratum corneum and the remainder of the epidermis, dermis, and adipose tissues to affect the target tissues. Thermal agents initially heat or cool this layer, and the underlying tissues lose or gain heat to each other through **conduction** •. Ultrasonic energy passes relatively easily through the stratum corneum. Because the cells of the stratum corneum are dead and dry, this tissue layer resists electrical stimulating currents and inhibits them from affecting the underlying tissues. **Transdermally** • applied medications must pass through the stratum corneum

---

Collagen: A protein-based connective tissue.
Conduction (thermal): The transfer of heat from a high temperature to a low temperature between two objects that are touching each other.
Transdermal (Transdermally): Introduction of medication to the subcutaneous tissues through unbroken skin.

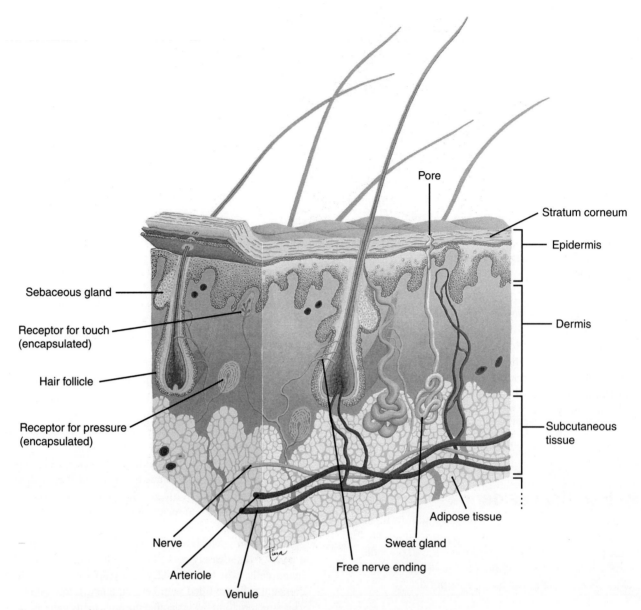

Figure 1-1. **Cross Section of the Skin.** Therapeutic modalities must first penetrate the epidermis, dermis, and subcutaneous adipose tissue before affecting the deeper tissues, including muscle. (From Scanlon, VC: Essentials of Anatomy and Physiology, ed 4. Philadelphia, FA Davis, 2003, with permission.)

by finding portals such as surrounding hair follicles and sweat glands.

Adipose Tissue

Immediately underlying the dermis is a layer of adipose tissue consisting of fat cells. Adipose tissues protects the underlying structures such as the heel and palm from hard blows (see Fig. 1-1). The high water content of adipose tissue makes it an ideal medium for ultrasound to pass through and it is selectively heated during some forms of **diathermy** •. Because the body's fat layering also serves as insulation against heat and cold (and retains heat in the core), the effectiveness of thermal agents such as cold packs or moist heat packs is reduced when they are applied over thick layers of adipose tissue. Therapeutic ultrasound is not significantly affected by the thickness of the adipose tissue layer.

Muscle

Muscle has the ability to actively shorten and to be passively lengthened. Muscles are classified by the function they

---

Diathermy: A classification of therapeutic modality that uses high-frequency electrical energy to heat subcutaneous tissues.

serve: smooth muscle, cardiac muscle, and skeletal muscle. Smooth muscle, which is not under voluntary control, is associated with the hollow organs of the body and the vascular system other than the capillaries. Cardiac muscle is responsible for the pumping of blood. Contraction of skeletal muscle results in the movement of the body's joints. Muscular tissue possesses little or no ability to reproduce duplicates of lost cells.

Skeletal muscle fiber is classified by the intensity and duration of the contraction it can produce or its proportion of contractile properties (Table 1-2). **Type I** muscle fibers are slow to fatigue and are prevalent in postural muscles (e.g., the spinal erector muscles, quadriceps femoris group, gastrocnemius and soleus muscles). **Type II** (fast-twitch) muscle fibers are capable of generating a high amount of force in a short amount of time. Type II fibers are predominant in explosive muscle contractions.

Voluntary muscle contractions are based on the size principle in which small-diameter type I **motor nerves** ● are recruited into the contraction first. When more tension within the muscle is needed, larger diameter type II motor nerves are activated, recruiting more motor units into the contraction. Increased muscular tension is produced by recruiting more **motor units** ● or increasing the frequency with which each unit is depolarized.

Skeletal muscle is frequently injured during athletics, work, or even by the activities of daily living. Despite this relatively high frequency of injury, muscle tissue only has limited ability to regenerate. Muscular tissues are heated or cooled through conduction with the overlying tissues. The flow of warm blood and increased cellular **metabolism** ●, such as that experienced during exercise, also increases the temperature of muscles. Therapeutic ultrasound heats muscle without heating the skin or adipose tissues. In some circumstances, an electrical current can directly cause muscle fibers to shorten, but at the cost of pain. Clinically, electrically induced muscle contractions are caused by depolarizing motor nerves.

Nervous Tissue

Nerves are classified as being in the central or peripheral nervous system. The central nervous system (CNS) includes the brain and spinal cord. The peripheral nervous system (PNS) is formed by all nerves leading to or from the CNS.

TABLE 1-2 Types of Skeletal Muscular Tissues

Type	Fiber Type	Energy Source	Contraction Type
Type I	Slow twitch	**Aerobic** ●	Long duration, low intensity
Type II	Fast twitch	**Anaerobic** ●	Short duration, high intensity
Type II-A	Mixture	Both	Characteristics of both type I and type II
Type II-X	Fast twitch	Anaerobic	Short duration, high intensity

Axon	Function	Diameter	Conduction Velocity m/sec
AFFERENTS			
Ia (A-alpha)	Muscle spindle afferent	12–20 **μm** ●	70–120
Ib (A-alpha)	Golgi tendon afferent	12–20 μm	70–120
II (A-beta)	Touch/pressure afferent Secondary muscle afferent	6–12 μm	30–70
III (A-delta)	Temperature afferent Sharp pain	1–6 μm	6–30
IV (C)	Temperature afferent Dull pain	<1.5 μm	0.5–2
EFFERENTS			
A-alpha	Skeletal muscle efferent	12–20 μm	70–120
A-gamma	**Muscle spindle** ● efferent	2–10 μm	10–50
A-beta	Muscle and muscle spindle efferent	8–12 μm	30–50

Motor nerve: A nerve that provides impulses to muscles.
Motor unit: A group of skeletal muscle fibers that are innervated by a single motor nerve.
Metabolism: The sum of physical and chemical reactions taking place within the body.
Aerobic: Requiring the presence of oxygen.
Anaerobic: Able to survive in the absence of oxygen.
μm: Micrometer, 1/1,000,000 of a meter.
Muscle spindle: An organ located within the muscular tissue that detects the rate and magnitude of a muscle contraction.

The nerves in the PNS are either traumatized during injury or send a signal—pain—that tissue damage has occurred. The pain system and CNS are described in Chapter 2.

Nerves conduct **afferent** ● and **efferent** ● impulses via action potentials. Individual nerve cells, neurons, form the basic functional unit of the nervous system, with three distinct segments forming each neuron: (1) dendrites, which transmit impulses toward (2) the nerve body, and (3) the axon, which transmits impulses away from the nerve body. Nerve impulses are transferred from one nerve to another through a synapse (Fig. 1-2). Although their anatomical and physiological structure and processes are similar, nerves

have specialized functions (Table 1-3). These differences can be exploited by different types of therapeutic modalities for purposes ranging from pain relief to developing stronger muscle contractions.

Synaptic junctions are either electrical or chemical. **Electrical synapses** have a gap junction that allows the nerve impulse to be transferred directly to the next nerve in sequence. Nerves that transmit information toward a synapse are presynaptic neurons; those that transmit the impulse away from the synapse are postsynaptic neurons. As shown in Figure 1-2, a nerve may be both presynaptic and postsynaptic.

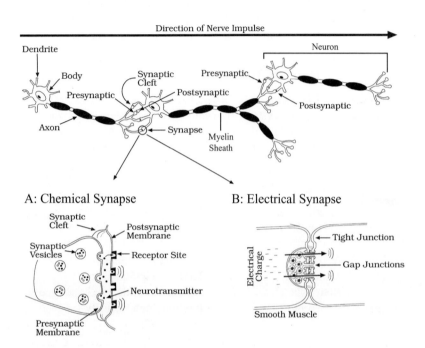

Figure 1-2. **Nerve Transmission.** Nerve impulses originate at the dendrite, pass through the body, and are transmitted along the axon (see Box 1-2 for a discussion of the propagation of nerve impulses). The junction between two nerves is called a *synapse*. Inset A depicts a chemical synapse in which the impulse is **propagated** ● by the release of a neurotransmitter from the presynaptic nerve that crosses the synaptic cleft and binds to a postsynaptic receptor site. Inset B portrays an electrical synapse in which the depolarization of the presynaptic nerve continues directly to the postsynaptic nerve.

TABLE 1-3   Types and Function of Various Peripheral Nerves

Axon	Function	Diameter	Size Group	Conduction Velocity m/sec	Receptor	Stimulus/Action
AFFERENT						
Ia (A-alpha α)	Muscle spindle afferent	12–20 μm	Large	70–120	Proprioceptive	Muscle velocity
Ib (A-alpha α)	Golgi tendon afferent	12–20 μm	Large	70–120	Mechanoreceptor	Length change
II (A-beta β)	Touch/pressure afferent Secondary muscle afferent	6–12 μm	Large	30–70	Cutaneous receptors Proprioceptive Mechanoreceptor	Touch Vibration Hair receptor Muscle length

------

Afferent: Carrying impulses toward a central structure, for example, the brain or spinal cord.

Efferent: Carrying impulses away from a central structure. Nerves leaving the central nervous system are efferent nerves.

Propagate (Propagation): To continue; transmit.

TABLE 1-3	Types and Function of Various Peripheral Nerves—cont'd					
Axon	*Function*	*Diameter*	*Size Group*	*Conduction Velocity m/sec*	*Receptor*	*Stimulus/Action*
III (A-delta δ)	Temperature afferent Sharp pain	1–6 μm	Small	6–30	Mechanoreceptor Thermoreceptors Nociceptor	Touch Temperature change Noxious mechanical and temperature
IV (C)	Temperature afferent Dull pain	<1.5 μm	Small	0.5–2	Nociceptor Mechanoreceptor Thermoreceptor	Noxious mechanical and temperature Touch Temperature change
EFFERENT						
A-alpha (α)	Skeletal muscle efferent	12–20 μm	Large	70–120	N/A	Innervate extrafusal muscle fiber
A-gamma (γ)	Muscle spindle efferent	2–10 μm	Small	10–50	N/A	Innervate intrafusal muscle fiber
A-beta	Muscle and muscle spindle efferent	8–12 μm	Large	30–50	N/A	Inntervate intra- and extrafusal muscle fiber

Most of the body's synapses are **chemical synapses** where a small gap, the synaptic cleft, separates the presynaptic and postsynaptic nerves. A chemical neurotransmitter is released from the presynaptic nerve, spills across the synaptic cleft, and binds into a receptor site on the postsynaptic neuron (Table 1-4). At an excitatory synapse, the neurotransmitter activates the postsynaptic nerve, making it easier for another action potential to occur (an excitatory postsynaptic potential). Activation of an inhibitory synapse makes the postsynaptic nerve more difficult to depolarize, potentially inhibiting its function.

The nerve cell's semipermeable membrane separates opposite electrical charges, creating a voltage difference across the membrane, the **resting potential.** The resting potential is approximately –70 **millivolts (mV)** ● between the inside and outside of the membrane. There is a higher concentration of positively charged particles outside of the membrane and a higher concentration of negatively charged particles inside the membrane. A high outflow of potassium (K+) ions and remaining negatively charged compounds inside the cell's membrane create a negative charge within the cell. Sodium (Na+) outside the membrane creates a positive charge. The cell membrane is more permeable to potassium than it is to sodium. So a greater amount of positively

charged potassium ions move out of the cell and fewer sodium ions move into the cell, resulting in the maintenance of a relatively negative interior. **Depolarization** of the nerve represents an increase in the cell membrane permeability to sodium that evokes an action potential. During depolarization, there is a loss of the negative internal charge when sodium gates in the membrane open and allow a large influx of positively charged sodium ions (Box 1-2).

Repolarization returns the electrical balance to the cell's resting potential. Using adenosine triphosphatase (ATP) for its energy source, the sodium-potassium pump actively transports two potassium ions from outside of the cell back to the inside for every three sodium ions moved from the inside to the outside; the duration of this process is the **refractory period** (Fig. 1-3).

Cells damaged in the CNS are not replaced through the natural human healing process, and their function is lost (although progress has been made in stimulating the regeneration of CNS cells). Nerve cells damaged in the PNS possess some ability to regenerate. Their functions may also be restored by a collateral system where intact nerves sprout toward the damaged tissues.[6] Muscular tissue can fail to heal if intramuscular nerves do not regenerate.[6]

Millivolt (mV): One millivolt equals 1/1,000 of a volt.

TABLE 1-4	**Common Neurotransmitters and Their Functions**

Neurotransmitter	Location	Functions
Acetylcholine	Motor nerves	Transmits motor impulses
Calcitonin gene-related peptide (CGRP)	Central nervous system	Causes vasodilation
		Activates leukocytes
		Reduces pain threshold
Dopamine	Brain stem	Absence results in motor dysfunction
		Increases blood pressure
		Increases cardiac output
		Causes vasoconstriction
Epinephrine	Brain stem	Behavior
		Bronchial dilation
		Emotions
		Mood
		Vasoconstriction
Norepinephrine	Autonomic nervous system	Arousal (flight-or-fight response)
		Dreams
		Mood regulation
		Vasoconstriction
Serotonin	Platelets	Sensory perception
	Mast cells	Sleep
		Temperature regulation
		Vasoconstriction
Substance P	Pain-transmitting nerve fibers	Transmits **noxious** ● impulses
		Produces inflammation-like responses in local tissues

Most therapeutic modalities have some affect on nerve function, primarily by affecting the sodium-potassium pump. Thermal agents and ultrasound influence nerve function by altering their conduction velocities. Slowing the rate of painful nerve transmission or activating touch and pressure but not pain impulses can decrease the perception of pain and can reduce muscle spasm. Most forms of electrical stimulation specifically target sensory, motor, or pain nerve fibers. The electrical stimulus causes a depolarization of these nerves in an orderly, predictable manner.

Connective Tissue

Connective tissues are the most abundant type of tissue in the body. Produced by fibroblasts, connective tissue is formed by **ground substance** ● and collagen fibers that serve as a cement to support and connect the other tissue types.[4,7] This tissue provides strength, structure, nutrition, and defense against trauma for the other tissues. The

fundamental types of connective tissue cells and their function are presented in Table 1-5.

Collagen, the predominant type of connective tissue, is found in high density in fascia, tendons, ligaments, cartilage, muscle, and bone. Eleven types of collagen are found in the body and, with the exception of meniscal cartilage, are highly vascular to aid in their repair (Table 1-6).

Connective tissues' elasticity is determined by the ratio of inelastic collagen fibers to elastic yellow elastin fibers. To illustrate the effect of collagen density and elasticity, consider the difference between muscle and tendon. Muscles are highly elastic and contain a much higher percentage of elastin fibers than collagen fibers. Tendons are relatively inelastic because 86% of their dry weight is collagen.[8] Collagen is also found in other inelastic tissues such as ligaments, fascia, cartilage, and bone.

The fascial network that interconnects the body is another abundant type of connective tissue. Superficial fascia, found between the skin and underlying tissue, normally has a relatively random, loose fibrous arrangement and is not

---

Noxious: Harmful, injurious, or painful. Capable of producing pain.
Ground substance: Material occupying the intercellular spaces in fibrous connective tissue, cartilage, or bone (also known as *matrix*).

Box 1-2. PROPAGATION OF NERVE IMPULSES

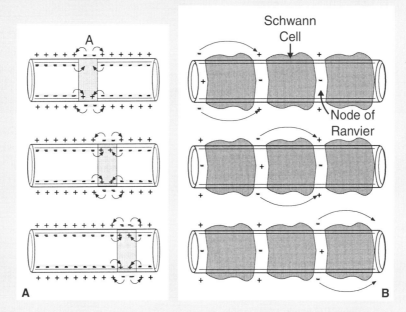

Nerve impulses are created by the depolarization of the nerve cell's membrane. At rest, the outside of the membrane has a positive charge, and the inside has a negative charge. When a stimulus that exceeds the nerve cell's threshold is received, that location in the nerve cell depolarizes and the sodium ions (Na^+) rush inside, causing a reversal of the membrane's polarity. This reversal moves along the membrane in a process called **propagation**. In a healthy nerve, this sequence repeats throughout the length of the nerve cell until the impulse reaches the synapse.

All excitable cell membranes have a different electrical charge between the inside and the outside of the membrane, the resting potential. Action potentials initiated at the nerve's receptor cause a depolarization in the naturally occurring direction (afferently for sensory nerves, efferently for motor nerves). Action potentials that are initiated along the axon will result in the impulse occurring in both directions.

Transmission of impulses in unmyelinated nerves (A) involves depolarization along the length of the axon, a slower and less efficient mechanism than the saltatory conduction mechanism found in myelinated nerves. (B) The axons of myelinated nerves are covered by a fatty myelin sheath (Schwann cells) that is interrupted by the nodes of Ranvier, gaps where the cell membrane is exposed. The myelin sheath, which is 80% fat and 20% protein, serves as an insulator. Depolarization occurs only at the nodes of Ranvier, jumping from one node to the next (*saltare* is Latin for "leap"). Because only selected areas of the axon are depolarized, transmission along myelinated nerves is faster, more efficient, and requires less metabolism than unmyelinated fibers (B).

The nerve's diameter also affects the speed at which the impulse is transmitted. Wider-diameter nerves transmit impulses faster than nerves having a smaller diameter, although small-diameter myelinated nerves have a faster conduction velocity than larger unmyelinated nerves. Small-diameter nerves also have longer refractory periods and lower discharge frequency than wider-diameter nerves.

Each impulse is followed by a refractory period, during which the sodium pathways close and the nerve is allowed to repolarize (see Fig. 1-3). Corresponding to the change in sodium permeability, there is an increased charge within the cell, hyperpolarization. The absolute refractory period represents the period of time (approximately 25% of the total refractory period) during which no additional stimulus, regardless of its magnitude, will trigger another action potential. The absolute refractory period ensures that the nerve can completely recharge before the next action potential is initiated. The length of this period determines the frequency at which the nerve can depolarize. Following the absolute refractory period, there is a relative refractory period during which a stimulus that is stronger than normal can initiate another action potential. A common local anesthetic, Novocain, works by decreasing the nerves' membrane permeability to sodium, preventing it from depolarizing.

The differences in nerve conduction velocities form the basis for the gate-control theory, a fundamental method of pain control.

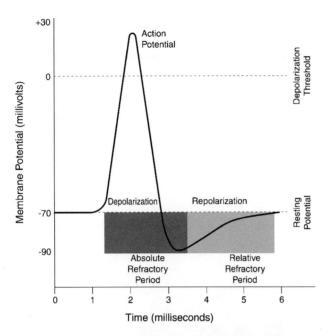

Figure 1-3. Nerve Depolarization and Repolarization. Once a stimulus reaches the depolarization threshold, the nerve will evoke an action potential. Following the depolarization there is a repolarization period. No further stimuli will cause depolarization during the absolute refractory period. During the relative refractory period, the membrane is capable of depolarizing, but it requires a more intense stimulus than the initial depolarization until the resting membrane potential is again reached.

TABLE 1-5	Types of Connective Tissue Cells and Their Function
Tissue Cell Type	*Function*
Fibroblasts	Secretes **extracellular** ● matrix components
Chondrocytes	Produces extracellular matrix components in cartilage
Myofibroblasts	Produces extracellular matrix components with contractile properties
Adipocytes	Stores lipids

as collagen dense and more elastic than deeper fascia. Superficial fascia contains adipose tissue, nerves, and blood vessels. Deep fascia has a high collagen content and the fibers are arranged along the lines of force. More inelastic than superficial fascia, deep fascia is responsible for transferring physical loads of force.

TABLE 1-6	Collagen Fiber Types
Type	*Location*
I	Skin, fascia, tendons, ligaments, bone, fibrous cartilage
II	Hyaline cartilage, elastic cartilage, vertebral disks, vitreous humor (eye)
III	Smooth muscles, nerves, bone marrow, blood vessels (often found with type I)
IV	**Basement membranes** ●
V	Smooth muscle, skeletal muscle
VI	Found in most, if not all, of the body's structures
VII	Basement membranes of skin
VIII	Endothelium
IX	Cartilage (primarily found during fetal development)
X	Mineralizing cartilage (growth plates)
XI	Cartilage, heart, skeletal muscle, skin, brain

✱ Practical Evidence

Superficial collagen can be heated using moist heat; deeper collagen can be heated by ultrasonic energy or diathermy. In both cases, mechanical stretching is required to permanently elongate (stretch) collagen.[9]

■ The Injury Process

The body's reaction to acute injury is divided into two distinct stages. The **primary injury** is associated with the tissue destruction directly resulting from the traumatic force. **Secondary injury** is cell death caused by a blockage of the oxygen supply to the injured area (**ischemia**) ● or caused by enzymatic damage and **mitochondrial** ● failure. Cells need oxygen to survive. If their oxygen supply is cut off they die. This death extends the injury response process. The damage done during the primary stage is irreversible. Treatment efforts used after trauma attempt to limit the amount of secondary injury.

Dead and damaged cells release their contents into the area adjacent to the injured site. The presence of these substances causes an inflammatory reaction from the body's tissues. As a result of both the primary trauma and the

---

Extracellular: Outside the cell membrane.
Basement membrane: Extracellular material that separates the base of epithelial cells from connective tissue.
Ischemia: Local and temporary deficiency of blood supply caused by obstruction of circulation to an area.
Mitochondria: The portion of the cells—the "power plant"—that generates a cell's energy in the form of adenosine triphosphate (ATP).

release of inflammatory **mediators** ●, **hemorrhage** ●, and **edema** ● occur. The buildup of fluids causes mechanical pressure on, and chemical irritation of, the nerve receptors in the area. Because of the clogging of blood vessels, further cell death results from a lack of oxygen being delivered to the surviving tissues. A subcycle occurs as a result of pain and ischemia, causing muscle spasm and increasing the possibility of atrophy over time (Fig. 1-4).

This sequence of events, the **injury response cycle**, is a self-perpetuating process. For the injury to resolve in the least amount of time, this cycle must be controlled to allow healing to occur.

The healing process is described in three phases: (1) the **acute inflammatory response,** (2) the **proliferation phase,** and (3) the **maturation phase.** Although the central events

of each of these phases are marked by distinct responses within a theoretical time frame, there is significant overlap between each phase (Fig. 1-5).

The acute inflammatory response involves the migration of **phagocytes** ● and fibroblasts to the area and the formation of **granulation tissue** ● to isolate and localize the trauma. During this time, **histamine** ● released from the traumatized cells increases capillary permeability, resulting in swelling as the proteins follow water out into the tissues. During the proliferation phase, the number and size of fibroblasts increases, causing ground substance and collagen to collect in the traumatized area in preparation to rebuild the damaged tissues. The injury process is completed during the maturation phase, when collagen and fibroblasts align themselves and attempt to adapt to the original tissue orientation and function, although this does not always occur (Table 1-7).[10]

Phagocytosis occurs in several distinct stages. Neutrophils dominate the first 6 to 24 hours following injury, releasing chemical "grenades" that are intended to destroy bacteria, but end up damaging even healthy tissues in the area. Although the release of neutrophils damages healthy tissues, their presence activates a process that triggers the release of macrophages.[11]

Macrophages, consisting of two types of cells, are responsible for restoring the tissues to their original state ("cleaning up the mess") by specifically targeting necrotic tissues.[6,11] They stimulate the proliferation stage by

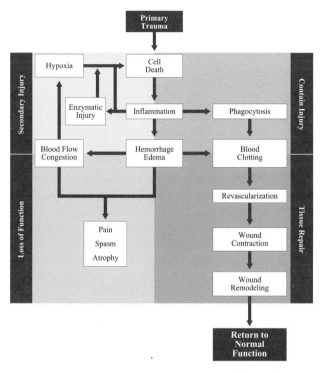

Figure 1-4. **The Injury Response Process.** In traumatic injuries, the primary trauma stems from an outside force and the physical damage inflicted is irreversible. Secondary injury occurs from deprivation of oxygen to the tissues and destructive enzymatic processes. This, combined with pain, spasm, or atrophy, leads to the tissues or body parts losing the ability to function normally. The body begins its road to repair by first containing the injury and then rebuilding the damaged tissue.

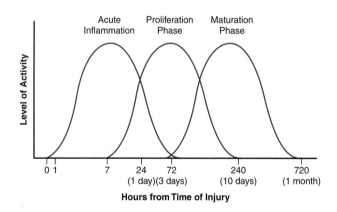

Figure 1-5. **Overlapping Stages of Wound Repair.** There is no clear delineation between the end of one stage of healing and the beginning of the next stage; it is possible for portions of all three stages to overlap. Phase I is the acute inflammatory response stage, phase II is the revascularization stage, and phase III is maturation.

Mediators: Chemicals that act through indirect means.
Hemorrhage: Bleeding from veins, arteries, or capillaries.
Edema: An excessive accumulation of serous fluids.
Phagocyte: A classification of scavenger cells that ingest and destroy unwanted substances in the body.
Granulation tissue: Delicate tissue composed of fibroblasts, collagen, and capillaries formed during the revascularization phase of wound healing.
Histamine: A blood-thinning chemical released from damaged tissue during the inflammatory process. Its primary function is vasodilation of arterioles and increased vascular permeability in venules.

TABLE 1-7	Phases of Wound Healing
Phase	*Events*
Inflammatory phase	Platelet accumulation, coagulation, leukocyte migration
Proliferation phase	Growth of new tissue (re-epithelization), development of new blood vessels (angiogenesis), development of fibrous tissue (fibroplasia), wound contraction, formation of collagen matrix
Maturation phase	Resolution of matrix, deposition of permanent tissues, return to function

releasing **growth factors** ⦁ that activate fibroblasts, increase the number of **satellite cells** ⦁, and stimulate the formation of myofibers.[4]

Acute Inflammatory Response

Inflammation is the body's natural physiological reaction to injury. Triggered by mechanical trauma such as spraining a ligament, bacterial invasion, or burns, the acute inflammatory response mobilizes the body's defensive systems and sets the stage for healing.[12] Inflammation has a bad reputation as an unwanted and unneeded part of the body's response to injury. Nothing could be further from the truth. Inflammation is a necessary part of the healing process. However, if the duration or intensity of the inflammation is excessive, the process becomes detrimental. Chronic inflammation can be a debilitating event. Therapeutic modalities influence the inflammatory response and help to deter its unwanted effects.

✱ Practical Evidence

RICE (rest, ice, compression, and elevation) and PRICE (protection, rest, ice, compression, and elevation) have long been the mainstays of the immediate treatment of musculoskeletal injuries (see Treatment Strategies: Preventing Secondary Injury, page 21. A new theory **POLICE** (protection, optimal loading, ice, compression, and elevation) reexamines this principle. While protection (immobilization) is

indicated immediately following injury, the POLICE method suggests that prolonged immobilization is detrimental to healing. Optimal loading is the early implementation of a "balanced and incremental loading program where early activity encourages early recovery."[13] The mechanical stresses of cyclic loading stimulate cellular responses that encourage tissue healing.

In the initial stages, the inflammatory response contains, destroys, and dilutes the injurious agents and attempts to localize the tissue damage. Pain caused by inflammation alerts the individual that tissue damage has occurred and, combined with **muscle guarding** ⦁ and splinting postures, protects the area from further insult. The movement of plasma and leukocytes to the involved area produces the cardinal signs of inflammation (Box 1-3).

The acute inflammatory response is characterized by the release of inflammatory mediators and the migration of fluids and **leukocytes** ⦁ from the blood into the extravascular tissues in the affected area. The inflammatory response can be divided into three phases, but the exact sequence of cellular events associated with these events depends on the number and type of cells involved; the tissue; and individual factors such as age, nutritional status, and general health status (Table 1-8).[2]

The body is armed with more inflammatory firepower than it normally needs. When physical trauma occurs, the immune system assumes that a bacterial invasion will also occur and triggers the release of neutrophils to counter this threat. Most musculoskeletal injuries do not have a bacterial component, so that portion of the inflammatory response that attempts to contain bacteria damages otherwise viable tissue.

The inflammatory response begins almost immediately following the trauma and persists until the stimulus is removed and the mediators are dissipated or their release into the tissues is inhibited. Acute inflammation may last only a few seconds or may extend for months. Chronic inflammation, discussed later, may persist from months to years. Inflammation, and its role in promoting tissue healing and repair, involves a fine balancing act between too much and too little of a response.

Following a traumatic injury, the cells undergo a primary reaction. This primary phase, also known as the reactive or acute inflammatory phase, is characteristic of the first 2 to 4 days after the injury, although the length of this phase varies. The inflammatory response occurs at two levels: (1) changes in local blood flow (hemodynamic changes) and (2) changes in cellular functioning that

---

Growth factors: Substances that stimulate the production of specific types of cells.

Satellite cell: Spindle-shaped cell that assists in the repair of skeletal muscle.

Muscle guarding: A voluntary or subconscious contraction of a muscle to protect an injured area.

Leukocytes: White blood cells that serve as scavengers.

Box 1-3. CARDINAL SIGNS OF INFLAMMATION

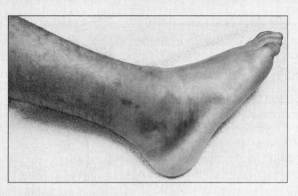

Sign	Associated Inflammatory Events
Heat	Increased blood flow, increased metabolic rate.
Redness	Increased blood flow, increased metabolic rate, histamine release.
Swelling	Leakage of inflammatory mediators into the surrounding tissues, hemorrhage, high concentration of proteins, **gamma globulins** ● and **fibrinogen** ● that block the venous return mechanism; in chronic conditions swelling may represent the proliferation of connective tissue.
Pain	Mechanical pressure on or chemical irritation of nerves, or both; triggered by the release of chemical irritants—bradykinin, histamine, prostaglandin, and other substances—in the inflamed area and increased tissue pressure caused by swelling or muscle spasm, or both.
Loss of function	Primary tissue damage, the sum of preceding signs, muscle guarding.

Five cardinal signs mark the acute inflammatory response. The result of inflammation is the loss of normal function. The magnitude of the patient's inflammation can be clinically quantified based on the amount of swelling, point tenderness, and loss of joint motion.[14] The amount of swelling and loss of range of motion can be measured relative to the uninvolved extremity. Tenderness can be loosely quantified by slight or severe discomfort during palpation, the inability to palpate because of pain, and pain caused by light touch.

TABLE 1-8	Stages of Inflammation After Injury	
Stage	*Process*	*Elapsed Time Since Injury (Days)*
Acute	Reaction to the injury	0–14
Subacute	Symptoms diminish	14–31
Chronic	Unwarranted inflammation	>31 days past the expected resolution

balance the presence of proinflammatory mediators and anti-inflammatory mediators of inflammation.

The primary effect of the inflammatory process is increased cell metabolism. Associated with this are changes in cellular function and the appearance of neutrophils and other granulocytes in the tissues. The outcome following injury is influenced by the balance between proinflammatory mediators and anti-inflammatory mediators of inflammation (Box 1-4).[15] We cannot control inflammation caused by the primary trauma, but we can influence the delivery of leukocytes and proinflammatory mediators by the use of thermal modalities or medications. The sequence of the cellular events differs from tissue to tissue.[16]

Neutrophils are the proinflammatory mediators. Normally flowing in the axial zone of the bloodstream (the middle of the vessel), platelets and neutrophilic leukocytes begin to tumble along the walls of the vessel (**margination**). In a process called **pavementing**, neutrophils adhere to the endothelial lining on the **venule** ● side of the capillary junction. They then escape to the extravascular space. With more severe trauma, red blood cells may also exit into the extravascular space (diapedesis).

Gamma globulin: An infection-fighting blood protein.
Fibrinogen: A protein present in the blood plasma and essential for the clotting of blood.
Venule: A small vein exiting from a capillary.

Box 1-4. MEDIATORS OF INFLAMMATION

Collectively known as mediators, chemicals are released to control a wide range of cellular and vascular events associated with inflammation. Mediators either perpetuate the inflammatory response (proinflammatory mediators) or inhibit the inflammatory response (anti-inflammatory mediators). These two types of mediators must be balanced to control the rate and duration of the inflammatory response.

Some mediators are released by the damaged cells. Other mediators are attracted to the area by **chemotaxis** ●. Some mediators cause **vasodilation** ● of the vessels, increasing the amount of blood, plasma proteins, and phagocytic leukocytes and the speed at which they are delivered to the area. Other mediators increase vascular permeability, allowing the movement of blood proteins and blood cells out of the vessels into the surrounding tissues.

- **Heparin:** Inhibits coagulation by preventing the conversion of prothrombin to thrombin.
- **Histamine:** Located in mast cells, basophils, and platelets. The primary function of histamine is vasodilation of arterioles and increased vascular permeability in venules.
- **Kinins:** A group of polypeptides that dilates arterioles, serves as strong chemotactics, and produces pain. They are primarily involved in the inflammatory process in the early stages of inflammatory hemodynamic changes.
- **Neutrophils:** Formed in the bone marrow, neutrophils are released into the bloodstream and serve the first line of cellular defense. Neutrophils are aggressive phagocytes that damage both insulting cells and viable, needed cells.
- **Prostaglandins:** Formed by **cyclooxygenase** (COX), prostaglandins are responsible for vasodilation and increased vascular permeability. These are synthesized locally in the injured tissues from fatty acids released from damaged cell membranes. Prostaglandins influence the duration and intensity of the inflammatory process. COX is only present in traumatized tissues.

    PGE$_1$: Increases vascular permeability
    PGE$_2$: Attracts leukocytes.

- **Serotonin:** Causes local vasoconstriction.
- **Leukotrienes:** Fatty acids that cause smooth muscle contraction, increase vascular permeability, and attract neutrophils. Includes slow-reacting substance of anaphylaxis (SRSA).

The presence of proteins changes the osmotic relationship between the blood and the adjacent tissues. During the inflammatory response, the protein content of the plasma decreases while the protein content of the **interstitial** ● fluid increases.[17] Water tends to follow the blood proteins out of the vessel through osmosis, resulting in edema. Edema, in turn, increases the tissue pressure, irritating the nerve receptors and blocking capillary flow.

One of the body's first responses to trauma is the localized release of norepinephrine in the traumatized tissues, causing vasoconstriction of the **arterioles** ● and venules to prevent blood loss in the affected area.[1] Capillaries are not formed by smooth muscle, so they do not constrict or dilate. Although the vessels are in the state of vasoconstriction, the **coagulation** ● process begins to repair the primary damage. This initial vasoconstriction is transitory, and in as little as 10 minutes after the injury, the vessels begin to dilate, increasing the volume of blood being delivered to the area.

During normal arteriole flow, blood cells travel in the center of the vessel (axial stream) and plasma flows along the vessel's walls (plasmatic stream), keeping the blood cells away from the walls. After the initial changes in vessel diameter, blood cells flow closer to the walls. As described in the coagulation section of this chapter, this movement of the blood cells toward the vascular walls leads to margination and pavementing of leukocytes.

Gaps form between the **endothelial cells** ● in the capillary beds. The increased space between the cells increases the blood vessel's permeability and allows fluids,

---

Chemotaxis: Movement of living protoplasm toward or away from a chemical stimulus.
Vasodilation: Increase in a blood vessel's diameter. This results in an increase in blood flow.
Interstitial: Between the tissues.
Arteriole: A small artery leading to a capillary at its distal end.
Coagulation: The process of blood clotting.
Endothelial cells: Flat cells lining the blood and lymphatic vessels and the heart.

proteins, and other substances to escape into the surrounding tissue.

As the volume of blood being delivered to the area increases, a protein-rich **exudate** ● is formed in the tissues. The prostaglandin PGE_1 increases vascular permeability, and prostaglandin PGE_2 attracts leukocytes to the area.[18] The fluids and proteins leak into the tissue through the newly formed gaps in the capillaries, depositing leukocytes along the site of the injury to localize and remove any harmful substances.

Swelling occurs as a result of the presence of fluids, proteins, and cell debris in the area. As the amount of swelling increases and the extravascular pressure increases, the vascular flow to and from the area is decreased. The venous and lymphatic networks are blocked, causing further clogging of blood flow to the area and perpetuating the process.

Prolonged inflammation damages the connective tissue by depriving it of nutrients, resulting in thickening of the synovial membrane. When unchecked, this condition can lead to the formation of joint adhesions that affect its **range of motion (ROM).** ● The release of cortisol, as described in the general adaptation syndrome, is effective in reducing the effects of chronic inflammation because of its cortisone-like anti-inflammatory effects.[19]

Hemorrhage

For hemorrhage to occur, one of two prerequisites must be met: the vessel must (1) lose its continuity (be ruptured) or (2) have a marked increase in permeability so that cells and fluids can escape, or said differently, a gradient must be present in which the pressure inside the vessel is greater than the external pressure.[20] For hemorrhage to stop, the reverse of the two conditions must be met: the vessel must be repaired or the pressure gradient must be equalized.

The primary injury inevitably tears the local blood vessels, resulting in hemorrhage. The release of certain inflammatory mediators may increase vascular permeability, also causing hemorrhage. This internal bleeding allows the inflammatory mediators to directly affect the injury site.[6]

Subcutaneous ● hemorrhage is easily recognized by **ecchymosis** ● of the skin associated with bruising. When hemorrhage occurs deeper in the tissues, a **hematoma** ● may form. Because of the depth of the bleeding, it may take hours or days for the discoloration to appear in the skin. In the short term, hematomas assist the healing process by equalizing the pressure gradient between the inside and the outside of the injured vessels, limiting the amount of blood

loss. However, the long-term presence of a hematoma in a muscle can restrict motion and hinder the repair process by perpetuating the inflammatory response.

Even in the best possible scenario, the treatment provided immediately after an injury does not affect primary hemorrhaging. By the time the initial injury occurs and the initial evaluation has occurred and ice is applied, several minutes have passed. In most instances, this time is sufficient for the coagulation process to seal the injured vasculature.[1] The application of cold treatments in this time frame helps limit the amount of secondary injury and decrease pain. External compression (wraps) and elevation helps equalize the pressures inside and outside the vessel, quickly reducing hemorrhage and minimizing the size of the hematoma.[21,22]

✱ Practical Evidence

During acute injury management, cold application has little effect on hemorrhage. As described in Chapter 5, the effects of cold are time- and depth-dependent. This means that the effects of cold will not be realized until approximately 10 minutes following application (at a minimum) as the effects penetrate the tissue layers. External compression may instantaneously reduce hemorrhaging in the traumatized tissues by equalizing the pressure gradients.[22,23]

Coagulation

The inflammatory process encourages the removal of debris and toxic substances from the injured area, and protects the tissues from further damage. Phagocytosis, the body's cellular defense system, involves ingestion of toxic organisms and other foreign particles, and their removal via the lymphatic system. In skin wounds, these wastes may be visible in the form of pus. During this process, scavenger cells, **monocytes** ●, **macrophages** ●, and leukocytes débride the area, devouring toxic and dead tissues by trapping them with arm-like appendages and engulfing them (Fig. 1-6). This entrapment occurs by random chance, but pain-free ROM exercises may increase the level of phagocytic activity.

The repair of the blood vessels, coagulation (blood clotting), involves a cascade of enzymes and consists of the formation of a **platelet** ● plug and the transformation of

---

Exudate: Fluid that collects in a cavity and has a high concentration of cells, protein, and other solid matter.

Range of motion (ROM): The distance, measured in degrees, that a limb moves in one plane (e.g., flexion-extension, adduction-abduction).

Subcutaneous: Beneath the skin.

Ecchymosis: A blue-black discoloration of the skin caused by movement of blood into the tissues. In the latter stages, the color may appear greenish brown or yellow.

Hematoma: A mass of blood confined to a limited area, resulting from the subcutaneous leakage of blood.

Monocyte: A white blood cell that matures to become a macrophage.

Macrophage: A blood cell having the ability to devour particles; a phagocyte.

Platelet: A free-flowing cell fragment in the bloodstream.

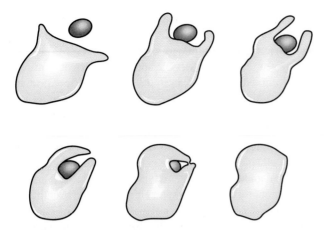

Figure 1-6. **The Process of Phagocytosis.** Scavenger cells randomly collide with vascular debris. Using arm-like appendages, the phagocytes surround, devour, and subsequently remove the waste.

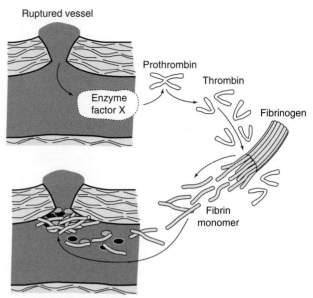

Figure 1-7. **The Process of Coagulation.** Activated by the presence of factor X, prothrombin is broken down into thrombin. In turn, the presence of thrombin causes fibrinogen to unwind into individual fibrin elements, fibrin monomer. Fibrin monomer adheres to the site in the damaged vessel, trapping platelets, red blood cells, and white blood cells. After contraction of the fibrin filaments, a permanent scar is formed.

fibrinogen into **fibrin** •. This is a complex process and is presented in this text only in its basic form.

When a vessel is ruptured, an initial seal is formed by platelets. The platelets and neutrophilic leukocytes flowing in the bloodstream begin to tumble along the walls of the vessel (**margination**). Eventually, these substances adhere to collagen exposed by the trauma, the process of **pavementing**. Because platelets cannot adhere to each other, they release adenosine diphosphate (ADP), which "glues" one layer of platelets to the other. This series of platelet depositions forms an unstable and leaky patch over the rupture site. Further events must occur to form a permanent repair.

The ruptured vessel releases an enzyme that acts as a distress signal, alerting the body that an injury has occurred. A subsequent set of reactions, combined with the platelet deposition, results in formation of a permanent seal. **Prothrombin** •, a free-floating element found in the bloodstream, reacts with the enzyme factor X, converting prothrombin into **thrombin** •. The presence of thrombin in the area then stimulates fibrinogen to unwind into its individual fibrin elements (Fig. 1-7).

Single, activated fibrin filaments, fibrin monomer, are split from fibrinogen and group together with fibronectin and collagen to form a fibrin lattice around the injured area. The fibrin threads trap red and white blood cells and platelets. As the fibrin lattice contracts, it removes the plasma and compresses the platelets, forming a patch to repair the damaged vessel.

Inflammation serves as both an aid and a deterrent to the coagulation process. In general, the inflammatory process encourages the delivery of prothrombin to the injured area by increasing blood flow. However, one of the chemical mediators, heparin, hinders coagulation by preventing prothrombin from being converted to thrombin. A

proper balance must be maintained between heparin and the other mediators. Too much heparin inhibits blood coagulation; too little heparin could result in unwanted blood clots in the vessels (thrombosis).

Proliferation Phase

The proliferation phase is marked by removal of the debris and temporary repair tissue formed during the inflammation stage and by the development of new, permanent replacement tissues. A temporary vascular framework is created to supply the repairing tissues with oxygen, nutrients, and the cells needed to restore the area. This framework remains in place until the wound contraction phase. The exact length of transition from the acute inflammatory response to proliferation is unclear, but it is thought to begin approximately 72 hours after the onset of trauma and may last 3 weeks.[24] The final outcome of the injury response process includes resolution, regeneration, or repair (Table 1-9).[6]

Healing occurs by primary intention or secondary intention. When the tissue damage is minimal, healing occurs by **primary intention**, where a minimal amount of granulation tissue and scar tissue are deposited across the gap. More significant tissue loss, or the involvement of more

---

Fibrin: A filamentous protein formed by the action of thrombin on fibrinogen.
Prothrombin: A chemical found in the blood that reacts with an enzyme to produce thrombin.
Thrombin: An enzyme formed in the blood of a damaged area.

TABLE 1-9	Possible Outcomes of the Injury Response Process

Outcome	Description
Resolution	Dead cells and cellular debris are removed by phagocytosis.
	The tissue is left with its original structure and function intact.
Regeneration	The damaged tissue is replaced by cells of the same type.
	The structure retains some or all of its original structure and function.
Repair	The original tissue is replaced with scar tissue.
	The original structure and function is lost.

complex tissues, requires healing by **secondary intention** that results in an increased amount of granulation tissue and substantial scar tissue formation.

Repair of an injured structure involves the interaction between two types of cells: (1) the cells belonging to the injured structure and (2) connective tissues' cells. In acute trauma, inflammation is an active process where the rate is controlled by the body's metabolism. In chronic conditions, inflammation is a passive process where the body forms new, and possibly unwanted, connective tissues.

Regeneration of tissues occurs when the new cells are of the same type and perform the same function as the original structure. Tissue replacement results when a different type of cell substitutes for the damaged cells, such as scar tissue. Excess scar tissue results in pain and/or loss of function. There is no clear delineation between "repair" and "regeneration." Most tissue trauma is eventually resolved through processes of both regeneration and repair.

The quality of healing is related to the number and type of cells that have been damaged. Labile cells (see Table 1-1), such as those found in the skin, have the best ability to produce a "clone" of the original tissues. In the case of skeletal muscles, the process involves the deposition of fibrous scar tissue that does not replicate the original structure. Evidence suggests that microregeneration can occur following minor skeletal muscle strains and microscopic meniscal tears.[24]

ATP regulates the rate and quality of healing. Serving as the cell's primary source of energy, ATP provides the metabolic energy needed to restore the cell's membrane properties by moving sodium and potassium into and out of the cell and to synthesize and build new proteins.

Soft tissue healing occurs through the proliferation of granulation tissue, requiring four separate but related processes: (1) fibroblast formation, (2) synthesis of collagen, (3) tissue remodeling, and (4) tissue alignment. The growth of granulation tissue requires the presence of fibroblasts, myofibroblasts, and endothelial cells, and is regulated by growth factors produced by platelets and macrophages. In healing muscle the regenerative function provided by satellite cells and myoblasts must be balanced against scar tissue formation and fibrosis mediated by fibroblasts.[4]

Revascularization

The process of repair begins at the periphery, where macrophages and **polymorphs** ●, both of which can withstand the low-oxygen environment, form granulation tissue and produce new capillary beds. These newly formed capillary beds grow around the margin of the wound and gradually work their way toward the center of the injured area, creating a scaffold around which new tissue will be formed. Skin wound repair involves the presence of mast cells. These cells release agents that stimulate fibroblasts and are involved in the remodeling of the extracellular matrix.[25]

Fibroblasts are attracted to the area by the presence of macrophages. Once in the area, fibroblasts begin laying down collagen over the injured structure to create the wound's extracellular matrix.[26] This deposition of collagen is random, with little order in the fibrous arrangement (Fig. 1-8). Stresses, in the form of gentle joint movements, may cause these fibers to arrange themselves in a more orderly fashion.[27]

Wound Contraction

Following revascularization, wound contraction decreases the size of the original fibrin clot. Myofibroblasts accumulate at the margins of the wound and begin to move toward the center. Possessing a high **actin** ● filament content, each new **myofibroblast** ● shortens to pull the ends of the damaged tissues closer together (Fig. 1-9).[25] Fibroblasts produce weak type III collagen, making the area vulnerable to tensile forces. Water is drawn to the area of repair, and blood vessels, proprioceptive nerves, and sensory nerves begin to develop. In superficial wounds, these events form the characteristic "scar."

As the scar tissue matures, it begins to resemble the tissue it is replacing. With time, the strength of the scar is increased by the replacement of the old collagen with a newer, stronger type. Wound contraction should not be confused with a *contracture*, where the tissues' loss of ability to lengthen causes limitation in a joint's ROM. With proper remodeling of the collagen, contractures are avoided.

Polymorph: A type of white blood cell; a granulocyte.
Actin: A contractile muscle protein.
Myofibroblasts: Fibroblasts that have contractile properties.

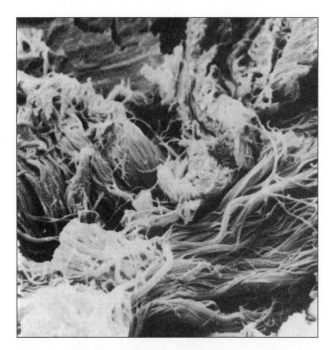

Figure 1-8. **Collagen Replacement.** Shown by means of an electron microscope, new, unorganized collagen can be seen interlacing with older, more densely packed collagen. (From Hunt, TK and Dunphy, JE [eds]: Fundamentals of Wound Management. Appleton-Century-Crofts, New York, 1979, p 38, with permission.)

Wound Remodeling

The body is always remodeling itself. Following trauma, the remodeling stage restores order to the previously deposited scar tissue. The presence of external stress causes the alignment of the fibers to remodel the wound.

Approximately 5 to 11 days following the injury, type III collagen begins to be replaced by stronger type I collagen, resulting in improved **tensile strength** ●.[28,29]

The use of early active ROM exercises can increase the tensile strength of healing ligaments and facilitate both the proliferation and maturation stages of healing.[6,30] Initially, collagen is deposited in a random matrix, causing the scar to be fragile. During remodeling, the fibers form a more organized matrix that increases its strength. However, scar tissue is never as functional as the tissue it replaces.[7] Consider a tear in one of the hamstring muscles. After a small tear, there is usually no residual strength or ROM deficit. After a massive tear in which a large amount of scar tissue is needed for repair, the muscle produces less strength and has decreased ROM.

Because scar tissue is inelastic, it is more similar in structure and function to ligaments and tendons than it is to muscle. Repair of muscular tissue is improved by a mechanism similar to what occurs when muscle hypertrophies in response to strength training. Muscle fiber contains satellite cells that remain dormant in certain muscular tissues. These cells lack the cytoplasm and proteins found in other muscle cells. After an injury, repair of muscular tissue occurs by recruiting satellite cells as the source of nuclei for new muscle cells (Figure 1-10).[31]

Maturation Phase

The maturation phase marks the conclusion of the proliferation phase and is characterized by "cleaning up" the area and increasing the strength of the repaired or replaced tissues. This is the final phase of the injury response process and may last a year or more.

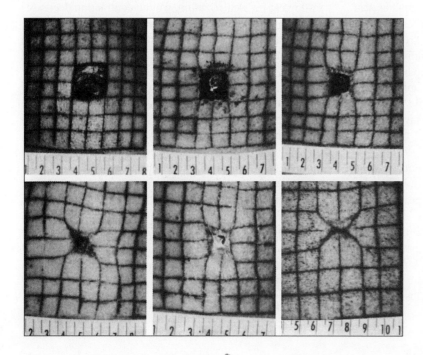

Figure 1-9. **Wound Contraction.** The outer margin of the wound moves toward the center, drawing the ends together. (From Fitzpatrick, TB: Dermatology in General Medicine. McGraw-Hill, New York, 1987, p 330, with permission.)

Tensile strength: The ability of a structure to withstand a pulling force along its length; resistance to tear.

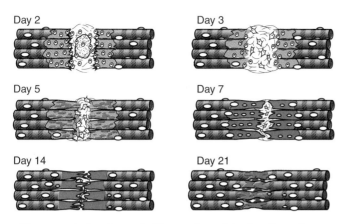

Day 2

Day 3

Day 5

Day 7

Day 14

Day 21

Figure 1-10. **A schematic illustration of the healing of skeletal muscle fibers.**

Day 2: The necrotized parts of the transected myofibers are being removed by macrophages. Fibroblasts have begun to form the connective tissue scar in the central zone (CZ).

Day 3: Satellite cells have become activated in the regeneration zone (RZ).

Day 5: Myoblasts have fused into myotubes in the RZ, and the connective tissue in the CZ has become denser.

Day 7: The regenerating muscle cells extend out of the old basal lamina cylinders into the CZ and begin to pierce through the scar.

Day 14: The scar of the CZ has further condensed and reduced in size, and the regenerating myofibers close the CZ gap.

Day 21: The interlacing myofibers are virtually fused with little intervening connective tissue (scar) in between. (Adapted from Järvinen, TAH, et al: Muscle injuries. Biology and treatment. Am J Sports Med 33:745, 2005.)

At the conclusion of the wound contraction, the number of fibroblasts, myofibroblasts, and macrophages is reduced to the preinjury level. Because these repair agents no longer need to be delivered to the area, the number of capillaries, the overall vascularity of the area, and the water content are reduced. In the case of superficial wounds, these events are indicated by the fading redness of the scar and the eventual return to near-normal skin color and texture.

The proportion of type I collagen continues to increase, replacing the existing type III collagen and other parts of the collagen lattice. As the amount of type I collagen continues to grow, the tissue's tensile strength increases. Because most musculoskeletal injuries are repaired by the replacement of tissues, ever increasing stresses must be applied to the collagen to encourage its proper organization and to allow maximum tensile strength.

Other Possible Consequences of Injury

Depending on the magnitude of the inflammatory response, the tissues involved, and the initial management of the injury, several other consequences of the injury are possible.

Secondary Injury

In the primary injury, cell death is the result of physical trauma and involves multiple types of tissues simultaneously. Cell death following the primary injury is the result of ischemia, a decreased oxygen supply to the area that suffocates the cells. This effect, metabolic or ischemic injury, is also known as secondary hypoxic injury.[32] Secondary enzymatic injury is caused by the release of certain inflammatory mediators.[33]

The primary injury results in ultrastructural changes within the tissues that damage the cell membrane, leading to a loss of homeostasis and **necrosis** ●. Hemorrhaging from damaged vessels, reduced blood flow caused by increased blood viscosity, **hydropic** ● swelling of damaged cells, and pressure from the hematoma and muscle spasm block the supply of fresh blood and result in ischemia. Capillaries in the adjacent areas rupture as the result of interstitial swelling, continuing the cycle by blocking the oxygen supply and killing additional cells. Subsequent cell death blocks more vascular structures, preventing more blood and oxygen from being delivered to the site.

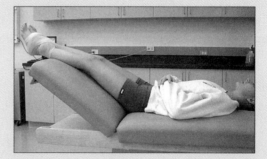

Treatment Strategies
Preventing Secondary Injury

Decreasing the need for oxygen in the injured area and decreasing the amount of blockage of arteriole and venous vessels will limit the amount of secondary injury. The need for oxygen is reduced by decreasing the rate of cellular metabolism through the use of cold application (see Chapter 5). Slowing

(Continued)

Necrosis: Cell death.

Hydropic: Relating to edema; an excessive amount of fluid.

cell metabolism also decreases the amount of secondary enzymatic injury. The blockage of the vasculature may be reduced by limiting the amount of fluids that collect in the area via the use of compression and elevation (see Treatment Strategies: Edema Reduction, page 23).

- Cold application: Reduces cell metabolism, which reduces the cell's need for oxygen that limits secondary hypoxic and enzymatic injury.
- Compression: Decreases hemorrhage and prevents swelling.
- Elevation: Encourages venous and lymphatic uptake and drainage from the extremity.

This phenomenon, metabolic injury, results in the cell's inability to use oxygen and places a dependence on the **glycolytic pathway** ● for ATP production. The inefficiency of this system and the unavailability of needed fuels create an ATP energy shortage that results in sodium-potassium pump failure. Secondary injury is first seen in the mitochondria within 30 minutes following the primary trauma.[32,33]

✳ Practical Evidence

The application of cold packs within 30 minutes following musculoskeletal trauma can decrease the amount of secondary injury.[32]

Enzymes released from the dying cells and the inflammatory mediators can cause secondary enzymatic injury.[33] The resulting changes in the cell membrane structure lead to the loss of the resting membrane potential and hydropic swelling, leading to the death of the cell.

Swelling and Edema

Although the line between swelling and edema is blurred, swelling is the increase in the volume of a body part as the result of fluid buildup. Edema is the buildup of excessive fluids and protein in the interstitial space resulting from the imbalance between the pressures inside and outside the cell membrane, or an obstruction of the

lymphatic return ● and venous return mechanisms. This collection of fluids causes the tissues to expand. The amount of edema that accumulates in the injured area is proportional to:[16]

- The severity of the injury (the number and type of cells damaged)
- Changes in vascular permeability
- The amount of primary and secondary hemorrhaging
- High-pressure gradients
- The presence of chemical inflammatory mediators

Starling's law describes the movement of fluids across the capillary membrane that results in the formation or removal of swelling.[34] Starling's law can be stated as:

1. The vascular hydrostatic pressure and the interstitial fluid colloid osmotic pressure force the contents from the capillary outward to the tissues
2. The plasma colloid osmotic pressure moves fluids from the tissues into the capillaries
3. The limb's hydrostatic pressure is altered by changes in the position of the limb

Normally, the vascular hydrostatic pressure and the plasma colloid pressure are approximately even, keeping the inflow and outflow equal (some return occurs through the lymphatic system). Capillary permeability increases after injury, making it easier for fluids and solid matter to leave the vessels (Fig. 1-11). If the pressure inside the vessels (vascular hydrostatic pressure) exceeds the pressure outside the vessels (plasma colloid osmotic pressure), fluids are forced out of the capillaries into the tissues, and swelling results. Likewise, if the pressure outside the vessels is greater than the pressure inside the vessel, fluids are forced into the vessels to be removed from the area. Most fluids are removed by the venous system, and solids are removed by the lymphatic system.

A limb's hydrostatic pressure depends on its position. When your arm is hanging at your side, its hydrostatic pressure is increased because gravity is pulling the blood distally (toward your fingers). The resulting pressure forces fluids into the interstitial space. When your arm is lifted above your head, the limb hydrostatic pressure decreases, forcing fluids back to your heart. The limb hydrostatic pressure is used to help control and reduce swelling in the extremities. This mechanism is discussed in the following sections.

Glycolytic pathway: A complex series of chemical reaction that yields adenosine triphosphatase from glucose.
Lymphatic return: A return process similar to that of the venous network but specializing in the removal of interstitial fluids.

Treatment Strategies
Edema Reduction

The key to managing edema is preventing it from occurring. Ice, compression, and elevation immediately following trauma discourage the formation of edema (see Chapter 5). The injured structure must be treated with a compression wrap (see Clinical Techniques: Compression Wraps, page 25) between treatment sessions. The patient must be educated regarding the importance of continually wearing the wrap, keeping the extremity elevated whenever possible throughout the day, and sleeping with the limb elevated.

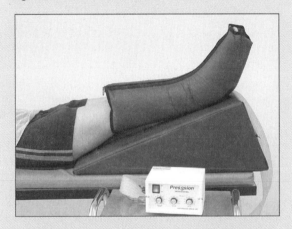

Unfortunately, even the best immediate care does not totally prevent the formation of edema. Once swelling forms, an early treatment goal must be to reduce edema and prevent its other detriments such as pain and decreased range of motion.

The following strategies can be used individually or in tandem to help reduce edema:

- Voluntary muscle contractions
- Elevation
- Compression devices
- Massage
- Electrically induced muscle contractions (muscle milking)
- Passive range of motion
- Compression wraps

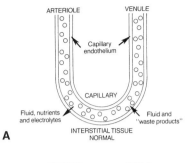

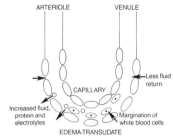

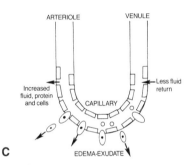

Figure 1-11. **The Formation of Edema.** (A) The normal pressure inside and outside the vessel causes an outward flow of fluids and nutrients at the arteriole end and absorption of wastes at the venule end. (B) The transudate stage. Following an injury, inflammatory mediators cause the arterioles to dilate. The increased capillary filtration pressure moves proteins and fluids into the tissues. (C) The exudate stage. Increased inflammation forces neutrophils and other blood cells out to the tissues, resulting in a thick, edematous fluid formation. (From Michlovitz, SL [ed]: Thermal Agents in Rehabilitation, ed 2. FA Davis, Philadelphia, 1990, p 7, with permission.)

Lymphatic flow is disrupted by edema. The tissues expand to cause the flap valves between the endothelial cells in the capillaries to become separated. The incomplete closure of the valves renders them ineffective by allowing the fluids to drain back into the injured area, increasing pressure within the vein that further decreases the venous return mechanism.[35] The expansion of tissues causes further hypoxic injury by clogging the vascular pathways, preventing the delivery of fresh oxygen-carrying blood.[36] When the limb is placed in a gravity-dependent position, interstitial pressure increases to the point where the lymphatic vessels collapse, further obstructing outflow from the area (Fig. 1-12).[21] Blood that leaves the veins must then be returned via the lymphatic system.

When the delivery of fresh blood and oxygen to the injured structures is blocked, venous and lymphatic return from the site is also inhibited, causing the cycle to continue.[36] The pressure caused by the fluid buildup also causes pain by stimulating mechanical nerve receptors in the area and chemically induced pain by depriving the tissues of oxygen.

Edema contributes to the continuation of the injury response cycle. Exudate clogs the vascular and cellular spaces, increasing tissue pressure and preventing oxygen from reaching the tissues and causing further cell death, pain,

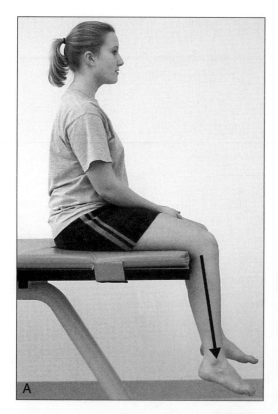
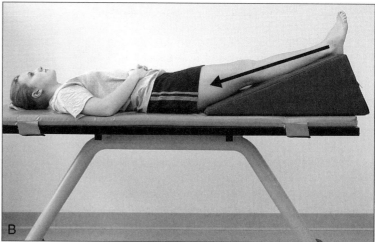

Figure 1-12. **Gravity-Dependent and -Independent Positions.** (A) Gravity-dependent position. Gravity works against venous return. (B) Gravity-independent position. Gravity assists venous return.

and restricted joint motion (Table 1-10).[37] The healing process itself is slowed by delayed cellular regeneration and improper collagen formation. Collagen deposition is increased in the edematous area and, when uncontrolled, leads to **fibrosis** ●, joint contractures, and delayed muscle healing.[38] These factors lead to a decrease in joint ROM, decreased muscular strength, loss of normal function, and eventually, atrophy and fibrosis in the afflicted body part.[37]

A primary goal during early injury management is to decrease the formation of edema and remove swelling from the injury site. Ice application reduces edema formation. Edema is removed by increasing venous and lymphatic return, gravity, increased blood circulation, and compression. The primary mechanism for removing protein from the interstitial space is through the lymphatic system.

✱ Practical Evidence

Compression wraps and stockings primarily serve to reduce acute hemorrhage and prevent venous stasis (pooling) and have little effect on venous return relative to active muscle contractions or intermittent compression.[22,41,42]

TABLE 1-10	Types of Exudate
Type	*Composition/Characteristic*
Serous	Watery consistency common following burns. Also referred to as transudate
Fibrinous	Plasma-rich fluid, especially high in plasma proteins; contains fibrinogen
Suppurative (purulent)	Pus containing dead neutrophils and target organism; abscess
Ulcer	Shredded inflamed tissue and shredded epithelia, leave a crater (ulcer)

Fibrosis: An abnormally large formation of inelastic fibrous tissue.

CLINICAL TECHNIQUES: COMPRESSION WRAPS

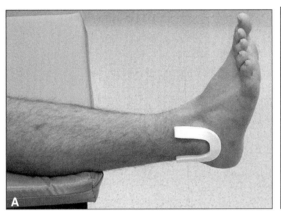

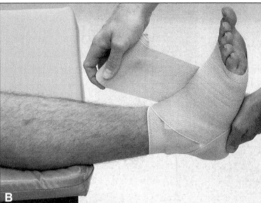

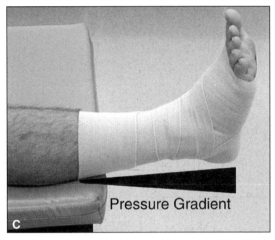

Pressure Gradient

Focal Compression to the Lateral Ankle Ligaments.
(A) A U-shaped "horseshoe" pad is placed around the lateral malleolus. (B) Starting at the metatarsophalangeal joints, apply the compression wrap and work proximally. (C) More pressure is applied at the distal end than at the proximal end, creating a pressure gradient.

Apply the compression wrap starting at the distal extremity and working proximally, gradually decreasing the pressure with each turn. Wraps applied with even pressure throughout their length are often counterproductive because they form a kind of tourniquet, inhibiting flow both to and from the area. Too much compression over superficial veins, such as the popliteal vein in the posterior knee, can elevate peripheral venous pressure and increase the risk of deep vein thrombosis[39,40] Compression is the quickest method to limit hemorrhaging in the injured tissues.

Compression may be applied to an injured area through three different techniques:

1. **Circumferential compression** provides an even pressure around the entire circumference of the body part. The cross-sectional area remains circular, but the diameter of the body part decreases. This type of compression is used for evenly shaped body areas, such as the knee or thigh. Elastic wraps and pneumatic or water-filled sleeves are common forms of circumferential compression.

2. **Collateral compression** produces pressure on only two sides of the body part, so that the cross-sectional area deforms elliptically. The soft tissues are compressed between the device and the bone. A common form of collateral compression is found in air-filled stirrup braces.

3. **Focal compression**, applied with U-shaped "horseshoe" pads, provides direct pressure to soft tissue surrounded by prominent bony structures (e.g., the lateral ligaments of the ankle or the acromioclavicular joint). The pad is placed over the area so that it is in contact with the injured soft tissue while avoiding the bone. A circumferential or collateral compression wrap is then used to apply pressure (see illustration above).

Check capillary refill in the distal extremity (fingers, toes) to ensure that adequate circulation is maintained.

Compression should be applied up to 30 to 40 mm Hg of pressure.[41] To develop a feel for how much pressure is being applied during a compression wrap, inflate a blood pressure cuff to 20 mm Hg and place it on the skin. Then apply an elastic wrap over top of the cuff. When you are finished, observe the value on the sphygmomanometer. Subtract the original value (e.g., 20 mm Hg) from the final value to determine how much pressure was applied. See Chapter 14 for more information on the effects of compression.

Venous or Lymphatic Return

Swelling and edema are reduced by transporting the fluid and solid wastes away from the area through the venous and lymphatic system (the contents of the lymphatic system eventually return to the venous network through the **thoracic duct** ●.[43] Because the mechanisms of these systems are similar, the function of the venous return system is used to describe the process of returning the contents of the lymphatic system from the extremities to the thorax.

The lymphatic and venous return process is passive relative to the arterial system. Changes in blood flow, blood pressure, and heart rate do not affect flow within these systems.[35] In contrast to its influence on arterial blood flow where pressures commonly exceed 80 mm Hg, blood pressure has little effect on returning venous blood to the heart, exerting approximately 15 mm Hg of pressure on the venous system.[20] Pressures working against the venous system increase 1 mm Hg for every millimeter in distance between the right atrium and the extremity.[44,45]

Once the blood passes through the capillaries, the body must rely on respiration, muscle contractions, and gravity to return the blood to the heart. The respiratory process causes venous return during both inspiration and expiration. When we take a breath of air, the diaphragm descends and creates a negative pressure gradient in the chest, causing a siphon-like effect that pulls the blood up the venous system, much like sucking on a straw.

During skeletal muscle contraction, the veins are compressed, reducing their diameter. Because of the function of one-way valves, the blood is forced to move out of the extremity toward the heart. As the force of the contraction is reduced, the one-way valves close, preventing the blood from moving back to its original position (Fig. 1-13).[35,44] During walking, for instance, contraction of the calf muscles, the soleus in particular, increases the local venous pressure to as high as 200 mm Hg.[44,46,47] Certain therapeutic modalities and rehabilitation exercises also can increase venous blood flow (Table 1-11).

The fluids within the venous return system are affected by gravity. Placing the extremity in a gravity-dependent position increases the limb's hydrostatic pressure within the peripheral blood vessels and forces fluids into the tissues (see Fig. 1-12). When the extremity is placed in a gravity-nondependent position (elevated) there is a natural downward flow of the fluids in the vessels. The effectiveness of gravity in returning blood to the heart is based on the angle of the extremity relative to the ground, the diameter of the veins, and blood **viscosity** ●.

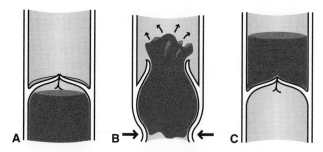

Figure 1-13. Function of One-Way Valves in Veins.
(A) The position of fluids within the vein when the muscle is relaxed. (B) As the muscle contracts, pressure causes the distal portion of the vein to collapse, opening the one-way valves and forcing blood toward the heart. (C) As the muscle relaxes, the valves close, preventing blood from moving back into the area.

	Rate of Femoral Vein Flow Affected by the Application of Various Modalities	
TABLE 1-11	

Technique	Femoral Vein Blood Flow (mL/min)
Passive straight-leg raises	1524
Anatomical CPM	1199
Nonanatomical CPM	836
Active ankle dorsiflexion	640
Pneumatic sleeve	586
Manual calf compression	532
Passive dorsiflexion	385

Adapted from Von Schroeder, HP, et al: The changes in intramuscular pressure and femoral vein flow with continuous passive motion, pneumatic compression stockings, and leg manipulations. Clin Orthop 218, May, 1991.

The maximum effect of gravity occurs when the limb is perpendicular (90 degrees) to the heart and least effective when the limb is horizontal. The effect of the limb's position on gravity influencing venous return is determined by the angle of the limb to the horizontal (Fig. 1-14). Gravity is an impediment to venous return when the long axis of the limb drops below horizontal.

The resistance to blood flow is inversely proportional to the fourth power of the vessel's radius ($1/radius^4$) (Fig. 1-15).[20] Consequently, small changes in the vessel's

---

Thoracic duct: A central collection point for the lymphatic system. The contents of the thoracic duct are routed into the left subclavian vein, where they return to the blood system.
Viscosity: The resistance of a fluid to flow.

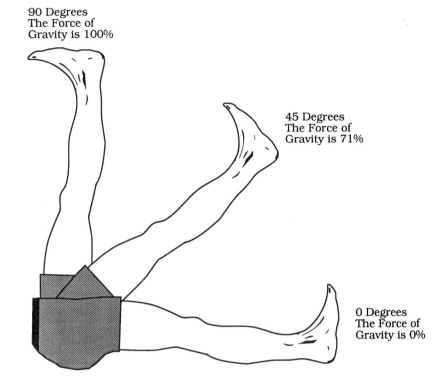

Figure 1-14. **Effect of Gravity on Venous Drainage at Various Limb Positions**. Gravity is most effective when the limb is at 90 degrees and is essentially nonexistent when the limb is parallel to the ground. A compromise between c omfort and function is found when the limb is elevated at a 45-degree angle.

90 Degrees
The Force of
Gravity is 100%

45 Degrees
The Force of
Gravity is 71%

0 Degrees
The Force of
Gravity is 0%

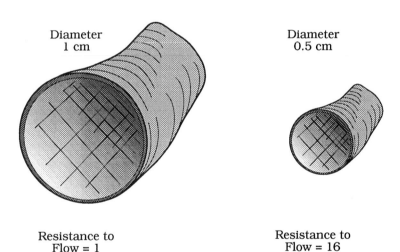

Diameter
1 cm

Diameter
0.5 cm

Figure 1-15. **Vessel's Diameter Relative to Resistance to Blood Flow.** Decreasing the diameter of a vessel by one-half increases the resistance to blood flow 16 times.

Resistance to
Flow = 1

Resistance to
Flow = 16

diameter result in big changes in its resistance to flow. Increasing the diameter decreases the resistance; decreasing the diameter increases the resistance to flow. Venules have a smaller diameter than veins; therefore, more resistance to flow occurs closer to the capillary-venule interface, but the rate of blood flow to the tissues cannot exceed the rate of flow at this interface.

Viscosity is a fluid's resistance to flow. Normally, the viscosity of blood remains constant. However, after injury, the viscosity of blood increases because of the loss of plasma into the surrounding tissues, and the ratio of liquids to solids decreases. Although this change in viscosity is not large enough to affect the systemic flow

of blood, it can cause clogging the area adjacent to the injury.

Lymphatic reabsorption is enhanced when the edema is spread over a larger area than when it is concentrated locally (see Chapter 14). Elevation, edema massage, and compression wraps and pads act to distribute edema and increase the rate of reabsorption.

Muscle Spasm
Muscle spasm, the involuntary contraction of muscle fibers, is the body's intrinsic mechanism for splinting and protecting the injured area and can result from direct trauma, decreased oxygen supply, or neurological

dysfunction.[48] Muscle spasm causes pain by stimulating mechanical and chemical pain receptors. Trigger points are localized areas of muscle spasm (Box 1-5).

Tension produced by the shortened fibers stimulates mechanical pain fibers while the decreased oxygen supply irritates chemical pain fibers. As muscle spasm persists, the associated ligaments and tendons are irritated.[52] As a result, the amount of muscle spasm increases to further protect the structures. This becomes a self-perpetuating cycle that is continued by pain, decreased oxygen supply, and a decreased amount of positive stress (in the form of movement).

Box 1-5. TRIGGER POINTS

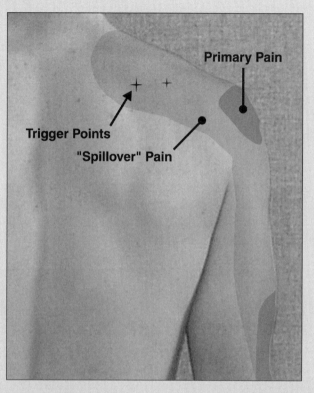

Trigger points of the supraspinatus muscle. The primary pain areas (the diagnostic criteria) are the darkened areas shown in the lateral deltoid and over the lateral epicondyle. Pain may spill over to the surrounding areas (light-shaded area).

Localized areas of muscle spasm, trigger points, can be caused by acute trauma, ischemia, inflammatory, or psychological stress.[49] Clinically, trigger points present themselves as discrete, localized, **hypersensitive** • areas located in taut bands of skeletal muscle.[50] Local tenderness and referred pain are produced during palpation and can result in limited motion and weakness in the affected muscle. A cross-friction type of massage can produce a local twitch muscle contraction. Trigger points usually form along the long axis of postural muscles. Most patients have multiple trigger points.[51] Trigger points are often confused with **fibromyalgia** •, and are part of the diagnostic criteria for fibromyalgia. However, trigger points can occur in the absence of fibromyalgia.[50,51] Trigger points are either active or latent.[50] Active trigger points are painful when the body part is at rest. Palpation reproduces the patient's symptoms of referred pain. When palpated or otherwise irritated, active trigger points can activate satellite trigger points.[51] Latent trigger points do not produce pain while at rest, but are painful during palpation and may limit range of motion and muscle strength. Common locations of trigger points and the resulting pain distribution are presented in Appendix B.

Hypersensitive: Abnormally increased sensitivity, a condition in which there is an exaggerated response by the body to a stimulus.

Fibromyalgia: Chronic inflammation of a muscle or connective tissue.

Treatment Strategies
Muscle Spasm and Trigger Points

Treatment strategies approach both the symptoms associated with the trigger point and correcting the behavioral, biomechanical, pathological, or ergonomic cause or causes that produce the trigger point or muscle spasm. Relieving pain will decrease the spasm, which will then stop the pain trigger. Massage, cryostretch, electrical stimulation, ultrasound, active exercise, injection of the site, and **iontophoresis** ● have been successfully used to decrease spasm.

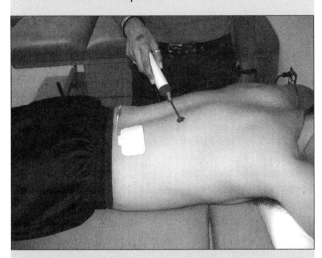

Cold application through ice packs or ice massage is an effective way of desensitizing the local nerve endings. Moist heat packs are effective with superficial spasm. Elongating the tissues along the lines of the muscle fibers also helps decrease the amount of spasm.

Muscle spasm may also be caused by impingement of spinal nerve roots or peripheral nerves. In this case, the treatment approach must be to relieve the pressure at the point on the nerve. For nerve roots, this may take the form of cervical or lumbar traction. For peripheral nerves, it could require the reduction of edema that is placing pressure on the nerve or the surgical removal of a bony outgrowth or fibrous sheath that forms around the nerve.

Muscle Atrophy and Weakness

When a muscle is not used, its fibers become progressively smaller as their actin and **myosin** ● contents decrease.

Disuse atrophy results when a body part is immobilized by an external splint, is partial weight-bearing, or when the individual consciously or unconsciously refuses to use the extremity because of pain.[53] **Denervation atrophy** occurs when there is no intact nerve supply to the muscle group. In either case, the resulting changes are similar.

✳ Practical Evidence

Postural muscle fibers begin to show physiological (microscopic) changes in as little as 24 hours after immobilization[55,57] and may appear clinically within 1 week following immobilization.[58]

Early immobilization assists the early stages of inflammation and repair by reducing the accumulation of macrophage, especially at the tendon-bone interface.[54] However, the size and function of the cells decrease in response to a prolonged lack of physical stress and afferent information sent from the injured area.[55] Accordingly, synthesis of protein, energy production, and contractility of the tissues begin to dwindle to the point of degeneration, at which time the muscle's ability to generate force decreases. The postural muscles, composed of slow-twitch (type I) fibers, are the first to show clinical and laboratory signs of atrophy.[56,57]

Treatment Strategies
Retarding Atrophy

Atrophy occurs when the muscle no longer receives the functional loads to which it is accustomed. The inability to contract the muscle, bear weight, or move the associated joints all decrease the amount of tension that the muscle experiences. When this is prolonged, the absence of this stress sends a signal to start taking away some of the muscle mass because the body (incorrectly) deduces that it is no longer needed.

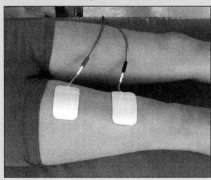

(Continued)

Iontophoresis: Introduction of ions into the body by use of electric current.
Myosin: Noncontractile muscle protein.

Rest is a double-edged sword in the treatment and rehabilitation of musculoskeletal injuries. Immobilization is necessary to protect the injured structures, but the lack of physical stress can inhibit proper remodeling of the tissues.[56] If you have ever seen an arm or leg that has been immobilized for a long time, you know that the adverse effects of immobilization are readily apparent.

The atrophy process may be deterred by several methods. Muscles immobilized in a lengthened position are more resistant to atrophy than those immobilized in a shortened position.[57] However, depending on the body part, the structures involved, and the type of injury, it is not always practical to immobilize the muscle in a lengthened position. Isometric contractions or electrical muscle stimulation, or both, can delay the atrophy process (see Chapter 13).

The injury response process accelerates the rate of atrophy. Edema and inflammation stimulate Golgi tendon organs, increasing the rate of atrophy (Box 1-6). As a muscle atrophies, the blood supply to the remaining fibers decreases, and the innervation of the muscle is hindered.[20,57] The continuing process of atrophy leads to reflex inhibition where the effusion and painful impulses create an inhibitory loop that essentially causes the person to "forget" how to contract the muscle, **arthrogenic muscle inhibition (AMI)**.

AMI is a presynaptic, reflex inhibition of a muscle caused by joint effusion.[16,59] Impulses from inhibitory **interneurons** ● interfere with the recruitment of the motoneurons of muscles crossing the involved joint.[16] In addition to causing atrophy, AMI hinders the rehabilitation process by delaying strength gains and interrupting joint proprioception.[59]

■ Chronic Inflammation

Chronic inflammation is often provoked by the long-term presence of low-intensity irritants. It is possible for the body to develop chronic inflammation without first going through an acute inflammatory stage significant enough for the patient to seek treatment. The inflammation was there, but at a level insufficient to call attention to it. Often, only when the tissue is near the point of failure does the patient seek assistance. The presence of chronic inflammation is a strong predictor of future disability.[60]

During chronic inflammation, the body is attempting to heal and repair itself. The magnitude of chronic inflammation is based on the balance between the underlying causes such as improper biomechanics and the body's attempt to resolve it. Low concentrations of inflammatory mediators are drawn to the area and, over time, weaken the connective tissue. When it is allowed to persist, chronic inflammation can result in permanent tissue damage.

The inflammatory response is primarily marked by the loss of function of the body part. During chronic inflammation, the body is still reacting to a stimulus from a delayed hypersensitivity that prolongs healing and repair, but is doing so in a slower manner. The cardinal signs of acute inflammation have given way to the hallmarks of chronic inflammation: production of fibrous connective and granulation tissue and the infiltration of mononuclear cells. The vascular changes associated with acute inflammation, vasodilation and exudation of fluids, are less pronounced or absent during chronic inflammation.

Mononuclear cells, leukocytes, lymphocytes, macrophages, and fibroblasts replace the infiltration of neutrophils seen during acute inflammation. Prolonged chronic inflammation also leads to the increased role of plasma cells. Tissue destruction associated with chronic inflammation is caused by cytokines produced by the mononuclear cells. Tissue healing is promoted by fibroblasts.

Tissue necrosis caused either by the original pathology or the inflammatory process itself occurs and further perpetuates the inflammatory response. The continual deposition of fibrous connective tissue can lead to a hardening of the tissue, **induration.** Fibroblastic activity continues to the point at which large quantities of collagen envelop the affected area, forming a **granuloma** ●. This granuloma affects the function of the involved part, leading to a loss of full function and to development of secondary reactions in associated structures.

Chronic inflammation can also self-perpetuate by altering the body's biomechanics. Pain, restricted motion, or loss of muscular strength can cause the body to substitute compensatory motion for normal motion. The newly acquired mechanics place new loads on the structures and activate an inflammatory response. A baseball pitcher with chronic rotator cuff inflammation may demonstrate this. The presence of a granuloma in the supraspinatus may decrease the ROM and strength of the muscles. By continuing to pitch, the athlete is further irritating the tendon. By changing the pitching motion, forces are distributed to tissues that are not accustomed to this stress, reactivating the inflammatory process.

Active, controlled exercise is beneficial in managing and controlling chronic inflammation.[60]

Interneuron: A neuron connecting two nerves.

Granuloma: A hard mass of fibrous tissue.

Box 1-6. MISGUIDED INTENTIONS

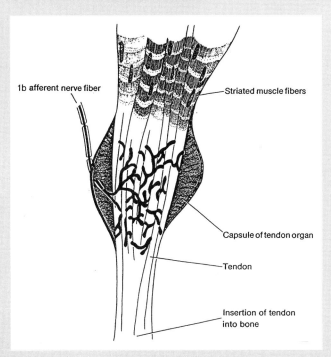

Golgi tendon organs (GTOs) function closely with muscle spindles in monitoring the amount of tension placed on a muscle and its tendon. Located within the muscle belly, projections from the spindle twine around individual muscle fibers. When the muscle contracts, the spindles monitor the rate and magnitude of tension produced.

GTOs divide into several branches, with the highest density being located at the muscle-tendon junction. When the muscle contracts, it places varying amounts of force on the tendon. The GTOs monitor the amount of strain placed on the tendon to prevent damage resulting from too much tension. If the rate of stimulation of GTOs or muscle spindles becomes too great, a nerve impulse is generated that inhibits the muscle contraction. The opposite antagonistic muscle may be facilitated to contract.

During the process of injury response, these nerves can be mechanically stimulated by pressure resulting from muscle spasm or edema, or they can be chemically stimulated by inflammatory mediators. Regardless of the nature of the stimulation, an inhibitory influence is placed on the muscle. If this process is allowed to continue the muscle atrophies.

Illustration from Ham, AW and Cormack, DH: Histology, ed 8. JB Lippincott, Philadelphia, 1979, p 584, with permission. JB Lippincott.

Chapter 2

The Physiology and Psychology of Pain

Brian G. Ragan, PhD, AT

Of all the components of the injury response, none is less consistent or less understood than an individual's response to pain. The perception of pain is a primal property of the nervous system and inherent to all people. Pain is more than a sensation. It is an "experience" involving the interaction thoughts, emotions, and past experiences leading to sensory and motor responses.[61] Acute pain is the primary reason people seek medical attention and the major complaint that they describe on initial evaluation. Chronic pain may be more debilitating than the trauma itself and may become emotionally and physically debilitating.[62,63]

● The expression "I have pain" is often uttered and is the main reason people seek medical attention. The term and concept of "Pain" has been defined by the International Association for the Study of Pain as "an unpleasant sensory and emotional experience associated with actual or potential tissue damage or described in terms of such damage."[64]

While humans have experienced pain since the beginning, our understanding of pain remains lacking. This is due to the complex interaction of the many factors that can affect pain. Our understanding of pain as it is defined today is less than 50 years old. In addition to the physiological component, pain also has psychological, emotional, and behavioral components.[65] It is described as an individual, highly variable experience and is affected by mood, culture, and past experiences as well as by age and personality.[66] What one individual interprets as pain may not be the same for another person in the identical situation.

✱ Practical Evidence

Rather than just being a sensation, pain is a *process* that involves sensory, motor, and emotional responses. Pain is formally defined as:

> an unpleasant sensory and emotional experience associated with actual or potential tissue damage, or described in terms of such damage. Each individual learns the application of the word through experience related to injury in early life. It is unquestionably a sensation in a part of the body but is also always an emotional experience.[64,67]

By definition, acute pain is unpleasant and has an identifiable cause and a limited duration.[61]

Pain, referred to as the fifth vital sign, serves as the body's line of self-defense.[68] It warns us that our tissues are in immediate jeopardy or have already been damaged. Pain, caused by mechanical forces or inflammatory mediators, activates protective reflexes and motivates behaviors that help to avoid—or at least decrease—physical trauma. Although we may not like pain, it is crucial to our survival. Loss of pain sensation leaves the body, or a body area, unprotected against serious damage and, potentially, unaware that trauma has occurred.[69] Pain loses its value when its defensive meaning is no longer needed. In this case pain may become more debilitating than the actual pathology and becomes a problem in and of itself.[61]

In order to best understand pain and the theories of pain **modulation** ● we first must understand the difference between pain and nociception. Pain is the unpleasant sensation. Nociception (from the Latin word *nocere*, "to harm") is the neural processes of encoding and processing noxious stimuli.[64] The important difference is that pain must be interpreted by higher brain centers as *pain* and nociception is the neurophysiological processes that may be interpreted as pain.

■ Dimensions of Pain Perception

Because of the complexity of pain and the involvement of both physiological and psychological components, the perception of pain varies from person to person and from day to day in the same person. The **cerebral cortex** is responsible for altering the perception and reaction to pain.

There are three dimensions of pain perception: sensory-discriminative, cognitive-evaluative, and affective-motivational (Table 2-1).[20,70,71]

There are some situations where pain perception is altered due to more important issues, a condition termed "battlefield conditions" by Melzak and Wall where, in the heat of battle, information regarding pain is ignored because of the distracting serious circumstances.[70] A good example of this is the typical movie portrayal of British soldiers just after a fierce battle:

"I say old chap, that was a nasty one, wasn't it? Too bad about your leg."

"My leg?"

"Your leg. You've been hit."

"Oh, bloody 'ell. Cup of tea, then?"

In this case, the soldier was so happy to make it out of combat alive, and his brain was so focused on analyzing the situation, that he did not realize an injury had occurred. This same type of processing also occurs in athletics. An athlete may be so focused on the competition that, when an injury occurs, its magnitude may not be immediately recognized.

Pain Threshold and Pain Tolerance

Nociceptors depolarize at a threshold below that required to cause tissue damage.[72] **Pain threshold** is the level (intensity) of noxious stimulus required to alert the individual to a potential threat to tissue. The pain threshold can be measured experimentally by introducing a painful stimulus such as cold water, pressure, or heat and gradually increasing the intensity until the individual reports "pain."[73] You can perform a simple experiment on yourself by squeezing your fingernail. The point at which you first experience pain could be quantitatively measured as your pain threshold by recording the amount of pressure exerted. Pain threshold is often based on the recruitment of A-delta fibers, a type of nerve that carries painful information.[67]

TABLE 2-1 Dimensions of Pain Perception

Component	Description
Sensory— Discriminative	Localizes the area (source) and type of pain.
Cognitive— Evaluative	Interprets sensations based on past experiences and expected outcomes.
Affective— Motivational	Influenced by the limbic system, affects internal (e.g., fear, anxiety) and outward response (e.g., screaming, crying) to the stimulus.

Modulate (Modulation): To regulate or adjust.

Pain tolerance, on the other hand, is a measure of how much pain a person can or will withstand.[67] In an experimental model, pain tolerance is measured by the amount of pain or "quantity" of exposure (cold water, pressure, heat) that an individual can or will endure before physically withdrawing from the painful stimuli.[73]

In assessing the physiological model of pain transmission, pain tolerance is associated with activation of C fibers, the **limbic system** ●, and the cortex.[67] Several synaptic interactions occur between these structures, and various levels of cognition influence the maximum level of noxious stimulation that can be tolerated. Examination of the physiology of noxious transmission and experimental research indicate that pain threshold and pain tolerance are not strongly correlated.[74] Therefore, a person who reports feeling excessive pain immediately after an injury may be able to endure the pain and continue to participate because of a high level of pain tolerance. An individual having a low pain tolerance may declare that an otherwise minor injury is preventing normal activity.

Pain threshold and pain tolerance are variable. The same person will have different levels of pain thresholds and pain tolerance at different times. They are also locally influenced by therapeutic modalities. Cold application, for example, can increase pain threshold 89% and pain tolerance by 76%.

Influences on Pain Perception

To understand the patient's pain and the response to pain, factors that influence the processing and interpretation of pain information must be understood. The patient's past experiences, expectations, and sociocultural background factor together to create a "pain filter" that increases or decreases the pain response. These factors will affect the assessment of pain and the patient's response to treatment.

Past Experiences

Past experiences can influence both the perception of pain and, probably more important, the response to it. The perception of pain from an injury can be influenced by a person's past experience with that injury and the consequences or the association it has with a location such as a hospital that increases anxiety.[73] The pain could also elicit fears of ending the patient's athletic career or having to undergo a long rehabilitation program. For example a person may alter the pain from a chronic shoulder injury because of fear about the diagnostic process, surgery, or treatment because of a fear of needles. These memories of past experiences come from the **limbic system**, which is responsible for the affect or emotional component of pain.

Expectations

A person's expectations can influence the perception and response to pain. These expectations can come from athletic participation and influence an individual's response to pain.[75–78] Pain tolerance is higher in athletes participating in contact sports.[79] For younger athletes, the situation influences response to pain wherein children tend to "tolerate" more pain when they are observed by their peers than when alone.[80]

Sociocultural

The sociocultural background of the individual influences both the perception of pain and the response to it.[81,82] Pain perception has been linked to ethnicity, socioeconomic status, and religious affiliation.[81,83–86] The concept of the cultural component is an important one in understanding the influences culture has on clinician-patient communication, impact on the quality of information used for diagnosis, and treatment outcome. Understanding what an individual values is important in understanding, assessing, and managing the injury/illness.

Personality, Age, and Gender

Personality, age, and gender can influence the perception and responses to pain. Likewise, extroverts express pain more freely than introverts, but introverts are more sensitive to pain.[87] As with most body systems, there is degeneration in neuronal circuitry that occurs with aging that lowers pain threshold. It is also this aging process that increases the ability to handle pain.

There are well-documented differences between men and women in their pain thresholds. Men typically have higher tolerance and thresholds.[72,82,88,89] These can be attributed to biological, psychological, or social influences. It is uncertain whether women are simply more willing to report and express pain than are men.[90] Clinicians should understand and account for the possible differences in pain threshold and pain tolerance when assessing, treatment planning, and documenting progress in the patient.

■ The Somatosensory System

The somatosensory system, the body's sensory systems, allows for our interaction with the external world by receiving input from receptors in the periphery and sending it to the higher centers.[91] One of the most important functions of the body's sensory systems is a warning system for self-protection. For example, we look both ways before crossing the street and freeze at the sound of a rattlesnake thanks to input from our visual and auditory systems. Our somatosensory system provides feedback regarding potentially injurious forces.

Specialized Sensory Receptors

A major advancement in our understanding of pain was the identification of specialized nerve receptors in the periphery. Stimulation of these receptors results in depolarization and the creation of action potentials that are transmitted to the brain, where the type and intensity of the stimulus is decoded (Box 2-1).

Limbic system: System in the brain that controls emotion.

Box 2-1. MECHANORECEPTORS

Superficial Somatosensory Receptors. Receptor organs for touch, temperature, and pain in the skin and the peripheral fibers that connect the receptor organs to the central nervous system.

Most receptor organs that detect pressure are surrounded by a connective tissue capsule, **encapsulated receptors** •. Superficial receptor organs are located in or just beneath the skin and are responsible for detecting stimuli that contact the body. Deep receptor organs are located in muscle and tendons and normally provide proprioceptive information about the state of muscle contraction and limb position. They activate peripheral processes that are large-diameter well-myelinated **A-beta** fibers. Varying levels of pressure (touch), movement, and vibration of the skin and texture (rough versus smooth) are detected by these receptor organs. Pain receptors (nociceptors) activate **A-delta** and **C fibers**.

Although the mechanisms that mechanoreceptors use to convert pressure applied to the skin into action potentials are complex, the presence of mechanically gated ion channels in the nerve membrane at least partially explains the process.[92] Mechanically gated ion channels are large protein molecules that pass through the neuronal membrane of the receptor. Extensions from the receptors act like a lever so that when the disk is compressed, the channel is stretched open, allowing sodium ions to flow into the receptor. This depolarizes the receptor and generates action potentials in the primary afferent fiber. As more pressure is applied, the frequency of action potentials increases proportionately.

Receptor Type	Function
Thermal receptors	Detect skin temperature; may be encapsulated or unencapsulated (free nerve endings)
Merkel's disks	Sensitive to low threshold mechanical pressure, but slowly adapt to stimuli.
Meissner's corpuscles	Sensitive to low threshold mechanical pressure, but rapidly adapt to constant pressure.
Pacinian corpuscles	Located deeper in the skin, react to higher levels of mechanical pressure; most responsive to varying pressure levels
Ruffini corpuscles	Located in the subcutaneous tissues, this organ is sensitive to stretching of the skin and changes in joint position and helps provide proprioceptive and kinesthetic feedback.
Nociceptors	Similar to some thermal receptors, nociceptors may be unencapsulated. Activated by mechanical, thermal, or chemical antagonists.

Encapsulated receptor: A sensory receptor formed by a nerve fiber and surrounding connective tissue cells.

Nociceptors must be stimulated to initiate pain. There are four primary mechanisms that can trigger peripheral nociceptors: mechanical, thermal, chemical, and polymodal stimulation (Fig. 2-1). Examples of mechanical stimuli are direct force trauma from an injury and pressure from swelling. Nociceptors also respond to extreme thermal conditions including the thermal changes associated with an active inflammatory response (or cold or heat therapeutic modalities). Chemical triggers are most associated with the inflammatory response and release of inflammatory prostaglandins and other algesic substances from the initial trauma and subsequent inflammatory processes (Table 2-2). Mild nociceptive stimuli (irritants) are used therapeutically to decrease pain, such as with capsaicin analgesic creams (or other over-the-counter pain-relieving creams). Polymodal stimulation is the combination of mechanical, thermal, and chemical stimuli.

Hyperalgesia

The peripheral nerves undergo sensitization that lowers the pain threshold. Nociceptors are normally activated as the result of the destruction of tissue cells. Following tissue damage, normally nonpainful stimuli such as light touch or warmth will easily activate these receptors, especially the C-fiber polymodal nociceptors. This is called **hyperesthesia,** pain produced by normally nonpainful stimuli (also known as allodynia), such as gentle touch or the pressure from sheets when a patient is trying to sleep. Furthermore, a pinprick that would normally be described as mildly painful can generate considerable pain, hyperalgesia. In both instances, damage to tissue not only activates nociceptors, it also makes the nociceptors more sensitive to all other forms of stimulation (Fig. 2-2). At the site of the damage, this change in threshold is called **primary hyperalgesia.** Over time, the hyperalgesia may spread to adjacent tissues, producing **secondary hyperalgesia**—increased pain in the area around the injured tissue.[93] Hyperesthesia and hyperalgesia are chemically mediated responses initiated by tissue damage.

First-Order Neurons

After action potentials have been generated from a stimulated receptor they travel on the corresponding afferent

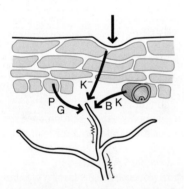

Figure 2-1. **Damage to tissue produced by mechanical or thermal stimuli releases chemicals from tissue cells.** These chemicals (K—potassium; BK—bradykinin; PG—prostaglandin) activate nociceptors, producing action potentials in primary afferent fibers (A-delta).

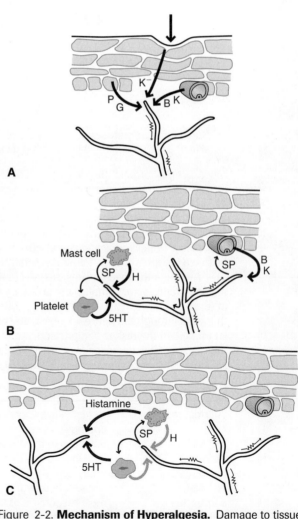

Figure 2-2. **Mechanism of Hyperalgesia.** Damage to tissue releases chemicals that activate nociceptors and also affects adjacent tissue. (A) The initial damage activates the nociceptor. (B) The branches of the primary afferent fibers stimulate adjacent connective tissue and vasculature. (C) The threshold of nociceptors in undamaged tissue is altered. (K—potassium; PG—prostaglandin; BK—bradykinin; SP—substance P; H—histamine; 5HT—serotonin)

TABLE 2-2	Select Inflammatory Pain Mediators
Mediator	*Action*
Bradykinins	Directly stimulates nociceptors
Prostaglandin	Sensitization of the nerve fibers so that other mediators can enhance nociception
Substance P	Neurotransmitter released centrally to produce the pain response and peripherally producing hyperalgesia and inflammatory responses
Histamine	Released by mast cells to directly stimulate nociceptors

nerve fiber for that receptor to be relayed to the dorsal horn of the spinal cord. All sensory input from peripheral receptors below the head are organized by dorsal roots that correspond to an area of skin, called a **dermatome** ● (Fig. 2-3).

The specific type of first-order afferent nerve fiber can be described in multiple ways. There are two main classifications for all afferent and efferent nerve fibers. Because it often is used to describe cutaneous input, the more well-known system is the Erlanger and Gasser's classification of peripheral nerve fibers. This system is based on the size and conduction speed (A, B, and C fibers). It includes all types of peripheral nerves including muscle, joint, cutaneous, and visceral. The other classification system for nerve fibers is the Lloyd's classification. This system is routinely used to describe muscle afferents and is organized similarly to Erlanger and Gasser's system by nerve size and conduction speed (see Table 1.3).

The afferents responsible for transmitting pain are the A-delta (A-δ) (group III) and C fibers (group IV). A-delta fibers are small-diameter, lightly myelinated nerves that transmit mechanical pressure, temperature extremes, or ischemic pain.[94,95] These fibers are responsible for what is known as the "fast" pain associated with an injury, often described as "rapid" and "sharp." The other important aspect of these afferents is their ability to localize the pain to a specific spot (epicritic pain).[96] C fibers are small-diameter, unmyelinated afferent fibers that also respond to mechanical pressure, extreme temperature, and chemicals (inflammatory markers). The pain originating from these fibers is referred to as "slow" pain that is characterized by a dull, nonlocalized, and diffuse pain sensation (protopathic pain). C fibers are the most abundant primary afferents in the human body and are the body's monitors for potential problems. The C fibers are well suited to accomplish this task

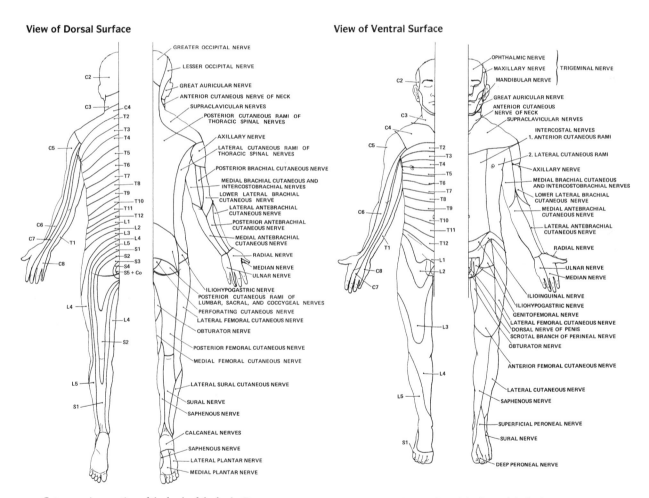

View of Dorsal Surface

View of Ventral Surface

Cutaneous innervation of the back of the body. Dermatomes are on the left, and peripheral nerves are on the right.

Cutaneous innervation of the front of the body. Dermatomes are on the left, and peripheral nerves are on the right.

Figure 2-3. **Peripheral Nerves and Dermatomes.** The right side of the body shows the innervation patterns of peripheral nerves. Spinal nerve and root patterns are shown on the left side of the body. (From Gilman, S and Newman, SW: Manter and Gatz's Essentials of Clinical Neuroanatomy and Neurophysiology, ed 10. FA Davis, Philadelphia, 2003, pp 43–44.)

Dermatome: A segmental skin area supplied by a spinal nerve root.

because they are polymodal and respond to painful and non-painful stimuli.

Afferents' Entrance in the Dorsal Horn

The first-order afferent nerve enters the dorsal horn of the spinal cord at the corresponding spinal level. The afferent nerve ends and synapses continue the signal along to higher centers for processing. The type of afferent will dictate where the synapse occurs in the dorsal horn. The gray matter of the spinal cord is divided into segments, each corresponding to the function of nerves (e.g., nociceptive, motor) that synapse there, either afferent or efferent. This organization of the gray matter is referred to as Rexed laminar organization (Fig. 2-4). Note that the gray matter consists of right and left segments

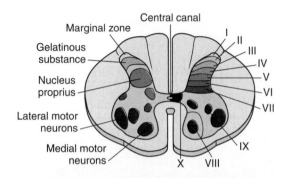

Figure 2-4. **Reflexed Laminar Organization.** The laminae are located in the gray matter of the spinal cord. Various synapses occur in each lamina. The spinal gate is located in lamina 2.

and is then organized from 1 to 9, where 1 is located in the dorsal horn and progressing to 9 in the ventral horn.

The impulses from first-order nerves can be polysynaptic and involve multiple **interneurons** ●. Interneurons allow for the divergence of the original stimulus to other pathways in the nervous system. It is common for the terminating first-order neurons to synapse with segmental interneurons that spread the impulse to other neighboring spinal levels. Interneurons play an important role in relaying reflex activity to motoneurons and spinal inhibition (Fig. 2-5). The original signal also synapses with the corresponding second-order neuron linked to the type nerve and stimulus.

The A-delta and C fibers are primary afferents that are responsible for transmitting nociceptive information and synapse at certain locations in the dorsal horn of the spinal cord. C fibers enter the dorsal horn and synapse primarily on lamina I and II. The A-delta fibers synapse a little further in on the dorsal horn at lamina V. **It is important to remember that all nociceptive and thermal signals travel on these two first-order, small-diameter afferents.**

Second-Order Neurons

The second-order neurons are primarily responsible for transmitting the stimuli (initially started from the receptor) up the spinal cord to higher centers. These neurons synapse with the first-order neurons. Nociceptive impulses typically cross the midline of the spinal cord to the specific ascending tracks to the higher centers via the spinothalamic or spinoparabrachial

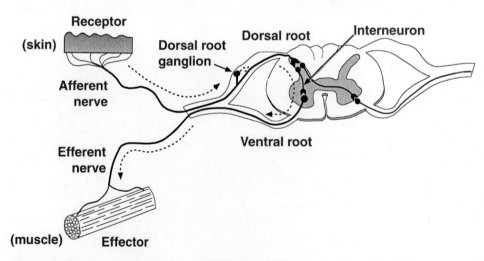

Figure 2-5. **Polysynaptic Loop.** The **withdrawal reflex** ● is a basic example of a polysynaptic relay. Stimulation of superficial pain receptors in the skin produces action potentials that travel along the afferent nerve fiber to the spinal cord. This fiber forms synapses with interneurons that project to motor neurons in the ventral horn. These motor neurons project back to muscle and generate protective movements that withdraw the limb from further damage. The interneurons also activate tract neurons that project to higher levels of the nervous system and produce the sensation of pain. Thus, activation of pain receptors normally produces both a reflexive and cognitive response.

Interneuron: A CNS neuron that forms an intermediate synaptic connection between other neurons.
Withdrawal reflex: A multisynaptic spinal reflex that is normally elicited by a noxious stimulus. Muscle groups are activated so that the body is moved away from the damaging stimulus.

pathways (Fig. 2-6). These tracts contain both nocio-specific or **wide dynamic range** • second-order neurons, which transmits both nociceptive and non-nociceptive impulses. The spinothalamic tract's destination is the **somatosensory cortex** •, while the spinoparabrachial tract passes through the pons to reach the hippocampus and the amygdala, where affective response to pain (unpleasantness) is evoked.[97]

Higher Centers

For sensory information to be processed and perceived, the stimulus must reach the cerebral cortex. The second-order neurons synapse with higher-order neurons through the **thalamus** •, which is responsible for transmitting the signal to higher centers, the amygdala and the cerebral cortex, specifically to the sensory homunculus. The sensory homunculus is the area in the brain responsible for processing sensory information throughout the body (Fig. 2-7). The amount of space in the sensory homunculus devoted to a body area is directly related to the density of sensory receptors in the periphery. It is important to remember that the nervous system must be intact for the sensory stimulus to be perceived. Once the higher centers perceive the sensory information, then the efferent impulses that produce motor, behavioral, and inflammatory responses may be produced by the brain.

In some cases sensory nerves other than nociceptors contribute to the pain response. The lower depolarization

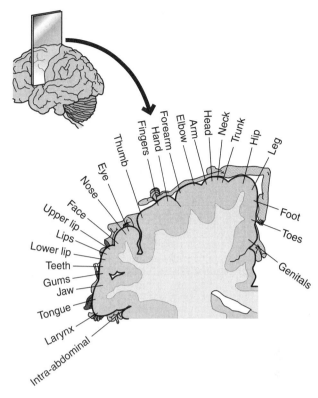

Figure 2-7. **Sensory Homunculus.** Each area of the somatosensory cortex interprets sensory input from specific body parts.

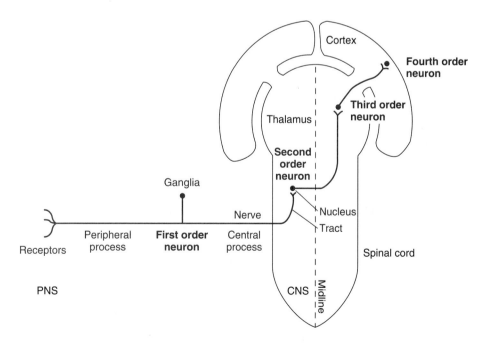

Figure 2-6. **Sensory Neurons, Nerves, and Tracts.** Primary afferent fibers connect the sensory receptor to second-order neurons in the CNS. The cell bodies of the primary afferent fibers are located in ganglia within the vertebra or skull but outside the CNS. Second-order neurons are located in nuclei within the spinal cord or brain stem and project across the midline to reach higher order neurons.

Wide dynamic range (neurons): Neurons in the spinal cord and thalamus that respond to a broad range of mechanical pressures. They respond to both touch and pain.
Somatosensory cortex: An area in the cerebral cortex, located in the postcentral gyrus of the parietal lobe, that is important in the perception of touch and proprioception and in the localization of pain sensation.
Thalamus: Gray matter in the center of the brain.

threshold of sensory nerves and the increased excitability of the CNS can make an otherwise nonpainful stimulus, such as light touch, be interpreted as pain.[97]

Pain Control Theory

The methods of pain control discussed in this section are based on the input in the system that is required and the location of the mechanism that is thought to be responsible for the pain control. Primary pain control techniques involve resolving the physiological pain triggers: decreasing mechanical and/or chemical irritation. Secondary pain control approaches target the transmission and perception of pain. In complex cases, multiple approaches to primary and secondary pain control are required.[98]

Melzak and Wall's Gate Control Theory

The Gate Control Theory of pain control can be described in terms of ascending and descending parts. The classic example of the ascending mechanism is rubbing the painful area to reduce the pain for some injuries. For example, a batter is struck with a pitch in the arm and immediately starts rubbing the area on the arm that was struck. The batter starts to feel a reduction in pain perception. This example represents the simple ascending component to Gate Control Theory (stimulus up and into the spinal cord). There are descending mechanisms that involve higher centers that are responsible for pain attenuation (stimulus sent down from higher centers). A simple approach to understanding which mechanism is likely at work starts with understanding what type of input is entering the system, usually from the periphery.

Ascending Mechanism

The ascending mechanism of the Gate Control Theory is based on increasing non-nociceptive input (stimuli) from the periphery into the spinal cord to elicit pain relief. This theory holds that the receptors of A-beta fibers (carrying nonpainful stimulus) can decrease the input of nociceptive stimuli from continuing to the second-order neuron. This mechanism occurs in the dorsal horn of the spinal cord, specifically in lamina II (substantia gelitinosa).[70,99–103]

The small diameter C and A-delta afferent fibers enter the dorsal horn and synapse directly on the second-order afferent neurons (T cells). This stimulus also facilitates a spinal inhibitory interneuron associated with those afferents allowing the small-diameter nociceptive stimuli to produce strong activation of the **tract cells** • when activated alone (Fig. 2-8).

When stimuli from large, myelinated A-beta fibers enter the dorsal horn it also synapses with both second-order neurons (T cells) and spinal interneurons. The "closing of the

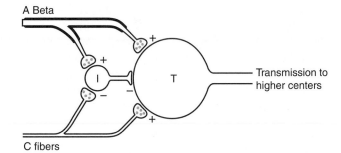

Figure 2-8. **Opening and Closing the Gate.** The Gate Control Theory models the interaction of nonpain-carrying fibers (e.g., A-beta) and nociceptors (C fibers and A-delta) at their synapse with the secondary afferent neurons. The substantia gelatinosa monitors the activity on both of these tracts, allowing the one that is more active to pass to the tract cell (T) and on to higher centers. If the nonpain tract is more active, these impulses are allowed to pass, thereby "closing the gate" on pain transmission.

gate" occurs from the spinal interneurons, which have an inhibitory effect on small-diameter afferent traffic. The role of the interneurons is to open or close the gate depending on the type of input the system receives from the peripheral receptors. A similar response is seen when large-diameter afferents are the only input into the system. It synapses directly with the second-order neuron and inhibits small-diameter afferent traffic, allowing for stronger transmission of the stimuli.

Large and Small Afferent Interaction

Nociceptive input from small-diameter afferents entering the system at the same time as mechanical input from large-diameter afferents is received forms the heart of the ascending mechanism. The two different afferents have antagonist effects on the gate. The large-diameter afferents are trying to inhibit or "close" the gate to small-diameter traffic, preventing continuation of the signal to the second-order neuron (T cell). The small-diameter afferents are trying to keep the "gate" open to allow for the nociceptive impulses to continue. The basic principle is that the tract with the most activity will prevail and be "allowed" to continue up the spinal cord. This means if the rate of large-diameter afferent traffic is greater than small-diameter traffic, the gate will close. Likewise if small diameter traffic is greater than the gate will remain open. The speed of transmission of the afferent fibers has nothing to do with the opening and closing of the gate.

In the example of the batter who was hit by a pitch. Immediately after the ball struck the batter, nociceptive stimuli were produced from the mechanical force and the associated inflammatory mediators. Initially, the only input into the system is small-diameter nociceptive afferent stimuli. This

---

Tract cells: Second-order neurons of the pain and temperature pathways. The axons of these cells cross the midline of the spinal cord and ascend in the anterior lateral fasciculus. Tract cells are sometimes called T cells, but they should not be confused with the T cells of the immune system.

is interpreted in the brain as pain. The batter then begins to rub the painful area. The batter is now adding mechanical (non-pain) stimuli into the system that is transmitted on large-diameter A-beta afferent nerves to the dorsal horn. Now we have competing stimuli into the system: the initial small-diameter afferent ("pain") and large-diameter afferent traffic (non-painful stimulus). The batter begins to rub the painful area intensely, increasing the rate of mechanical input into the system. The rate is now greater than the rate of small-diameter nociceptive stimuli and the batter starts to feel a decrease in pain because the gate has been closed by the intense rubbing (large-diameter traffic).

✳ Practical Evidence

Most therapeutic modalities that are applied for the purposes of assisting tissue healing also activate the gate mechanism. For example, ice applied to decrease cell metabolism and limit secondary injury initially decreases pain by stimulating sensory receptors.[66,104,105]

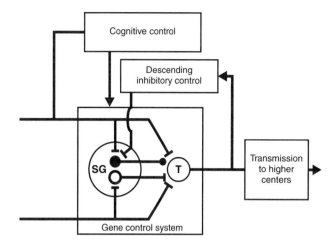

Figure 2-9. **Descending Pain Control Theory.** The original Gate Control Theory was modified to add "higher centers" and their influence on pain control. The higher centers decrease the perception of pain by sending impulses to the spinal level that trigger enkephalin interneuron and the release of epinephrine and serotonin that directly and indirectly decrease pain transmission.

The release of spinal opioids has been linked to the closing of the gate. The large-diameter afferents synapse with spinal **enkephalin** • interneurons, which release enkephalin at the spinal level, having an inhibitory effect of small-diameter afferents. This is most likely responsible for the attenuation of small-diameter traffic and reduction in pain. Clinical treatments such as TENS, massage, whirlpools, or gentle range-of-motion activities activate non-nociceptive receptors, which produce large-diameter afferent input and elicit this pain modulation.

Descending Pain Modulation

While the ascending mechanism formed the entire original Gate Control Theory, researchers concluded that the initial theory was incomplete. However, it could not explain all examples of pain control. Because pain is a complex interaction of physiological and psychological components, the role of the brain's ability to elicit pain control was recognized and included. The Gate Control Theory was updated to include higher centers with the addition of cognitive control and descending inhibitory control (Fig. 2-9).

With the descending mechanisms for pain control it is important to acknowledge that the small-diameter nociceptive pathway and stimuli are transmitting to higher centers. The influence of stimulating non-nociceptive large-diameter afferents is not part of these mechanisms. Remember that all thermal information is carried by small-diameter A-delta and C fibers. These descending mechanisms are initiated by specific higher-center structures.

Endogenous Opiates

The influence of the endogenous opiate system contributes to the higher centers' descending mechanism of pain control. The hypothalamus can also control pain caused by prolonged intense stimulation. The hypothalamus controls the release of beta-endorphins from the pituitary gland. These powerful endogenous opiates then enter the bloodstream and circulate. This contribution results in strong inhibition of pain perception. Enkephalin is another endogenous opiate, triggered by the descending mechanism, originating in the raphe nucleus.

Central Biasing

The basic descending mechanism is that certain higher-center (brain) structures can facilitate the closing of the gate or inhibition of small-diameter afferent traffic through descending connections in the dorsal horn. The portions of the cerebral cortex responsible for emotion facilitate the periaqueductal gray region, starting a descending pain control mechanism. This portion of the descending mechanism is often referred to as "central biasing." The periaqueductal gray region activates the **raphe nuclei** • that have descending connections to the spinal level. The stimulation of the raphe nucleus has been linked to the endogenous opiate system (Fig. 2-10). This mechanism synapses with the spinal

---

Enkephalin: A substance released by the body that reduces the perception of pain by bonding to pain receptor sites.

Nucleus (Nuclei): A cluster of neurons in the CNS.

Raphe nuclei: Cluster of nuclei found in the pons that regulate serotonin.

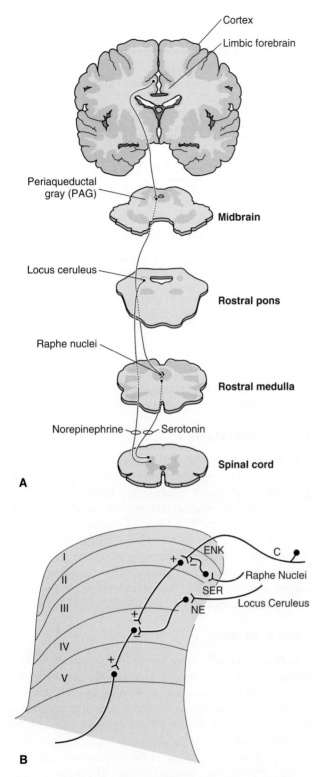

A

B

Figure 2-10. **Descending Modulation Pathways of Pain.**
(A) The cerebral cortex can decrease pain transmission in the ascending pain pathways through a series of descending connections with brain stem nuclei. (B) Descending modulation of dorsal horn neurons. Descending fibers from the raphe nucleus and locus ceruleus modulate the activation of dorsal horn neurons by C fibers. ENK-enkephalin; SER-serotonin; NE-Norepinephrine

enkaphalin interneurons, thus closing the gate, decreasing afferent traffic, and thereby reducing pain. There is an addition spinal mechanism produced by this portion of the descending mechanism. Serotonin is released locally at the spinal level, inhibiting the second-order neuron directly and indirectly activating the spinal enkaphalin interneuron. In addition to the periaqueductal gray region, descending contributions from descending fibers originate in the locus ceruleus nucleus in the pons. These are also part of the descending pain control mechanism because they trigger the release of norepinephrine, which has an inhibitory effect on pain transmission at the spinal level.

■ Common Pain Syndromes

Pain is a vital warning system that an injury has—or will—occur. Unfortunately, pain sometimes misinforms us about the location of the damage, especially when the actual damage is to a visceral organ. Pain sometimes persists for weeks, months, or even years after healing should have taken place, sending an alarm when no such warning is needed. Treatment of such pathological pain symptoms can be difficult, and the effects can be severely incapacitating.

Chronic Pain

Acute pain may be an indication that something is wrong within the body. It forces us to do something to fix the problem—let go of the hot pan, stay off the sprained ankle, or seek medical advice. But sometimes pain persists long after the healing process has been completed, the amount of pain perceived is much greater than the detectable tissue damage would seem to produce, or pain is being produced without the same triggers seen in acute pain. This is chronic pain—pain that extends beyond the normal course of injury or illness.

Chronic pain involves the prolonged changes in the peripheral nervous system described so far in this chapter.[93] Hyperalgesia becomes maladaptive, meaning that there is a pain response in the absence of actual tissue damage. In this case the pain becomes the pathology.[97] In some types of chronic pain, such as rheumatoid arthritis, the **contralateral** ● joint will also become painful. This response, symmetrical pain, may be caused by neurological and/or circulatory factors.[93]

Chronic pain is difficult to treat and takes a serious toll on the lives of sufferers and eventually becomes integrated into an individual's life, having physical, psychological, and socioeconomic consequences (Table 2-3).[81] Some people become habituated to chronic pain. In such cases the pain is still there, but there are fewer outward signs of it.[61] Chronic pain can be incapacitating and lead the afflicted person to take increasingly drastic actions to obtain even temporary relief. Depression is a common consequence and depression itself may increase the level of perceived pain in

---

Contralateral: Pertaining to the opposite side of the body. The left side is contralateral to the right.

TABLE 2-3	Characteristics of Chronic Pain

Symptoms last longer than 6 months
Few objective medical findings
Medication abuse
Difficulty in sleeping
Depression
Manipulative behavior
Somatic preoccupation

a vicious cycle that produces great anguish for patients and their families.

Chronic pain may reflect an ongoing disease that continually activates nociceptors. The pain is produced by activation of nociceptors by the mechanisms discussed in the Pain Threshold and Pain Tolerance section, but the pain persists because the condition persists. For example, arthritis produces chronic inflammation of the joints, resulting in increasingly severe pain when the affected joints are moved. Although cancerous tumors may initially grow painlessly, considerable pain is produced when they begin to compress nerve fibers. Other chronic diseases produce pain because tissue is destroyed as the disease progresses.

In cases of nociceptive chronic pain, the primary goal of treatment is to stop the underlying inflammatory process. If the inflammation can be controlled, the pain should be resolved. Unfortunately, treatment of chronic, progressive conditions is often difficult or unsuccessful. Too much attention paid to the treatment of the disease with inadequate treatment of pain symptoms can lead to considerable unnecessary suffering by the patient.

If no persistent disease can be identified as the source of chronic pain, the problem is likely to be an abnormality in the neurons of the pain system, **neuropathic chronic pain**. The problem may be in the peripheral nerves or in neurons within the CNS. We have only a very minimal understanding of the changes that occur to produce neuropathic chronic pain. And because there is no identifiable disease to treat, providing effective therapy is challenging. Even the development of a consistent way of naming the different clinical syndromes has proved difficult.[96] Successful treatment of neuropathic chronic pain requires more research into the neuroscience of pain. Some research suggests that synaptic reorganization at higher levels, even in the cerebral cortex, may play a role in neuropathic chronic pain.[106]

Complete severance of a peripheral nerve, a **neuropathy** ●, normally abolishes all **somatic** ● sensation the nerve provides. If nerves are partially damaged, however, neuropathic pain can develop. The initial damage can be caused by trauma that compresses the nerve, damaging some of the nerve fibers inside. Entrapment of the nerve or repetitive

small injuries over time, as in carpal tunnel syndrome, may also produce this syndrome. The key distinction between this and nociceptive chronic pain is that the pain persists after the damaged tissue has completely healed. There is no ongoing disease that is activating the nociceptors. Instead, the nociceptors are spontaneously active.

Referred Pain

Pain is normally well localized to the site of injury. If you have been stung by a bee, you know exactly where to look for the stinger. This is the result of the precise topography of the ascending pain system from the surface of the body all the way to the homunculus in the cerebral cortex. However, pain originating from the **visceral** ● organs is difficult to localize. Imagine taking a drink of very hot coffee. We can distinguish clearly if the coffee burns the lips, tongue, or cheeks. But if we ignore these warning signals and hastily swallow the burning brew, we feel pain on the inside but will have a difficult time localizing this internal pain to the esophagus versus trachea or stomach. Even damage to deeper muscles may sometimes seem to originate from the skin or muscles at some distance from the actual damage. Frequently, pain originating from visceral organs is perceived as originating from an area of the skin far removed from the organ. For example, damage to the diaphragm is normally not felt as pain at the base of the thorax but rather as an ache in the skin and muscles of the neck and shoulder. Pain from the heart may be felt in the chest, but also may seem to radiate down the arm. Pain caused by appendicitis is normally felt as originating diffusely from the abdomen (McBurney's point). Trauma to the spleen will cause pain in the upper left shoulder (Kerr's sign). This is referred pain—pain originating from inflamed structures producing pain elsewhere in the body.

In addition to the misinterpretation of the location of pain (or the source of the pain), referred pain also produces hyperalgesia in the affected skin area. Careful examination shows that the patterns of hyperalgesia after damage to different organs are fairly consistent across patients and are responsive to clinical tests such as the cervical compression test.[95]

By mapping the area of hyperalgesia, insight into the identity of the damaged organ is obtained. These patterns also suggest a possible explanation for referred pain (Fig. 2-11). During fetal development, the visceral organs migrate from their original location in the embryo. For instance, the diaphragm originates at cervical levels in the neck, but then relocates to its adult position in the lower thorax. Owing to this migration, the branches of the primary afferent fibers innervate both organ and skin (Fig. 2-11A). Because the skin area is more exposed, we learn to associate pain due to damage to the skin with activation of the cutaneous branch. Later, if the visceral organ is damaged, the same afferent fibers are activated and we misinterpret the origin of the pain.

Neuropathy: Destruction, trauma, or inhibition of a nerve.
Somatic: Pertaining to the body.
Visceral: Pertaining to organs of the body.

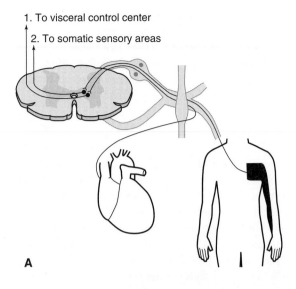

1. To visceral control center

2. To somatic sensory areas

A

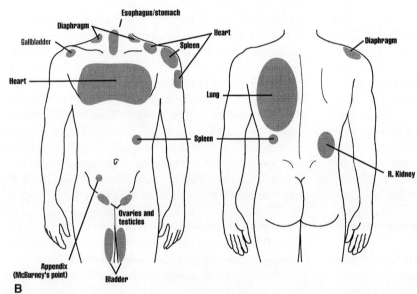

Esophagus/stomach

Diaphragm

Gallbladder

Heart

Heart

Spleen

Spleen

Lung

Diaphragm

R. Kidney

Ovaries and testicles

Appendix (McBurney's point)

Bladder

B

Figure 2-11. **Referred Pain.** Pain originating from visceral organs is poorly localized and may seem to originate from the surface of the body some distance from the site of injury. (A) Possible mechanism of referred pain as the result of a heart attack. (B) Common patterns of experienced pain after damage to different organs.

Patients who are suffering from pain of unknown origin may be experiencing referred pain. Careful, thorough history and evaluation are required to identify the actual cause of the patient's discomfort. Ultimately, the underlying pathology of the pain should be clear before treatment is prescribed. In cases in which the true cause of the pain is suspect, or if there is uncertainty of the nature of the pain, the patient should be referred for further examination.

Peripheral Nerve Root and Spinal Cord

The most common pattern of sensory loss occurs when peripheral nerves are damaged. Damage to a peripheral nerve normally destroys all fibers in the nerve—sensory and motor—producing a complete loss of function distal to the site of damage. The affected area is confined to the region of the body innervated by the damaged nerve. For example,

damage to the musculocutaneous nerve results in loss of motor and sensory function in the peripheral distribution. If damage occurs more centrally, affecting spinal nerves or dorsal roots, the pattern of sensory loss changes to a dermatome pattern (see Fig. 2-3). For example, damage to the sixth cervical dorsal root (C6) produces loss of all sensation in a narrow region of skin that includes innervation patterns of three peripheral nerves: the radial, median, and musculocutaneous nerves.

When the spinal cord itself is damaged, a much more complex pattern of sensory loss occurs. For instance, a patient who suffers spinal cord damage at the C6 level may lose sensation of touch and proprioception in the C6 dermatome and all the lower dermatomes on the **ipsilateral** • side of the body. From the patient's perspective, it would seem that the ipsilateral side of the body was "missing" from the C6 dermatome inferiorly with one notable exception: the

---

Ipsilateral: On the same side of the body.

patient would still experience pain when stuck with a sharp needle. Pain would still be processed but with no apparent source of the stimulus. While touch and proprioception are intact on the contralateral side of the body, pain sensation on that side of the body would be absent below the C6 dermatome.

Myofascial Pain Syndrome

Muscle aches and pains are certainly a common occurrence and normally are self-resolving. Pain emanating from muscle and connective tissues that is persistent and shows no indication of being caused by arthritis or other nociceptive process may result from myofascial pain syndrome or trigger point pain. Muscles in the painful area often have very high tone—the muscles feel very tense and are quite sore. A key sign of this syndrome is the presence of trigger points. Even though the pain is felt over a large area, the trigger point may be confined to a small part of just one of the affected muscles.

The anatomical and physiological identification of trigger points and the mechanism of the pain generation are unknown, but one hypothesis holds that trigger points exist in many muscles but are inactive. If the muscle is damaged, even slightly, in the area of a trigger point, the trigger point produces a reflexive muscle contraction that further activates the trigger point. The process becomes self-sustaining. This hypothesis is supported by treatment approaches that relax the muscle by stretching or directly inactivate the trigger point by injection of anesthetic. This breaks the self-sustaining loop, and can produce permanent relief (see Treatment Strategies: Muscle Spasm and Trigger Points, page 29).

Sympathetically Maintained Pain Syndrome

Perhaps the most disabling of all chronic pain syndromes is pain that is produced by action of the sympathetic nervous system, also known by other names such as "complex regional pain syndrome" or "reflex sympathetic dystrophy." This syndrome often starts with trauma, possibly minor trauma, to the soft tissues or bones. Despite appropriate treatment for the trauma, the wound or fractured bone does not heal well. The affected area reddens and may sweat profusely—signs of sympathetic activation. Nerve blocks provide temporary relief, but the pain continues to increase over time and can reach severe levels. Even cutting the sensory nerve proximal to the affected area may provide only temporary relief.

The key sign is that blockade of sympathetic innervation to the affected area provides profound and even permanent pain relief. This may be done by injecting local anesthetic into the sympathetic **ganglia** ● or by infusing the affected area with drugs that block sympathetic activity. Furthermore, this blockade allows healing of the damaged area to progress. The mechanisms of this syndrome are unknown, but it does appear to be due in part to the development of sensitivity of nociceptors to norepinephrine—the neurotransmitter released by sympathetic nerves.[96]

It is important to note that sympathetically maintained pain is best treated early. Poorly healing injuries that show signs of increased sympathetic activation in the damaged area should be carefully evaluated for signs of this syndrome and treatment should be started before the pain becomes severe. In some cases, once the pain reaches severe levels, no treatment is effective.

■ Clinical Pain Control

As discussed in the Pain Control Theory section, primary pain control involves removing or reducing the mechanical and/or chemical stimuli that trigger the nociceptor by encouraging healing and return of normal function. Secondary pain control techniques involve interrupting the transmission of noxious impulses and/or the interpretation of these impulses in the brain. Secondary pain control techniques are often used for patient comfort between interventions or to remove pain to allow for active exercise.

Pain is sometimes indirectly decreased as the result of the **placebo effect**. In experiments to determine a therapeutic modality's or drug's **efficacy** ● as an analgesic, two control groups are often used to compare results with the experimental group of patients who receive the actual treatment. One group receives the treatment and a "**sham** ● control" group is given a "treatment" cleverly disguised as indistinguishable from the intervention that is being tested (Box 2-2). Researchers take particular care to make sure that the participants do not know which group they are in. In many experiments, the placebo results in a measurable reduction in pain compared with the sham control group. While placebo treatments are not a recommended option, the fact that the patient believes that there will be pain reduction often does result in pain reduction.

Therapeutic Modalities

Therapeutic modalities are used for both primary and secondary pain control techniques, often during the same application. Energy applied to the body for the purposes of influencing tissue healing often stimulates sensory receptors that activate the ascending or descending (or both) components of the Gate Control Theory.

Ganglia: A cluster of neurons in the peripheral nervous system.

Efficacy: The ability of a modality or treatment regimen to produce the intended effects.

Sham: A device or "drug" that has no physiological effect on the body (e.g., an ultrasound unit with the output intensity set to zero).

Box 2-2. THE PLACEBO EFFECT

Placebo, stemming from the Latin word for "I shall please," is the term used to describe pain reduction obtained through mechanisms other than those related to the physiological effects of the treatment. The placebo effect is linked to a psychological mechanism: the patient thinks that the treatment is beneficial, then a degree of pain reduction occurs. The physiological mechanisms of the placebo effect are not well understood.

All therapeutic modalities have some degree of placebo effect. This effect may be increased when the modality is applied with a sense of enthusiasm and faith. Indeed, most studies comparing pain reduction between a sham therapeutic modality and an actual treatment have shown decreased levels of pain in both groups. The placebo effect is so powerful that, in one instance, patients who receive placebo pills may even display some side effects of the presumed medication.[81]

The placebo effect can be exploited in the application of therapeutic modalities. Changing modalities and new approaches in the treatment of an injury can positively influence the patient's perception and result in decreased pain.

This section provides an overview of the mechanisms by which therapeutic modalities affect the pain process. Additional detail is provided in the corresponding chapters.

Thermal Agents

Cold first acts as a counterirritant that triggers descending pain control via the release of enkephalin. By slowing the sodium-potassium pump, the rate of nerve depolarization is decreased and the nerve's depolarization threshold is increased. Small-diameter, myelinated nerves are the first to exhibit this change.

Heat also initially acts as a counterirritant to reduce pain via the gate mechanism. The stimulation of sensory nerve fibers, including polymodal thermoreceptors, increases the depolarization threshold of the peripheral nerves, and acts centrally in the thalamus. Heat also reduces muscle spasm, thereby eliminating a mechanical pain trigger.

Therapeutic Ultrasound and Shortwave Diathermy

Thermal therapeutic ultrasound and shortwave diathermy provide many of the analgesic effects of moist heat. The unique aspect of these devices is their ability to alter cell membrane permeability that alters (slows) the nerves' rate of depolarization. Increasing cell membrane permeability opens the sodium channels and congests the area with sodium (Na^+), thereby inhibiting the sodium-potassium pump.[107] This, in turn, increases the pain threshold.[108,109]

Because these are deep heating agents, they are capable of increasing blood flow within the muscles. Restoring blood flow reduces pain caused by ischemia and hypoxia.

Electrical Stimulation Pain Control

Electrical stimulation (ES) can affect pain transmission at the sensory, motor, and noxious levels. Sensory-level ES uses a submotor intensity and a high number of pulses per second (pps) to activate A-beta nerves, inhibiting pain at the spinal level via the ascending mechanism of the Gate Control Theory. Motor-level ES uses a low number of pps to evoke moderate to strong muscle contractions that, in addition the ascending Gate Control Theory, activate the release of endogenous opiates via the gate's descending component. Noxious-level ES activates C fibers and results in pain control via the central biasing mechanism.

Mechanical Modalities and Exercise

This family of therapeutic agents, including active intermittent compression, continuous passive motion, cervical/lumbar traction, and active exercise, primarily provides mechanical pain reduction by removing swelling, restoring joint motion, decreasing pressure on nerve endings, and restoring blood flow. Restoring normal joint and muscle function decreases swelling, restores joint mechanics, and improves muscle function. There is also secondary pain relief by activation of sensory nerves.

Medications

Therapeutic medications can decrease pain through one of three mechanisms: decreasing the inflammatory response, blocking the transmission of noxious impulses, or altering the perception of pain.

Analgesics and Anti-Inflammatory Medications

Nonsteroidal anti-inflammatory drugs (NSAIDs) cover a wide spectrum of over-the-counter (e.g., aspirin, acetaminophen) and prescription medications (e.g., Naproxen). The NSAID family's primary function is inhibiting the cyclooxygenase enzymes COX-1 and COX-2. When COX-2 is inhibited, prostaglandin production is blocked, thereby preventing (or decreasing) the sensitization peripheral nerves (see Hyperalgesia, page 36).[110]

Regarding pain control, the primary action of NSAIDs is to block the action of prostaglandin. Because prostaglandin sensitizes polymodal nociceptors, aspirin counteracts their effect and thereby reduces pain and inflammation. Acetaminophen inhibits synthesis of cyclooxygenase and nitric oxide to decrease pain, but has little effect on inflammation.[98]

Local Anesthetics

Local anesthetics temporarily block nerve conduction, resulting in the loss of sensation in the area. Anesthetics such as lidocaine block the action of voltage-gated sodium channels and very effectively shut down action potential production in nerve fibers.

Opioid Analgesics

Although much maligned because of its many negative physiological, psychological, social, and political attributes, opium and its chemical derivatives, opioids, are one of the best pure analgesics. Opioids block the affective component of pain—the unpleasantness—with little effect on touch or proprioception. Like many drugs derived from plants, opioids act by interacting with neurotransmitter receptors on cells in the nervous system to alter pain perception. These cells are normally regulated by a family of neurotransmitters sometimes called the endogenous opioids or, collectively, endorphins.

Most opioids are highly addictive and are usually prescribed for severe acute pain or pain that does not respond to nonopioid medications and other interventions. Examples of opioid medications include morphine, hydrocodone, propoxyphene, tramadol, and codeine. Often these opioid medications are combined with nonopioid medications such as acetaminophen or ibuprofen. Because of the addictive nature of these medications, these drugs are used for the shortest possible duration.

■ Pain Assessment

The integrative process of perception of pain is variable and subjective. The nebulous nature of pain makes it difficult to assess and quantify. The perceived pain level is a personal expression of what one person feels. The feeling is based on a discriminative, affective, and evaluative process. Pain assessment should encompass both the subjective and objective evaluations to properly document the level and amount of pain that the patient is experiencing (Table 2-4). Although quantifying from person to person (and even within the same person from day to day) is challenging, pain descriptors can accurately diagnose injury and disease and document improvement in the patient's functional status.

Pain measurement consists of several measurable objective parameters that place the patient's pain experience in context.[68] During the clinical examination you may ask a patient how he or she feels today; the response you may receive is usually "better," "worse," or "the same." By asking, you are requiring the person to measure the pain and compare it to the way it felt yesterday. The patient is then usually asked about the location, duration, and type of

TABLE 2-4	Measures of Pain Assessment[61]	
Dimension	*Examples*
Sensory	Intensity, duration, location, frequency
Cognitive/Affective	Unpleasantness
Behavior Interference	Physical, social, emotional

pain being experienced (Table 2-5). The responses to these questions allow the clinician to chart a subjective baseline of the patient's present pain status. In turn, these responses can also help in further evaluation of the underlying pathology.

The person's behavior and movement patterns also provide subjective, nonverbal cues regarding the level of pain. Guarding a joint (self-immobilization), facial expression, voice intonation, and posture are all indicators of pain-related dysfunction.[61] Improvement in these cues should be seen over the course of the patient's treatment sessions.

Several standardized methods are available to measure the amount of pain in relatively objective terms. Through the use of these tools, the location, intensity, and duration of the pain may be ascertained. Other methods exist that assess activities, emotions, and/or personality traits that influence the perception of pain.

Patient Self-Reporting of Pain

Once the subjective evaluation is made, the patient's pain should be objectively evaluated using a standardized pain scale. As pain is a personal experience, the patient's self-reported measures and description of pain are often the most meaningful.[61] Documentation of pain allows decreases or increases in the levels or types of pain experienced by the patient to be quantified.

TABLE 2-5	Subjective Clinical Assessment of Pain

- What causes pain?
- What relieves pain?
- Where is your pain?
- When did your pain begin?
- What is the duration of your pain?
- Have you ever experienced this pain before?
- Can you describe how the pain feels?
- Is the pain getting better or worse?
- Does your pain increase with activity?
- Do you have more pain after activity?
- Do you have pain at night?

During follow-up pain testing, there is disagreement about whether the patient should have access to the prior results. One school of thought is that seeing these scores may bias the results of the current score, but this technique does provide an absolute pain score at that point in time. However, if the goal is to determine relative change in pain levels, the trend is to allow the patient to see the score history so that the current level of pain may be placed in context.[68] Regardless of which approach is taken, it must be used throughout the measurement of the patient's pain.

The measurement of pain is classified into two types of tools, multidimensional and unidimensional. Multidimensional scales often incorporate various components of pain including affective and behavior, whereas unidimensional scales reflect one dimension of pain, usually its intensity.

McGill Pain Questionnaire

The McGill Pain Questionnaire is a multidimensional scale. It is well researched and considered by many to be the gold standard of pain measures.[111,112] The questionnaire consists of four parts: body location, verbal descriptors, change in pain, and strength of pain. Part 1, marking on a body diagram, identifies the location of the pain. Part 2 consists of 18 word sets of descriptive words representing characteristics of pain. The individual is instructed to mark the words that best describe his or her pain. Only words that best fit the pain should be marked and subsets that aren't appropriate should be left unmarked. An example of a subset of words consists of the following; 1 jumping, 2 flashing, and 3 shooting. In Part 3, the person's pain changes are dimension measured. Characteristics of the pain's duration, such as whether the pain is continuous, rhythmic, brief, or transient, are measured. Part 4 measures the intensity of the pain: mild, discomforting, distressing, horrible, or excruciating. The intensity is also measured at its worst, least, and current levels. The individual is also asked to rate the intensity compared to the worst toothache, headache, and stomachache pain ever experienced. The reliability and validity of the McGill scale is well established.[113–115] Also available is a short form of the McGill Pain Questionnaire (Box 2-3), containing 15 word descriptors, a visual analog scale, and a present pain intensity item. The short form has been highly correlated to the long form and is considered an adequate alternative to the original.[116]

There are both advantages and drawbacks to using the McGill scale. The obvious advantage is that it is a multidimensional scale, capable of measuring many aspects of pain. The scale depicts changes in its four sections. This allows the clinician to evaluate more comprehensive changes over the course of treatment. Some researchers have questioned the scale's practicality because it takes approximately 20 minutes to complete and another 5 minutes to score.[117]

Visual Analog Scale

The visual analog scale (VAS) is a horizontal or vertical line, usually 10 centimeters in length, with verbal descriptors at the extremes indicating No Pain and Worst Imaginable Pain. The participant is instructed to place a mark on the line indicating the amount of pain experienced (Box 2-4). The distance from the far left is measured and scored either out of a 101-point scale or rounded to the nearest full or half centimeter and then scored between 0 to 10 or 0 to 20. The scale is commonly utilized because of its ease of use and simple construction.[65] However, it should be used and interpreted with caution because of the large amount of error associated with the scale of up to 40%.[118] Be aware of this limitation when interpreting changes in pain from day to day.

The VAS has high test-retest reliability and is recommended for patients older than 8 years.[61,68] Photocopied scales may produce significant variations in the length of the instrument, reducing its reliability.[68]

Variations of the visual analog scale include the **numeric rating scale** (NRS) and the **faces pain scale**. The NRS uses a system that uses numbers to rate the pain. Most scales use an 11-point system (0 to 10), but variants include 21- and 101-point scales.[68] The faces pain scale uses expressive drawings (similar to emoticons) to communicate pain and is useful with young children.[61]

✱ Practical Evidence

The visual analog scale is a commonly used method of identifying change in the level of pain, but has a large error range. Patients prefer the verbal rating scale, but this instrument does not produce consistently sensitive results because of the low number of levels used. Clinically, the numeric rating scale has good sensitivity and is a valid and reliable instrument.[68]

Numeric Rating Scale

With the numeric rating scale the patient selects a number to represent his or her level of pain. The numbers usually range from 0 to 10 for an 11-point numeric scale (Box 2-5). Numerical scales are typically quick and easy to administer.[119,120] People also may have a problem conceptualizing pain as a number. The same caution should be used with these types of scale as with the visual analog scales.

Verbal Descriptor Scale

The verbal descriptor scale is an easy method of measuring the patient's pain. These scales are often preferred over the visual analog scale for populations with hearing, visual, and psychomotor deficits.[121] Verbal descriptor scales are typically divided into categories that provide very general descriptions of pain such as mild, moderate, and severe. These types of scales provide a good description of the pain but are unable to quantify pain. Using an ordinal scale, the verbal rating scale (VRS) associates point values with pain descriptors (Box 2-6). The relatively

Box 2-3. MCGILL PAIN QUESTIONNAIRE (SHORT FORM)

A. Where Is Your Pain?

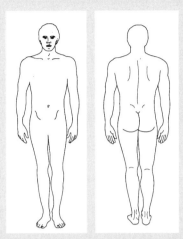

Using the above drawing, please mark the area(s) where you feel pain. Mark an "E" if the source of the pain is external or "I" if it is internal. If the source of the pain is both internal and external, please mark "B."

B. Pain Rating Index

Many different words can be used to describe pain. From the list below, please circle those words that best describe **the pain you are currently experiencing**. Use only one word from each category. You do not need to mark a word in each category. Only mark those words that most accurately describe your pain **now**.

1. Flickering Quivering Pulsing Throbbing Beating Pounding	2. Jumping Flashing Shooting	3. Pricking Boring Stabbing Drilling	4. Sharp Cutting Lacerating
5. Pinching Pressing Gnawing Cramping Crushing	6. Tugging Pulling Wrenching	7. Hot Burning Scalding Searing	8. Tingling Itchy Smarting Stinging
9. Dull Sore Hurting Aching Heavy	10. Tender Taut Rasping Splitting	11. Tiring Exhausting	12. Sickening Suffocating
13. Fearful Frightful Terrifying	14. Punishing Grueling Cruel Vicious Killing	15. Wretched Blinding	16. Annoying Troublesome Miserable Intense Unbearable
17. Spreading Radiating Penetrating Piercing	18. Tight Numb Drawing Squeezing Tearing	19. Cool Cold Freezing	20. Nagging Nauseating Agonizing Dreadful Torturing

The McGill Pain Questionnaire (MPQ) is used during the patient's first visit to identify painful areas and quantify the intensity of the pain. In part A the patient is asked to localize the area(s) of pain and indicate if the source of the discomfort is superficial (external) or deep (internal). To score the Pain Rating Index, add up the total number of words chosen, up to the maximum of 20 words (one for each category). The level of the pain intensity is determined by assigning a value to each word by its order (first word equals 1, second word equals 2, and so on). Therefore, a patient could have a high MPQ score of 20 (selecting a word in each group), but have a low-intensity score by selecting the first word in every group.

Box 2-4. THE VISUAL ANALOG SCALE

Pain as
bad as it —————————————————————————— No pain
could be

Using a 10-cm line labeled as above, the patient places a mark on the line at the point that best represents the current pain intensity. The distance from the right side of the line to the "mark" is measured in centimeters and represents the pain "score." The VAS is consistent, reliable, and easy to use. It can be used before and after treatments to measure the effectiveness of treatment or day to day to measure a patient's progress.

Box 2-5. THE NUMERIC RATING SCALE

No Pain   **Worst Pain Imaginable**

0	1	2	3	4	5	6	7	8	9	10

Similar to the visual analog scale (see Box 2-4), the numeric rating scale has descriptors such as No Pain on the 0 end of the scale and Worst Pain Imaginable on the high end. The patient then marks the number that best represents the level of pain. The results of this numeric rating scale should be a whole number. For instance, 7 is an acceptable result, 7.5 is not.

Box 2-6. THE VERBAL RATING SCALE

0	No pain
1	Mild pain
2	Moderate pain
3	Severe pain

The patient is presented with descriptors such as those presented above, either in writing or read aloud to the individual. The patient then selects the number that best describes the intensity of pain at that moment.

few levels of pain and, therefore, the misinterpretation of the intervals between the pain levels is more probable than with other methods, but valid and reliable results may be obtained.[68]

✱ Practical Evidence

Although popular and easy to use, single-item pain scales are inadequate for accurately measuring a patient's pain. One item cannot precisely measure the entire spectrum of the pain response and the responses are easily altered by extrinsic factors such as mood and emotional state.[121]

PROMIS Pain Scales

The Patient Reported Outcomes Measurement Information System (PROMIS) is an NIH blueprint initiative to build a system of highly reliable, precise measures of patient-reported health status for physical, mental, and social well-being. PROMIS tools measure a variety of health-related domains by asking what patients are able to do and how they feel (Fig. 2-12).[123] One goal of the PROMIS system was to create universal measures so that clinical and research data could be interpreted across sites and studies, including across a wide variety of disease and health conditions. While most PROMIS scales have been validated in other disease populations, the scales do hold promise for use in athletic training.

PREVIEW OF SAMPLE ITEMS

Figure 2 is an excerpt from the paper version of the seven-item short form. This instrument is also available for online administration. There are a variety of formatting options for the online version.

In the past 7 days....	Had no Pain	Never	Rarely	Sometimes	Often	Always
PAINBE2 When I was in pain I became irritable............................	☐ 1	☐ 2	☐ 3	☐ 4	☐ 5	☐ 6
PAINBE3 When I was in pain I grimaced........	☐ 1	☐ 2	☐ 3	☐ 4	☐ 5	☐ 6

A

PREVIEW OF SAMPLE ITEMS

Figure 2 is an excerpt from the paper version of the six-item short form. This instrument is also available for online administration. There are a variety of formatting options for the online version.

In the past 7 days....	Not at all	A little bit	Somewhat	Quite a bit	Very much
PAININ9 1 How much did pain interfere with your day to day activities?	☐ 1	☐ 2	☐ 3	☐ 4	☐ 5
PAININ22 2 How much did pain interfere with work around the home?	☐ 1	☐ 2	☐ 3	☐ 4	☐ 5
PAININ31 3 How much did pain interfere with your ability to participate in social activities?	☐ 1	☐ 2	☐ 3	☐ 4	☐ 5

B

Figure 2-12. **The PROMIS Pain Scales.** (A) The Pain Behavior scale and (B) the Pain Interference scale.

The domain of pain is one area in which PROMIS has built scales for use across patient populations. PROMIS currently has two completed pain scales: the PROMIS Pain Behavior and the PROMIS Pain Interference. It also has a PROMIS Pain Quality that has not yet been completed.

PROMIS Pain Behavior

The pain behavior measures focus on the external manifestations of pain: behaviors indicating that an individual is experiencing pain. These behaviors can be verbal or nonverbal, involuntary or deliberate. These behaviors include displays of sighing, crying, guarding, facial expressions, and asking for help. This pain behavior measure has a total of 39 items assessed over the past 7 days. Each item is measured on a 6-point Likert scale from Had No Pain to Always. This measure is available from PROMIS free of charge and is available in both computer adaptive form and a paper-and-pencil short form.

PROMIS Pain Interference

Pain interference measures the consequences of pain on relevant aspects of one's life. It evaluates the effect pain has on social, cognitive, emotional, physical, and recreational activities as well as asking about sleep and enjoyment in life. The pain interference measure includes 41 items that ask patients to rate how their amount of pain hindered various activities over the past 7 days using a 5-point Likert scale from Not at All to Very Much. This measure is available in both computer adaptive form and a paper-and-pencil short form.

Sensitivity of Pain Scales

Changes in pain levels can be compared in the same individual using only the same instrument. Scores between the NRS and VAS, for example, cannot be meaningfully compared. The error associated with each scale must be determined for the amount of change needed to identify a "real" change. When an 11-point scale (0 to 10) is used, the amount of change in the person's pain needed at the extreme scores (e.g., 1 to 3, 8 to 10) must be greater than those in the middle (4 to 7) to see the same change in scores in the middle of the range. Therefore, changes in raw scores and percentage of change can be useful when interpreted with caution. For instance, a 3-point change from 9 to 6 on the NRS is a 33% decrease in pain. A change from 6 to 4 is two points, but also represents a 33% decrease.[68]

Percentage of change is calculated as:

(Pre-test score – post-test score)/Pretreatment score $\times$ 100

The role of pain scales in uses other than monitoring an individual patient's change in pain intensity is debatable. Some researchers argue that statistical comparisons between groups is meaningless, while others maintain that there is validity in this approach.[124]

Chapter 3

Development and Delivery of Intervention Strategies

Sara D. Brown, MS, LAT

This chapter presents an overview of the decision-making process used in developing treatment plans and modality selection based on the best available evidence. A case study is used to help reinforce the problem-solving approach presented in this chapter.

● The problem-solving approach (PSA) is a logic-based technique that uses the clinical examination findings, the patient's long-term goals (including the resolution of participation restrictions), and the best available evidence to develop an intervention strategy. We practice logical thinking as a part of our daily routine, involving basic skills such as getting dressed in the morning or more complicated tasks such as finding your way around an unfamiliar city. The PSA extends this logical thinking to the care of the patient.

This text began by explaining that therapeutic modalities are used to create the proper environment for healing to occur. The components of the injury response process are interrelated. For example, swelling causes pain, pain causes spasm, and spasm causes pain (Fig. 3-1). Although pain may be the patient's primary complaint, simply focusing the treatments on pain relief does little to resolve the underlying cause of the discomfort and the associated dysfunction. Approaching the patient's problems on a purely symptomatic basis often produces short-term benefits but unsatisfactory long-term results.

Treatment and rehabilitation (collectively known as "intervention") program planning is among the most complex skills that must be mastered. This process integrates clinical examination skills, knowledge of pathology, and identification of the patient's level of function and participation restrictions with knowledge of the physiological effects of therapeutic techniques, goal setting, and patient motivation and education. The body of knowledge is continuously progressing, and the efficacy of interventions is being established or refuted.

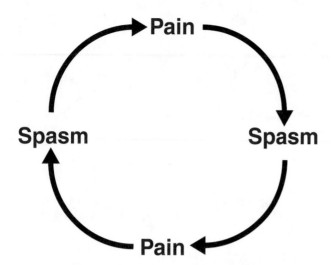

Figure 3-1. **The Pain-Spasm-Pain Cycle.** This represents a self-perpetuating process in which pain causes muscle spasm and muscle spasm produces pain. This cycle continues until either pain or muscle spasm is resolved.

✱ Practical Evidence

Obtaining a correct diagnosis is important for identifying the current indications and **contraindications** ● to a specific treatment. Intervention planning depends on the patient's goal (level of activity) and must address those impairments that limit activity.[2,125]

■ International Classification of Function

The result of injury or disease often focuses on what the patient is unable to do—disability. In 2002 the World Health Organization (WHO) implemented a new classification system that emphasizes what the patient is able to do, the International Classification of Functioning, Disability and Health (ICF).[125] This model synthesizes parts of two disability models: the medical model and the social model. The medical model centers on resolution of the pathology. The social model focuses on the impact of the condition on the patient's quality of life. Termed a **biopsychological model,** the ICF system integrates the biological, social, and individual components of health (Box 3-1).

■ Intervention Outcomes

The interventions such as surgery, therapeutic modalities, and therapeutic exercises used to resolve the patient's activity limitations and participation restrictions are collectively known as outcomes (Table 3-1).[126,127] Historically, interventions have primarily focused on resolving pathology

(a disease-oriented approach) rather than addressing those factors that are meaningful to the patient (a patient-oriented approach). Clinician-based measures primarily assess impairments. Patient-based measures are self-evaluations of activity limitations and participation restrictions.[127]

Measuring Outcomes

Patient-oriented evidence that matters (POEM) identifies the effect that the condition has on the patient's health status and health-related quality of life (HRQOL). While the physical examination is used to identify impairments, treating only those impairments will result in an ineffective treatment if the patient's physical, psychological, and social needs are not considered. For example, a 10-degree improvement in knee range of motion may be measurable but not change the patient's ability to walk up the three steps to his apartment, leaving his functional limitations (and perception of progress) unchanged. As we saw in Chapter 2, the patient's past experiences, expectations, and perceptions have profound influence on pain, function, and quality of life.[128]

Each outcome scale should have values that assist in determining improvement in the patient's condition. Depending on how well the instrument has been validated the following measures may be available for interpreting scores[127]:

Minimum Detectable Change (MDC): The smallest detectable difference accounting for measurement error. Useful in determining the efficacy of an intervention.

Minimally Clinically Important Change (MCID): A measure of responsiveness, the MCID identifies the smallest change that is important or beneficial to the patient.

✱ Practical Evidence

The Global Rating of Change is a simple, patient-based outcome measure that asks the patient, "With respect to your _____ [insert condition here], how would you describe yourself now compared to immediately after your injury?" The patient then marks his or her perception on a scale such as that below:

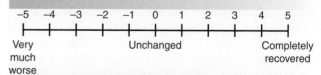

The Minimum Detectable Change is 0.45 points (on 11-point scale). The Minimally Clinically Important Change is 2 points (on 11-point scale).[129]

Contraindications (Contraindicate): To make inadvisable.

Box 3-1. WORLD HEALTH ORGANIZATION INTERNATIONAL CLASSIFICATION OF FUNCTION

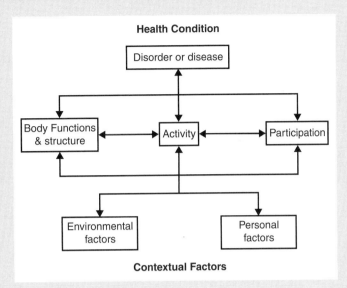

A patient's level of function/disability is the result of the interactions between **health conditions** and **contextual factors.** Health conditions include injury and disease. Contextual factors consist of external environmental factors such as social attitudes and the physical characteristics where the person lives and works, and personal factors including gender, profession, and life experiences.

Focusing on the patient, the ICF system identifies[125]:

- The individual's level of function
- Those interventions that maximize function
- The desired outcomes of the intervention, leading to an evaluation of the intervention's effectiveness
- The individual's assessment of improvement

The language of the ICF:

Term	Definition
Body functions	The body's physiological and psychological systems
Body structures	The body's limbs and organs (includes the musculoskeletal system)
Impairment	Dysfunction of the body's functions and/or structures
Activity	The ability of an individual to perform tasks or actions
Participation	Involvement in work, social, recreational, and leisure activities
Activity limitations	Challenges in performing tasks associated with daily life
Participation restrictions	Challenges in experiencing life situations
Environmental factors	The physical, social, and attitudinal environment in which people live their lives

Adapted from World Health Organization: Towards a common language for functioning, disability, and health. ICF. Geneva, Switzerland. 2002. Available online: http://www.who.int/classifications/icf/training/icfbeginnersguide.pdf

■ Incorporating Evidence Into Decision-Making

Often the therapeutic modalities used are selected out of habit rather than based on a plan. The decision to use a device or technique is frequently based more on fad or tradition than science. The goal of **evidence-based practice** is to provide the most efficient, effective treatment, thereby maximizing the patient's outcomes and making effective use of the clinician's time.

Diagnostic tests, such as those used for orthopedic examination, produce a "positive" or "negative" result, thereby making the measurement of their usefulness relatively easy.

Evaluating the evidence for therapeutic modalities is more convoluted because of the number of factors that influence the outcomes.

Much of the research regarding the efficacy of therapeutic modalities is contradictory or inconclusive. Differences in tissue type (ligaments versus tendons versus muscle, for example), tissue depth (superficial versus deep, for example), the age of the patient, the effect of the natural healing progression, and variations in application protocol make it difficult to evaluate the effectiveness of these devices. Other stumbling blocks relate to poorly designed studies and the inappropriate application of animal studies to a clinical (patient-based) population.

TABLE 3-1	Clinician- and Patient-Based Outcome Measures
Measure	*Description*
Clinician-based outcomes	Measures used to assess the results of interventions from the clinician's perspective; can include objective measures of strength, range of motion, edema, etc., or clinician-report instruments.
Patient-based outcomes	Measures used to assess concerns important to the patient that often relate to symptoms, functional ability, or health-related quality of life. **Condition-specific measures:** Specific to a joint (e.g., Cincinnati Knee Rating Scale) or body area (e.g., Disability of the Arm, Shoulder, and Hand). These scales use multiple questions to assess the patient's level of function and may also include clinician-based measures. **Generic measures:** Global Rating of Change: A single question to determine improvement over time.

When determining if a therapeutic modality would be effective in treating a specific condition, three factors should be considered (Table 3-2). First, can the energy produced by the modality either directly or indirectly affect the target tissues? Assuming that the energy can affect the tissues, the next layer is whether or not the modality produces the physiological response required to promote healing. If the response to either of these questions is "no," then the therapeutic modality should not be used.

Once we can substantiate that energy can penetrate the tissues and affect the physiology, we get to the big question: "Does this device improve patient outcomes?" More specifically, does this device produce better outcomes versus a placebo/sham treatment or better than other treatment techniques or no treatment at all?

Asking Clinical Questions

An age-old adage states that to get the right answer you must ask the right question. This concept is especially true when developing a clinical question to determine the best course of care for a patient. PICO, a mnemonic for **P**atient, **I**ntervention, **C**omparison, and **O**utcomes, provides structure for developing clinical questions.

Patient: 21-year-old female college soccer player; works part-time as a restaurant server

Condition: 1 week status post-ACL reconstruction; bone-patellar tendon-bone autograft

Consider the example of the above patient who is 1 week post-operative for a bone-patellar-bone reconstruction of the anterior cruciate ligament. A manual muscle test for extension is graded 1/5 (cannot produce movement but a muscle contraction is palpable) and the girth around the femur 4 cm proximal to the knee joint line is 2 cm less than the uninvolved extremity. The PICO development of a clinical question would involve the following elements:

	Patient	**Intervention**	**Comparison**	**Outcome**
Description	Identify the patient's demographics	The therapy or therapies being considered	Other therapies being considered (optional)	The desired results and the time frame to obtain those results.
Example	In a 21-year-old female soccer player 1 week post–ACL reconstruction	does neuromuscular electrical stimulation	or no stimulation	restore quadriceps function?
Plain language	In a 21-year-old female soccer player 1 week post–ACL reconstruction, does neuromuscular electrical stimulation or no stimulation function better to restore function?			

TABLE 3-2	Types of Evidence for Therapeutic Modalities
Type of Evidence	*Description*
Physical (Physics)	Is the energy produced by the device capable of directly or indirectly stimulating the target tissues?
Physiological	Does the direct or indirect stimulation of the target tissues produce the intended physiological effects?
Clinical	Do the physiological effects result in positive patient outcomes?

Direct stimulation = the energy applied to the body has a focused effect on the traumatized tissues; indirect stimulation = the energy applied to the body produces a cascade effect that will affect the target tissues.

This clinical question then drives the literature review seeking the best available evidence. Figure 3-2 presents an overview of the process used in determining if an intervention should be used based on the available evidence.

Finding Evidence

Personal experience and expertise carry weight in evidence-based practice, but they carry the least amount of weight. To be considered effective, the use of therapeutic modalities must be validated through published research. Clinical experience is often the foundation of these studies. The ability to critically review published papers—which is beyond the scope of this text—makes interpreting the evidence easier.

✱ Practical Evidence

Systematic reviews are a critical assessment of published research that addresses a focused research question. These reviews synthesize the best evidence and make recommendations for clinical application. Clinical trials involve research conducted on humans who are affected by a condition. PEDro rates the scientific strength of the research design on a scale of 0 to 10, with 10 representing the strongest methodology.

Several databases are available to help find the answers to clinical questions. Search engines such as pubmed.com and sportdiscus.com specifically target peer-reviewed health and medical journals. Other engines such as the Cochrane and PEDro databases incorporate publications from multiple databases and are specifically designed to help answer clinical questions (Box 3-2).

The Problem-Solving Approach

People respond to trauma differently and have different post-injury goals, necessitating individualized treatment plans. When based on **normative data** ● , generalized treatment guidelines provide a reference point for determining where the patient "should be" and what treatment approaches should be considered. Individual treatment plans differentiate the specifics of each patient's case and lead to a more efficient and successful outcome.

The PSA is an ongoing process of evaluation, analysis, and planning consisting of seven steps: (1) obtain a medical history, (2) identify the patient's activity limitations and participation restrictions and then identify the underlying impairments contributing to those limitations (problems), (3) prioritize the problems, (4) set treatment goals, (5) review the evidence, (6) plan the interventions, (7) and reexamine the patient and assess outcomes (Table 3-3). To illustrate these components, case studies also appear at the

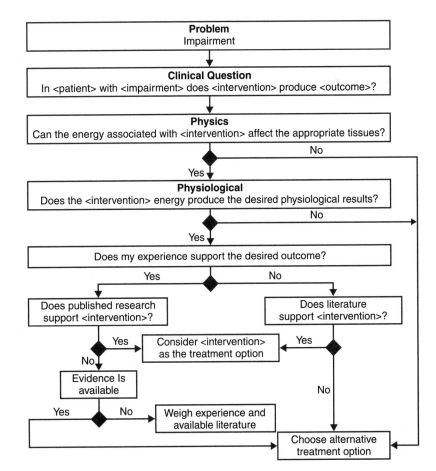

Figure 3-2. **Evidence-Based Decision Tree.** Starting with the problem, a clinical question (PICO) is developed and a therapeutic modality (intervention) is selected. If the physics are sound and the device is capable of eliciting the appropriate physiological effects, the question then focuses on the patient outcomes. Personal experience is the first filter in making this determination, but if the published research does not support its use another option should be determined. If the research supports the intervention, proceed with the treatment. (Adapted from Ragan, BG with permission.)

Normative data: Information that can be used to describe a specific population.

Box 3-2. SEARCHING FOR EVIDENCE USING THE PEDro DATABASE

PEDro
PHYSIOTHERAPY EVIDENCE DATABASE

Change font size: A- A A+

🏠 Home   🔍 New Search (Simple)   🔍 New Search (Advanced)   ❓ Search Help

Simple Search

Search term (or terms): [   ]

[Search]

THE GEORGE INSTITUTE
for Global Health

Affiliated with

THE UNIVERSITY OF SYDNEY

The database was last updated on 4 October 2011 (this includes records added or amended since 5 September 2011). The next update is planned for Monday 7 November 2011. The total number of records on the database is 20,286.

A

Contact us   **Accessibility statement**   **Fair use statement**

PEDro
PHYSIOTHERAPY EVIDENCE DATABASE

Change font size: A- A A+

🏠 Home   🔍 New Search (Simple)   🔍 New Search (Advanced)   ❓ Search Help

Simple Search

Search term (or terms) [**knee electrical stimulation muscle function**]

[Search]

THE GEORGE INSTITUTE
for Global Health

Affiliated with

THE UNIVERSITY OF SYDNEY

The database was last updated on 4 October 2011 (this includes records added or amended since 5 September 2011). The next update is planned for Monday 7 November 2011. The total number of records on the database is 20,286.

B

Contact us   **Accessibility statement**   **Fair use statement**

Box 3-2. SEARCHING FOR EVIDENCE USING THE PEDro DATABASE—cont'd

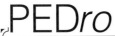
PHYSIOTHERAPY EVIDENCE DATABASE

Change font size: A- A A+

🏠 **Home**   🖥 **Display Selected Records**   🔍 **New Search (Advanced)**   🔍 **New Search (Simple)**   🔍 **Continue Searching (Simple)**   ⑦ **Search Help**

Search Results

Click on a title to view details of that record. If your search has returned many records you may need to click on *Next* (at the top or bottom of the list of records). To display a list of records from one or a series of searches, click on *Select* and then *Display Selected Records* (at the top of the page).

Record 1 - 25 of 41 **Next Last**

Title	Method	Score (/10)	Select Record
Philadelphia Panel evidence-based clinical practice guidelines on selected rehabilitation interventions for knee pain [with systematic review]	practice guideline systematic review	N/A	Select
Effects of neuromuscular electrical stimulation after anterior cruciate ligament reconstruction on quadriceps strength, function, and patient-oriented outcomes: a systematic review	systematic review	N/A	Select
Surface neuromuscular electrical stimulation for quadriceps strengthening pre and post total knee replacement (Cochrane review) [with consumer summary]	systematic review	N/A	Select
Physical therapy interventions for patients with osteoarthritis of the knee: an overview of systematic reviews	systematic review	N/A	Select
(Therapeutic methods for knee osteoarthrits: randomized controlled trial and systemic evaluation) [Chinese - simplified characters]	systematic review	N/A	Select
A critical review of electrical stimulation of the quadriceps muscles	systematic review	N/A	Select
Randomised controlled trial of electrical stimulation of the quadriceps after proximal femoral fracture	clinical trial	7/10	Select
Home based neuromuscular electrical stimulation as a new rehabilitative strategy for severely disabled patients with chronic obstructive pulmonary disease (COPD)	clinical trial	7/10	Select
Does electric stimulation of the vastus medialis muscle influence rehabilitation after total knee replacement?	clinical trial	6/10	Select
Effects of long term resistance training and simultaneous electro-stimulation on muscle strength and functional mobility in multiple sclerosis	clinical trial	6/10	Select

C

The Physiotherapy Evidence Database (pedro.org.au) provides a list of current published research relating to orthopedic medicine (A). The search is conducted using basic search terms, similar to that used for other internet search engines; PEDro has advanced search options as well.

Recall the patient in the above case (21-year-old female; 1 week post-operative ACL reconstruction; MMT extension = 1/5; measurable atrophy). Because the patient is unable to voluntarily contract the muscle and elicit movement, you are considering using electrical stimulation to help retrain the muscle.

To assist you in making this decision, you will use a review of the PEDro database (or similar search engine) to determine if electrical stimulation can help improve muscle function and, if so, which parameters appear to be most effective.

To begin the search, start with general terms such as "electrical stimulation" and "muscle function" and "knee" (B). In this case, the search yielded 41 articles, each of which is identified as a systematic review or clinical trial. A manual review of the articles is needed to identify the most appropriate ones. If too few articles are returned, broaden your search terms; if too many are returned, use more restrictive terms.

TABLE 3-3   **Components of the Problem-Solving Approach**

Component	*Purpose*
Patient Examination: Obtain a medical history	Determine past medical history and history of the present condition to:
	Recognize the indications for the use of therapeutic modalities and other interventions such as exercise
	Recognize any contraindications to the use of therapeutic modalities or other interventions
	Recognize the demands a patient's current and desired activity level places upon the tissues
Patient Examination: Recognition of the problem	Identify impediments (e.g., prior surgery) or comorbidities (e.g., diabetes) that present clinical challenges in developing the treatment plan.
	Via the clinical examination identify:
	The pathology and impairments
	The stage of healing
Prioritization of the problem	Activity limitations
	Participation restrictions
Goal setting	Develop the logical treatment order based on a cause-and-effect relationship between the pathology, impairments, and functional limitations.
	Develop structure and sequence in the treatment plan
	Establish benchmarks to determine efficacy of the treatment plan as determined by the patient's definition of success
	Long-term goals: Identify the desired outcomes of the plan
	Short-term goals: Describe the patient's expected progress during a given time.
Review of the best available evidence	Using available published research combined with personal experience, identify those interventions that have demonstrated efficacy in assisting in the resolution of the patient's problem.
Treatment planning	Determine the modalities and exercises (interventions) to be used and their sequence based on the prioritized patient's problems and treatment goals
	Clinician-based measures are used to determine the course of treatment[127]
Reexamination	Evaluation of the patient's current physical status:
	Reassessment of previously identified problems
	Examination techniques that are no longer contraindicated
	New problems that have developed since the previous examination
	The findings are used to:
	Assess the effectiveness of the current treatment plan
	Reassess the short- and long-term goals
	Determine changes that are needed in the treatment plan
	Outcome measures are used to determine the effectiveness of the interventions used[127]

end of each section. Although the focus of this text is on therapeutic modalities, the role of these interventions is to prepare the patient for therapeutic exercise, manual techniques, and functional activities. Therapeutic modalities are also used after these treatments as a way of controlling exercise-induced inflammation.

■ Patient Examination

To provide proper care to the patient, the pathology, impairments, activity limitations, and participation restrictions must be identified. The problem-recognition stage is designed to identify the type of tissues involved and the stage of the healing process, followed by the impact of the condition on the patient's function and the impairments that cause these functional limitations (Table 3-4).

Medical History

Recognition of the problems begins by reviewing the patient's existing medical records. Diagnostic test reports, operative reports, the physician's prescription, and referral notes are all good sources. Prior treatment notes describe the interventions that have been used, the parameters used in their application, and how effective they were. Other sources of information include preparticipation medical examinations and notes pertaining to prior examinations and treatment of unrelated conditions. Identify any medical

TABLE 3-4 **Information Gained During the Patient Examination**

Segment	Description
Patient's narrative	The patient's description of the problems and resulting impact on activity and participation
Medical history	Any significant medical condition that may affect the current course of treatment
Medications	Current use of prescription, nonprescription, or recreational medication that may alter the findings of the examination or present a contraindication to the use of therapeutic modalities or other therapeutic interventions
Mechanism of injury	The description of how the injury occurred or the onset of symptoms
Normal level of activity	Identifies the patient's current and desired activity lifestyle
Type of tissues involved	Anatomy, function, size, depth of trauma
Nature of the trauma	For example, sprain, strain, fracture, contusion, improper biomechanics
Stage of injury response	Acute inflammation, proliferation, maturation, chronic inflammation
Impairments	Pain, decreased range of motion, decreased strength
Patient goals	Long-term, short-term
Contraindications	Modalities, exercises, manual techniques, and medications that cannot be used

contraindications to the use of specific interventions during the patient interview (Box 3-3).

Subjective • information is obtained during the formal patient interview and during informal discussion (Fig. 3-3). Good clinical skills require keen listening skills and the ability to identify and solicit pertinent information from the patient. For instance, a patient's comment such as "My knee feels as if it is going to give out" may identify quadriceps muscle weakness, pain, or rotational instability. Complaints of feeling "worse" after therapy may indicate

Box 3-3. MEDICAL CONTRAINDICATIONS TO THERAPEUTIC MODALITY USE

The use of certain therapeutic modalities or other therapeutic interventions may be contraindicated based on the patient's current stage of healing or the body area being treated, or because of unrelated medical conditions. Identifying regional contraindications requires knowledge of the modality being used. The clinical examination should identify the indications and contraindications to the use of specific therapeutic modalities. However, underlying medical contraindications against the use of certain therapeutic modalities must be identified prior to beginning any treatments.

Contraindications are either absolute or relative. An **absolute contraindication** means that the modality or protocol must not be used under any circumstance. **Relative contraindications** mean that the treatment can be modified to accommodate the patient's condition, decreasing the temperature of a warm whirlpool for example. **Precautions** identify how misuse of the modality can cause harm to the patient.

Medical contraindications can be identified through a comprehensive medical questionnaire and be confirmed during the history taking/patient interview process. The medical questionnaire should be administered at the start of the academic year in the case of institutional sports medicine facilities or at the time of the first visit for other outpatient facilities.

The following is a partial list of common medical contraindications and methods to identify them. Health care providers are legally, morally, and ethically responsible to be familiar with the contraindications of the device, technique, or procedure being administered. In the case of therapeutic modalities, the manufacturer's user's guide lists the precise contraindications and precautions for that device.

Contraindication	Identified By	Example
Acute injury/ inflammation	Written Questionnaire	"When did this injury occur?"
	Clinical Examination	Assess the cardinal signs of inflammation
Implanted metal	Written Questionnaire	"Have you had a fracture that required surgery?"

Continued

Subjective: Symptoms stated by the patient that are not externally apparent, such as pain. Personal beliefs and attitudes may alter subjective symptoms.

Box 3-3. MEDICAL CONTRAINDICATIONS TO THERAPEUTIC MODALITY USE—cont'd

Contraindication	Identified By	Example
	Clinical Evaluation	"Do you have implants such as plates or screws?" Observe the area to be treated for surgical scars
Hypertension	Written Questionnaire	"Are you currently taking medication for high blood pressure?" "Have you been told you had high blood pressure?"
Circulatory impairment	Clinical Examination	Assess blood pressure
	Written Questionnaire	"Have you been diagnosed as having circulatory problems such as peripheral vascular disease, blood clots, or Raynaud's phenomenon?" "Are your hands or feet sensitive to heat or cold?" "Have you been diagnosed as having a heart condition?"
	Clinical Examination	Assess capillary refill Observe the feet and ankles for edema
Cardiorespiratory insufficiency	Written Questionnaire	In addition to findings for high blood pressure and circulatory impairment: "Are you taking medication for your heart?" "Have you ever suffered a heart attack or stroke?" "Do you regularly suffer from shortness of breath or have difficulty breathing?"
	Clinical Examination	Inspect the nailbeds for cyanosis or enlargement Check capillary refill in the nailbed
Thrombophlebitis ●	Written Questionnaire	"Have you been diagnosed as having blood clots?" "Do you suffer from unexplained swelling in the feet and ankles?"
	Clinical Examination	Warmth, redness, swelling, and tenderness in the affected area
Sensory impairment	Written Questionnaire	"Do you suffer from tingling, burning, or numbness in your arms or legs?" "Do you have diabetes or is there a history of diabetes in your family?" (Diabetes often leads to decreased sensory function.)
	Clinical Examination	Perform a sensory (dermatome) screen
Infection	Written Examination	"Are you currently taking prescription antibiotic medications?"
	Clinical Examination	Inspect the area for signs of infection including pustules, increased temperature, and red streaks
Cancer	Written Questionnaire	"Have you ever been diagnosed with cancer?" "Do you have constant unexplained pain at night?"
Pregnancy	Written Questionnaire	"Are you pregnant or is there the chance that you might be pregnant?"

Thrombophlebitis: Inflammation of the veins.

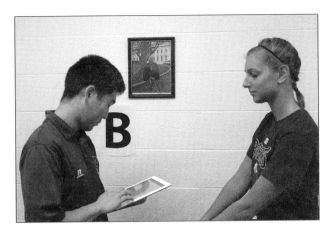

Figure 3-3. **The Patient Interview.** Much of the success in treatment planning lies in effective communication between the patient and the clinician.

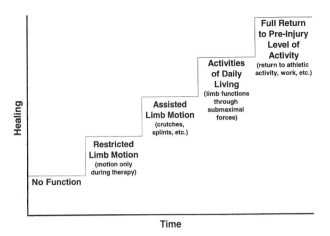

Figure 3-4. **Return to Function After Injury.** The return to the pre-injury level of activity follows a progressive sequence in which one level of function must be obtained before progressing to the next level. Although this figure shows a linear and steady progression, there is overlap and setbacks between stages.

that the exercise and/or treatment parameters were too intense. The Global Rating of Change, or similar outcome measure, should also be incorporated into the patient interview (see Table 3-1). Remarks indicating improvements may determine the best patterns of modality use and parameters selected. When applicable, these remarks should be noted in the patient's medical file.

It is easy to focus your attention solely on observable impairments such as swelling, discoloration, decreased range of motion, and the reported symptoms of pain and numbness. Although the short-term objective of a treatment session is to provide symptomatic relief or objective improvement in one of these parameters, the long-term goals of proper healing and return to a normal lifestyle will not be met until the underlying pathology is identified and managed (Fig. 3-4).

If we consider the case of a patient who complains of pain during shoulder elevation, permanent pain relief will not be obtained until the underlying biomechanical dysfunction of abnormal arthrokinematics is addressed. As we will see in the following sections, **palliative treatments** ● may be required in the early treatment phases but only as a transition or adjunct to curative treatments.

Problem Recognition

The participation restrictions described by the patient may result from a culmination of multiple pathologies and

Case Study Part 1: The Patient's Medical History

A 22-year-old woman diagnosed with patellofemoral pain syndrome of the right knee has been referred by an orthopedic surgeon. The following information has been obtained:

Report: Intermittent pain "under the right kneecap" that increases when she goes up or down stairs and occasionally after long periods of sitting. The pain and intermittent "giving way" prohibit the patient from participating in strenuous activity.

Medical history: The patient has been diagnosed with exercise-induced bronchospasm (EIB), which is triggered by exercise in a cold environment.

History of present condition: While participating in soccer, the patient twisted her knee with her foot planted, resulting in a tear of the anterior cruciate ligament (ACL) and medial meniscus. She underwent

ACL reconstruction with a bone–patellar tendon–bone autograft and a partial medial meniscectomy. She returned to play soccer 6 months after the surgery. One month later, she developed her present symptoms that have persisted for 6 months.

Diagnostic tests: Radiographic studies demonstrate normal findings associated with ACL repair. No evidence of degenerative changes.

Activity limitations: Must climb stairs leading with the uninvolved leg.

Participation restrictions: Unable to participate in soccer; describes difficulty in attending classes secondary to pain with prolonged walking.

General medical conditions: No significant illnesses.

Continued

Palliative: Pain relief without addressing the cause of the pain. Treatment only of the symptoms.

Case Study Part 1: The Patient's Medical History—cont'd

Medications: Patient reports taking 200 mg ibuprofen as needed for pain with moderate relief. Uses albuterol when EIB is symptomatic.

Contraindications to modality use: None.

Contraindications to therapeutic exercise: None.

Patient goals: Pain-free activities of daily living (ADLs). To return to recreational soccer.

Examination findings:

Participation restrictions:	Cannot participate in soccer.
Activity limitations:	The patient cannot climb or descend stairs without pain. Feet excessively pronate (bilaterally) with early heel rise during walking gait secondary to the inability to extend the knee. The patient cannot sit for more than 30 minutes without developing knee pain.
Observation:	Healed incision over the patellar tendon. **Keloid** • formation is present.
Palpation:	Pain is produced during palpation along the medial **retinaculum** • and at the inferior patellar pole.
Patellar mobility:	The patella is **hypomobile** • superiorly and medially.
Patellar tracking:	Increased lateral tracking relative to the opposite side.
Range of Motion:	**Involved:** **Active:** 10 degrees of extension to 135 degrees of flexion (0 − 10 − 135 degrees) **Passive:** 3 degrees of hyperextension to 140 degrees of flexion (3 − 10 − 135 degrees) **Uninvolved:** **Active:** 5 degrees of hyperextension to 145 degrees of flexion (5 − 0 − 145 degrees)

	Passive: 1 degree of hyperextension to 150 degrees of flexion (1 − 0 − 150 degrees)
Girth:	Girth is 1 cm greater than that of the uninvolved knee as measured over the joint line. Mild effusion is present.
Tone:	The patient displays poor control of the quadriceps muscle group. The vastus medius oblique (VMO) lacks tone and mass compared with that on the uninvolved side.
Muscle Function Assessment:	Hip muscle groups are 5/5 bilaterally. Quadriceps are 5/5 bilaterally, with pain elicited at the patellofemoral joint on the involved side. Hamstring groups are 5/5 bilaterally. Ankle groups are 5/5 bilaterally.
Joint Function Assessment	Passive prone knee flexion: 0 to 120 degrees on R; 0 to 140 degrees on L Both knees lack 10 degrees of extension with the hip at 90 degrees. Passive ankle dorsiflexion with knee extended: 0 to 10 degrees bilaterally.
Pain rating:	Patient describes pain as 5/10 when she is descending stairs, 1/10 while sitting.
Stress tests:	All within normal limits as compared bilaterally.
Selective tissue tests:	Thessaly for meniscus: unremarkable.

This introduces the patient, her relative medical history, and reports from which we can build our problem list. The problem recognition uses this patient history to identify functional deficits and those conditions that should be the focus of the patient's treatment goals.

impairments (see Box 3-1). Using valid and reliable tools, correct measurement techniques, consistency during re-examination, and proper documentation of the results contribute to the accumulation of documented evidence of the patient's progress (Table 3-5). These tools are not appropriate for every condition, and the patient may have one or more contraindications to their use.

Conduct formal patient examinations and reexaminations regularly. Before each treatment session, interview the patient to evaluate the effectiveness of the prior interventions and home treatments and determine the patient's physical and mental/emotional status.

The patient's mental and emotional states and motivation to return to activity are important in determining

---

Keloid: A nodular, firm, movable, and tender mass of dense, irregularly distributed collagen scar tissue in the dermis and subcutaneous tissue. Common in the African American population, keloid scarring tends to occur after trauma or surgery.

Retinaculum: A fibrous membrane that holds an organ or body part in place.

Hypomobile: An abnormal limitation of normal motion.

TABLE 3-5	Select Tools Used in the Examination of Orthopedic Conditions		
Tool	*How Measured*	*Information Gained*	*Contraindications to Use*
Active range of motion	Goniometric measurement or a percentage of full movement in the case of the spine.	Ability to move actively or passively with reference to specific motions.	Acute unstable musculoskeletal injuries.
Muscle function assessment	Measurement by manual muscle test using a grading scale, a hand-held **dynamometer** ●, or an isokinetic device.	Indication of muscular strength or neurological deficits. Can also determine injury to a muscle or tendon by eliciting pain and/or weakness associated with contraction of the muscle or muscle group.	Acute unstable injuries to ligaments, tendons, or bones. Any orthopedic test that would directly stress unstable or recently repaired structures. Recent repairs of ligaments or tendons.
Swelling	Circumferential measurement with a tape measure around specific landmarks or **volumetric measurements** ●.	Indication of the presence of swelling or edema relative to the opposite extremity.	None.
Weight-bearing status	Measurement as full, partial, or non–weight bearing. Can also be described as a percentage of full weight bearing.	Ability of the patient to bear weight in the presence of pain, swelling, weakness, and/or decreased range of motion.	Conditions that preclude weight bearing.
hypertrophy ●	Circumferential measurement with a tape measure and result compared with that for opposite extremity.	Determination of the decrease or increase of tissue mass. Note that there is little correlation between limb girth and strength.	None.
Pain	Pain rating scale of 0 to 10, with 0 being no pain and 10 being the worst pain imaginable.	Presence of pain with a specific functional activity (squatting), movement (shoulder flexion), stress test (valgus stress to the elbow), or at rest.	Caution should be exercised not to use a functional activity to assess pain that may compromise unstable or recently repaired tissues.
Sensation	Light touch to bilateral areas of the body having the same dermatomal or specific nerve distributions.	Assessment of the sensory nervous system. Note that dermatomal distributions may vary greatly from person to person.	**Dementia** ● or disorientation.
Flexibility	Assessment of muscle length by fixing one end of the muscle and moving the other end until maximum	Determination of whether a muscle or muscle group is functioning at a normal length or if it is producing	Acute injuries to musculotendinous tissues. Any test that would directly stress unstable or

Continued

Dynamometer: A device used for measuring muscular strength.
Volumetric measurement: Determination of the size of a body part by measuring the amount of water it displaces.
Hypertrophy: To develop an increase in bulk, for example, in the cross-sectional area of muscle.
Dementia: The progressive loss of cognitive and intellectual functions without impairment of perception or consciousness. Symptoms include disorientation, memory impairment, impaired judgment, and impaired intellectual ability.

TABLE 3-5   Select Tools Used in the Examination of Orthopedic Conditions—cont'd

Tool	How Measured	Information Gained	Contraindications to Use
	length is reached. Can sometimes be measured goniometrically or assessed as normal or restricted compared with the uninvolved limb.	abnormal stresses because of tightness.	recently repaired structures.
Functional Assessment			
Activity	Measurement as the capability of a patient to perform desired and necessary tasks or actions, including sport-specific functions.	Determination of the patient's level of function with regard to executing a specific task or action.	Any functional task that would directly stress unstable or recently repaired structures.
Biomechanical assessment	Observation and measurement of biomechanical problems that can alter function. It may be performed as a specific measurement (leg length) or observed as a part of a functional activity (gait analysis).	Determination of the causes of abnormal stresses placed on the body by inherent biomechanical problems. Sometimes the effects of these problems can be decreased or eliminated with exercise, a change in footwear, or the use of **orthotics** ● .	Any analysis that would directly stress unstable or recently repaired structures.
Posture	Inspection and observation of posture and comparison with normative information.	Assessment of abnormal tissue stress caused by poor postural control or habits.	None.

treatment interventions. To maximize participation, educate the patient about the nature of the injury, intervention goals and plan to meet these goals, and the expectations for recovery. The pace of the recovery is affected by the patient's motivational level.[130] Some patients need to be held back because of their high motivation level. Other patients have to be continuously motivated to reach their treatment goals. Patients who consistently lack motivation or display behavioral signs of disinterest in their recovery may need the assistance of a mental health care provider.

✳ Practical Evidence

A depressed mood is associated with higher disability in patients with specific and nonspecific chronic low back pain.[131]

The information collected during examination and the treatment sessions should be identified and recorded in the patient's file using measurable and objective terms. Although each treatment session should begin with a patient interview, a full reexamination of the patient's condition should be conducted regularly (e.g., at the end of a goal period). Ongoing reexamination and comparison of outcome measures allow the patient's current state to be compared with baseline information. A determination can then be made about whether the patient has improved as expected or if the treatment plan must be modified because of a lack of patient progress.

Prioritization of the Problems

Prioritizing the patient's problems assists in developing the logical treatment progression. This step requires an understanding of pathophysiology, the events associated with each stage of the healing process, and the beneficial

---

Orthotics: Orthopedic devices for correcting deformity or malalignment.

effects (and the potentially hazardous effects) that each modality has on the injury response process. Prioritizing the problems based on their cause-and-effect relationship to the patient's functional limitations helps to develop a logical treatment sequence, defines the focus of **self-treatment** ●, and maximizes the use of available treatment time.

The key to resolving the patient's functional deficit is to identify the problem or problems that trigger the other signs and symptoms. A question that can be used in prioritizing the treatment plan is "What other impairments will be reduced if this problem is resolved?"

Consider a patient who cannot bear weight secondary to pain, decreased range of motion (ROM), and swelling in the left ankle. Which one of these problems should receive the highest treatment priority? If our treatment approach focused solely on pain, the patient would still be unable to walk properly because of the swelling, decreased joint ROM, and a lack of strength. The ROM exercises could not be adequately conducted because of the patient's pain and joint swelling, leaving reducing swelling as our highest treatment priority.

Swelling places mechanical pressure on the nerve endings, inhibits blood flow to and from the area, and expands the tissues in the area. A treatment plan that emphasizes swelling reduction would decrease pain and increase ROM, enabling the return of normal gait. The treatments used to reduce swelling (e.g., compression and elevation) also have a direct effect on suppressing pain transmission by lessening the pressure on nerve endings and activating sensory receptors (compression and elevation). Although ice does not decrease swelling (it only prevents it), cold does slow nerve conduction velocity and decreasing pain. Prescription or over-the-counter anti-inflammatory or pain medication may also be prescribed.

Once inflammation has been controlled, swelling reduced, and limited pain-free motion restored, more functional exercises can be initiated. ROM exercises, stretching, balancing, proprioception, and strengthening protocols would be introduced into the treatment plan, followed by weight-bearing exercises leading to normal gait.

Case Study Part 2: **Problem Recognition**

The following problems were identified from the case study scenario:

1. Decreased ability to function without pain
2. Poor patellar mobility and tracking secondary to muscular weakness and soft tissue adhesions, including the presence of a keloid
3. Increased swelling of the right knee as compared with the uninvolved knee
4. Decreased active range of motion of the right knee
5. Decreased flexibility of the quadriceps, hamstrings, and calf muscles on the involved side
6. Improper biomechanics of both feet (pathological subtalar **pronation** ●

Commentary

- The pain ratings are important because pain indicates pathology and affects the individual's quality of life. Even though this patient is active, attention must be paid to the disability affecting her daily life and work. Her relatively sedentary occupation contributes to her discomfort. She spends more time sitting and performing more sedentary activity than she does exercising. Pain experienced during palpation should not be used to determine improvement because the amount of pressure applied to the area is not well controlled.
- The finding of joint effusion is significant. Accumulation of 20 to 30 mL of fluid within the knee joint capsule may cause inhibition of the VMO, altering patellofemoral biomechanics leading to chronic inflammation.
- The ability to restore ROM this long after surgery is challenging, but scar and tissue remodeling can remain active for 12 to 24 months. The chronic pain and swelling could indicate that the inflammation and remodeling phase is still active, increasing the possibility of restoring the tissue. Scarring, decreased patellar mobility, and muscle tightness negatively affect ROM. The VMO cannot contract.

The loss of even a few degrees of ROM is problematic because of the biomechanical changes at the patellofemoral joint. This can lead to other biomechanical changes in both lower extremities caused by a functional length discrepancy that is created when the patient is weight bearing.

Continued

Self-treatment: Treatment or rehabilitation performed by the patient without direct supervision including home treatment programs.

Pronation: An inward flattening and tilting of the foot, resulting in the lowering of the medial longitudinal arch.

Case Study Part 2: The Patient's Medical History—cont'd

- Findings of a hypomobile patella, decreased ROM, and chronic swelling may be indicative of hypertrophic scarring of the **infrapatellar** ● area. Abnormal patellofemoral joint biomechanics and patellofemoral pain are common complications after ACL reconstruction. Normal tissue biomechanics must be restored before normal joint biomechanics return and pain decreases.
- Decreased flexibility of the quadriceps and hamstrings may cause increased stress on the knee joint capsule, retinaculum, and patellofemoral joint. The most common compensatory motion caused by tightness of the gastrocnemius and soleus is foot pronation, leading to increased tibial rotation and increased lateral forces on the patellofemoral joint.

Even though the patient mentions that her knee "gives out," it is not listed as a problem because the results of stress testing and selective tissue tests were negative and may be the result of pain. In this case, the "giving out" sensation is most probably indicative of pain, quadriceps inhibition, or muscle weakness and will be resolved as these individual problems are addressed, although muscle strength needs to be addressed. If the patient continues to report this problem after strength has returned and swelling has decreased, ligamentous stability should be reevaluated and/or the patient referred back to the physician.

Goal Setting

Clear, concise, and measurable goals translate the prioritized problem list into a well-structured treatment plan (Box 3-4). Short-term and long-term goals guide the rehabilitation program by establishing timelines, identifying outcomes, and providing a benchmark to measure the effectiveness of the intervention. The patient meeting the established goals with improving outcome measures indicates that the program may advance to the next stage. A lack of progress may indicate that the treatment approach needs to be modified. Properly written and documented goals are also used for insurance and legal purposes and demonstrate the criteria used to decide when to discharge the patient from care. When based on outcome measures, treatment goals can be used as the basis for research on treatment efficacy.132

Treatment goals are estimates of the patient's progress at specific points in time and should be consistent with the patient's priorities, lifestyle, and participation expectations.[130] The patient and, when applicable, the patient's family should participate in setting the treatment goals.[133] Patient motivation is another important function of treatment goals. Motivated patients will most likely be more compliant in actively participating in their recovery.

✱ Practical Evidence

Patient compliance with the treatment plan is increased and the outcomes improved when the patient's family helps develop the goals and completely understands the progression.[134,135,136]

Case Study Part 3: Prioritization of the Problem

The patient's problems ranked in terms of treatment priority are:

1. Improper foot biomechanics and decreased patellar mobility
2. Decreased flexibility and range of motion of the quadriceps, hamstrings, and calf muscles
3. Swelling of the right knee
4. Poor patellar tracking
5. Pain during stair climbing, sitting, and contraction of the right quadriceps
6. Inability to play soccer

Commentary

Correcting the biomechanical causes for the patient's pain and dysfunction takes the highest priority in this treatment program. The patient may excessively pronate to compensate for the lack of dorsiflexion arising from tightness of the calf muscles. This places increased stress on the patellofemoral joint and contributes to decreased knee and ankle ROM. To prevent further compensation in the kinetic chain, the gastrocnemius and soleus flexibility must be increased.

- If, after normal gastrocnemius-soleus flexibility is restored, hyperpronation of the feet is still believed to

---

Infrapatellar: The distal portion of the patella including the patellar tendon.

Case Study Part 3: Prioritization of the Problem—cont'd

be contributing to the pathology, a trial use of orthotics or a change of footwear is warranted. Treating the symptoms of pain and swelling without addressing the possible causes will provide only temporary relief of the symptoms. The plan must contain therapeutic exercises to correct the patient's biomechanical problems.

- The effusion causes pain and inhibition of the quadriceps. Eliminating the swelling will improve the quadriceps tone, ability to improve strength, and the ability to control patellar tracking within the femoral groove. If the treatment does not eliminate the swelling, the patient should be referred back to the physician.
- The hypomobile peripatellar tissues are important in the patellofemoral joint's overall health. Before the quadriceps can properly track the patella through active muscle contraction, the patella must be able to move freely. Hypomobility of the

peripatellar tissues hinders normal tracking and places pathological stresses on the joint. Along with restoring normal movement, neuromuscular reeducation of the muscle group to provide active control must be emphasized.

- The pain and dysfunction caused by tendinopathy contributed to the patient's problems; these are often ranked as the highest priority. In this case, the focus is eliminating the stresses that cause the inflammation and purposefully avoiding strengthening exercises through painful arcs of motion; strengthening will occur only within the patient's pain-free ROM.
- The functional problems of this patient have not been given the highest treatment priority. The treatment is prioritized to eliminate and correct those problems that contribute to the symptoms. We would expect to see improved function as the patient's symptoms are decreased.

The treatment goals and outcomes are relative to the pathology being treated. Ideally, the optimal goal is a full recovery or "100%." In some cases, "98%" may be the highest possible outcome but would be sufficient for a full return to activity and high patient satisfaction. Clinically, full function may never be restored, but the final outcomes may still be sufficient to remove the disability.

Consider the two goals presented in Table 3-6: a loosely defined goal, "To increase active dorsiflexion," and a more measurably stated goal, "To increase active dorsiflexion to allow the patient to climb stairs unassisted." In the first example, the patient may show improvement by increasing active dorsiflexion from 0 to 8 degrees, but because 10 degrees of dorsiflexion is required for a normal

gait, normal walking gait probably will not be restored. The ability to climb stairs unassisted is quantifiable and measures function.

Long-Term Goals

Long-term goals provide direction to the treatment plan by identifying and quantifying the final outcomes of the program. In most cases, the long-term goal is to return the patient to the pre-injury level of participation, but this is not always feasible (Table 3-7). Although long-term goals are modified throughout the treatment process, they are revised less often than short-term goals. There are fewer long-term goals than short-term goals. Most important, long-term goals focus on restoring participation rather than addressing the individual pathologies afflicting the person.

TABLE 3-6 Measurable Goals

Problem	The patient has an inversion ankle sprain, limiting his ability to walk to school and participate in baseball.
	Dorsiflexion active range of motion is 0 to 2 degrees, resulting in an abnormal walking gait and an inability to walk up stairs without support.
Nonobjective goal	To increase active dorsiflexion.
Objective goal	To increase active dorsiflexion that allows unassisted stair climbing
Reexamination	**Clinician-based measures:** The patient has 0 to 8 degrees of active dorsiflexion.
	Patient-based measures: The patient must rely on the handrail to climb stairs.
Assessment	The patient has not yet met the goal of climbing stairs unassisted, but is progressing toward that goal. The clinician-based measure indicates that the patient is lacking the minimum of 10 degrees of dorsiflexion required for normal gait.

Box 3-4. DEVELOPING WRITTEN GOALS

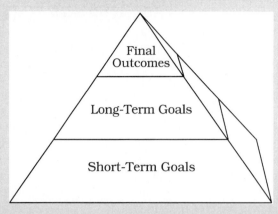

Short-term (1 to 14 days) and long-term (more than 14 days) goals should be stated in objective, measurable terms that describe the quality and quantity of the desired outcome. Not only should the question "Has this goal been met?" be answered with a "Yes" or "No" response; goals should also describe the magnitude of the performance. Suppose you must obtain a score of 73 to pass an examination on your ability to write patient goals. A qualitative measure of your success would be a grade of "Pass" or "Fail" when your examination was returned. Although this scoring system informs you (and your instructor) if you scored above or below the passing point, it does not indicate by how much. If the examination is returned with a grade of 99 or 66, you can base your performance relative to the passing point.

Start the goal writing process by taking all of the prioritized problems and, in an orderly fashion, formulate the final treatment outcome, a list of long-term goals, and the list of short-term goals. Some short-term goals may apply to more than one long-term goal. The final step is to determine a reasonable time frame for the accomplishment of each goal.

Goals can be written using the ABCD format and should be stated in terms of what will be accomplished rather than what limitations will still be present (e.g., "Shoulder elevation = 0 to 140 degrees" versus "Shoulder elevation limited 30 degrees"). This serves to motivate the patient and also keep the clinician focused on how the plan must be altered to facilitate the patient's progress.[130] Goals should be written in precise versus general terms for each problem. For example, a general short-term goal stating that "All ROM will increase 50 degrees" may not be clear if some motions are increased by only 30 degrees, whereas others are increased greater than 50 degrees.

The ABCD Goal Writing Structure

Segment	Purpose	Example
Audience	Person who will perform the task	"The patient will." "The patient and coach will modify practice to . . ." "The patient and employer will alter . . ."
Behavior	Description of task to be performed using action verbs	The patient will obtain enough active knee flexion to allow comfortable sitting . . ."
Condition	Definition of tools, devices, or techniques used in obtaining the goal	"The patient will balance on the involved side for 30 seconds using one hand for support."
Degree	Quality with which the task will be performed, usually described in numerical terms	"The patient will achieve 0 to 90 degrees of active knee range of motion."

Adapted from Kettenbach, G: Writing Patient/Client Notes: Ensuring Accuracy in Documentation, ed 4. , Philadelphia, FA Davis, 2009.

TABLE 3-7	Feasible Goals
Problem	The patient has degenerative disk disease of the lumbar spine, resulting in an inability to sit for longer 30 minutes or play golf.
Nonfeasible goal	The patient will be pain free.
Feasible goal	The patient's symptoms will be controlled with therapeutic exercise so that he or she is able to return to full participation.
Assessment	With a chronic condition such as degenerative disk disease, the patient will most likely have a continuation of the symptoms or have intermittent symptoms. A feasible goal is to control the patient's symptoms to the point at which the individual can function within the limits of pain and limit recurrences.

Although every attempt should be made to make long-term goals measurable, they should also be functional. Goals such as "To return to full competition in college football" or "To return to the pre-injury level of activity at work" define the final outcome of the patient's therapy, and successful completion of the activity is measurable.

Short-Term Goals

Short-term goals describe the patient's projected progress in a specific time and focus on the specific problems identified during the examination that, if met, will achieve the long-term goals. The length of time set to achieve the short-term goals depends on the pathology. In general, the time established for meeting the short-term goals is an estimation of the time required to produce a measurable change in the patient's condition. These typically are in terms of 2 weeks or less.

Short-term goals serve as measuring sticks for the treatment plan. Subsequent patient reexaminations will determine if the patient is meeting the goals. If they are not being met, the treatment program should be reevaluated and appropriate changes made.

Once the patient's problems have been identified and prioritized, and the appropriate goals have been established, treatment planning naturally follows. Treatment planning is the application of your knowledge of the physiological effects of the therapeutic modalities and exercise to resolve the problems required to achieve the patient's goals. The stage of the healing process and the choice of therapeutic techniques largely determine what types of modalities will resolve the pathology (Fig. 3-5).

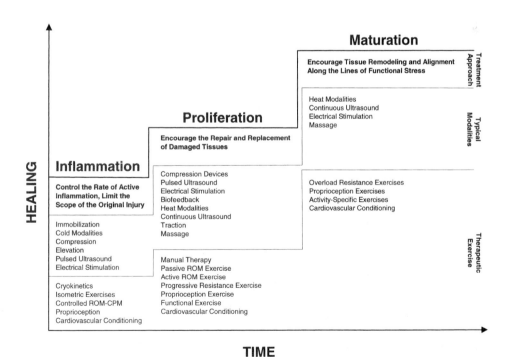

TIME

Figure 3-5. **Modality Boilerplate.** Each stage of the injury response has specific treatment goals that best respond to certain modalities or therapies. When the patient is in the "overlap" phase between two plateaus, the modalities and other interventions from the advanced stage on the right are commonly followed by the modalities of the lesser stage on the left. For example, a patient may use a hot whirlpool and perform active range-of-motion exercises followed by the use of an ice pack. CPM = continuous passive motion.

Case Study Part 4: Long-Term Goals

At the time of discharge, the patient will have met the following long-term goals:

1. The ability to perform normal ADLs (e.g., climbing stairs, prolonged sitting) without pain.
2. Demonstrate normal strength in the right leg.
3. Achieve normal ROM in the right leg.
4. Full return to soccer and other recreational activities.

Commentary

Long-term goals 1 and 2 reflect the patient's expected treatment outcomes as derived from the patient interview.

The remaining goals describe the functional behaviors that would be necessary for the patient to return to full athletic activity (goal 2). Each of these long-term goals will be addressed by one or more short-term goals. Notice that not all of the patient's problems are specifically cited in the long-term goal list. These issues, such as swelling, are addressed by the short-term goals.

Case Study Part 5: Short-Term Goals

The following short-term goals have initially been established for this patient:

1. Excessive pronation will be moderated by stretching the calf muscles.
2. Edema will be decreased by 1.0 cm around the joint line.
3. Medial patellar glide will improve to two out of four quadrants.
4. Flexibility will increase to:
   Quadriceps: Knee flexion to 0 to 140 degrees.
   Hamstrings: Knee extension to 0 degrees.
   Calf muscles: Dorsiflexion to 0 to 15 degrees.
5. The ROM of the knee will be from 0 to 140 degrees.
6. Pain free quadriceps contraction.
7. Compliance and independence in a home exercise program.
8. The patient will not participate in soccer at this time.

Commentary

It will take approximately 2 weeks to observe progress toward the short-term goals. The goals can be measured or easily answered as met or not met and are a reasonable expectation of what the patient's condition should be after 2 weeks. All the goals represent progress in the condition and, if met, will signify that the plan is working.

- The patient's excessive pronation must be controlled to achieve a normal gait pattern. The physical examination findings indicate tightness of the calf muscles that prohibits an appropriate amount of dorsiflexion, resulting in an early heel rise during stance. Orthotics can assist in restoring normal biomechanics. Decreasing the amount of swelling within the joint capsule will prevent inhibition of the VMO, improving biomechanics by assisting in terminal knee extension and patellar tracking. Flexibility and ROM for the entire lower extremity will be emphasized.

- Decreasing adhesions associated with functional shortening of the lateral patellar retinaculum will increase medial patellar glide. This goal will probably not be achieved in 2 weeks, but we expect to see improvements in patellar mobility as swelling decreases and VMO strength increases. Exercises must be conducted to improve patellar tracking. The pain associated with quadriceps contraction should decrease as patellar tracking is improved.

- Goal 8, "The patient will not participate in soccer at this time," is different from the others in that it describes a behavior the patient must avoid. In this case, the rest from the aggravating activity is important for the rest of the treatment plan to be effective. The patient must remain compliant with her home treatment program and stay within her prescribed limits of physical activity.

The decision process regarding the type of therapeutic modality to use (e.g., heat, cold, electrical) is based on the tissue characteristics, their **conductive properties** ● , the stage of healing, the depth that the modality penetrates, and the desired physiological responses for the stage of healing (Fig. 3-6). Once the modality type has been determined, the method of application is determined based on physical characteristics such as the size and shape of the surface area being treated. For example, if a chronic lateral ankle sprain is being treated and there is little or no swelling, the modality type of choice would probably be heat. In this scenario, the physical characteristics of the

---

Conductive properties: The ability of a tissue to transfer heat (from a high temperature to a low temperature) or electrical energy.

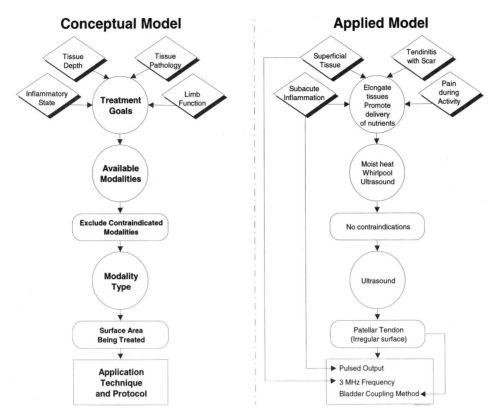

Conceptual Model   **Applied Model**

Figure 3-6. **Decision-Making Scheme for the Selection of Therapeutic Modalities.** The model on the left shows the factors used when deciding what therapeutic modality to use. First, the treatment goals are considered, along with the types of tissues that are injured and the current inflammatory state. Contraindicated modalities are excluded from the modalities available to the clinician and the most appropriate modality type is selected. The contour and size of the body area are then considered in deciding the best application technique. Note that often more than one modality can be considered the best to use. The applied model demonstrates the decision making for a patient with subacute patellar inflammation.

lateral ankle (an irregular surface) would most likely call for the use of a warm whirlpool rather than a moist heat pack because a heat pack would not fit the contour of the area being treated.

A common frustration is that there is often no single "best" choice of modality, although some choices are better than others. The final decision of what modality to use should be based on the prevailing scientific evidence, personal comfort of the modality, and patient input. If satisfactory results are not being obtained from the selected modality, modify the treatment plan to incorporate an alternate modality.

Considerations of the Healing Stage

Each stage of the injury response process has special responses that must be addressed during treatment. Although the time needed to reach each healing stage differs from case to case, the healing process and the associated treatment strategy follow an orderly sequence (see Fig. 3-5).

A common goal among these treatment approaches is to maintain, and in some cases improve, the patient's cardiovascular level. Except in conditions where cardiovascular exercise is impractical or medically contraindicated, some form of cardiovascular exercise should be incorporated into the treatment plan. Patients who are suffering from lower extremity injuries may be able to exercise with an upper body **ergometer** ● or perform pool or wheelchair exercises (Fig. 3-7). For upper extremity injuries, stationary bike exercises, pool exercise, or jogging may be used for cardiovascular maintenance or improvement.

Active Inflammatory Stage

Initially following the onset of acute trauma or after surgery, the treatment approach should decrease the amount of active inflammation and contain the scope of the original injury by reducing secondary hypoxic injury and controlling edema and spasm. The inflammatory response is necessary, but controlling its secondary effects is critical to reducing the healing time. Cold modalities reduce the amount of secondary hypoxic injury, decrease pain, and reduce spasm. Compression devices and elevation encourage venous and lymphatic return, and immobilization

---

Ergometer: A device used to measure the amount of work performed by the legs or arms.

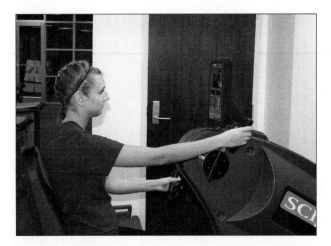

Figure 3-7. **Upper Body Ergometer.** Used to maintain cardio-vascular endurance in patients suffering from lower extremity injury or other conditions that would prohibit running.

devices limit the limb's ROM. Electrical stimulation may be used to help to reduce pain and restore muscle function.

Exercise may take the form of gentle, pain-free ROM and possibly **ergometer** • exercises within the patient's pain tolerance. In some acute injuries or postsurgical conditions, continuous passive motion may be prescribed to maintain joint mobility. Obtaining this motion should not come at the expense of compromising tissue integrity. Cardiovascular maintenance programs should be implemented as soon as possible.

Proliferation Phase

The proliferation stage overlaps portions of the inflammatory and maturation stages (see Fig. 1.5). During the proliferation stage, the treatment goal is to assist the body in delivering oxygen and nutrients necessary to repair the injured tissues and to remove the inflammatory waste products. This goal is met by increasing blood flow to and from the injured tissues.

ROM is needed to prevent functional shortening of the fibers and to encourage the alignment of collagen along the lines of stress.[13] Low-intensity tension is placed on the structures to slowly increase their tensile strength and to assist in the formation of proprioceptive receptors. Proprioceptive activities and muscle reeducation exercises are begun to help protect the limb during **activities of daily living (ADLs)** •. Newly formed capillary buds are fragile, and must not be damaged by excessive joint movement or increased tissue tension.

Early in the proliferation stage, these needs may conflict with the residual effects of acute inflammation. As the signs and symptoms of acute inflammation are resolved, the patient should report decreased pain. Edema may continue to congest the delivery of fresh blood and

the modalities used during the proliferation stage may increase swelling, so a balance must be maintained among the treatment approaches. A common example of this is the use of heat before rehabilitation exercises, followed by ice application afterward.

Maturation Phase

Therapeutic modalities used during the maturation phase should increase tissue extensibility and control post-exercise inflammation because the tissue is still remodeling to form a strong, permanent repair. Usually, this scar tissue does not have the same functionality as the tissue it replaces, so the fibers must be arranged along the lines of functional stress to prevent the scar from creating limitations in ROM or strength.

Proprioceptive activities and muscle strengthening are used to protect the limb during exertion. These exercises should follow a functional progression from that of ADLs to sport- or work-specific activities (e.g., walking, jogging, running in a straight line, running, and cutting).

Patient Self-Treatment

The patient's compliance with the program determines the return to full, unaltered activity in the least possible time. The time spent between treatment visits is the most important factor in determining the return-to-activity time frame. A kind of "protective custody" is formed when the clinician is working directly with the patient. In this situation, the clinician ensures that the patient complies with the prescribed routines. However, the patient's behavior after leaving this structured care will either reinforce or hinder the healing process, especially considering that a patient is under a clinician's direct care for a very small proportion of time.

Most rehabilitation plans include home treatment components where the patient self-administers treatments (e.g., an ice pack), performs exercise routines (e.g., straight-leg raises), and adheres to modified activity (e.g., the use of crutches). Noncompliant patients reduce their therapeutic activities to the time spent with the clinician and may deteriorate their condition by not following the prescribed plan (e.g., not using crutches as prescribed). Compliance with the rehabilitation program can be increased by educating the patient about the nature of the injury being treated, the benefits of complying with the home treatment program, and the potential consequences of straying from the plan.

To help maintain compliance, self-treatment plans should include no more than three treatments or exercises at any one time. Instruct the patient on how to perform the self-treatments and exercises before being allowed to leave the treatment facility. These instructions should be given to the patient in writing, and illustrations that depict the exercises to be performed are also helpful.

Activities of daily living (ADLs): Fundamental skills that are required for a certain lifestyle, including mobility, self-care, and grooming.

Reexamination

Reexamination determines the patient's progress toward meeting the short- and long-term goals. If the short-term goals are met, new short-term goals are established, and any necessary adjustments to the plan are made. If the goals are not met, identify the reasons for the deficiency. After identifying why the goals were not met, reestablish short-term goals and develop a new treatment plan based on the reexamination of the patient (Table 3-8). Reexamination also provides an opportunity to readminister outcome measures.

This portion of the problem-solving approach should assess the initial decision-making and planning process. Asking yourself questions such as "Were the original goals too aggressive or too conservative?" and "What other factors that I didn't anticipate affect the patient?" helps build proficiency in treatment planning. Making notations of your strengths, weaknesses, and common errors (and everybody makes them) in treatment planning serves as a good self-assessment tool.

■ Influences on Patient Care

The physical setting where the treatment is provided influences the patient's treatment plan. Possible clinical settings include acute care hospitals, subacute settings, home care, outpatient rehabilitation, and athletic training facilities. The focus of treatment and the criteria for discharge vary from setting to setting. In many instances, a patient is discharged from one rehabilitation setting to enter a different setting. For example, an athlete who re-ceives hospital-based therapy after surgery is then discharged to the college's sports medicine staff. An industrial worker who has suffered a back injury would receive outpatient therapy and then participate in a **work hardening** ● program before returning to work.

The treatment plan is affected by both internal and external factors. Internal factors include the experience and expertise of the staff and the type of equipment available. External influences include time and financial constraints imposed by insurance companies, the time the patient is able to dedicate to the supervised and home programs, the support the patient receives from friends and family, and the patient's motivation.

Treatment plans for patients hospitalized in acute care settings will focus on stabilizing the patient in preparation for discharge to subacute care, home, or outpatient rehabilitation. The goals of treatment are more immediate, focusing on short-term goals such as wound healing, restoration of ROM, and maximal independence in **transfers** ● and mobility.

Patients who can be discharged from hospital care but require further rehabilitation may be discharged to a subacute care facility, such as a skilled nursing facility or rehabilitation hospital. The treatment goals focus on attaining maximal functional independence so the patient may return home. The focus of the plan will be developing the ROM, strength, and mobility required to allow the patient to perform unassisted ADLs.

Home rehabilitation is more cost effective than inpatient care. This is an ideal alternative for patients who no longer require inpatient care but cannot attend outpatient rehabilitation. Patients may lack the resources to get to the

TABLE 3-8	**Reasons for Not Obtaining Goals**
Unrealistic goals	Initial patient goals were too ambitious given the time established.
Unobtainable goals	Established goal was not physically possible.
A plan that is too conservative	Protocol used did not evoke the physiological responses required for healing to occur in an appropriate time frame.
A plan that is too aggressive	Protocol increased unwanted inflammatory reactions or otherwise delayed the healing process.
Incorrect treatment used	Treatment used was not appropriate for the patient's healing stage or was inappropriately applied.
Problem missed during the examination	Treatment plan cannot address problems that were not identified.
Problem not addressed in the plan	Treatment plan did not adequately address all of the patient's problems or were incorrectly prioritized during the treatment plan.
Lack of patient compliance	Patient did not follow the home care program, did not give full effort during rehabilitation sessions, or did not follow activity recommendations.
Unexpected and unavoidable setbacks	Uncontrollable events in the patient's life (e.g., illness, accident, family matters) delayed the patient's progress and prevented a regular treatment schedule.

Work hardening: Job-specific exercises used to prevent work-related injuries or to rehabilitate injured workers.

Transfers: Assisted patient mobility, such as moving from a wheelchair to a bed.

Case Study Part 6: Treatment Planning

The following treatment approaches have been selected to meet the short-term goals:

1. Orthotics to Control Excessive Pronation

Theory
Permanent control of foot motion is needed to decrease recurrent stress on the patellofemoral joint.

2. Thermal Ultrasound Application to the Lateral Retinaculum

Output of 3 MHz; 6 minutes; high intensity.

Theory
Ultrasound is applied over the lateral retinaculum while patellar mobilization is being performed. Stretching the tissues during heating is more effective than mobilization alone.

3. Patellar Mobilization

Theory
Increase patellar motion by stretching the peripatellar tissues before performing ROM and neuromuscular reeducation techniques.

4. Electrical Stimulation

Motor-level stimulation targeting the quadriceps femoris muscle group.

Theory
Electrical stimulation will help restore normal neuromuscular function. Encourage the patient to voluntarily contract the muscle during stimulation to maximize muscle recruitment. Once the patient can voluntarily contract the muscles, biofeedback is used to improve muscle function during exercise.

5. Flexibility Exercises: Quadriceps, Hamstrings, and Gastrocnemius-Soleus Muscle Group

Minimum of 30 seconds, five repetitions each.

Theory
Increasing flexibility will improve the joint mechanics and decrease abnormal stress on the joint capsule. Flexibility techniques should produce a gentle stretch in the involved muscle but not cause pain in the patellofemoral joint. A 10-minute pain-free warm-up on a stationary bicycle could be used to physiologically elevate tissue temperatures before stretching.

6. Strengthening of the Hip, Hamstring, and Gastrocnemius-Soleus Muscle Group

Theory
Strengthening exercises can be performed immediately, avoiding pain at the patellofemoral joint.

7. Cardiovascular Exercise

Theory
The patient's cardiovascular fitness must be maintained. An upper body ergometer or free-style swimming for cardiovascular endurance could be used to meet this need.

8. Ice

Theory
The patient's program may create inflammation in the patellofemoral joint. Application of ice would be effective in decreasing cell metabolism.

9. Home Exercise Program: Patella Mobilization, Flexibility Exercises, and Ice

Theory
The home program should include no more than three exercises or modalities, selected based on the time available to the patient to perform the exercises, the motivation of the patient, and the activity level of the patient.

outpatient setting or may lack the physical mobility required to travel to and from the clinic. The goals and plan for the home care are more long term in their scope, similar to those of outpatient settings, focusing on the maximum relief of symptoms and restoration of function. If the patient will eventually attend outpatient rehabilitation, the home rehabilitation plan will focus on restoring the patient's ability to travel to the clinic.

Outpatient rehabilitation focuses on obtaining maximum patient independence. Areas that enter into the treatment plan are relief of symptoms, restoration of ROM, strength, balance, and return to ADLs. Although the goals and plan focus on these areas, the ultimate goal is the restoration of function.

Historically, patients may have received outpatient care until all aspects of their condition had been alleviated or they had reached a plateau. Insurance industry restrictions on the reimbursement amount paid for outpatient rehabilitation factor into the planning process. For example, an insurance company may establish a limit of 60 consecutive days of treatment, regardless of the severity of the injury. With less severe injuries, the treatment goal is

Case Study Part 7: Changes in the Program

Changes in the program are based on the patient reexamination. These findings indicate which treatment goals have been met. If goals have not been met, then the treatment program must be modified accordingly.

1. Ultrasound can be used before patellar mobilization until the tissue extensibility is restored.
2. Modalities other than ice may be used to treat the patellar tendinopathy. Heat may be used when active inflammation subsides.
3. Electrical stimulation and biofeedback may be discontinued as the patient demonstrates control of the patella during functional activity.
4. Strengthening exercises are progressed based on the clinician's judgment. Using pain-free exercise as a guide, any strengthening exercise may be performed throughout the rehabilitation.
5. ROM exercises would be eliminated as full motion is restored. The patient would be encouraged to continue active-assisted ROM.
6. As soon as the patient could tolerate standing on one leg without symptoms, proprioception exercises would be added to improve function in the surgically reconstructed leg. The patient would be taken through a functional progression of running, agility training, and sport-specific skills to return to full activity.

to return the patient to normal activity, but in instances of greater pathology, the focus may be for the patient to recover to the point at which self-treatment could be conducted in a safe manner.

Patient care in athletic training facilities presents unique circumstances for treatment planning. In most situations care is provided on a **capitated** ● basis. The patients in this case tend to be in better physical condition, younger, and oriented to intense exercise. Patients may be available for multiple treatment sessions per day, but there is no evidence that increasing the number of treatments decreases the amount of time lost.

All of these factors allow for more aggressive goal setting and planning. Because the circumstances are unique, clinicians must keep in mind that the expectations for return to sports activity are also unique. The patients in this setting will be returning to activities that place them under great physical stress and require psychological confidence, and these factors must be considered when formulating a treatment program.

Capitated: The provision of health care services for a fixed cost or flat fee.

Chapter 4

Administrative Considerations

This chapter discusses administrative concerns as they relate to the delivery of interventions, maintaining a safe facility, and the role of medical records. Issues relating to billing and third-party reimbursement are also discussed.

● The actual application of therapeutic modalities is only part of the rehabilitation process. Health care is bound by governmental regulations and fraught with areas of potential liability. Federal, state, and institutional regulations are meant to ensure safe, effective, and efficient patient care. Further administrative needs are required when the services provided are billed to a third party for reimbursement.

■ Legal Considerations in Patient Care

During therapeutic interventions, your minimum legal duty is to prevent further injury or harm to the patient by practicing in a safe and professional manner. Professional ethics and responsibility mandate that the care provided be in the best interest of the patient, be safe and effective, and progress toward meeting the patient's goals.

Before using a therapeutic modality, you must be familiar with the effects and side effects of the device or protocol being used and be able to recognize contraindications that prohibit use (see Box 3-1). Proper use also requires knowledge of the device's characteristics, maintenance requirements, and safety considerations.

This section primarily addresses legal considerations pertaining to patient intervention routines. It does not represent all aspects of liability that you may be exposed to in the daily routine of professional practice.

Scope of Practice

The legal boundaries that define the manner in which clinicians may practice, the scope of practice, are established on a state-by-state basis through regulation such as licensure, registration, or certification (Table 4-1). Professional regulation protects the public from unqualified health care providers. There are differences in the scope of practice from one profession to another and differences in the scope of practice for the same profession from state to state.[137,138] The scope of practice may define the standard of care used in liability cases.

Professional practice statements, such as the National Athletic Trainers' Association Position Statements or the American Physical Therapy Association Guide to Physical Therapy Practice, and professional best practice statements further define appropriate professional behavior. The institutional or facility **Policies and Procedures Manual** should

TABLE 4-1	Types of Professional State Regulation
Type	*Description*
Licensure	The highest level of regulation that establishes the scope of professional practice, sets the minimal education standards for licensure eligibility, and protects professional titles.
Certification	A state-based certification test is often required; defines the scope of professional practice, but does not protect professional titles.
Registration	A person must register with the state board prior to practicing the profession. Registration has minimal (if any) prerequisites. Only registered professionals can use the given title.
Exemption	Allows one profession to perform some of the skills and roles of another profession without infringement.

reflect both state practice acts and professional **standards of practice** ●.

Knowing the legislation that regulates professional practice in your state is a part of your professional responsibility. This information can be obtained through the state board overseeing your field of practice.

Medical Prescriptions

State regulation may require that a physician directly refer all patients or require a physician's direction of the care given. Professions granted **direct access** ● by state regulation do not require a physician's referral. However, third-party payors will often not provide reimbursement for services unless the care is prescribed by a physician. In cases where the patient is prescribed a specific protocol for treatment, you are bound to abide by the prescription unless the physician grants a verbal or written change.

In states where direct access is not granted, the use of some therapeutic modalities such as electrical stimulation, ultrasound, and traction may also require a physician's prescription. Cold packs, moist heat packs, and whirlpools typically do not require a prescription.

Protocol such as **phonophoresis** ● (Chapter 7) or iontophoresis (Chapter 13) that use prescription medications require that each patient being treated have a prescription for the medication being used. State pharmacy practice acts may further restrict the use of these protocols. "Blanket prescriptions" where the medication is prescribed to the facility and then administered at the practitioner's discretion may be common practice, but its legality is precarious.

Informed Consent

Except in cases of emergency care, patients must grant their consent to be treated. Otherwise, an act of criminal **battery** ● and professional negligence may have been committed. A patient seeking care is a form of implied consent, so simply treating someone without formal consent being granted is normally not sufficient to determine professional negligence. For negligence to be determined for a lack of informed consent, the patient must suffer harm from the care rendered.[139,140]

Before beginning the treatment, educate the patient about the modality and/or exercise, the sensations to be expected during the session, and any adverse signs or symptoms that indicate that the intervention should be modified or discontinued. Inform the patient about any potential hazards associated with the use of the device and any residual side effects (Table 4-2). Informed consent is not a waiver of the patient's right to pursue claims of negligence or liability against the facility or clinician.

Each patient should have a signed informed consent form or documentation of verbal consent on file. If the patient is younger than the age of 18 years, this document (and all other consent forms) must be signed by the patient's parent or **legal guardian** ●. This document notwithstanding, patients have the right to refuse any form of care or modality.

TABLE 4-2	Elements of Informed Consent for Treatment

Description of the modalities and/or exercises to be used
An overview of how the device works
Benefits provided by the device (physiological responses)
Expected normal sensations
Adverse sensations to be reported
Potential hazards associated with the device
Residual effects

Standards of practice: The criteria against which an individual's performance is measured.
Direct access: Health care services can be provided without physician referral. Note that a physician referral is often required for third-party reimbursement.
Phonophoresis: The introduction of medication into the body through the use of ultrasonic energy.
Battery: The unwanted touching of one person by another.
Legal guardian: An individual who is legally responsible for the care of a minor.

Patient Confidentiality

All medical records are confidential documents. The patient must grant written permission before these records are released to an outside individual (e.g., physicians, college recruiters, employers). The authorization to release medical information should explicitly state to whom the information is being released and for what purpose it will be used (Table 4-3). Additionally, if this information will be used to assist in determining the patient's medical clearance for an athletic college scholarship or employment, the release form should include a disclaimer noting that the information found in the medical records will be used as a part of the decision-making process and may either aid or hinder the patient's cause.[140]

The unauthorized release of medical records not only breaks the bond of patient–caregiver confidentiality but may also be outside the parameters of state and professional codes of conduct. Liability may be found through **defamation of character.** When this occurs by the spoken word, it is termed **slander;** when it occurs through print or electronic media it is termed **libel.**

Individuals who are in the public eye, athletes for example, have a lower privacy threshold than "private" figures. Health care providers must still maintain a high standard of ethical and moral conduct to protect the patient's right to confidentiality.

The patient should be allowed to review his or her medical records on request. Whenever the patient's medical records are removed from the facility, the date the records were sent, the purpose of the release, and the date of the return should be documented.

The duration of time that medical records must be kept is established by each state. The records of current and past patients must be stored in a manner conducive to maintaining their confidentiality.

The **Health Insurance Portability and Accountability Act** (HIPAA), created by the U.S. Health and Human Services Department to ensure that workers have continual health care coverage while changing jobs, has affected the maintenance and transmittal of patient records and information.[141] The HIPAA regulations affect past, present, and future medical records, but state regulation can override the HIPAA requirements.

In addition to standardizing the electronic exchange of medical information, HIPAA also seeks to ensure patient confidentiality by controlling the security of **Protected Health Information** (PHI).[142] HIPAA also increases the importance of informed consent and release of information documents, which must be written using understandable terms.[141]

✱ Practical Evidence

Secondary schools, colleges, and universities that use public sign in logs that reveal the nature of the patient's visit (injury or illness, interventions, etc.) are in apparent violation of FERPA regulations.[143] This method allows public access of medical records. The best approach is to document each visit in the patient's file.

Any school—regardless of the age of the students taught—that receives federal funds is also subject to regulation from the **Family Education Rights Privacy Act** (FERPA).[143] FERPA protects education records, including medical files, from unauthorized release. With the rare exception of schools that do not receive federal funds, institutions must adhere to both HIPAA and FERPA privacy requirements.

Negligence

Patients have the right to receive safe and proper treatment without exposure to undue hazards. This implies that care is provided in a professionally competent and accepted manner. This standard covers not only the physical act of applying therapeutic modalities and implementing rehabilitation routines, but also means that the devices being used must be in safe operating condition and the facility free of foreseeable hazards (Box 4-1).

Professional negligence is loosely defined as providing care that falls below the minimally accepted standard (substandard care), although there are many factors and influences leading into the final determination.[144] Professional standards of practice, the facility policies and procedure manuals, best practice, and state practice acts form the benchmark for determining if the care provided was standard or substandard.

Possessing state-based practice credentials such as licensure may change the threshold for negligence and remove certain institutional protections. Licensed professionals may be considered independent practitioners, placing an increased onus of responsibility on the caregiver and lessening the burden on the caregiver's employer.

TABLE 4-3   Medical Information Release Authorization

Description of the information to be released

The individual or individuals who will receive the information

For what purpose or purposes the information will be used

The date that the authorization will expire

The person granting the authorization's signature. If someone other than the patient authorizes the release, the relationship between the two (e.g., parent, guardian) must be documented.

The release of information form should also note that the patient has the right to revoke the authorization, consequences of failing to sign the authorization, and that the potential exists that the recipient of the information may be redisclosed.

Box 4-1. NEGLIGENCE

Negligence implies unintentional harm. Ordinary negligence is the failure to act as a reasonable and prudent person would in the same situation. Gross negligence is the complete failure to foresee and act on a situation to prevent harm from occurring (e.g., not having a fence around a swimming pool). Professional negligence occurs when the individual provides substandard care or acts outside of the professional norms or acts out of carelessness, thus breaching the duty of care (see below).

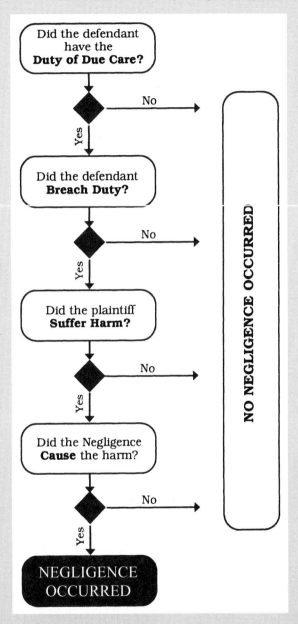

For a court to find a person guilty of negligence, a clear relationship between the alleged act of negligence and the harm suffered by the individual must be established. A court must first establish if the defendant had a **duty** to act on behalf of the plaintiff. Then, if a duty exists, the court asks, "Did the defendant **breach this obligation?"** The breach of duty is determined by comparing the actions that the defendant did (or did not) take with those that a reasonable and prudent person having a similar level of education and experience would have taken under similar circumstances (see Box 4-2). If the defendant had no duty to respond or was determined to have acted in a reasonable and prudent manner, no negligence can be found.

If the defendant was obliged to respond but failed to act in a reasonable and prudent manner, the court must determine if plaintiff actually suffered physical or **financial harm.** The final link in

(Continued)

Box 4-1. NEGLIGENCE—cont'd

determining negligence is that of **causation.** A direct relationship between the actions of the defendant and the harm suffered by the plaintiff must be established.

Ordinary torts can be classified as:

Malfeasance: The performance of an unlawful or improper act.
Misfeasance: The improper performance of an otherwise lawful act. (commission)
Nonfeasance: The failure to act when there is a duty to act. (omission)
Malpractice: Negligence on the part of a professional serving in the line of duty.

Not all negligence that occurs in the patient care setting is professional negligence. Hazards that are not relevant to the care being rendered, tripping on an upturned carpet in a clinic, for example, could be determined as being ordinary negligence. Because this event has no bearing on patient care, professional negligence would not be considered.[145]

A supervisor can be held liable for ordinary or professionally negligent acts performed by employees or students, or their failure to supervise, under the doctrine of **vicarious liability** (sometimes called **respondeat superior,** Latin for "let the master answer").[145] In cases in which physician supervision is required, the physician can be liable for the acts of the health care provider, especially when Food and Drug Administration (FDA)–regulated modalities or medications are involved.

Negligent Delivery of Treatment

Negligent professional behavior occurs when a health care provider departs from the accepted standard of care.[144] In performing unnecessary or detrimental acts, liability for failure to use **due care** ● may be determined. Reckless or careless treatment may result in professional negligence.[140] Negligence may be classified into two types on the basis of behavior: (1) omission and (2) commission.

Omission occurs when an individual fails to respond to a given situation when a response is necessary to limit or reduce harm. Consider the following example: a patient goes to the physician with complaints of an injury. If the physician fails to evaluate, treat, or refer the injury, an act of omission may have occurred. In this case, the negligent act stems from the physician's failure to properly respond to a medical condition.

Commission occurs when an individual acts on a situation but does not perform at the level that a reasonable and prudent person would (Box 4-2). In the rehabilitation process, an act of commission could occur if a clinician treats a stress fracture with ultrasound. In this example, negligence occurred because the individual acted, but with an improper technique (stress fractures are a contraindication to ultrasound application).

The relationship between the patient's goals and professional negligence is remarkably ambiguous. Goals can be construed as a "professional promise" to the patient. However, goal setting is generally a professional judgment rather than a contractual obligation between the clinician and patient, especially when the patient is included in setting the goals. What is of concern is the manner in which the goals are communicated to the patient. Presenting the goals as ". . . to obtain 90 degrees of knee flexion" is much different from the clinician stating, "I will be able to make you walk again." If miscommunicated or overstated, therapeutic promises can be interpreted to be a binding legal contract that could result in a breach of contract or fraud if they are not met.[145]

Negligent Care of Facilities

The design of patient care facilities must guarantee that patients receive care in the safest environment possible. The facility must also conform to state codes governing health care facilities.

Ensuring safety is an ongoing process involving thorough intervention planning, patient evaluation, and equipment and facility maintenance. Injury sustained from improper or unsafe facilities can result in negligence being found against the staff or institution. The hydrotherapy area and areas where electrical modalities are used are of special concern regarding the facility's physical design (Table 4-4).

Knowingly using an unsafe therapeutic modality or other equipment reflects negligence on the part of the clinician or facility administrator. All therapeutic equipment must be inspected and calibrated by a qualified service technician at least yearly. More frequent service should be performed on intensive-use equipment. Manufacturer and/or local regulation pertaining to equipment in a health care facility may also mandate shorter inspection and maintenance cycles. The inspection or service date, the technician, and the services performed should be documented and kept on file.

Proper daily care is needed to help maintain the equipment in safe working order. Wear and tear through normal use is to be expected, and proper care of the equipment will keep this to a minimum. Logical precautions, such as avoiding liquid spilling into the equipment, proper positioning of

---

Due care: An established responsibility for an individual to respond to a given situation in a certain manner.

Box 4-2. SO WHO IS THIS REASONABLE AND PRUDENT PERSON?

When an individual is charged with negligence, the person's actions are measured against those that a reasonable and prudent person would have taken in the same situation. So who is this reasonable and prudent person?

The reasonable and prudent person is a fictitious individual who is created by the courts. Variables such as the defendant's age, physical condition, education, professional experience, and mental capacity are factored together to determine what actions would be considered reasonable.[144] Because the criteria for determining what is reasonable and prudent change based on the situation, and because juries are not qualified to determine what the proper standard of care would be in a given situation, a mechanism exists that identifies what is "reasonable and prudent" for any given type of situation.

Through the testimony of expert witnesses, professional position statements, and other accepted (documented) protocols such as Best Practices, a standard of care is established that describes what actions should be expected of an individual in a given situation. The standard of care is determined by the professional standards of practice, state practice acts, and the testimony of experts. Profession-specific documents such as the Guide to Physical Therapist Practice can also be used to judge or to determine the appropriateness of the individual's actions.

If a practitioner exceeds his or her scope of practice and enters another field, for example, a health care professional who performs a task that falls within a physician's domain, that practitioner would be held to the standard of that profession.

TABLE 4-4 Considerations for Safe Facilities

- All electrical modalities should be connected to a ground-fault interrupter. Whirlpools and jacuzzis must be connected to these devices (see Box 4-5).
- Patients must not be permitted to turn whirlpools or jacuzzis on or off while they are in the water. Ideally, the switches should be located so that they cannot be reached from these tubs.
- Hydrotherapy areas must have an adequate line of sight to monitor patients.
- All modalities should be inspected and calibrated by a licensed professional at intervals prescribed by the manufacturer.
- Flooring should be made of a nonslip material.
- A policies and procedure manual for describing the use, inspection, and maintenance of the equipment should be maintained.

---

electrical cords, and regular inspection of plugs, assist in maintaining the longevity of equipment.

Food and Drug Administration Oversight

The United States Congress established the U.S. Food and Drug Administration (FDA) to provide oversight to ensure that medical devices (and medications) are safe and effective. The FDA's Center for Devices and Radiologic Health regulates a wide range of therapeutic devices to ensure patient safety, to evaluate claims regarding their efficacy, and to eliminate unnecessary exposure to **radiation** ● emitted from the device. Other FDA regulations relate to those devices that produce electrical interference or are controlled by microprocessors. The FDA also is the major regulator of over-the-counter and prescription medications.

The FDA's definition of a medical device is quite lengthy, but can be summarized as relying on a mechanism other than chemical action to diagnose, treat, or prevent conditions in humans and animals.[146] Medical devices are assigned to one of three classifications based on their potential harm to the individual in the event of their failure. A class I device carries little risk to the patient; class III presents the greatest risk. The device may also be restricted to sales to, or under the orders of, a licensed physician or health care practitioner.

Before being marketed, devices controlled by the FDA, such as electrical stimulators, and therapeutic ultrasound must undergo a rigorous Premarket Review Application Process (PMA), an investigational status that evaluates the product's inherent safety, efficacy, and manufacturing processes.[146]

Devices having the investigational status designation are not eligible for reimbursement and a strict clinical protocol must be used. Devices in the PMA must be granted an Investigational Device Exception by the **Institutional Review Board** ● before being applied to humans.

Radiation: The transfer of electromagnetic energy that does not require the presence of a medium (see Chapter 5).

Institutional Review Board: An institutional agency that oversees medical investigations involving humans or animals by assuring compliance with federal regulations. In research involving humans, the IRB functions to protect the rights and health of the subjects.

The FDA also regulates product labeling, information, and instruction manuals.[147] Regulated therapeutic modalities must minimally include the information presented in Table 4-5 and, when possible, the device description, indications, and contraindications should appear together on the first page of the product information. If the device is being marketed on the basis of clinical data, the information presented is expanded to include supporting clinical studies. Depending on the complexity of the device, an operator's manual, patient's manual, and references may also have to be included with the device.[147]

Occupational Safety & Health Administration Regulations

The Occupational Safety & Health Administration (OSHA) is a division of the U.S. Department of Labor that is charged with protecting the health of most of the United States workforce. OSHA develops codes—safety standards and regulations—to prevent work-related injuries and illnesses and, through an enforcement branch, fines or prosecutes employers who do not comply with the standards. Many states also have departments that work cooperatively with OSHA.

OSHA has developed a series of rules that require institutions to protect workers from blood-borne pathogens such as the hepatitis B virus (HBV). These rules apply to all employees who may be exposed to biological hazards (biohazards) including blood, synovial fluid, and saliva as a part of their job requirements.

The **Universal Precautions** ● are a set of standards that help prevent against accidental contact with biohazards. Exposure control plans focus on personal protection (and, when applicable, protective equipment), proper disposal of medical wastes including hypodermic needles and scalpels ("sharps"), and proper handling of soiled laundry. Institutions must develop an exposure control plan to protect its employees and conduct an annual in-service training program that describes these policies and procedures.

■ Medical Documentation

Medical records serve several functions (Table 4-6). Within the context of this text, documentation assists in the planning and evaluation of the intervention program. Documentation provides a method to determine the program's effectiveness and records describe the quantity and quality of the services provided. Failure to maintain accurate, legible medical records may result in professional negligence and the absence of these records places the caregiver in an indefensible position. From both a legal

TABLE 4-5 U.S. Food and Drug Administration (FDA) Device-Labeling Minimal Requirements	
Information	*Description*
Description	A brief description of how the device functions, physical characteristics, and performance characteristics.
Indications	Describe the intended use and the specific types of conditions (e.g., injuries, diseases) that warrant the use of the device.
Contraindications	Describe conditions where the risk of use outweighs the anticipated benefits.
Warnings	Warnings describe hazards (serious effects or death) other than those described in the contraindications. An example of this would be a device such as diathermy that also emits radiation.
Boxed warning	The FDA may require that especially concerning or hazardous warnings be placed in a box close to the device description. Warning boxes are generally issued when clinical human data, or in some instances animal data, show a high probability of adverse effects.
Precautions	Alert the user to special care necessary for safe and effective use of the device. Precautions is used as the plural of "Caution."
Adverse effects	An undesirable side effect stemming from the use of the device that is not presented in the Contraindications, Warnings, or Precautions sections.
Conformance to standards	If applicable, this section refers to the FDA medical device, materials, or standards used in the evaluation and/or manufacture of the device.
Operator's manual	A brief description of the contents of the unit's operator's manual.
Patient's manual	A brief description of the contents of the unit's instruction/informational packet for use by the patient.

Universal Precautions: A series of steps, established by OSHA, that individuals should take to avoid accidental exposure to blood-borne pathogens. Universal precautions are also referred to as "Standard Precautions."

TABLE 4-6 Purpose of Medical Records

Serve as a communication tool among health care
  providers
Document the intervention
Assist in the continuity of care given
Provide a basis for developing future intervention plans
Document informed consent
Serve as a legal document to show that the medical staff
  provided reasonable care
Memory aid in legal cases
Meet professional requirement and standards
Serve as a basis for reimbursement decisions
Basis for discharge/discontinuation of care
Provide a database for research

and third-party reimbursement perspective, remember that
"if it wasn't documented, it wasn't done."

Medical records document the course of the patient's care from the initial visit to discharge or return to activity. As described in Chapter 3, specifically stated goals and objective measurements should be used.

Several different record-keeping systems are used for clinical documentation (e.g., SOAP, HOPS), and desktop computers and personal digital assistants (PDAs) have taken on an increased role (Table 4-7). Many multi-modalities allow patient treatment data to be stored on a data card (see Chapter 12). Third-party reimbursement places unique and increased demands on the documentation process. The following sections describe the role and purpose of medical records.

The state's **statute of limitations** ● determines the length of time that medical records should be kept after the patient is no longer receiving care. However the computerization of these records allows them to be stored indefinitely.

Continuity of Care

Document the examination findings and the intervention plan as specifically and clearly as possible so that continuity of care can be maintained when more than one clinician is involved in the patient's care. The medical record should include all communication to and from other health care providers (including referral forms), the patient, and the patient's family members.

Treatment Rendered and Patient Progress

Documentation of the day's treatments should describe the date, time, individual or individuals providing the care, the pathology being treated, the therapeutic modalities and exercises that were used, and the parameters used. These treatments must help meet the goals documented in the patient's plan. Each treatment session should begin with an interview and reexamination to determine the patient's current status. That is, did the prior treatment improve the patient's condition, worsen it, or was there no appreciable change? (See Chapter 3.)

Following the conclusion of the treatment, reinterview the patient, and note any necessary adjustments to the patient's medical record. Even seemingly minor changes in a modality's application parameters can produce significantly different physiological effects. A lack of continuity of treatment is a

TABLE 4-7 Types of Medical Records

Document	Purpose
Medical history	Details prior medical conditions. Identifies conditions that contraindicate the use of certain modalities, although the patient should be specifically questioned before applying any device (e.g., a person with a history of cardiovascular disease requiring medication would be excluded from full-body warm whirlpools).
Preparticipation examination	Used with athletes to identify the status of any existing condition physical examination and to determine the current status of preexisting conditions.
Consent form	Indicates that the patient (or the parent[s] if the patient is under the age of 18 years) has granted permission to be treated. Consent forms do not protect the clinician from liability stemming from acts of negligence.
Injury report	Used in athletics to document the onset of an acute injury or the aggravation of a chronic condition.
Referral form	Allows for feedback from the physician regarding the level of activity and prescribed course of rehabilitation.
Prescription record	For modality use (if required) and medications (e.g., phonophoresis, iontophoresis) if indicated.
Treatment record	Provides an ongoing record of the patient's intervention plan and notes.

Statute of limitations: A legal time limit allowed for the filing of a lawsuit.

pitfall that may delay the patient's progress. Well-documented examination and treatment records help to ensure that all involved understand the patient's current **disposition** ●.

A facility treatment log is a beneficial administrative tool. Documentation of facility usage and the demands placed on the staff and equipment can be used to justify the need for more clinicians or the purchase of new equipment.

Legal Record

Medical records protect both the caregiver and the patient. Well-documented records assist in proving that the staff exercised reasonable patient care. If a liability case were to come to trial, the medical staff may use these records to refresh their memories when testifying about the case, and the documents themselves may be admitted as evidence. Standardized terminology and medical short hand are found in Appendix C.

Professional Standards of Practice and most state practice acts require that complete and accurate medical records be maintained. Medical records correlate the care given with that prescribed by the physician. Different work settings such as high schools, colleges, for-profit clinics, and hospitals may also have additional record-keeping requirements.

Reimbursement Documentation

Although the primary role of documentation is to improve patient care by ensuring treatment continuity among caregivers, when seeking third-party reimbursement medical records are business documents. Insurance companies require the use of goal-based treatment plans for reimbursement. Therapeutic services billed for this purpose will be reimbursed only if they meet the patient's treatment goals.

Third-party payors, insurance companies, may review these documents to determine if reimbursement for the services is warranted. When the bill for service appears excessive or the amount of care provided seems prolonged, the documentation may undergo peer review for determination of reimbursement.

In the case of possible excessive billing, the documentation is compared with the billing during the treatment session. The documentation must be clearly and concisely written so that someone reviewing the chart can gain a full understanding of the care provided so a fair determination of the reimbursement may be made.

The claim reviewer will evaluate the objective measures such as range of motion, pain rating scales, and strength in the patient's record. Patient-based outcome measures will also be considered. If the patient continues to show no improvement or if the treatment protocol does not appear to match the patient's goals, payment for services can be declined. Further investigation may be initiated

to determine if care was truly needed or if it was unnecessarily extended.

■ Third-Party Reimbursement

The **Centers for Medicare & Medicaid Services (CMS),** formerly the Health Care Finance Administration (HCFA), oversees the two largest medical payors, Medicare and Medicaid. Other third-party insurance companies use the Medicare and Medicaid standards for establishing their own guidelines in determining the rate for reimbursable services.

The rate of reimbursement, the amount paid, is frequently based on the usual, customary, and reasonable (UCR) system. Changes in health care financing and insurance coverage are resulting in the increased use of capitation methods (fixed payment rate per patient) and the resource-based relative value scale (RBRVS) system.

Receiving reimbursement for services rendered requires documentation of the condition being treated and documentation of the treatment services that are being billed. The individual or individuals rendering the treatment must be state licensed in their area of practice and the treatment provided must meet the patient's treatment goals. The decision to provide reimbursement for a claim is ultimately left to the individual insurance company.[148]

Billing Codes

Receiving third-party reimbursement for services rendered requires the submission of two forms of documentation: diagnostic codes using the **International Classification of Diseases (ICD)** and the **Current Procedural Terminology (CPT)** codes.

The ICD codes describe the patient's pathology. The CPT codes describe the care provided to the patient. The CPT codes must correlate with the ICD codes to be reimbursed. Medicare has established treatment and rehabilitation guidelines for most ICD conditions.

Improper coding can result in a claim being rejected. In the worst case, improper coding can result in facility audits, loss of provider status, or fines.

International Classification of Diseases Codes
The ICD codes were developed by the American Hospital Association (AHA) to describe pathology and surgical procedures arranged by relevant groups. The National Center for Health Statistics developed the Clinical Modification (CM) of the ICD codes; most relevant to this text is the addition of a classification system for surgical, diagnostic, and therapeutic procedures (Box 4-3). The coding scheme is regularly updated and is now in its tenth edition, carrying the name ICD-10-CM (ICD: International Classification of Disease; 10: Tenth edition; CM: Clinical Modification); however, the Ninth edition is still widely used.[149]

Disposition: The patient's current physical status and projected course of recovery.

Box 4-3. ICD-9-CM CODING SYSTEM EXAMPLES

ICD-9-CM	Description
Knee Bursitis	
726.60	**Enthesopathy** ● of knee, unspecified
844.20	Pes anserinus tendinitis or bursitis
844.21	**Prepatellar** ● bursitis
Knee Sprains	
844.20	Old disruption of the lateral collateral ligament
844.21	Old disruption of the medial collateral ligament
844.22	Old disruption of the anterior cruciate ligament
844.23	Old disruption of the posterior cruciate ligament
844.00	Acute lateral collateral ligament sprain
844.20	Acute medial collateral ligament sprain
844.21	Acute anterior cruciate ligament sprain/tear
844.30	Acute posterior cruciate ligament sprain/tear

The ICD-9-CM code is a five-digit string (trailing zeros are often dropped) that describes the pathology and structure involved. The evolution of this system has, at times, made the codes relatively disjointed. The first three digits identify the body area, although the progression is not always sequential. The second two digits describe the pathology. In addition to reimbursement purposes, these data are used for record keeping, **epidemiology** ●, and other research purposes. ICD codes change regularly.

The information above is presented for informational purposes only.

Current Procedural Terminology Codes

The CPT codes were established by the AMA Department of Coding and Nomenclature to define those treatments rendered by health care providers who are licensed by the state to perform the service.[148] The AMA uses the term "therapist" generically, but certain codes, such as evaluation and reevaluation, are specific as to the type of professional providing the service.

Physical medicine codes include both therapeutic modalities and therapeutic exercise. Although therapeutic modalities are reasonably well defined, therapeutic exercise is not. In just over 20 years the definition of "therapeutic exercise" was changed by Medicare and insurance companies 10 times, 3 times in an 18-month period.[150]

Therapeutic modalities fall under the CPT's **Physical Medicine Codes** category. The reimbursement rate for most procedures is based on 15-minute **time units** that are rounded up or down from the halfway point. Each procedure has a unique CPT code, although on first glance there appears to be overlap between them. For this reason, CPT coding is usually performed by someone with expertise in this area.

Most therapeutic procedures are covered by the CPT physical medicine code (Box 4-4). However, cold packs and moist heat packs are not eligible for reimbursement unless they are used in conjunction with another therapeutic procedure (e.g., range-of-motion exercises).

Phonophoresis, another technique described in this text, is not billable as well. However, the application of ultrasound is billable or the treatment could be coded as 97039 (unlisted modality), although there is the potential of having the claim denied.

■ Evidence-Based Practice

Changes in the health care system have caused third-party payors to reexamine those services that are performed for reimbursement. As a consequence, to control costs, third-party payors are requiring documentation and evidence that the treatments being rendered are beneficial to meeting the patient's treatment goals.[151] Treatments rendered must conform with the patient's treatment plan and the devices used must be beneficial to the patient's condition. Proof that therapeutic treatments and, by extension, therapeutic modalities produce the effects that we believe is termed evidence-based practice.

Patient- and clinician-centered outcome measures determine the quality of the end result of medical care (see Chapter 3). The determination is made based on the procedures used in patient care and the resulting patient satisfaction and quality of life. Documentation of the results of your interventions is a large piece of the evidence puzzle. If a patient is positively responding in the

---

Enthesopathy: Pathology of the bony attachment of tendon, ligament, or joint capsule.

Prepatellar: Around the patella.

Epidemiology: The study of the distribution, rates, and causes of injuries and illness within a specified population. This information may then be used to prevent future occurrence.

Box 4-4. CPT CODING SYSTEM (SELECTED ENTRIES)

Code	Procedure	Time Unit	Comment
Evaluation			
97001	Physical Therapy Evaluation	Per-service	For use by a licensed physical therapist with a new patient
97002	Physical Therapy Reevaluation	Per-service	Follow-up evaluation by a physical therapist
97003	Occupational Therapy Evaluation	Per-service	For use by a licensed occupational therapist with a new patient
97004	Occupational Therapy Reevaluation	Per-service	Follow-up evaluation by an occupational therapist
97005	Athletic Training Evaluation	Per-service	For use by a licensed athletic trainer with a new patient
97006	Athletic Training Reevaluation	Per-service	Follow-up evaluation by an athletic trainer
Therapeutic Modalities			
97010	Moist heat pack	Per-visit	For payment, must be used in conjunction with another procedure
97010	Ice bag/ice massage	Per-visit	For payment, must be used in conjunction with another procedure
97014	Electrical stimulation (unattended)	Per-visit	For those treatments which do not require constant clinician involvement (e.g., sensory-level pain control, edema reduction)
97016	Vasopneumatic therapy	Per-visit	Compression for edema reduction
97018	Paraffin bath	Service-based	
97022	Whirlpool therapy	Per-visit	For restoration of range of motion
97022	Fluidotherapy	Service-based	Sterile application for wound debridement
97024	Diathermy	Service-based	Only shortwave diathermy is approved for clinical use
64550	TENS application	Service-based	For pain reduction
97032	Electrical stimulation (manual)	Time-based	Requires constant clinician-patient contact (e.g., trigger point therapy)
97033	Iontophoresis	Time-based	Covers the cost of the technique, medication, and electrodes
97034	Contrast baths	Time-based	
97035	Ultrasound	Time-based	Minimum of 8 minutes billable time required
97039	Unlisted therapeutic modality	Time-based	Requires constant attendance
Manual Techniques			
97012	Manual traction	Per-visit	
97124	Massage therapy	Time-based	
97140	Manual therapy, one or more regions	Time-based	Used to code myofascial release and edema reduction
Therapeutic Exercise			
90901	Biofeedback	Service-based	Used for neuromuscular reeducation or relaxation
97110	Therapeutic exercise	Time-based	Used for establishing range of motion, strength, and endurance for one or more joints. Requires one-on-one clinician/patient interaction

Box 4-4. CPT CODING SYSTEM (SELECTED ENTRIES)—cont'd

Code	Procedure	Time Unit	Comment
97112	Neuromuscular reeducation	Time-based	Used for reeducation of function, motion, proprioception, balance, etc.
97113	Aquatic therapy	Time-based	Clinician constantly oversees two or more patients
97150	Group therapeutic procedure	Service-based	
97750	Physical performance test	Time-based	Functional evaluations

The above represents common Current Procedural Terminology evaluation and Physical Medicine codes. Evaluation codes are service based and are not included in time-based treatment services.

These codes change regularly and are presented as an example and, as presented here, should not be used for billing purposes. Refer to the current CPT coding documents for an up-to-date reference on these codes and their interpretation.

anticipated amount of time then it can be assumed that the intervention(s) are working. If the result of the patient's record indicates that positive outcomes are not being obtained, the intervention strategy must be rethought.

Each therapeutic modality or classification of modalities (e.g., cold agents, heating agents) presented in this text includes a section titled **Controversies in Treatment.** This section provides an overview of questions and concerns regarding the general efficacy of the device or specific concerns with individual application techniques.

■ Facilities

The physical facility where care is given must be free of potential hazards and be conducive to patient care, including access by disabled patients or clinicians. The hydrotherapy area, treatment area, plumbing, and electrical systems are of special concern. Hospital-based clinics and some outpatient clinics are accredited by agencies such as the Joint Commission (JC) or state regulatory boards. These organizations may have specific safety guidelines that must be met and the facility may be subject to inspection.

Electrical Systems

The health care facility's electrical system deserves special scrutiny. The presence of water and the potential for accidental patient contact with electrical sources are potential hazards. Therapeutic modalities operate on 110-volt "household" current, while some equipment may operate on rechargeable or replaceable batteries. Other equipment, such as large icemakers, may require 220 volts. Some

equipment, such as isokinetic devices, whirlpools, or electrodiagnostic equipment, may require a dedicated circuit, where there is only one outlet. Extension cords should never be used to operate therapeutic equipment.

Electrical outlets leading to whirlpools and other modalities where water is a concern must be served by a ground-fault interrupter (GFI), although GFIs are recommended for all outlets that will serve patients (Box 4-5). Outlets in the treatment area should be located 2 to 3 feet above the floor; in the hydrotherapy area, 4 feet or higher (and out of the reach of patients using the tub). Microprocessor-controlled modalities, such as electrical stimulators, may also require a surge protector. State building and/or health codes may also prescribe other requirements.

Treatment Area

The patient treatment area should be spacious and well lighted. Treatment tables should be approximately 30 inches high, although adjustable tables are useful for certain types of treatments and meet **Americans With Disabilities Act** ● (ADA) specifications for access by patients or clinicians with disabilities. Split-leg tables allow for the body part to be elevated during the treatment (Fig. 4-1). If shortwave diathermy treatments are to be used in the facility, all-wood tables are required.

Tables should be no less than 30 inches apart. Even using this minimum figure, one or two treatment tables should have more space on the side to allow for range-of-motion exercises, massage, myofascial release, and other procedures.

Fixtures should provide a lighting power of 50 to 75 **footcandles** ● at a height of 4 feet above the floor. In

---

Americans With Disabilities Act: Legislation passed in 1990 (Public Law 101-336) that protects the right of disabled individuals by creating standards to ensure access and prohibit discrimination in transportation, accommodation, public services, and so on.

Footcandle: A measure of light equal to 1 lumen per square foot. One lumen is the amount of light emitted by one international candle.

Box 4-5. GROUND-FAULT CIRCUIT INTERRUPTERS

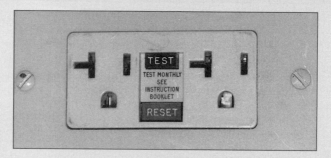

Ground-fault interrupters (GFIs, or GFCIs for ground-fault circuit interrupters) are used to guard against hazardous currents by continuously monitoring the amount of current entering a circuit compared with the amount of current leaving it. If there is a discrepancy of more than 5 milliampere (mA), current leakage has been detected, and the GFI will stop the flow of electricity to the unit in as little as 1/40 of a second.

Always seeking the course of least resistance, electrical currents tend to stay within the insulation of the path formed by the circuit, but because of condensation, microscopic imperfections in the circuitry, or even dust, some current leakage inevitably occurs. Only two leads are required to complete an electrical circuit; however, most outlets contain a third conductor that leads to the ground. As this name implies, the grounded wire literally leads to a pipe or other conductor that is buried in the ground. Normally, when current leaks into the **chassis** •, it will follow the ground wire back to the earth. This leakage is termed a "ground fault" and occurs to some degree in all electrical equipment.

Any leaked current must find an alternate path back to the ground. Ideally, this route is through a grounded circuit, but if the circuit is not properly grounded or the leakage is too great, the current must find an alternate route back to the ground. A person who is in contact with an ungrounded device while touching a grounded source (e.g., a whirlpool and a pipe) can easily form this alternate route for the current to take. In this case, the current would leak from the chassis of the ungrounded device and flow through the person to the ground, producing potentially fatal results.

Ground-fault interrupters must be distinguished from standard circuit breakers. Although GFIs stop the current flow at very low amperages, standard circuit breakers require a much larger discrepancy (up to 25 A) to be activated. Circuit breakers are not adequate for use in athletic training rooms, physical therapy clinics, or hospitals, especially in hydrotherapy areas. The 1991 National Electric Code requires the use of GFIs in all health care facilities that use therapeutic pools.[152] A GFI may be housed in either the wall outlet or in the circuit breaker box. In either case, GFIs are easily recognizable by their TEST and RESET buttons. Each GFI should be tested at regular intervals, with monthly intervals being considered ideal. Each testing date should be documented.

In the event that the GFI trips, disconnect the patient from the unit, and turn off the power to the unit. Check all connections, depress the RESET button on the GFI, restart the equipment without the patient being in contact with it, and ensure that a ground fault does not reoccur. If the GFI trips again, disconnect the unit, label the unit and the outlet "Out of Order," and call for service.

other areas of the facility, the power of the lighting can be reduced to 30 to 50 footcandles at a height of 4 feet above the floor.

Hydrotherapy Area

The hydrotherapy area possesses unique safety concerns. Here, perhaps more than in any other portion of the health care facility, the greatest potential for hazards exists. The hydrotherapy area typically houses whirlpools, rehabilitation "swim tanks," ice machines, hot and cold water supply (for whirlpools, immersion tubs, and coolers), sinks, refrigerator, freezer, and ice machine.

Ideally, the on-off switches controlling the whirlpool motors should be located so that the patient who is in the tub cannot reach them. If the whirlpool has this switch mounted on the motor, patients are not to turn the unit on or off while in the water. It is a good practice to post signs stating rules for the use of these devices in the hydrotherapy area.

The hydrotherapy area itself should be in full view of the staff. Because of the noise associated with this modality, this area is normally "glassed off" from the rest of the rehabilitation facility (Fig. 4-2). A closed door will help reduce the noise in the rest of the treatment facility.

Enclosing the hydrotherapy area increases the amount of humidity; ice machines, refrigerators, freezers, and other ap-

---

Chassis: The framework to which electrical components are attached.

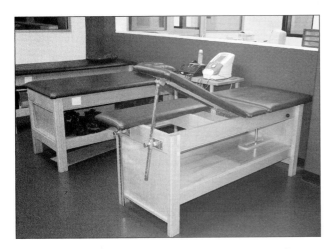

Figure 4-1. **Split-Leg Table**. These tables assist in venous return from the lower extremity by being elevated during treatment.

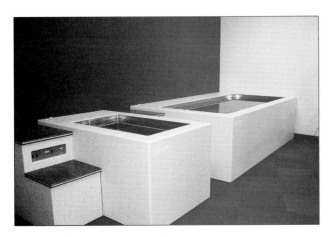

Figure 4-2. **The Hydrotherapy Area.** The hydrotherapy room is a high-risk area. This room should be in full view of the staff and is therefore usually enclosed in glass to prevent humidity and noise from affecting the rest of the facility.

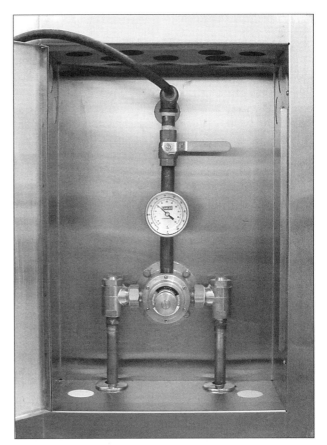

Figure 4-3. **Hot/Cold Water Mixing Valve.** A mixing valve helps prevent scalding by safely controlling the flow of water (bottom control). A thermostat indicates the temperature of the water flow (middle dial) that is controlled by the handle on the top. The thermometer must be calibrated annually. The hose to the whirlpool has been moved out of the way.

pliances produce heat. The combination of heat and humidity encourages the growth of fungi, bacteria, and viruses. To thwart this problem, the hydrotherapy area should be well ventilated and air-conditioned to maintain 40% to 50% humidity and air recycled 8 to 10 times per hour.[153]

Each whirlpool should have its own fill faucets, although a hose may be used to fill multiple tubs. Each tub should have a hot and cold control or a mixing valve that regulates the temperature of the water entering the tub (Fig. 4-3). Whirlpool temperature gauges must be annually calibrated. A large swan neck faucet should be available for filling immersion tubs, coolers, and so on.

The floor should be covered with a nonslip surface and should be gently sloped toward one or more floor drains. Each whirlpool should have a dedicated drain.

■ Product Maintenance

All therapeutic equipment must be kept in its optimum working condition. Knowingly using an unsafe therapeutic modality is negligent professional behavior. Maintenance requires regular inspection for defects or hazards, periodic cleaning, and professional calibration according to the manufacturer's recommendations.

Electrically operated modalities such as electrical stimulators, therapeutic ultrasound, and shortwave diathermy are required to be regularly (e.g., annually or biannually) inspected and calibrated by a qualified service technician. The date of these inspections must be documented on the unit and the type of work performed should be recorded in an equipment maintenance logbook.

Normal wear and tear of equipment is expected. Proper care of the equipment will help to reduce the long-term toll of use. Logical precautions such as avoiding spills into the equipment, keeping electrical cords neatly stored, and regular inspection of electrical plugs and leads will assist in maintaining the longevity of the equipment.

If a defect is found in the plug or cord, the GFI continues to trip, or the unit fails to function properly, unplug it, label it as being inoperative, and remove it from the treatment area. A qualified technician should then service the unit. Operators must not attempt to perform maintenance or repairs beyond those that are described in the operator's manual.

Policies and Procedures Manual

A policies and procedures manual delineates the facility's scope of service, operational plans, and standard operating procedures. Policies are used to guide administrative decision making. Procedures describe the processes used to carry out the policies. The standards and procedures described in the policies and procedures manual can be used to determine if professional negligence has occurred. The depth and breadth of policies and procedure manuals cannot be covered here, but the implications of treatment and rehabilitation must be discussed.

A primary purpose of the policies and procedure manual is defining the roles and lines of reporting amongst administrators and the clinical staff. **Job descriptions** define the roles, responsibility, and minimum expectations for each employee. An **organizational chart** describes the relationships between all of the individuals involved in the delivery of services.

Standard operating procedures describe the procedures that are to be followed in various situations and may include **standing orders** •. Standing operating procedures or standing orders are not prescriptive "cookbooks" that dictate the patient's treatment. Rather, they present a conceptual framework for the procedures to be implemented. Procedures for medical emergencies should also be described in this section.

Medical documentation procedures are another portion of the reporting structure that should be addressed in the policies and procedures manual, including annotated examples of how to complete each document and any applicable routing. An appendix of the manual should also include the approved medical shorthand and abbreviations for the facility.

Sections of the manual should be dedicated to how the facility meets the compliance requirements of governmental regulations (including OSHA) and educational or facility accreditation requirements agencies.

Standing orders: A "blanket prescription" from a physician describing how injuries are to be managed when the physician is not present.

End of Section

Case Study: The Patient's Medical History

A 42-year-old man sprained his left ankle 2 days ago while participating in a tennis tournament. He was evaluated by his primary physician and was diagnosed with a grade 1 lateral ankle sprain. He has been referred to you for evaluation and treatment of his injury. The following information has been obtained directly from the patient and from the patient's medical records.

Medical history: The patient reports that he has pain on weight bearing, located along the lateral aspect of the left ankle.

History of present condition: The patient reports that he "rolled" on his left foot while playing tennis. He was able to continue playing, but the pain increased and the ankle began to swell later in the day. The patient has a history of bilateral ankle sprains.

Diagnostic tests: Radiographs demonstrate a previous avulsion fracture of the lateral malleolus.

Activity limitations: Antalgic gait •, pain climbing stairs.

Participation restrictions: Unable to perform weight-bearing ADLs, unable to participate in tennis.

General medical conditions: The patient has a history of insulin-dependent diabetes.

Medications: Insulin. The doctor prescribed acetaminophen for the pain because the patient does not tolerate nonsteroidal anti-inflammatory drugs as a result of his peptic ulcer.

Contraindications to interventions: The patient has diabetes. Caution must be used with heat modalities if sensory exam of feet is not normal.

Patient goals: To play in the tennis tournament in 5 days. Pain-free ADLs.

Examination findings:

Participation Restrictions:	Unable to participate in tennis
Activity Limitations:	Patient cannot walk without assistance (crutches). Unable to climb stairs
Observation:	Swelling and discoloration are present along the distal aspect of the lateral malleolus.
Palpation:	Pain over the anterior talofibular ligament
Range of Motion:	Active ROM: Left (inv) Right Dorsiflexion 7°-0-32° 15°-0-37° (knee extended)

	Dorsiflexion (knee flexed)	10°-0-32° 15°-0-37°
	Inversion/	5°-0°-3° 15°-0°-5°
Girth:		Left Right
	Figure eight technique	21.25 in. 19.5 in.
	Base of the fifth metatarsal	12.25 in. 12.0 in.
Tone:	The patient demonstrates the ability to elicit muscle contractions, but is limited by pain.	
Muscle Function Assessment:	Dorsiflexors: 5/5, but painful Plantarflexors: 5/5 Invertors: 5/5 Evertors: 5/5, but painful	
Joint Function Assessment:	Left Right One-leg stance for 20 seconds	2 deviations 0 deviations
Pain rating:	2/10 with level walking	
Stress tests:	All tests for laxity negative	
Selective tissue tests:	All tests for laxity negative	

The patient's history of regular participation in competitive tennis indicates that he is a good candidate for relatively aggressive rehabilitation. His history of diabetes could be an influence on the selection of therapeutic modalities and exercises, but this condition appears to be well controlled. Because he is sensitive to non-steroidal anti-inflammatory medications, his level of discomfort and swelling may be beyond that expected. There is noticeable swelling and range-of-motion restrictions in the left ankle, but strength is within normal limits. Proprioception is a problem, but the fact that the patient is within normal limits for the right leg indicates that this disruption is probably related to the pathology. Pain is slight and there are no other significant findings.

Problem Recognition

The following problems have been identified based on the information presented in the case study scenario:

1. Decreased function secondary to pain, including the ability to participate in tennis.
2. Decreased ROM of the left ankle.
3. Swelling of the left ankle.
4. Decreased balance and proprioception of the left ankle.

Antalgic gait: A gait resulting from pain on weight bearing. The stance phase of gait is shortened on the affected side.

Commentary

- The pain rating given by the patient is consistent with an acute grade 1 lateral ankle sprain. It is significant that he does have pain with weight bearing and must compete again in 5 days. In many instances the course of treatment for this injury would consist of rest, but because he desires to play in a tournament, it is prudent to attempt to return him to safe activity. The ramifications and risks with an aggressive treatment approach must be explained to the patient so that he may make a reasonable, informed decision as to continuing to participate.
- The ROM deficits are probably related to pain and swelling. Running requires a minimum of 15 degrees of dorsiflexion to maintain a normal biomechanical pattern.
- Although swelling is minimal, it may reduce the overall ankle motion. The patient's balance difficulties may be affected by swelling disrupting the joint receptors responsible for proprioception.
- The dorsiflexors and evertors evoke strong contractions, but pain is experienced. The pain does not arise from the muscles; therefore, a strength rating of 5/5 is given.
- The patient's balance deficit is a key factor in his return to activity in a safe and timely manner. Balance and proprioception during functional activities related to tennis must be obtained prior to clearing him to play.
- The patient's diabetes could have an influence on the course of care, but the diabetes appears to be well controlled. If present, decreased sensation or ulceration associated with diabetes would affect the modalities used.

Prioritization of the Problem
The patient's problems ranked in terms of treatment priority are:

1. Swelling of the left ankle.
2. Decreased ROM of the left ankle.
3. Decreased balance and proprioception of the left ankle.
4. Decreased function secondary to pain, including the ability to participate in tennis.

Commentary

- Most of the patient's activity limitations are related to swelling within the ankle joint, increasing pain, decreasing ROM, and decreasing weight-bearing ability. The treatment goals should address edema removal as the highest priority. Caution must be used to prevent additional swelling formation.
- The decreased ROM is a significant deterrent to the patient's ability to play tennis in 5 days. To return to safe activity, ROM must be restored to provide an adequate amount of ankle plantarflexion and dorsiflexion. Strength and flexibility will most likely be restored to normal as the swelling and pain are reduced.
- Balance and proprioception are essential to most activities. In the case of this patient, balance is required because he will be called on to quickly stop, start, and change direction. Proper proprioception is needed for the patient's muscles to protect the joint from potentially injurious forces. Be respectful of any pain that the patient reports while performing balance exercises. These exercises cannot be performed at the expense of any harm they may do to the injury.
- The inability to function in a safe, pain-free manner is the biggest problem facing the patient and clinician because of the time constraints in this scenario. By addressing these problems, the rehabilitation will lead to a return to safe function.

Long-Term Goals
At the time of discharge, the following long-term goals will be achieved:

1. Regain a normal gait pattern within 5 days.
2. Be able to play in a tennis match using a protective support in 5 days.

Commentary

- The goals are reasonable and obtainable within the 5-day time frame. However, the patient must be carefully examined at the end of 5 days to verify that it is safe for him to compete. Withhold the patient from competition if these goals are not met.
- The ability to return to competition does not imply that the patient is totally healed. After the match, the patient will need to resume therapy so that the rehabilitation program can be completed.

Short-Term Goals
The following short-term goals have initially been established for this patient:

1. Swelling will decrease to within 1/4 inch relative to the right ankle within 3 days.
2. The patient will be able to walk without pain (0 to 1/10) within 3 days.
3. The patient's ROM in the left ankle will be 10 degrees of dorsiflexion, 35 degrees of plantarflexion, 8 degrees of inversion, and 4 degrees of eversion within 4 days.
4. The patient will be able to display equal balance between the left and right ankle within 4 days.
5. The patient will not participate in tennis at this time.

Commentary

A 3-day period was established for reaching the first short-term goal. Referring back to the commentary for prioritizing the problems, note that swelling must be reduced before any improvement can be seen in the remaining problem areas. If the first goal is met early, the remaining time frames can be accelerated. The fifth goal is different from the rest in that it describes a behavior that is to be avoided. In this situation, the patient must avoid placing harmful stresses on the involved joint.

Intervention Planning

The following treatment approaches have been selected to meet the short-term goals:

1. Intermittent Compression With Elevation Sixty minutes. Pressure setting of 60 mm Hg with an ON-OFF cycle of 30 seconds "ON" to 15 seconds "OFF."

Theory

Intermittent compression and elevation assists in the venous and lymphatic return of edema. Edema reduction will decongest the area and allow nutrients and oxygen to reach the damaged tissues. As the edema becomes stabilized, this intermittent compression may be used post-treatment to control the edema.

2. Retrograde Massage Effleurage strokes from the toes to the lower leg to "milk" edema proximally. "Uncorking" the leg proximal to the ankle precedes the effleurage strokes.

Effleurage massage will aid the venous and lymphatic system in transporting edema proximally. Movement of this material out of the injured area will decrease pain and help to improve ROM.

3. Range of Motion and Flexibility Exercises

Theory

The patient will need specific exercises to promote increased ROM to achieve functional limits. Cryokinetics may initially be used to speed the reacquisition of motion.

4. Resistance Exercises

Theory

The patient will need to maintain strength in the injured area and return the surrounding musculature to proper function. He may start out with isometric contractions and progress to isotonic contractions or resistance tubing as tolerated.

5. Balance Exercises

Theory

The patient demonstrated balance deficits during the initial evaluation that will decrease optimal function. The patient can use a balance system or one-leg stance exercises, progressing from stable to less stable surfaces as tolerated.

6. Maintain Cardiovascular Conditioning

Theory

Cardiovascular and musculoskeletal endurance must be maintained so that the patient is ready to return to strenuous physical activity.

7. Progressive Return to Activity

Theory

The capability of the injured ankle to withstand progressively more difficult stresses must be addressed to allow the patient to return to activity in a safe manner. The functional progression would include jogging, running, and progressively harder agility, as well as sport-specific drills to tax the injured area.

8. Ice, Compression, and Elevation Twenty minutes after exercise and during home treatments.

Theory

Cold will decrease the metabolic rate in the treated tissues, helping to limit further damage secondary to anoxia and will assist in decreasing pain. The patient will be educated about how to apply a compression wrap and instructed to keep his leg elevated as much as possible, including at work, at rest, and during sleep.

9. Home Exercise Program: ROM, Strengthening, Balancing Exercises, and Ice With Elevation

Theory

To achieve the goals in a short time, the patient must have an inclusive home program addressing the areas of deficits. Patient compliance is imperative because of the goal of return to activity in 5 days.

Case Study: The Patient's Medical History

A 16-year-old basketball player has been referred to you by his primary care physician for evaluation, treatment, and rehabilitation. The following information has been obtained Directly from the patient and from the patient's medical records.

Medical history: The patient reports pain and muscle spasm in his cervical musculature that limits his motion. Basketball practice is scheduled to begin in 1 week.

History of present condition: The patient was involved in a motor vehicle accident and has been given a diagnosis of a cervical strain and sprain.

Diagnostic tests: Radiographs were negative for bony involvement.

Activity limitations: Decreased cervical spine range of motion.

Participation restrictions: To be able to sleep through the night and begin basketball practice as soon as possible.

General medical conditions: The patient suffers from asthma; otherwise, he is healthy.

Medications: The patient uses an inhaler for his asthma. Muscle relaxants have been prescribed for his cervical injury.

Contraindications to interventions: None.

Patient goals: To participate in basketball practice within three weeks.

Examination findings:

Participation Restrictions:	Unable to participate in soccer.
Activity Limitations:	Unable to sleep soundly secondary to pain and discomfort. Full cervical spine range of motion is lacking.
Observation:	The patient wears a soft cervical collar for comfort. The patient has a guarded posture.
Palpation:	Increased tone is present in the left upper trapezius due to muscle spasm. Trigger points are palpated in both upper trapezius muscles, with the left more tender than the right.
Range of Motion:	A ROM : Flexion: 50%
	(C-spine) Extension: 40%
	Right rotation: 50%
	Left rotation: 50%
	Right-side bending: 25%
	Left-side bending: 50%
	(% relative to uninvolved side)

	PROM: Flexibility of cervical musculature cannot be assessed due to pain and guarding.
Tone:	Increased tone (muscle spasm) is noted in the left trapezius.
Muscle Function Assessment:	Testing of all cervical musculature elicits pain—no grades given because of pain.
Joint Function Assessment:	Vertebral joint glides are negative for laxity, but yield pain.
Upper-Quarter Neurological Screen:	Deep tendon reflexes are 2/2 bilaterally. Sensations are intact to light touch bilaterally. Result of manual muscle test is 5/5 throughout.
Pain Rating:	Pain with right-side bending is 7/10. Patient reports constant pain of varying intensity with all ADLs.
Selective Tissue Tests:	Cervical compression: No radicular pain; increased cervical pain. Cervical distraction: No radicular pain; increased cervical pain.

This patient suffered a "whiplash"-type injury and now has significant deficits in cervical mobility. Cervical fracture, dislocation, and trauma to the spinal cord have been ruled out. The patient's primary complaints are related to muscle spasm that is most likely caused by cervical nerve root impingement.

Note that the patient's physical examination could not be completed because of pain and range-of-motion restrictions. These procedures should be performed as permitted during subsequent reexaminations.

Problem Recognition

The following problems have been identified based on the information presented in the case study scenario:

1. Inability to play basketball.
2. Inability to sleep undisturbed secondary to pain.
3. Decreased cervical ROM.
4. Inability to assess strength and flexibility of the cervical musculature because of pain.
5. Pain is rated 7/10 during right-side bending.
6. Increased tone because of muscle spasm of the left upper trapezius.
7. Patient wears a soft cervical collar for comfort.

Commentary

- The inability to function is the result of the pain, spasm, and loss of ROM of the cervical muscles. Although all of these are significant problems, the primary reason why someone seeks and needs rehabilitation is to reduce pain and restore function.

- The decreased cervical ROM is most likely a result of pain and spasm versus true joint restriction of the connective tissues about the joint. In an otherwise healthy 16-year-old patient, you would not see changes in the joint structures so quickly after an injury of this type.
- The inability to complete any portion of the patient assessment should be noted, and the reason for the omission should be explained. This documentation serves as a reminder to assess these at a future date and informs other clinicians who are not familiar with the patient's history that these tests were not performed. By noting that these examinations were not conducted, other clinicians will not assume that areas were not assessed or were assessed and were normal.
- The increased muscle tone of the trapezius is caused by the pain-spasm-pain cycle and is typical after acute musculoskeletal injury, secondary to a reflexive protective mechanism. Although this mechanism is protective during the acute stages of an injury, the clinician must work to relieve the pain-spasm-pain cycle so that healing may take place. The spasm will restrict blood flow and the delivery of nutrients and oxygen to the injured tissues and surrounding areas.
- The soft cervical collar is not a problem itself; it is a reasonable treatment option at this time. Although this collar serves an important protective purpose, it does not allow normal function.

Prioritization of the Problems

The patient's problems ranked in terms of treatment priority are:

1. Pain is rated 7/10 during right-sided bending.
2. Increased muscle tone secondary to muscle spasm of the left upper trapezius.
3. Decreased cervical ROM.
4. Inability to assess strength and flexibility of the cervical musculature because of pain.
5. Inability to play basketball.
6. Inability to sleep undisturbed because of pain.
7. Patient wears a soft cervical collar for comfort.

Commentary

- This patient's pain and spasm are given the highest priority because they cause the patient's restricted motion. The pain-spasm-pain cycle is a protective response that, when prolonged, can delay the return of the patient to full activity. The decreased cervical ROM will limit the ability of the patient to perform ADLs, will prohibit him from competing in basketball, and will hinder rehabilitation exercises. The clinician must use modalities and exercise to reduce the pain-spasm-pain cycle and increase blood flow to the area.
- Assigning a low priority to the functional problems should not be interpreted as indicating that these concerns are trivial. These functional problems are

a result of the patient's other problems. By correcting the problems of pain, spasm, ROM, and any inadequacies of strength and flexibility, the clinician will be able to return the patient to functional activity.
- Wearing the soft cervical collar is not of great concern at this time. Although a patient should not be allowed to rely on this orthosis, it is prudent to allow him to wear it for comfort. He should be weaned from it as tolerated.

Long-Term Goals

At the time of discharge, the following long-term goals will be achieved:

1. The patient will return to full activity playing basketball.
2. The patient will be able to sleep undisturbed without use of the cervical collar.
3. The patient will have normal ROM, flexibility, and strength.
4. The patient will be symptom free.

Commentary

The long-term goals have been established for a 3-week period. The goals address basic ADLs such as sleep as well as more strenuous activities (e.g., sports, fitness, and work). Note that the patient will have normal ROM, flexibility, and strength. This goal is certainly feasible in this period and essential if this patient is to return to activity, predisposing himself to further injury.

Short-Term Goals

The following short-term goals have initially been established for this patient:

1. The patient's pain with right-side bending will be reported as 3/10 or less.
2. The patient's muscle spasm will decrease to the point at which the cervical collar will be worn only at night.
3. The patient's cervical ROM will improve to:

Flexion:	75%
Extension:	60%
Right rotation:	75%
Left rotation:	75%
Right-side bending:	50%
Left-side bending:	75%

4. The clinician will be able to assess the strength and flexibility of the patient's cervical musculature.
5. The patient will be able to sleep throughout the night undisturbed by pain.
6. Patient will not participate in basketball at this time.
7. Patient will be compliant and independent in a home exercise program.

Commentary

- A 1-week period for attaining the short-term goals is initially set. In a young, active, otherwise healthy person this period should be adequate to note changes in the patient's condition. Because this patient has a short time frame before the start of basketball season, the clinician will want to evaluate the patient more frequently so that changes can be expediently made to the rehabilitation program.

- The first three goals are set to measure the efficacy of the program in relieving the patient's pain and spasm. Goal 4 is information that could not be determined during the initial evaluation because of the patient's pain.
- The goals concerning sleep and the use of the collar are reasonable. If they are met, the patient will be less dependent on the collar and function better. The patient should not be participating in basketball because he is likely to aggravate the injury and may be at risk for reinjury.
- The final goal is always important because we should always strive to make our patients independent through compliance with their home program, which will expedite the rehabilitation process.

Treatment Planning

The treatment plan for this case study is presented at the end of Sections 2 through 5. The plan outlined in each chapter focuses on modalities discussed in that chapter. Although the various chapters present a wide range of treatment strategies, this is not to imply that all of these modalities would be used during the same treatment session. Care must be taken to avoid overtreating the patient, especially when the patient is billed per modality used. All of the possible treatment approaches are not necessarily presented, and your instructor may describe other treatment plans or challenge you to devise your own strategy. The following would also be incorporated into the patient's treatment plan:

1. Cardiovascular Exercise Stationary bicycle riding for 30 minutes, maintaining the patient's heart rate at 122 to 163 beats per minute.

Theory

Cardiovascular exercise would be incorporated early to maintain the patient at a high level of conditioning. The patient must maintain his heart rate in the target range to achieve aerobic conditioning. The patient could progress to other forms of cardiovascular conditioning as his healing permits.

2. Weaning From the Cervical Collar

Theory

The patient should be allowed to wear the cervical collar as needed as long as he does not become dependent on it. He should be encouraged to wean himself from its use, wearing it less during waking hours, only at night for sleep, and then not at all as long as he can sleep undisturbed and perform normal ADLs without increasing his symptoms.

3. Strengthening Exercises Progressive resistance exercises (PREs) for the lower extremities, upper extremities, and spinal musculature as the patient's cervical ROM becomes normal and there is no pain with ADLs.

Theory

Strengthening of the injured area and maintaining peak muscular strength are needed so that the patient may return to full activity in the shortest possible time. Exercise for the lower extremities could be started almost immediately; PREs for the upper extremities and spine should be started after the pain begins to subside and the ROM begins to increase.

4. Progressive Return to Basketball The patient would first progress through individual basketball drills and then to one-on-one drills. After successful completion of these, he could progress to scrimmaging and then full competition.

● ● ● **Section 1 Quiz**

1. An example of an injury caused by macrotrauma is:
   A. Stress fracture
   B. Sprain
   C. Tendinopathy
   D. Pes planus

2. This phagocyte is released immediately following trauma to contain bacteria, but in the process destroys viable tissues:
   A. Serotonin
   B. Kinin
   C. Neutrophil
   D. Leukotriene

3. Which of the following cell types is anaerobic and therefore is able to withstand a low-oxygen environment?
   A. Fibrocyte
   B. Granuloma
   C. Macrophage
   D. Anerocyte

4. After depolarization of the nerve, the period during which a stronger-than-normal stimulus is required to initiate another action potential is the:
   A. Absolute refractory period
   B. Relative refractory period
   C. Silent refractory period
   D. Latent refractory period

5. The removal of debris and temporary tissue and the growth of new, permanent tissue occur during:
   A. Acute inflammation phase
   B. Maturation phase
   C. Proliferation phase

6. The rate of atrophy is accelerated through the stimulation of:
   A. Golgi tendon organs
   B. Phasic stretch receptors
   C. Actin and myosin filaments
   D. Blood flow

7. The healing process begins with:
   A. Inflammation
   B. Coagulation
   C. Phagocytosis
   D. Repair phase

8. All of the following aid in venous return *except:*
   A. Gravity
   B. Muscular contractions
   C. The sodium-potassium pump
   D. One-way valves

9. Which of the following structures has the poorest blood supply?
   A. Muscle
   B. Fascia
   C. Meniscal cartilage
   D. Bone

10. During early stage of intervention, which type of muscle fibers should be targeted to reduce the development of atrophy?
    A. Slow twitch (type I)
    B. Slow twitch (type II)
    C. Fast twitch (type I)
    D. Fast twitch (type II)

11. According to the Gate Control Theory of pain modulation, what monitors the activity of the incoming nerves and subsequently opens or closes the gate?
    A. T cell
    B. Dorsal horn
    C. Paleospinothalamic tract
    D. Substantia gelatinosa

12. The perception of, and the subsequent reaction to, pain occurs in the:
    A. Medulla
    B. Cerebellum
    C. Cerebral cortex
    D. Thalamus

13. The amount of stimulus required to trigger the pain response is termed:
    A. Pain threshold
    B. Pain tolerance

14. Pain produced by irritation of the brachial plexus due to entrapment of its roots will be felt in the arm or hand instead of the armpit. This mislocalization is closely related to a phenomenon called:
    A. Phantom limb pain
    B. Referred pain
    C. Chronic pain
    D. Epicritic pain

15. Indicate those nerve fibers responsible for nociception:
    A. A-beta
    B. A-delta
    C. A-gamma
    D. C fibers

16. According to the World Health Organization's International Classification of Function, dysfunction of the body's functions and/or structures is termed:
    A. Disability
    B. Participation restriction
    C. Activity limitation
    D. Impairment

17. A functional outcome scale's responsiveness to change that is important or beneficial to the patient is described by the:
    A. Minimum detectable change (MDC)
    B. Minimally clinically important change (MCID)

18. Strength, range of motion, and girth are examples of:
    A. Clinician-based outcomes
    B. Patient-based outcomes

19. Which type of state regulation establishes the scope of professional practice, sets the minimal education standards, and protects professional roles and titles?
    A. Certification
    B. Exemption
    C. Licensure
    D. Registration

20. Whirlpools and other electrical devices that may be used in the presence of water must be connected to a:
    A. Hospital-grade plug
    B. Three-pronged outlet
    C. Circuit breaker
    D. Ground-fault circuit interrupter

21. Employers or clinical instructors can be held liable for negligent acts of their employees or students through the doctrine of:
    A. Contributory negligence
    B. Vicarious liability
    C. Gross negligence
    D. Omission

22. The intentional and unwanted touching of one person by another is termed:
    A. Nonfeasance
    B. Slander
    C. Battery
    D. Assault

23. _____ is the coding system used to identify the type and nature of care provided to the patient.
    A. CPT
    B. ICD
    C. OSHA
    D. PMC

24. Which of the following would be considered when determining the actions that a "reasonable and prudent person" would have taken under similar circumstances?
    A. Testimony of expert witnesses
    B. The defendant's age, education, and mental capacity
    C. State practice regulations
    D. All of the above

References

1. Knight KL: Cryotherapy in Sport Injury Management. Human Kinetics, Champaign, IL, 1995.
2. Mueller MJ, Maluf KS: Tissue adaptation to physical stress: A proposed "physical stress theory" to guide physical therapist practice, education, and research. *Phys Ther.* 82:383, 2002.
3. Allen RJ: Human Stress: Its Nature and Control. Burgess, Minneapolis, MN, 1983.
4. Ho AM, Bedair H, Fu FH, et al: The role of non-steroidal anti-inflammatory drugs (NSAIDS) after acute exercise-induced muscle injuries. *Int SportMed J.* 5:209, 2004.
5. Bryan JM, et al: Altered load history affects periprosthetic bone loss following cementless total hip arthroplasty. *J Orthop Res.* 14:762, 1996.
6. Järvinen TAH, Järvinen TLN, Kääriäinen M, et al: Muscle injuries. Biology and treatment. *Am J Sports Med.* 33:745, 2005.
7. Lamme EN, et al: Allogenic fibroblasts in dermal substitutes induce inflammation and scar formation. *Wound Repair Regen.* 10:152, 2002.
8. Enwemeka CS: Inflammation, cellularity, and fibrillogenesis in regenerating tendon: Implications for tendon rehabilitation. *Phys Ther.* 69:816, 1989.
9. Sawyer PC, Uhl TL, Mattacola CG, et al: Effects of moist heat on hamstring flexibility and muscle temperature. *J Strength Cond Res.* 17:285, 2003.
10. Gross MT: Chronic tendinitis: Pathomechanics of injury, factors affecting the healing response, and treatment. *J Orthop Sports Phys Ther.* 16:248, 1992.
11. Butterfield TA, Best TM, Merrick MA: The dual roles of neutrophils and macrophages in inflammation: A critical balance between tissue damage and repair. *J Athl Train.* 41:457, 2006.
12. Wilkerson GB: Inflammation in connective tissue: Etiology and management. *J Athl Train.* 20:298, 1985.
13. Bleakley CM, Glasgow P, MacAuley DC: PRICE needs updating, should we call the POLICE? *Br J Sports Med.* 46:220, 2012.
14. Starkey C, Brown S, Ryan J: Examination of Orthopedic and Athletic Injuries, ed 3. FA Davis, Philadelphia, 2010.
15. Ward PA, Lentsch AB: The acute inflammatory response and its regulation. *Arch Surg.* 134:666, 1999.
16. Hopkins JT, Ingersoll CD: Arthrogenic muscle inhibition: A limiting factor in joint rehabilitation. *J Sport Rehabil.* 9:135, 2000.
17. Voight ML: Reduction of post-traumatic ankle edema with high-voltage pulsed galvanic stimulation. *J Athl Train.* 19:278, 1984.
18. Salter RB, et al: The biological effect of continuous passive motion on the healing of full thickness defects in articular cartilage. *J Bone Joint Surg.* 62:A1232, 1980.
19. Denegar CR, et al: Influence of transcutaneous electrical nerve stimulation on pain, range of motion, and serum cortisol concentration in females experiencing delayed onset muscle soreness. *J Orthop Sports Phys Ther.* 11:100, 1989.
20. Hall JE: Guyton and Hall Textbook of Medical Physiology. Saunders, New York, 2010.
21. Rucinski TJ, et al: The effects of intermittent compression on edema in postacute ankle sprains. *J Orthop Sports Phys Ther.* 14:65, 1991.
22. Kraemer WJ, French DN, Spiering BA: Compression in the treatment of acute muscle injuries in sport. *Intl SportMed J.* 5:200, 2004.
23. Knobloch K, Grasemann R, Spies M, et al: Midportion Achilles tendon microcirculation after intermittent combined cryotherapy and compression compared with cryotherapy alone. A randomized trial. *Am J Sports Med.* 36:2128, 2008.
24. Houglum PA: Soft tissue healing and its impact on rehabilitation. *J Sports Rehabil.* 1:19, 1992.
25. Hebda PA, et al: Mast cell and myofibroblast in wound healing. *Dermatol Clin.* 11:685, 1993.
26. Olsen L, Sherratt JA, Maini PK: A mechanochemical model for adult dermal wound contraction and the permanence of

the contracted tissue displacement profile. *J Theor Biol.* 177:113, 1995.

27. Kirsner RS, Eaglstein WH: The wound healing process. *Dermatol Clin.* 11:629, 1993.

28. Rosenbaum AJ, Wicker JF, Dines JS, et al: Histologic stages of healing correlate with restoration of tensile strength in a model of experimental tendon repair. *HSS J.* 6:164, 2010.

29. Lechner CT, Dahners LE: Healing of the medial collateral ligament in unstable rat knees. *Am J Sports Med.* 19:508, 1991.

30. Kannus P, Parkkari J, Järvinen TLN, et al: Basic science and clinical studies coincide: Active treatment approach is needed after a sports injury. *Scand J Med Sci Sports.* 13:150, 2003.

31. Russell B, et al: Repair of injured skeletal muscle: A molecular approach. *Med Sci Sports Exerc.* 24:189, 1992.

32. Merrick MA, McBrier NM: Progression of secondary injury after musculoskeletal trauma—a window of opportunity? *J Sport Rehabil.* 19:380, 2010.

33. Merrick MA, et al: A preliminary examination of cryotherapy and secondary injury in skeletal muscle. *Med Sci Sports Exerc.* 31:1516, 1999.

34. Vanudevan SV, Melvin JL: Upper extremity edema control: Rationale of the techniques. *Am J Occup Ther.* 33:520, 1980.

35. Myrer WJ, et al: Cold- and hot-pack contrast therapy: Subcutaneous and intramuscular temperature change. *J Athl Train.* 32:238, 1997.

36. Capps SG: Cryotherapy and intermittent pneumatic compression for soft tissue trauma. *Athl Ther Today.* 14:2, 2009.

37. Gilbart MK, et al: Anterior tibial compartment pressures during intermittent sequential pneumatic compression therapy. *Am J Sports Med.* 23:769, 1995.

38. Shillinger A, et al: Effect of manual lymph drainage on the course of serum levels of muscle enzymes after treadmill exercise. *Am J Phys Med Rehabil.* 85:516, 2006.

39. Merrick MA, et al: The effects of ice and compression wraps on intramuscular temperatures at various depths. *J Athl Train.* 28:236, 1993.

40. Dervin GF, et al: Effects of cold and compression dressings on early postoperative outcomes for the arthroscopic anterior cruciate ligament reconstruction patient. *J Orthop Sports Phys Ther.* 27:403, 1998.

41. Stöckle U, et al: Fastest reduction of posttraumatic edema: Continuous cryotherapy or intermittent impulse compression? *Foot Ankle Int.* 18:432, 1997.

42. Partsch H: Intermittent pneumatic compression in immobile patients. *Int Wound J.* 5:389, 2008.

43. Stöckle U, et al: Fastest reduction of posttraumatic edema: Continuous cryotherapy or intermittent impulse compression? *Foot Ankle Int.* 18:432, 1997.

44. Shoemaker JK, et al: Failure of manual massage to alter limb blood flow: Measures by Doppler ultrasound. *Med Sci Sports Exerc.* 29:610, 1997.

45. Silverberg SM: Trouble in the vascular periphery. *Emerg Med.* 19:22, 1987.

46. McCulloch J, Boyd VB: The effects of whirlpool and the dependent position on lower extremity volume. *J Orthop Sports Phys Ther.* 16:169, 1992.

47. Goddard AA, Pierce CS, McLeod KJ: Reversal of lower limb edema by calf muscle pump stimulation. *J Cardiopulm Rehabil Prev.* 28:174, 2008.

48. Kisner C , Colby LA: Therapeutic Exercise: Foundations and Techniques, ed 5. FA Davis, Philadelphia, 2007.

49. Niddam DM: Brain manifestation and modulation of pain from myofascial trigger points. *Curr Pain Headache Rep.* 13:370, 2009.

50. Alvarez DJ, Rockwell PG: Trigger points: Diagnosis and management. *Am Fam Physician.* 65:653, 2002.

51. Pollard LC, Kingsley GH, Choy EH, et al: Fibromyalgic rheumatoid arthritis and disease assessment. *Rheumatology.* 49:924, 2010.

52. Cailliet R: Soft Tissue Pain and Disability. FA Davis, Philadelphia, 1977.

53. Urso ML: Disuse atrophy of human skeletal muscle: Cell signaling and potential interventions. *Med Sci Sports Exerc.* 41:1860, 2009.

54. Dagher E, Hays PL, Kawamura S, et al: Immobilization modulates macrophage accumulation in tendon-bone healing. *Clin Orthop Relat Res.* 467:281, 2009.

55. Urbancova H, et al: Bone fracture influences reflex muscle atrophy which is sex-dependent. *Physiol Res.* 42:35, 1993.

56. DeVahl J: Neuromuscular electrical stimulation (NMES) in rehabilitation. In Gersh MR (ed): Electrotherapy in Rehabilitation. FA Davis, Philadelphia, 1992, pp 218–268.

57. Clark BC: *In vivo* alterations in skeletal muscle form and function after disuse atrophy. *Med Sci Sports Exerc.* 41:1869, 2009.

58. Urso ML: Regulation of muscle atrophy: Wasting away from the outside in: An introduction. *Med Sci Sports Exerc.* 41:1856, 2009.

59. Hopkins JT, et al: Cryotherapy and transcutaneous electric neuromuscular stimulation decrease arthrogenic muscle inhibition of the vastus medialis after knee joint effusion. *J Athl Train.* 37:25, 2001.

60. Beavers KM, Brinkley TE, Nicklas BJ: Effect of exercise training on chronic inflammation. *Clinica Chimica Acta.* 411:785, 2010.

61. Huguet A, Stinson JN, McGrath, PJ: Measurement of self-reported pain intensity in children and adolescents. *J Psychosom Res.* 68:329, 2010.

62. Lester D, Yang B: An approach for examining the rationality of suicide. *Psychol Rep.* 79:405, 1996.

63. Orbach I: Dissociation, physical pain, and suicide: A hypothesis. *Suicide Life Threat Behav.* 24:68, 1994.

64. International Association for the Study of Pain: Taxonomy. http://www.iasp-pain.org/AM/Template.cfm?Section= General_Resource_Links&Template=/CM/HTMLDisplay. cfm&ContentID=3058. Retrieved October 11, 2011.

65. Ho K, Spence J, Murphy M: Review of pain-measurement tools. *An Emerg Med.* 27:427, 1996.

66. Ahles T, Blanchard, E, Ruchdeschel J: The multidimensional nature of cancer-related pain. *Pain.* 17:277, 1983.

67. Giles BE, Walker JS: Sex differences in pain and analgesia. *Pain Rev.* 7:181, 2000.

68. Williamson A, Hoggart B: Pain: A review of three commonly used pain rating scales. *J Clin Nurs.* 14:798, 2005.

69. Biswal N, et al: Congenital indifference to pain. *Indian J Pediatr.* 65:755, 1998.

70. Melzack R, Wall PD: The gate control theory of pain. In Soulairac, A, Cahn, J and Carpentier, J (eds): Pain: Proceedings of the International Symposium on Pain. Academic Press, London, 1968.

71. Fulbright RK, et al: Functional MR imaging of regional brain activation associated with the affective experience of pain. *AJR Am J Roentgenol.*177:1205, 2001.

72. Criste A: Gender and pain. *AANA J.* 70:475, 2002.

73. Robinson ME, Wise EA: Prior pain experience: Influence on the observation of experimental pain in men and women. *J Pain.* 5:264, 2004.

74. Scott V, Gijsbers K: Pain perception in competitive swimmers. *BMJ.* 282:91, 1981.

75. Hall EG, Davies S: Gender differences in perceived intensity and affect of pain between athletes and non-athletes. *Percept Mot Skills.* 73:779, 1991.

76. Jarmenko ME, et al: The differential ability of athletes and non-athletes to cope with two types of pain: A radical behavioral model. *Psychological Rec.* 31:265, 1981.

77. Walker J: Pain distraction in athletes and non-athletes. *Percept Mot Skills.* 33:1187, 1971.

78. Yamaguchi AY, et al: Difference in pain response and anxiety between athletes and non-athletes. *J Athl Train.* 32:S45, 1997.

79. Ryan ED, Kovacic CR: Pain tolerance and athletic participation. *Percept Mot Skills.* 22:383, 1966.

80. Lord RH, Kozar B: Pain tolerance in the presence of others: Implications for youth sports. *Phys Sports Med.* 17:71, 1989.

81. Green CR, Ndao-Brumblay SK, Nagrant AM, et al: Race, age, and gender influences among clusters of African American and white patients with chronic pain. *J Pain.* 5:171, 2004.

82. Unruh AM: Gender variations in clinical pain experience. *Pain.* 65:2, 1996.

83. Zombroski M: Cultural components in response to pain. *J Soc Issues.* 8:15, 1952.

84. Zola I: Culture and symptoms: An analysis of patients presenting complaints. *Am Soc Rev.* 31:615, 1966.

85. Edwards CL, et al: Race, ethnicity and pain. *Pain.* 94:133, 2001.

86. Defrin R, Eli I, Pud D: Interactions among sex, ethnicity, religion, and gender role expectations of pain. *Gend Med.* 8:172, 2011.

87. French S: Pain: Some physiological and sociological aspects. *Physiotherapy.* 75:255, 1989.

88. Karchnick KL, et al: Gender differences in pain threshold, tolerance and anxiety. *J Athl Train.* 32:S44, 1997.

89. Walton DM, Macdermid JC, Nielson W, et al: Pressure pain threshold testing demonstrates predictive ability in people with acute whiplash. *J Orthop Sports Phys Ther.* 41:658, 2011.

90. Vallerand AH: Gender differences in pain. *Image J Nurs Sch.* 27:235, 1995.

91. Gilman S, Newman SW: Pain and temperature. In Essentials of Clinical Neuroanatomy and Neurophysiology, ed 9. FA Davis, 1996, pp 48–57.

92. Takahashi A, Gotoh H: Mechanosensitive whole-cell currents in cultured rat somatosensory neurons. *Brain Res.* 869:225, 2000.

93. Shenker N, Haigh R, Roberts E, et al: Pain, neurogenic inflammation and symmetry in medical practice. *Pain Rev.* 8:27, 2001.

94. Taylor DCM, Pierau F-K: Nociceptive afferent neurons. In Winlow W (ed): Studies in Neuroscience, vol 14. Manchester University Press, Manchester, UK, 1991.

95. Smart KM, Blake C, Staines A, et al: Clinical indicators of "nociceptive," "peripherial neuropathic" and "central" mechanisms of musculoskeletal pain. A Delphi survey of expert clinicians. *Man Ther.* 15:80, 2010.

96. Fields HL: Pain. McGraw-Hill, New York, 1987.

97. Scholz J, Woolf CJ: Can we conquer pain? *Nat Neurosci.* Nov(S):1062, 2002.

98. Langford RM: Pain management today—what have we learned? *Clin Rheumatol.* 25(S):S2, 2006.

99. Melzack R, Wall, PD: Pain mechanisms: A new theory. *Science.* 150:971, 1965.

100. Melzack R: Neurophysiology foundations of pain. In Sternbach, RA (ed): The Psychology of Pain. Raven Press, New York, 1986, pp 1–24.

101. Melzack R: The Puzzle of Pain. Basic Books, New York, 1973.

102. Melzack R, Wall PD: The Challenge of Pain. Basic Books, New York, 1983.

103. Dickenson AH: Gate control theory of pain stands the test of time. *Br J Anaesth.* 88:755, 2002.

104. Mendiguchia J, Brughelli M: A return-to-sport algorithm for acute hamstring injuries. *Phys Ther Sport.* 12:2, 2011.

105. Denegar CR, Dougherty DR, Friedman JE, et al: Preferences for heat, cold, or contrast in patients with knee osteoarthritis affect treatment response. *Clin Interv Aging.* 5:199, 2010.

106. Juottonen K, et al: Altered central sensorimotor processing in patients with complex regional pain syndrome. *Pain.* 98:315, 2002.

107. Baker KG, et al: A review of therapeutic ultrasound: Biophysical effects. *Phys Ther.* 81:1351, 2001.

108. Lehmann JF, et al: Effect of therapeutic temperatures on tendon extensibility. *Arch Phys Med Rehabil.* 51:481, 1970.

109. Reed BV, et al: Effects of ultrasound and stretch on knee ligament extensibility. *J Orthop Sports Phys Ther.* 30:341, 2000.

110. McCormack K: The evolving NSAID: Focus on lornoxicam. *Pain Rev.* 6:262, 1999.

111. Masedo AI, Esteve R. Some empirical evidence regarding the validity of the Spanish version of the McGill Pain Questionnaire (MPQ-SV). *Pain.* 85:451, 2000.

112. Drewes AM, Helweg-Larsen S, Petersen P, et al: McGill Pain Questionnaire translated into Danish: Experimental and clinical findings. *Clin J Pain.* 9:80, 1993.

113. Snell CC, Fotherhill-Bourbonnais F, Durocher-Hendriks S: Patient controlled analgesia and intramuscular injections: A comparison of patient pain experiences and postoperative outcomes. *J Adv Nurs.* 25:681, 1997.

114. Herr K, Mobily P: Comparison of selected pain assessment tools for use with the elderly. *App Nurs Res.* 6:39, 1993.

115. DeConno F, Caraceni A, Gamba A: Pain measurement in cancer patients: A comparison of six methods. *Pain.* 57:161, 1994.

116. Wright KD, Asmundson GJ, McCreary DR: Factorial validity of the short-form McGill pain questionnaire (SF-MPQ). *Eur J Pain.* 5:279, 2001.

117. Davis GC: The clinical assessment of chronic pain in rheumatic disease: Evaluating the use of two instruments. *J Adv Nurs.* 14:397, 1989.

118. Deloach LJ, Higgins MS, Caplan AB, et al: The visual analog scale in the immediate postoperative period: Intrasubject variability and correlation with a numeric scale. *Anesth Analg.* 86:102, 1998.

119. Farrar JT, Young JP, LaMoreaux L, et al: Clinical importance of changes in chronic pain intensity measured on an 11-point numeric pain rating scale. *Pain.* 94:149, 2001.

120. Dalton J, McNaull F: A call for standardizing the clinical rating of pain intensity using a 0 to 10 rating scale. *Cancer Nurs.* 21:46, 1998.

121. Anderson KO. Assessment tools for the evaluation of pain in the oncology patient. *Curr Pain Headache Rep.* 11:259, 2007.

122. Echternauch J: *Pain,* vol. 12. New York: Churchill Livingstone, 1987.

123. PROMIS instruments available for use. http://www.nihpromis.org/Documents/Item_Bank_Tables_Feb_2011.pdf. Accessed October 11, 2011.

124. Gridley L, van den Dolder PA: The percentage improvement in pain scale as a measure of physiotherapy treatment effects. *Aust J Physiother.* 47:133, 2001.

125. World Health Organization: Towards a Common Language for Functioning, Disability, and Health. ICF. Geneva, Switzerland. 2002. http://www.who.int/classifications/icf/training/icfbeginnersguide.pdf.

126. Snyder AR, Parsons JT, McLeod TCV, et al: Using disablement models and clinical outcomes assessment to enable evidence-based athletic training practice, part II: Clinical outcomes assessment. *J Athl Train.* 43:437, 2008.

127. Michner LA: Patient- and clinician-rated outcome measures for clinical decision making in rehabilitation. *J Sport Rehabil.* 20:37, 2011.

128. Snyder AR, Parsons JT, McLeod TCV, et al: Using disablement models and clinical outcomes assessment to enable evidence-based athletic training practice, part I: Disablement models. *J Athl Train.* 43:428, 2008.

129. Kamper SJ, Maher CG, Mackay G: Global rating of change scales: A review of strengths and weaknesses and considerations for design. *J Man Manip Ther.* 17:3, 163–170, 2009.

130. Monsma E, Mensch J, and Farroll J: Keeping your head in the game: Sport-specific imagery and anxiety among injured athletes. *J Athl Train.* 44:410, 2009.

131. Lundberg M, Frennered K, Hägg O, et al: The impact of fear-avoidance model variables on disability in patients with specific or nonspecific chronic low back pain. *Spine.* 36:1547, 2011.

132. Deyo RA, Carter WB: Strategies for improving and expanding the application of health status measures in clinical settings: A researcher-developer viewpoint. *Med Care.* 30:176, 1992.

133. Baker SM, et al: Patient participation in physical therapy goal setting. *Phys Ther.* 81:1118, 2001.

134. Northern JG, et al: Involvement of adult rehabilitation patients in setting occupational therapy goals. *Am J Occup Ther.* 49:214, 1995.

135. Nelson CE, Payton OD: A system for involving patients in program planning. *Am J Occup Ther.* 45:753, 1991.

136. Randall KE, McEwen IR: Writing patient-centered functional goals. *Phys Ther.* 80:1197, 2000.

137. State Regulatory Agencies. Board of Certification, Inc. http://www.bocatc.org/index.php?option=com_content&view=article&id=92&Itemid=144.

138. Licensing Authorities. The Federation of State Boards of Physical Therapy. https://www.fsbpt.org/Licensing Authorities/index.asp.

139. Berger KJ: Health and sports law collide: Do professional athletes have an unfettered choice to accept risk of harm? *Med Law.* 30:1, 2011.

140. Kane SM, White RA: Medical malpractice and the sports medicine clinician. *Clin Orthop Relat Res.* 467:412, 2009.

141. Schwab NC, Pohlman KJ: Records—the Achilles' heel of school nursing: Answers to bothersome questions. *J Sch Nurs.* 20:236, 2004.

142. Kompanje EJO, Maas AIR: Is the Glasgow Coma Scale score protected health information? The effect of new United States regulations (HIPPA) on completion of screening logs in emergency research trials. *Intensive Care Med.* 134:313, 2006.

143. Bergren MD: HIPPA-FERPA revisited. *J Sch Nurs.* 20:107, 2004.

144. Anderson B, Parr A: Risk management: Determining the standard of care. *Athl Ther Today.* 11:6, 2006.

145. Scott RW: Legal Aspects of Documenting Patient Care, ed 2. Aspen, Gaithersburg, MD, 2000.

146. Park J, et al: Premarket approval (PMA) manual. HHS Publication, FDA, 1997.

147. Basile EM, Armentrout E, Reeves KN: Medical device labeling and advertising: An overview. *Food Drug.* 54:519, 1999.

148. Albohm MJ, et al: Reimbursement for Athletic Trainers. Slack, Thorofare, NJ, 2001.

149. Brown F: ICD-9-CM Coding Handbook, With Answers: 2002. American Hospital Association, Chicago, 2002.

150. National Athletic Trainers' Association: Understanding and Initiating the Reimbursement Process. NATA, Dallas, 2002.

151. Streator S, Buckley WE: Clinical outcomes in sports medicine. *Athl Ther Today.* 5:57, 2000.

152. Therapeutic pools and tubs in health care facilities. In National Electric Code. National Fire Protection Association. http://www.nfpa.org/assets/files/pdf/a680.pdf

153. Ray R, Konin J: Facility design and planning. In Ray R: Management Strategies in Athletic Training, ed 2. Human Kinetics, Champaign, IL, 2011, pp 155–186.

Therapeutic Cold and Superficial Heating Agents

This section describes the physics, biophysical effects, and the clinical application of cold modalities and superficial heating agents. Deep heating modalities, those that normally penetrate deeper than 2–3 cm, are presented in Section Three.

Chapter 5

Thermal Modalities

This chapter presents information regarding those modalities that rely on a gradient-based heat exchange that alters the body's physiology. The chapter consists of two sections, cold and heat. Each section describes the physics, physiological effects, and evidence that support or question their use. Use of specific thermal modalities and their unique effects are described in the next chapter.

● Based on a difference in temperatures, thermal modalities transfer energy (heat) to or from the tissues (Appendix A). Compared with the extreme range of temperatures found throughout the universe, there is a scant difference between the upper and lower temperature limits of thermal treatments. Within our tissues, the 65°F (18.3°C) that span the therapeutic upper limits of heat modalities and the lower limits of cold modalities elicit a wide range of cellular and vascular events (Box 5-1).

"Heat" is not an actual form of energy; rather, it is a term used to describe a type of energy transfer. Thermal therapeutic modalities transfer heat from the cooler surface to the warmer surface through the exchange of **kinetic energy** ●. Examples of this are a hot pack transferring energy to the skin or the skin transferring energy to an ice pack. This energy exchange requires one fundamental condition: one object must be hotter than the other. Energy carriers then transmit energy from the high temperature area to the cooler object. The greater the temperature difference, **the temperature gradient,** the more rapid the exchange **(the Fourier law).**[2] Heat is added to or removed from the body by one of five mechanisms: conduction, convection, radiation, evaporation, or conversion, although multiple mechanisms may occur at the same time (Box 5-2).

The skin contains receptors that are sensitive to temperature (thermoreceptors). The majority of these receptors are responsive to cold, while a lower number are responsive to heat.[3] Many thermoreceptors are wide dynamic range neurons that trigger a pain response when the temperature becomes too hot or too cold (see Chapter 2). Although the sensation of heat or cold is the most outwardly noticeable effect, often the primary benefit of these modalities is altering cell metabolism. The rate of the body's chemical (metabolic) processes is affected by changes in temperature. Every 1.8°F (1°C)

Kinetic energy: The energy an object possesses by virtue of its motion.

Box 5-1. HEAT AS A PHYSICAL ENTITY

Temperatures and their effects are relative. If the temperature outside is 60° today, but was 80° yesterday you would think, "It's cold." If it was 40° yesterday, you would think, "It's warming up." This concept holds true for the application of thermal modalities.

The classifications of "heat" and "cold" are based on the physiological response elicited by the temperature. Temperature is a measurement of the speed of molecular motion that describes the amount of kinetic energy, heat, in an object. Infrared energy is emitted from any object having a temperature greater than **absolute zero** ●. An increased rate of motion is identified as an increase in temperature.

The basic principle of thermal modalities is to transfer heat across a temperature gradient (i.e., one object is hotter than the other). Heat is lost from the warmer object and moved into the cooler object. The greater the temperature gradient, the more quickly energy is transferred. When a moist heat pack is placed on a patient, energy is transferred away from the pack and absorbed by the tissues. When an ice pack is applied heat is drawn away from the tissues and delivered to the pack, melting the ice.

Heat is measured in **calories.** The common definition of a calorie is the amount of energy needed to raise the temperature of 1 gram of water by 1°C (note that this calorie is different from the k-calories used to describe food energy). Scientists, however, changed this definition to be 1.0 calorie equals 4.1860 joules of energy.[1]

Different materials require different amounts of energy to increase their temperature. **Specific heat capacity** (often simply shortened to "specific heat") is the amount of energy needed to increase the temperature of a unit of mass by 1°C. A substance's specific heat varies with its temperature. **Thermal conductivity** is the quantity of heat (in calories per second) passing though a substance 1 cm thick by 1 cm wide separating a temperature gradient of 1°C. As it relates to therapeutic modalities, thermal conductivity is used to describe how well different tissues do (or do not) transfer thermal energy.

Box 5-2. THE TRANSFER OF THERMAL ENERGY

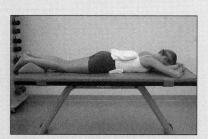

Conduction (e.g., ice pack, moist heat pack)

Conduction is the transfer of heat between two touching objects. Examples of therapeutic modalities that rely on conduction include moist heat packs and ice application. Within the body, the transfer of energy from one tissue layer to another occurs via conduction.

Some materials are better conductors of heat than others. Consider wooden and metal picnic tables that have been sitting in direct sunlight and have the same temperature. If you placed one hand on the wooden table and the other hand on the metal table, the metal table would feel "hotter" more rapidly. Even though you are touching two objects with equal temperatures, the greater ability of metal to conduct heat (compared with wood) warms your hand more rapidly (see Box 5-1).

Continued

Absolute zero: Theoretically, the lowest possible temperature, equal to –273°C or –460°F. At this point, all atomic and molecular motion ceases.

Box 5-2. THE TRANSFER OF THERMAL ENERGY—cont'd

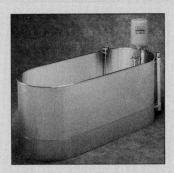

Convection (e.g., warm or cold whirlpool)

Convection is the transfer of heat by the movement of a **medium** ●, usually air or water. Of the three **states of matter** ●, gases are poor conductors of heat. Liquids are better conductors. Solids, generally speaking, are the best conductors. Circulating air or water increases its ability to transport heat. The actual transfer of energy from the medium to the body still occurs through conduction; the delivery of the energy occurs by movement of the medium. The circulation of the medium results in the cooling of one object and the subsequent heating of another object. Whirlpools are the most common example of therapeutic modalities that use convection.

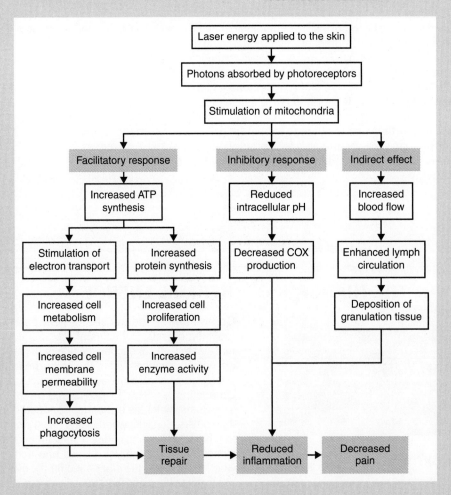

Radiation (e.g., infrared lamp)
Radiation (e.g., LASER, see Chapter 19)

Radiation is the transfer of energy without the use of a medium, and the heat gained or lost through radiation is termed "radiant energy." Radiant energy

---

Medium: A material used to promote the transfer of energy. An object or substance that permits the transmission of energy through it.

States of matter: Physical matter can take three forms: solid, liquid, and gas. Using H_2O as an example, we see the three states of matter as ice, water, and steam.

Box 5-2. THE TRANSFER OF THERMAL ENERGY—cont'd

diverges • as it travels, resulting in a reduction of the energy received at different distances along its path. All thermal therapeutic modalities provide radiant energy. For some, such as LASER and shortwave diathermy, radiation is the primary transmission mechanism. Conductive modalities, such as moist heat packs, lose some of their energy through radiation. This effect can be illustrated by placing your hand just above a moist heat pack. The heat you feel is being lost from the pack via radiation.

Some forms of energy must be changed to another form to have a thermal effect on the body. This process, **conversion,** is seen in modalities such as shortwave diathermy, where electrical energy is converted into heat, and therapeutic ultrasound, where acoustical energy is converted into heat.

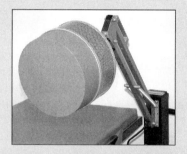

Conversion (e.g., shortwave diathermy, ultrasound)

Heat loss can also occur through **evaporation.** The change from the liquid state to the gaseous state requires that thermal energy be removed from the body. The heat absorbed by the liquid cools the tissue as the liquid changes its state into gas via conversion. Vapocoolant sprays are an example of a modality that operates by evaporation.

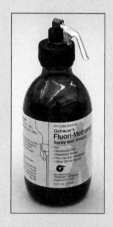

Evaporation (e.g., vapocoolant spray)

change in tissue temperature results in a 13% increase (heat) or decrease (cold) in the tissues' metabolic rate.[4,5]

Each type of tissue conducts heat at a different rate (Table 5-1).[6] This means that changes in skin temperature do not immediately reflect the changes in underlying temperatures.[7] Skin temperature is approximately 91°F (33°C), although there is a great deal of variability in this temperature, especially when compared to the core temperature. Skin temperature is influenced by such factors

TABLE 5-1	Tissue Thermal Conductivity
TISSUE	THERMAL CONDUCTIVITY (W/M°C)
Skin	0.96
Adipose Tissue	0.19
Muscle	0.64

W/m = Watts per meter; higher values indicate more transmission of energy.

Divergence: The spreading of a beam or wave.

as ambient temperature, humidity, exercise, time of day, and food and alcohol consumption. The deeper the tissue is within the body, the higher the temperature. Resting muscle temperature is approximately 95°F (35°C).

The adipose tissue layer limits the effective depth of penetration of thermal modalities (Box 5-3). Skin temperature is cooler than adipose tissue, which is cooler than muscular tissue. The temperature changes of deeper tissues are always less than those of the overlying tissues.[7]

Energy that is absorbed by one tissue layer cannot be transmitted to deeper layers: this is known as the **law of Grotthus-Draper** (see Appendix A). As the superficial layers absorb energy, there is less energy that can be transmitted to the deeper layers. This means that the applied energy must be able to affect the target tissues to be effective as a

Box 5-3. NATURE'S INSULATOR: ADIPOSE TISSUE

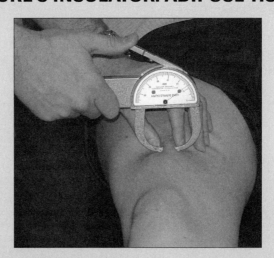

The thickness of the patient's adipose tissue layer can be calculated by determining the skinfold overlying the treatment area and then dividing that number by two (skinfold/2).[8]

Most mammals have a subcutaneous layer of adipose tissue. Those that live in cold climates have a thick layer of adipose tissue that serves as insulation, retaining body temperature by reducing the loss of heat to the surrounding environment. This principle also applies to humans and impacts the deep tissue response to thermal agents.

Thick, insulating layers of adipose tissue reduce the rate and depth of intramuscular cooling and require longer treatment durations to reach therapeutic treatment temperatures.[6,9,10,11] With less than 8 mm of subcutaneous adipose tissue, intramuscular cooling occurs at a rate of 1.30°F (0.72°C)/minute per 1 cm within the muscle. At 10 mm to 18 mm of adipose tissue, the rate of cooling decreases to 0.81°F (0.45°C)/min. When the amount of adipose tissue increases to over 20 mm in thickness, the rate of cooling slows to 0.45°F (0.25°C)/min.[9] Each of these rates decreases as the depth within the muscle increases; however, the adipose tissue layer only explains just over 20% of the total variation in intramuscular temperature decrease.[12]

Skinfold measurements can be used as a guide for determining treatment duration for intramuscular tissues located 1 cm below the adipose tissue:[11]

Skinfold Measurement	Treatment Duration
20 mm or less	25 min
20 to 30 mm	40 min
30 to 40 mm	60 min

If the facilities, time, or equipment are not available to measure the subcutaneous tissue thickness, such as the immediate management of an injury, treatment durations can be estimated based on the patient's body build and estimation of body fat: thin patients would be treated for 25 minutes; patients with a large amount of adipose tissue (i.e., obese patients) would be treated for 60 minutes.

Although it may take longer for intramuscular cooling to occur, adipose tissue also slows the rewarming process. If the patient remains still following the treatment, thicker layers of adipose tissues will result in longer rewarming times than thinner layers.[8,9,10,13]

Although most of the research has examined the relationship between adipose tissue and intramuscular cooling, this tissue layer also decreases effectiveness of superficial heating.[7]

treatment modality. Using a superficial heating or cooling agent for a deep injury affects the superficial sensory nerves and blood vessels but does not produce the needed metabolic changes in the traumatized tissues.

Cold application decreases cell metabolism and is used (1) when the acute inflammatory response is active, (2) before range-of-motion exercises (i.e., cryokinetics), and (3) after physical activity to reduce cell metabolism. When used for immediate treatment or during the active inflammation stage, use some form of ice pack. When used before rehabilitation exercises, a cold whirlpool or immersion should be used because of the latent cooling effects of these modalities.[8,9,14] Athletes and other highly motivated persons often return to physical activity before full healing of the tissues has occurred, thus perpetuating the inflammatory process. As a result, cold application is often used more frequently with athletes than with the general population.

Heat application is indicated in five conditions: (1) to control the inflammatory reaction in its subacute or chronic stages, (2) to encourage tissue healing, (3) to promote venous drainage, (4) to reduce edema and ecchymosis, and (5) to improve range of motion (ROM) before physical activity or rehabilitation.

■ Cold Modalities

Cryotherapy is the application of cold modalities that have a temperature range between 32°F and 65°F (0°C and 18°C). The term "cold" describes a relative temperature state characterized by decreased molecular motion and the relative absence of heat (see Box 5-1). "Cold" cannot be transferred because thermal energy always moves from a high energy concentration ("heat") to a lower concentration ("cold"). When a cold modality is placed on the skin, the heat transfer is from the skin to the cold modality until the temperatures are equal.

The effects of cryotherapy are related to the slowing of cell metabolism (Fig. 5-1). The body responds to the loss of heat with a series of local responses including vasoconstriction, decreased metabolic rate, decreased inflammation, and decreased pain. Cold can be safely applied to most musculoskeletal injuries throughout the healing process (Table 5-2). The primary benefit of cold application, especially in the treatment of acute injuries, is reducing cell metabolism.

Magnitude and Duration of Temperature Decrease

During cryotherapy the heat lost from the tissue to the modality must be greater than the heat gained from adjacent tissues, blood flow, and local metabolism.[15] The depth, magnitude, and duration of the effects of cryotherapy are based on the cold modality being used and the anatomical and physiological properties of the tissues being treated.[6,8–10,16–22] Because the skin is in direct contact with the modality, it is the first tissue to lose heat. As the skin cools, it draws heat from the underlying tissues, adipose tissue, fascia, and muscle in that order.

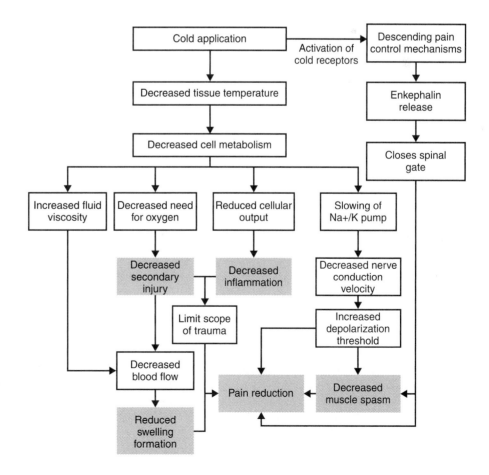

Figure 5-1. **Schematic of the Effects of Cold Application.** Physiological effects are derived from decreased cell metabolism as the result of decreased tissue temperature. This slows cellular reactions, decreases the cells' need for oxygen, and decreases blood flow. The sensation of cold also triggers descending pain control mechanisms.

TABLE 5-2   General Indications and Contraindications for Cold Treatments

Indications	Contraindications
Acute injury or inflammation	Circulatory insufficiency
Acute, chronic, or postsurgical pain	Deep vein **thrombosis** ●
Prevent edema formation	Cold hypersensitivity/Cold **urticaria** ●
Prior to or in conjunction with rehabilitation exercises	Anesthetic skin
Spasticity accompanying central nervous system disorders	Advanced diabetes
Acute or chronic muscle spasm	Chronic wounds
Neuralgia ●[131]	Uncovered open wounds
	Peripheral vascular disease ●
	Raynaud's phenomenon ●*
	Lupus ● or other conditions where cryoglobulins are present: may result in the aggregation of serum proteins, **cryoglobulinemia** ●.
	Hemoglobinemia ●
	Cold-induced myocardial ischemia (when large areas are treated)

Precautions
Over the carotid sinus
Over areas of infection
Near the eyes
Avoid treating large areas with individuals having:
Cardiac involvement
Respiratory involvement
Hypertension

*Although this is usually a benign condition, Raynaud's phenomenon may be a symptom of an underlying disease state, most commonly systemic sclerosis.[132]

✳ Practical Evidence

The depth and duration of cold application depend on the temperature gradient between the target tissues and the cold modality, the mass (area) of tissue treated, and the duration of the treatment.[14,18,19,20,21,22] Compression wraps also increase the effective depth of cooling.[14]

The potential for heat exchange depends on the temperature difference between the cold modality and the skin.

The greater the temperature gradient, the more rapid the energy exchange and the deeper the effects of the treatment because more energy is transferred. The cold modality will continue to remove heat from the body until the temperature of the modality and the skin are approximately equal. During this process, the modality also gains heat from the environmental temperature (atmospheric temperature) (Fig. 5-2).

The time between treatment bouts is unclear, ranging from a 1:2 ratio (2 minutes between treatments for every minute ice is applied) to a 1:6 ratio.[23] Overcooling the tissues may increase the risk of frostbite and may delay the healing process.

Neuralgia: Pain following the path of a nerve; a hypersensitive nerve.

Thrombosis: The formation or presence of a blood clot within the vascular system.

Urticaria: Skin vascular reaction to an irritant characterized by red, itchy areas; wheals; or papules. Commonly referred to as "hives."

Peripheral vascular disease: Actually, a syndrome describing an insufficiency of arteries or veins for maintaining proper circulation (also known as PVD).

Raynaud's phenomenon: A vascular reaction to cold application or stress that results in a white, red, or blue discoloration of the extremities. The fingers and toes are the first to be affected.

Lupus: A chronic disorder of the body's immune system that affects the skin, joints, internal organs, and neurological system.

Cryoglobulinemia: A condition in which abnormal blood proteins, cryoglobulins, group together when exposed to cold. This can lead to skin color changes, hives, subcutaneous hemorrhage, and other disorders.

Hemoglobinemia: An excessive proportion of hemoglobin in plasma.

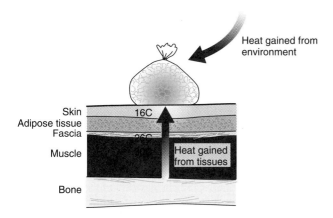

Figure 5-2. Conductive Cooling of the Skin and Subcutaneous Tissues. The deeper the tissues, the less cooling that occurs. The subcutaneous adipose tissue layer is the greatest barrier to deeper cooling.

Skin Cooling

During a 30-minute ice pack application skin temperature decreases 36°F to 45°F (20°C to 25°C).[14] The depth of cooling is related to the treatment duration and the size of the area being treated: as the treatment duration increases, the greater the temperature decrease and depth of cooling,

the larger the area being cooled, the deeper the cooling occurs (Fig. 5-3).

Local metabolic factors also affect cooling. Venous flow carries cold blood away from the area while the arteries deliver blood that warms the area. An intact sympathetic nervous system will better regulate cooling than an impaired one. Desensitized or denervated areas or areas lacking normal **vasomotor** ● function may be overcooled because of the inability to regulate the blood flow needed to maintain tissue temperatures, increasing the risk of cold injury.[9,10]

The type of cold modality being used also influences the amount of cooling. When applied directly to the skin, ice packs and ice massage produce the greatest temperature gradient. Although the temperature gradient is not as great, cold immersion treatments (including cold whirlpools) affect a larger surface area than ice packs. An ice pack results in a greater decrease in skin and subcutaneous tissue temperature than a 50°F (10°C) whirlpool, but each method is equally effective in reducing intramuscular temperature.[10]

Intermittent ice pack application involves the application of cold for 10 minutes, followed by 10 minutes of no cold application. This sequence is repeated for the duration of the treatment. By removing the ice pack, the skin is able to rewarm, thereby maintaining a temperature gradient between the pack and the skin. The muscle continues to cool

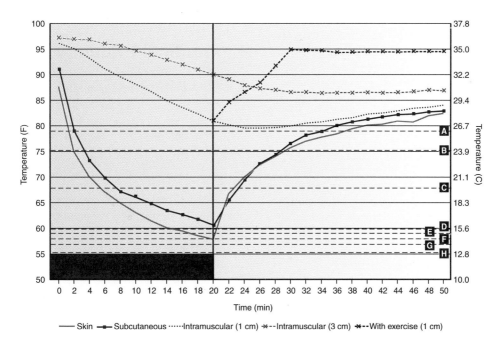

— Skin ▪— Subcutaneous ····· Intramuscular (1 cm) ✳-- Intramuscular (3 cm) ✳-- With exercise (1 cm)

Figure 5-3. Tissue Cooling During a 20-Minute Ice Pack Application. Notable benchmarks are the following: (A) 9°F skin temperature decrease: Sensitivity of muscle spindles is decreased. (B) 13°F skin temperature decrease: Motor nerve conduction velocity decreased by 14%; sensory nerve conduction velocity decreased by 33%. (C) 20°F tissue temperature decrease: Acetylcholine concentrations decrease 20%. (D) 60°F skin temperature: Previously inhibited sensory nerve transmission begins to return during rewarming from maximum cooling. (E) 59°F skin temperature: Permeability of lymph vessels is decreased. (F) 58°F skin temperature: Maximum analgesia occurs. (G) 57°F skin temperature: Maximum decrease in blood flow. (H) 55°F skin temperature: Risk of cold-related injury increases.

Vasomotor: Muscles and their associated nerves acting on arteries and veins that cause constriction or dilation.

when the ice is removed, but the skin rewarms. When compared to continuous ice application this method is more effective in decreasing pain, may decrease capillary blood flow and increase venous outflow in tendons,[24] but has no effect on function or limiting the formation of swelling relative to continuous application.[25]

Intra-articular Temperature Decrease

There is a moderate correlation between skin temperature and **intra-articular** • temperature.[26,27] As the temperature of the skin overlying a joint decreases, the temperature within the joint decreases proportionally (r = 0.65; decreasing the skin temperature 10°F [5.6°C] would result in a 6.5°F [3.6°C] decrease in the intra-articular temperature).[5,22,28] Intra-articular temperatures may decrease as much as 12.8°F (7.1°C) during a 60-minute ice pack application to the knee.[29] Ice packs intermittently applied to the shoulder following surgery result in significant decreases in the glenohumeral joint and the subacromial space temperature.[30]

Intramuscular Temperature Decrease

Intramuscular temperature decrease results from cooling the skin. Intramusclar heat is conducted toward the skin. However, unlike the skin, intramuscular temperatures continue to decrease for up to 30 minutes following removal of the modality (when the patient remains sedentary) (see Fig. 5-2). Muscle temperature 1 cm deep will decrease approximately 16.4°F (8.9°C), at 2 cm 16.2°F (9.0°C), and at 3 cm 11.0°F (6.1°C).[14] The amount of intramuscular cooling is increased following exercise because the muscle temperature is above normal, thereby increasing the temperature gradient.[31]

✱ Practical Evidence

Because of various physiological factors including adipose tissue layer thickness, skin density, vascularity, body temperature, and treatment duration, skin temperature is a poor indicator of underlying tissue temperature.[12] Underlying tissue temperatures will always be significantly warmer than skin temperature.

Using a compression wrap to secure the ice bag to the body part causes a significant decrease in subcutaneous tissue temperatures when compared with the use of an ice bag alone, as long as the wrap is not placed between the ice pack and the skin.[8,13] Although there are no differences between skin surface temperatures between ice applied with and without a wrap, the compression improves the contact between the ice pack and the skin and compresses the subcutaneous tissues, aiding in the exchange of heat away from the body.[14] Tight compression, greater than

30 to 40 mm Hg, may reduce blood flow and keeps the area from being rewarmed. Covering the ice pack also reduces the amount of heat lost to the surrounding environment and enhances the effectiveness of the treatment.[6,8,14] Insulation, such as an elastic wrap or terry cloth towel between the ice pack and the skin, decreases the temperature gradient and slows the transfer of heat, often rendering the treatment ineffective.[32]

Tissue Rewarming

Skin is rewarmed by the air, absorbing heat from the underlying tissues, and warm blood flow to the area. Subcutaneous tissues rewarm by drawing heat from underlying tissues while deeper tissues are rewarmed via the delivery of warm blood and increased cell metabolism. Initially, as the skin rewarms further cooling of intramuscular tissues occurs as heat is wicked away from the muscle.[33] Muscle cooling is prolonged when the patient remains sedentary.[8,9]

The continued cooling of the intramuscular tissues is enhanced by a delayed hormonal response that triggers vasodilation and the thermal conductivity of the target and overlying tissues.[6] Deeper tissues require a longer rewarming period than do superficial ones. Just as adipose tissue insulates deeper structures from the effects of the cold, adipose tissue also slows the rewarming process as its thickness increases.[8,9,10,13] Increasing the surface area being treated results in a longer rewarming period.

✱ Practical Evidence

If the patient remains sedentary following the treatment, intramuscular temperatures will continue to decrease for another 30 minutes and the temperature will remain decreased for approximately 20 to 60 minutes following treatment.[8,9,34]

Activity (muscle contractions) can counter the effects of cooling. In most settings patients do not remain sedentary following treatment. Moderate activity, such as walking or rehabilitation exercises, increases the rate of intramuscular rewarming by increasing local cell metabolism and blood flow,[18] but does not appear to affect the rewarming of capsular or ligamentous tissues.[35] At approximately 2 cm deep in the triceps surae muscle group, moderate walking results in a 7°F (3.9°C) increase at 20 minutes following treatment and 9.5°F (5.3°C) 30 minutes after treatment relative to remaining sedentary.[34]

Therapeutic Temperature Benchmarks

Cooling the skin activates a mechanism that is thought to conserve heat in the body's core, triggering a series of metabolic and vascular events that produce the beneficial

---

Intra-articular: Within a joint.

effects of cryotherapy. During treatment, the most rapid and significant temperature decreases occur in the skin and **synovium** •. The magnitude of skin temperature change varies with the method of cold application. However, the skin is rarely the target of the treatment, so the effects on the underlying tissues must be deduced from the changes in skin temperature (Table 5-3).[6] The thresholds of these events are discussed here, with more specific information being described in the following sections.

Superficial blood flow begins to decrease soon after a cold modality is applied and continues a relatively steady decrease for the next 13 minutes. At approximately 13 minutes into the treatment, the rate of blood flow decrease begins to level out and small fluctuations in blood flow begin to occur.[36] When the skin temperature decreases to approximately 57°F (13.9°C), the maximal decrease in local blood flow is obtained. Changes in the lymphatic system are slower to occur. Lymphatic vessels are relatively unaffected by cold treatment until the temperature reaches 59°F (15.0°C), at which point their cross-sectional area begins to decrease.

Tissue temperatures must reach to 50°F to 59°F (10°C to 15°C) to maximize the decrease in cell metabolism.[37] Neurological changes begin to occur when the skin temperature decreases 9.0°F (5°C). At this point, the sensitivity of muscle spindles is decreased. A 13.3°F (7.4°C) decrease in skin temperature results in a 14% decrease in motor nerve conduction velocity and a 33% decrease in

---

TABLE 5-3 Factors Influencing the Depth, Magnitude, and Duration of Cold Treatments

Factor	Influence
Modality	
Treatment temperature	Larger temperature gradients between the modality and the skin increase the rate of exchange. The treatment temperature is often directly related to the type of cold modality used.
	Lower skin/cold modality temperatures result in deeper cooling and longer-lasting effects. Cooling larger areas at relatively warmer temperatures (e.g., ice pack vs. ice immersion) results in longer rewarming time.[33]
Type of cold	Ice that is melting or a bag that has a small amount of water mixed with the ice (wetted ice) results in more significant skin and intramuscular cooling than does using crushed or cubed ice.[22] The liquid medium allows the cold pack to be in better contact with the skin.
Specific heat	The modality's ability to transfer heat from the skin. The use of insulating materials (e.g., terry cloth towel) must also be considered.
Insulating medium between the modality and skin	Insulating medium slows the heat exchange from the skin to the modality (needed for reusable ice packs or patients who have precautions to cryotherapy).
Treatment duration	Longer treatment durations result in greater decreases in skin, subcutaneous, and intramuscular temperature and a longer rewarming time.
Area (size) of skin affected	Cooling larger areas of skin results in deeper tissue cooling relative to smaller areas.
Use of a compression wrap	The use of a compression wrap improves the conduction of energy, thus increasing the depth of cooling.
Post-treatment activity	Muscular exertion in the treated area increases the rate of rewarming.
Anatomical/Physiological	
Subcutaneous adipose tissue	An increased amount of adipose tissue reduces the effective depth of temperature decrease. The treatment duration should be increased as the amount of adipose tissue increases.
Depth of target tissues	Deeper tissues require longer treatment durations.
Vascularity of target tissues	Increased blood flow to and from the area decreases the rate of cooling. Arterial flow delivers warm blood to the area; venous blood carries away cool blood.
Cell metabolism	Active cell metabolism produces heat.
Sympathetic nervous system	An intact sympathetic nervous system is needed to maintain local temperature.
Resting muscle temperature	Increased muscle temperature, such as that after exercising, increases the amount of heat exchange from the muscle.[31]

Synovium: Membrane lining the capsule of a joint.

sensory nerve conduction velocity.[38] Tissue temperatures of 68°F (20°C) result in a 60% decrease in **acetylcholine** ● levels.[39]

Maximum analgesia is obtained when skin temperature is decreased to approximately 58°F (14.4°C) and sensation returns when skin temperature reaches 60°F (15.6°C).[16,40] These temperatures are reached after approximately 20 minutes of treatment time using ice packs. Tissues begin to lose their viscoelastic properties when their temperatures reach 64°F (18°C).[41]

If the temperature of circulating blood is decreased by 0.2°F (0.1°C), the **hypothalamus** ● responds by initiating several systemic events. Systemic vasoconstriction occurs and the heart rate is decreased in an attempt to localize the cold (see Fig. 5-1). If the proportion of the body area being cooled is large, the heart rate is reduced to maintain the body's core temperature by limiting the rate and volume of circulating blood. If the core temperature continues to decrease toward the point of **hypothermia** ●, shivering and increased muscle tone assist in keeping the body heat inward. This severe response is normal when the human body is exposed to extremely cold environments (e.g., falling into a near-frozen lake or a full-body cold immersion below 40°F [4.4°C]). It is not a common response in therapeutic cold application.

The risk of cold-related injury increases once skin temperature reaches 55°F (12.8°C) for approximately 2 hours. If the skin temperature reaches 32°F (0°C) **intracellular** ● fluids begin to freeze and result in **frostbite** (see the Frostbite section in this chapter).

Sensations Associated With Cold Application

The terms traditionally used to describe the sensations associated with cold application are "cold," "burning," "aching," and "numbness" (analgesia).[42] Analgesia, the absence of pain, is obtained after 18 to 21 minutes of cold application. Anesthesia, the result of decreasing the nerve conduction velocity and increasing the threshold required to fire the nerves,[43] is seldom achieved.[44]

Although these reactions are most pronounced during ice immersion, they can occur during other methods of cold application. The affective response during the initial treatment period (cold, burning, aching) may deter patient compliance. Not all people experience the same sensations during cold application, but educating the patient about the sensations to be expected during the treatment tends to make cold application, especially cold immersion, more tolerable.[45,46] Repeated exposures to cold treatments can decrease the sensory and affective response to cold application.[47]

● EFFECTS ON

The Injury Response Process

The cellular and **hemodynamic** ● effects of cold application are beneficial in the treatment of acute, subacute, and chronic conditions. Unlike heat modalities, cold is rarely contraindicated throughout the course of tissue healing. However, prolonged use of cold may extend the time required for healing.

During the treatment of acute injuries, the primary physiological effect of cold is the reduction of cell metabolism. Reducing cell metabolism limits the amount of secondary injury by decreasing the cells' need for oxygen. Immediate care of musculoskeletal injuries is augmented by the use of compression and elevation.

Cellular Response

The most beneficial effect of cold application for an acute injury is the decreased need for oxygen in the area being treated, thus limiting the scope of secondary injury.[12,43,48] Cold application slows cell metabolism and reduces the rate of damaging cellular reactions, thus decreasing the amount of oxygen the cells require to survive.[49] Maximum decrease in cell metabolism is reached when the temperature decreases to 50°F to 59°F (10°C to 15°C).[37] Reducing the cells' metabolic load also lessens the amount of cellular mitochondrial damage, keeping the cell viable.[49]

✱ Practical Evidence

Secondary injury is relatively slow developing. As described by Merrick[50] the maximum benefits of cold application in reducing secondary injury occur when treatment is initiated within 30 minutes following trauma.

During a 20-minute ice pack treatment, cell metabolism decreases by 19%.[16,19] By reducing the number of cells killed by a lack of oxygen, the amount of secondary hypoxic injury is limited. Because fewer cells are damaged from secondary hypoxic injury, decreased amounts of inflammatory mediators are released into the area, containing the scope of the injury (see Chapter 1).

The depth of penetration and magnitude of decreased cellular response is related to the subcutaneous tissues' temperature decrease, not the change in skin temperature.

Acetylcholine: Neurotransmitter responsible for transmitting motor nerve impulses.
Hypothalamus: The body's thermoregulatory center.
Hypothermia: Decreased core temperature.
Intracellular: Within the membrane of a cell.
Hemodynamic: The systemic and local characteristics of blood flow.

Traditional treatment durations of 20 to 30 minutes may not be sufficient to adequately cool deep target tissues, even with average amounts of overlying adipose tissues.[9,49]

Inflammation

Changes in cellular function and blood dynamics serve to control the effects of acute inflammation. Cold application suppresses the inflammatory response by:

- Reducing the release of inflammatory mediators[43]
- Decreasing prostaglandin synthesis[43]
- Decreasing capillary permeability[43]
- Decreasing *leukocyte/endothelial interaction*[51]
- Decreasing *creatine kinase* activity[52]

The secondary formation of edema and hemorrhage is limited because of the inhibitory effect on the mediators and decreased capillary permeability.

As we saw in the injury response cycle (see Fig. 1-4), limiting the amount of inflammation reduces the effects of the remaining components. Suppressing the release of inflammatory mediators decreases the amount of hemorrhage and swelling; decreasing the mechanical pressure on nerves decreases pain. As muscle spasm and edema are reduced, the area is less congested, limiting the amount of secondary hypoxic cell death.

Blood and Fluid Dynamics

The primary hemodynamic effects of cold application are local arteriole vasoconstriction (capillaries cannot constrict because their walls do not contain smooth muscle), increased blood viscosity, and reduced blood flow. Because cold application decreases the rate of cell metabolism and reduces the tissue's need for oxygen, it would seem that blood flow to the treatment area would be reduced. Despite this seemingly sound logic, the effect of cold application on blood flow still is a topic of investigation.

Vasoconstriction is mediated by the autonomic nervous system and the release of local proteins.[53] Rho kinase, accompanied by other mediators, inhibits skin vasoconstriction in both early- and late-stage skin cooling, but is most active during the late stages.[53]

Decreasing tissue temperatures stimulates thermoreceptors in the blood vessels and local soft tissues, triggering a response from the sympathetic nervous system instructing the vessels to constrict. The body then attempts to maintain intramuscular temperatures by releasing hormonal mediators from the hypothalamus and adrenal medulla.[6] Vasoconstriction is also influenced by a reduction in the release of histamine and prostaglandin, two inflammatory mediators that produce vasodilation.

As the molecular motion of the blood and tissue fluids slows, viscosity increases, increasing resistance to flow.

The reduction in blood flow occurs too late to affect the initial hemorrhage, but may prevent excessive hematoma formation.

Most studies have concluded that cold application causes decreased blood flow,[16,19,54,55] but the results are not universally conclusive.[16,56] Blood flow decrease begins to occur soon (within 10 minutes) after the application of cold and continues to steadily decrease for the next 13 minutes and begins to oscillate between 13 and 17 minutes of treatment (Table 5-4).[6,16,19,51,55,57] Because capillaries do not constrict, blood flow reduction at this level results from vasoconstriction and reduced perfusion of the arterioles, reducing local **perfusion** ●.[58]

Using a cold compression device, superficial oxygen saturation begins to reduce approximately 7 minutes into the treatment. Oxygen saturation in muscle does not appear to be affected by treatment.[57] In joints and tendons, cold compression therapy reduces congestion on the venule side of the capillary-venule junction, allowing for improved deep oxygen saturation.[59,60] Each of these findings supports the role of cold application in the reduction of secondary hypoxic injury.

✱ Practical Evidence

Although cold application appears to decrease blood flow, the oxygen concentration in the treated area does not appear to be affected.[57,59,60] Therefore the decreased blood flow does not increase hypoxia.

One school of thought suggests that the body will increase blood flow through local vasodilation to warm the treated area, but researchers generally no longer consider this to occur (Box 5-4). The treated skin turns red during treatment (erythema), an event that could be related to increased blood flow, but is more likely the result of local histamine release and an increased concentration of **oxyhemoglobin** ●.

TABLE 5-4	Blood Flow Changes Following a 20-Minute Ice Pack Application
VASCULATURE	BLOOD FLOW DECREASE (% REDUCTION)
Arterial	38
Capillary	25
Soft tissue blood flow	26
Skeletal blood flow	19

Perfusion: Local blood flow that supplies tissues and organs with oxygen and nutrients.
Oxyhemoglobin: Hemoglobin that is carrying oxygen found in the arterial system.

Box 5-4. HUNTING FOR PROOF OF COLD-INDUCED VASODILATION

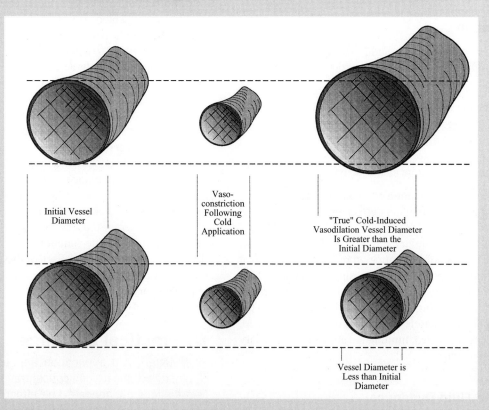

Vascular Response to Cold Application. (A) The concept of cold-induced vasodilation. After the application of therapeutic cold there is an immediate vasoconstriction. This is followed by vasodilation, resulting in a larger diameter than before the ice application. This event has not been substantiated. (B) Vascular reaction as suggested by Knight. After the initial vasoconstriction there is a dilation of the vessel, but its diameter is still reduced in comparison to the original diameter.

What effect does cold application have on local blood flow? In the early 1930s, Lewis[61] performed studies on skin temperature changes during cold treatments. When the fingers were immersed in cold water, alternating periods of cooling and warming were seen in the skin. Terming it the "hunting response," Lewis deduced that blood vessels underwent a series of vasoconstrictions and vasodilations in an attempt to adapt to the temperature (A). The magnitude and frequency of the hunting response varies with the body's core temperature. Cooler body temperatures lead to a reduced frequency and magnitude of this response.[62] However, the hunting response has been identified only in selected areas of the body (e.g., fingers, nose) and most often is associated with exposure to extreme cold environments.[54]

The concept of the hunting response influenced the manner in which cold was used clinically for several decades following Lewis's discovery (and still may be an influence today). Clinicians worked under the incorrect assumption that using a treatment duration that was too long (e.g., more than 20 minutes) would result in cold-induced vasodilation.

Many of the misconceptions of the hunting response were clarified by Knight, who identified that the degree of vasodilation only lessened the amount of initial vasoconstriction.[63,40] Despite the vasodilation, there was still a net vasoconstriction when compared with the vessel diameter before treatment (B).[21]

Contemporary thought suggests that cold-induced vasodilation does not occur during standard cryotherapy sessions. However, certain diseases and/or neurological deficits that affect the sympathetic nervous system or local thermal regulation could result in vasodilation.

Contemporary research using relatively healthy subjects and therapeutic temperature ranges and durations agree that reactive vasodilation does not occur during cold application in healthy subjects. Any increase in blood flow is transitory, remains significantly below the pretreatment level, and is probably related to another mechanism, such as increased heart rate or stroke volume, because the vessel diameter does not appear to increase.[54]

Swelling Formation and Reduction

There is a significant difference in the effect of cold application in the control of swelling formation and its role in edema reduction. The use of cryotherapy substantially limits edema *formation* and reduces the effects of arthrogenic muscle inhibition by increasing the responsiveness of the affected motor neuron pools.[64,65] Cold application alone does not promote the *removal* of swelling and potentially could hinder the venous and lymphatic return mechanism by increasing fluid viscosity. Compression and elevation during the cold treatment will assist in venous return.

Cryotherapy limits the formation of edema by reducing cell metabolism, thereby decreasing metabolic activity and limiting the amount of secondary hypoxic injury. The subsequent vasoconstriction decreases the permeability of the postcapillary venules and the reduced blood flow decreases the intravascular pressure. Both events discourage fluids from escaping into the tissues.[48] Although cryotherapy substantially reduces edema formation following musculoskeletal trauma, cold application does not prevent edema formation associated with disease states such as venous insufficiency.

Because lymphatic and venous return are not influenced by arterial blood flow, the hemodynamic changes associated with cold application have little, if any, effect on edema reduction. The mechanisms of compression, elevation (gravity), muscle contractions, and muscle milking must still be incorporated into the treatment plan to reduce edema.

It stands to reason that the vasoconstriction described for arteries would apply to both the venous and lymphatic vessels. However, whereas cold application results in constriction of the arterioles and venules, the amount of arteriole vasoconstriction is greater than that for venules. This effect occurs until tissue temperatures decrease more than 27°F (15°C). After this, the permeability of lymph vessels begins to decrease. The surface area of the venules relative to the arterioles increases the area for reabsorption and limits the formation of edema (Fig. 5-4).[58,66] This effect has also been substantiated in clinical studies.[55]

Overcooling the tissues can hinder the control of edema formation.[48,67] Prolonged, inappropriate cooling can increase the permeability of superficial lymphatic vessels and result in the lymph contents spilling back into the tissues.[67] This effect is increased when the limb is placed in a gravity-dependent position and no form of external compression is used.[48] Prolonged cold application can increase the viscosity of fluids in the area, increasing the fluid's resistance to flow and potentially hindering the venous return process.

Nerve Conduction

Cold application decreases the rate that nerve impulses are transmitted and increases the depolarization threshold required to initiate the impulse. Because tissues cool at different rates, changes in nerve depolarization and nerve

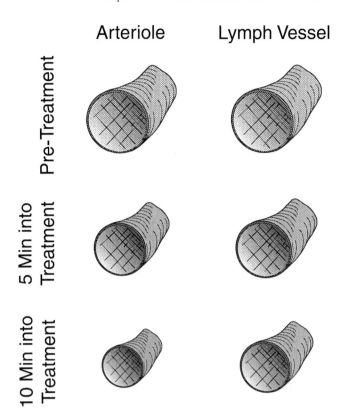

Figure 5-4. **Cross-Sectional Diameter of Arterioles and Lymph Vessels During Treatment.** As the tissue temperatures decrease, the cross-sectional diameter of both vessels decreases, but the change is greatest in arterioles, making the relative surface area of the lymph vessels larger.

conduction velocity do not occur simultaneously. Longer cooling times are required to effect changes in deep nerves. Superficial nerves will be affected before those nerves that are located deeper within the tissues.

✻ Practical Evidence

A 15-minute cold water immersion is more effective at decreasing sensory and motor nerve conduction velocity than is ice pack application or ice massage.[68]

Nerve conduction velocity is decreased by reducing the rate of synaptic transmission and increasing the time required for the nerve to depolarize and repolarize. As the temperature of the nerve decreases, its depolarization threshold increases. The nerve's resting potential is decreased, slowing the action potential and lengthening the refractory period. The time required for nerves to depolarize and repolarize is lengthened, decreasing the overall frequency of transmission.[69]

The decreased rate of nerve conduction is based on the exchange of calcium (Ca^{2+}) and sodium (Na^+) at the nerve's gated ion channel. Cold decreases membrane permeability and increases friction between Ca^{2+} and the gate, slowing the ion exchange and thereby decreasing the depolarization rate.[70]

The constant stimulation of the ice pack will also increase the depolarization threshold. With time receptors accommodate to the unchanging stimulus, further increasing the depolarization threshold and decreasing the conduction rate.[70]

All types of nerves are affected by cold application. Based on the type of nerve, the reduction of afferent impulses from muscles is proportionate to the amount of cooling (Table 5-5).[57,68,70] A 13.3°F to 18.0°F (7.4°C to 10°C) reduction in skin temperature reduces motor nerve conduction velocity by approximately 14% and sensory nerve conduction velocity by 33%.[70]

Each 1.8°F (1°C) drop in intramuscular temperature results in a 1.1- to 2.6-m/sec reduction in nerve conduction velocity.[38] Sensory nerve transmission is more affected by cooling than motor nerves, slowing by 2.6-m/sec while motor nerves slow by 1.5-m/sec.[68]

Cold also reduces the speed of nerve conduction by slowing communication at the synapse. Acetylcholine concentrations decrease approximately 60% as neuromuscular temperatures decrease by 36°F (20°C), further reducing the rate of transmission.[39] In certain cases, this can lead to **neurapraxia** ● and **axonotmesis** ●.[71]

During normal treatment duration and intensity, the largest decrease in nerve conduction velocity occurs immediately after the application of ice when the temperature gradient is the greatest.[72] As the tissue temperature continues to decline, nerve conduction rate will decrease to a point where impulses can no longer occur. Caution must be used to avoid cold-induced nerve palsy.

Pain Control

Cold application is useful in both primary and secondary pain control approaches.[73] Primary pain control occurs by removing the chemical and mechanical pain triggers by reducing inflammation and limiting swelling. Secondary pain control occurs at the application site by interrupting nerve transmission and decreasing nerve condition velocity. At the spinal cord level pain control occurs through neurological and vascular mechanisms.[4] On purely a sensory level, by stimulating the small-diameter neurons, cold inhibits pain transmission by acting as a **counterirritant** ●, triggering the descending pain control mechanisms that result in enkephalin release.[74] Cold increases the concentration of intracellular Ca^2, inhibiting potassium (K^+) channels and thereby slowing the depolarization and repolarization of sensory nerve membranes.[3] The net result of these effects is decreased pain transmission and perception.

Physiologically, the transmission of noxious impulses is reduced by lowering the excitability of free nerve endings and decreasing nerve conduction velocity resulting in an increased pain threshold (**cold-induced neuropraxia**).[4] Small-diameter, myelinated nerves are the first to exhibit a change in their conduction velocities. The last to respond to cold temperatures are unmyelinated, small-diameter nerves. During the course of treatment, pain threshold at the site of treatment is increased 89% and pain tolerance is increased 79% when the skin temperature is decreased by 18°F (10°C). Distal to the treatment site, pain threshold decreases 71%, and pain tolerance decreases 56% during treatment.[70]

Proprioception and Joint Position Sense

Changes in nerve conduction velocity of cutaneous sensory nerves and joint receptors interrupt the transmission and perception of pain and may affect proprioception (the ability to determine the joint's position and velocity of movement), balance, agility, and/or joint position sense.[17,75–84] These deficits may last up to 5 to 10 minutes following application.[82] Cold applied to the joint and surrounding muscle appears to interrupt joint position sense during and immediately following cooling, although the peroneal muscles appear to be less affected.[65,81,82,85] Joint proprioceptive response may depend on the type of injury being treated.

✻ Practical Evidence

Many, but not all, laboratory studies suggest that cryotherapy reduces joint position sense and proprioception in a healthy population.[78,80–86] However, the amount of research on this topic—especially with patients who have an active pathology or chronic lateral ankle instability—is limited. Exercise caution when having a patient participate in dynamic activities following cryotherapy, especially when the entire joint is cooled.[78,84,85] The dominant shoulders of throwing athletes may be particularly at risk.[80]

An adequate rewarming period should be allowed before the patient engages in proprioceptive-intensive exercises.[83,86,87] This can be achieved through progressive warm-up activities.

TABLE 5-5	Decrease in Muscular Afferent Nerve Transmission During Cryotherapy
NERVE	PERCENT DECREASE*
Ia receptor	56
Ib receptor	42
Golgi tendon organs	50

Per 18°F (10°C) decrease in intramuscular temperature.

Neurapraxia: A temporary loss of function in a peripheral nerve.

Axonotmesis: Damage to nerve tissue without physical severing of the nerve.

Counterirritant: A substance causing irritation of superficial sensory nerves so as to reduce the transmission of pain from underlying nerves.

Other mechanism may compensate for decreased proprioceptive nerve activity (Fig. 5-5). Proprioceptive nerves are low-threshold mechanoreceptors that have thick, myelinated axons. Their deep location within the tissues and myelin layer insulate these nerves from the full effects of cold therapy and, therefore, they may be less affected than superficial nerves.[17] Secondary spindles are possibly less affected by cold application than are primary spindles,[75] and different types of stretch receptors are activated at different points in the ROM.[76] Other nerve receptors may compensate for those receptors that are affected.[88] When the treatment targets the joint capsule but not the muscle, type II nerves may be inhibited and proprioceptive function is compensated for by other sensory input such as the brain interpreting the amount of effort needed to perform the movement.[17,75]

The shoulder may be more vulnerable to decreased proprioception following treatment. Shoulder joint position and reposition sense during slow movement do not appear to be negatively influenced by shoulder cryotherapy.[79] However, during functional high-velocity shoulder motions such as throwing, significant decreases in shoulder proprioception and throwing accuracy may occur.[80]

Muscle Spasm

Cold reduces muscle spasm by suppressing the stretch reflex by two mechanisms:

1. Reducing the threshold of afferent nerve endings.
2. Decreasing the sensitivity of muscle spindles.

A drop of 9°F (5°C) in surface skin temperature reduces the sensitivity of muscle spindles. Decreased muscle spindle activity, combined with the decreased rate of afferent nerve impulses, inhibits the stretch reflex mechanism, decreasing muscle spasm.[69,89] The activity of type Ia fibers decrease with cold application, type II fibers become more active, and type Ib fibers are less affected by cold.[69] Cold inhibits **gamma-motoneurons** ● and facilitates **alpha-motoneurons** ●. To reduce spasticity, gamma inhibition must exceed alpha facilitation.[69]

Because cold disrupts muscle spasm, pain is reduced by alleviating the mechanical stimulation placed on the nerve receptors in the area of spasm. A short-term break in the pain-spasm-pain cycle may result in long-term relief of muscle spasms secondary to decreasing the amount of mechanical pressure placed on the nerves and other tissues. A brief disruption in pain may also break the injury response cycle and allow tissue healing and repair to proceed unhindered.[43]

Muscle Function

Decreased nerve conduction velocity and the neurophysiological effects that result in decreased muscle spasm also affect the limb's muscular ability. Decreased nerve conduction velocity, decreased sensitivity of muscle spindles, and increased fluid viscosity leads to a decreased ability to perform rapid muscle movements and obtain maximum force.[67,86,90] The time required for the muscle contraction and relaxation cycle decreases, increasing the time for muscle to develop its maximum tension.[90,91] These detrimental effects are negated if a warm-up period is added prior to exercise.[91]

After a 20-minute cold application, the quadriceps femoris muscle group produces decreased concentric and eccentric strength and decreased isokinetic strength, power,[84,91–96] and endurance[92–95] for up to 30 minutes after the treatment. For this reason, provide the patient with adequate rewarming time (approximately 30 minutes) before beginning intense work or athletic activities. A 3-minute ice application between exercise bouts has demonstrated the ability to increase exercise work, velocity, and power, possibly the result of slowing the increase of intramuscular temperatures.[97] Following ice massage there is no resulting increase or decrease in muscle strength.[98]

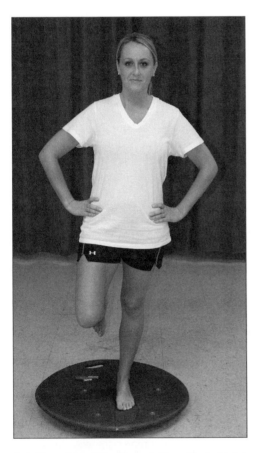

Figure 5-5. **Proprioception Board.** The effect of joint cooling appears to decrease proprioception immediately following cryotherapy, but is regained as the joint and surrounding muscles rewarm.

Gamma-motoneurons: Efferent motor nerves that innervate the intrafusal fibers of a muscle spindle.

Alpha-motoneurons: Efferent motor neurons that innervate muscle fibers.

Effect on Inhibited Muscle

Cooling a swollen joint helps to reduce edema-induced neuromuscular inhibition. Following ice pack application of swollen knees, muscular activity returned to baseline or preinjury levels.[65] However, joint cooling causes a stiffening of the capsule and other structures surrounding the joint, potentially limiting its ROM.[84,86]

Changes in temperature increase motoneuron pool excitability, indicating that these nerves are active and will contribute to the muscle contraction.[78] During a 20-minute cold application neuron excitability is inversely correlated with temperature. As the temperature decreases, the motoneuron pool excitability increases, making more motor units available. During the rewarming phase, the reverse effect occurs and the two variables become positively correlated: as temperature increases, the motoneuron pool excitability continues to increase.[99]

■ Effects of Immediate Treatment

Immediate treatment—rest, ice, compression, and elevation (RICE)—counteracts the body's initial response to an injury, including postsurgical care (Fig. 5-6). **Rest** limits the scope of the original injury by preventing further trauma. In acute trauma, "rest" may take the form of immobilizing the body part, the use of crutches, or other methods of avoiding additional insult to the injured tissues. Crushed **ice** is the ideal form of cold application during immediate treatment because it produces the most rapid and significant temperature decrease relative to other forms of cold application, while conforming to the body part being treated.[100]

During immediate treatment the purpose of ice application is to decrease cell metabolism, thereby decreasing the need for oxygen in the injured area. This effect reduces the amount of secondary hypoxic injury and secondary enzymatic injury by enabling the cells to survive on the limited amount of oxygen they are receiving. Thicker layers

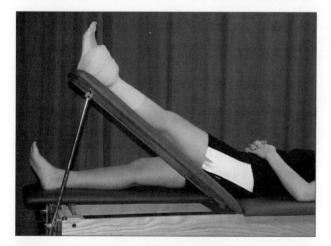

Figure 5-6. Ice, Compression, and Elevation. An ice bag is secured in place with an elastic wrap and the body part is elevated. This technique decreases the pressure gradient, lessening the amount of fluids that escape into the tissues and encouraging venous and lymphatic return.

of adipose tissue require a longer treatment duration than the "traditional" 20 to 30 minutes to obtain the desired cooling (see Box 5-3).[49]

Ice application also provides secondary benefits in the immediate treatment of an injury by reducing pain. Because of the other factors surrounding the injury (e.g., the severity of the injury or the person's emotional state), the effects of ice on limiting pain cannot be accurately predicted for every case. The combination of ice, compression, and elevation has been shown to decrease the amount of time lost due to acute musculoskeletal injury.[101]

Compression decreases the pressure gradient between the blood vessels and tissues. This discourages further leakage from the capillary beds into the interstitial tissues while also encouraging increased lymphatic drainage. Compression wraps must be applied so that a pressure gradient is formed between the distal end of the wrap and the proximal end (see Clinical Techniques: Compression Wraps, Chapter 1)

✳ Practical Evidence

External compression using an elastic wrap or plastic wrap to secure a cold pack improves skin and subcutaneous tissue cooling. In acute conditions the cooling, combined with compression and elevation assist in preventing swelling.[13,14] Once swelling has occurred, compression and elevation assist in reducing swelling. Cold application alone has little effect on reducing swelling. Walking with the ice wrapped on the lower extremity can negate deep cooling effects by increasing cell metabolism and increasing blood flow.[34] Plastic wraps may encourage walking more so than elastic wraps.

Using an elastic wrap to secure the ice bag to the body part produces a significant reduction in subcutaneous tissue temperatures as compared with simply placing the ice pack on the skin.[13] However, placing the wrap between the pack and the skin reduces the amount of skin temperature drop because the wrap acts as an insulator.[8,13]

The combination of ice and compression results in reduced cell metabolism deeper within the tissues, helping to limit the scope and severity of secondary injury. An additional benefit of using an elastic wrap is increased joint proprioception secondary to stimulating the afferent receptors in the skin and superficial subcutaneous tissues.[102] This effect can serve to protect injured joints by assisting the body's awareness of the joint's position. The compression wrap also helps to decrease pain by stimulating sensory and proprioceptive nerve endings that override noxious stimuli.

Compression and **elevation** decrease the vascular hydrostatic pressure within the capillary beds, reducing capillary outflow to the tissue. The difference in pressures encourages absorption of edema by the lymphatic system. The force of gravity acting on the elevated extremity encourages venous and lymphatic return. This effect is greatest when the extremity is at 90 degrees perpendicular to the ground; however, this position is not necessarily practical. The limb should be elevated as high as possible while still maintaining a comfortable position. Mechanical implements such as split-leg tables can effectively raise the lower extremity to a 45-degree angle, at which point the effect of gravity is 71% of that in the vertical position (see Fig. 1.14). The effects of elevation in reducing edema are short lived. Edema returns to pretreatment volumes within 5 minutes of returning the limb to the gravity-dependent position.[64]

◼ Cryokinetics

Cryokinetics involves the use of cold therapy in conjunction with movement (*cryo* = "cold"; *kinetic* = "motion") and is used to improve ROM by eliminating or reducing the element of pain. Early, safe, pain-free motion through the normal range results in a more pronounced macrophage reaction, quicker hematoma resolution, increased vascular growth, faster regeneration of muscle and scar tissue, and increased tensile strength of healed muscle.[27]

Cryokinetics may be initiated in cases in which the underlying soft tissue and bone are intact and in which pain is limiting the amount of functional movement. Although cryokinetics is useful in increasing ROM, care must be taken to prevent masking pain that would otherwise alert the individual to further tissue damage.

◼ Cold-Related Injury

Two factors associated with cryotherapy can increase the risk of cold-related injury during treatment: the skin temperature decrease and the amount of pressure used to secure the ice pack. Extreme temperatures, those not normally reached during properly applied treatments, can result in frostbite. Cold and the pressure associated with a compression wrap can traumatize superficial nerves.

Cold-Induced Neuropathy

Securing an ice pack with an elastic wrap increases the depth and magnitude of the treatment. When too much pressure is applied to an elastic wrap that is securing an ice pack over large, superficial nerves, the resulting overcooling can result in neuropathy, causing the loss of sensory or motor function, or both. The common peroneal nerve (located just superior to the fibular head) and the ulnar nerve (posteromedial aspect of the elbow) are most prone to this condition. Decrease the amount of pressure used when securing an ice pack over any superficial nerve.

✳ Practical Evidence

To avoid cold-induced neuropathy of large superficial nerves (e.g., the common peroneal n, ulnar n), do not apply tight compression wraps[103] and limit the treatment duration to 10 to 15 minutes.[23]

Compression wraps should not be used when treating **compartment syndromes** ●. The external pressure from the wrap can significantly increase the amount of pressure within the compartment and result in neurological or vascular insufficiency in the distal extremity. During any treatment, regularly check the patient for signs of nerve dysfunction, such as tingling in the distal extremity, and normal blood flow in the fingers or toes, by observing the capillary refill in the nailbed.

Frostbite

Under normal conditions there is little chance of developing frostbite when frozen water is used as the means of cold application.[89] Picture these forms of ice application: an ice bag, ice massage, and ice immersion. During the course of each of these treatments, water is present. An ice bag fills with water as the ice melts, ice massage leaves a trail of water with each stroke, and water is the medium used during an ice immersion.

The presence of water indicates that ice is melting and the water is in its **change of state** ●; therefore, the temperature of the ice pack is slightly above 32°F (0°C). Frostbite occurs when the skin temperature falls below freezing. When the subcutaneous temperature falls below 55°F (12.8°C), the risk of cold-related tissue damage increases. During the course of a 20-minute treatment, cold modalities that have water present cause a decrease in skin temperature to 56°F (13.3°C).[89]

The risk of frostbite increases when using reusable ice packs. These devices contain water mixed with antifreeze and are stored at temperatures below freezing. Because the surface temperature of the pack may be below freezing, a medium such as a wet towel must be placed between the pack and the skin in order to reduce the risk of frostbite.

After approximately 5 minutes of cold application, the skin is marked by erythema, redness indicating that the circulatory system is continuing to deliver warm blood, even though the skin temperature has dropped substantially. If the area displays signs of **pallor** ●, the circulatory system has been unable to maintain tissue temperatures within normal physiological limits, increasing the risk of frostbite. If the tissues become **cyanotic** ●, the treatment should be discontinued.

Compartment syndrome: Increased pressure within a muscular compartment, causing decreased blood flow to and from the distal extremity, and decreased distal nerve function and decreased local muscular blood profusion and pain.

Change of state: Transformation from one physical state to another (e.g., ice to water).

Pallor: Lack of color in the skin.

Cyanosis (cyanotic): A blue-gray discoloration of the skin caused by a lack of oxygen.

If the treatment is colder than the recommended temperature, if the treatment duration is too long, or if the patient suffers from significant circulatory insufficiency or decreased sensation, the risk of frostbite (or cold injury) increases (Box 5-5). Prolonged exposure to intense cold decreases circulation throughout the body. Because of the proximity of arteries (flowing to the area) and veins (flowing out of the area), venous blood cools the incoming arterial blood. Significant decreases in core temperature increase the amount of systemic vasoconstriction and further lower the heart rate. If the treated area is ischemic, warm blood cannot reach the tissues. Clinically, this effect would be seen only during full-body immersion in a tank that is too cold.

■ Contraindications and Precautions in the Use of Cold Modalities

The primary contraindications to the use of cold modalities are conditions in which the body is unable to cope with the temperature because of allergy, hypersensitivity, or circulatory or nerve insufficiency (see Table 5-2). Most of the disease states that contraindicate cold application affect the blood or nerve supply.

Some people do not tolerate cold exposure well. In some cases, cold intolerance can be related to neurovascular disorders such as Raynaud's phenomenon, an arterial spasm that blocks blood flow and results in cyanosis. This condition most frequently occurs in the toes, fingers, nose, and ears. Although often benign and painless, Raynaud's phenomenon can indicate underlying cold-induced myocardial ischemia.[104] In other cases the individual may have a true allergy to cold. This condition is characterized by urticaria, the outbreak of hives, itching, and, in rare cases, anaphylactic shock.

Recall that arterial blood warms the treated area and venous blood carries cold away. Local (to the area being treated) or systemic circulatory impairments can produce unwanted effects such as cold-induced injury. Disease states such as lupus are also contraindications to cold application. Abnormal blood proteins, cryoglobulins, adhere

Box 5-5. SIGNS AND SYMPTOMS OF FROSTBITE

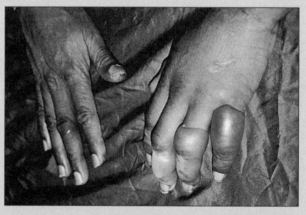

Even the most minor case of frostbite is accompanied by extreme pain. This pain is so severe that patients who have normal sensory function will not allow the treatment to continue. The primary concern is for patients who have sensory and/or circulatory impairment or those on whom reusable ice packs are applied.

The first physical sign of frostbite is the fading of the redness normally associated with cold application. This color is replaced by a waxy white sheen. If frostbite is allowed to continue, the skin will blister or molt and lead to an obvious buildup of edema.

Even though the chance of frostbite is slim, patients with impaired circulation are at a higher risk. The use of elastic wraps and cold further decreases skin temperature and requires that the skin reaction be more closely monitored. During any physical procedure, the circulation to the extremities can be checked by monitoring the flow of blood to the nailbeds. Gently squeezing the nail removes the blood, making it turn white or pale. When the force is removed, the original color should return. If it fails to return, circulatory impairment should be suspected.

If frostbite is suspected, immediately remove the patient from the source of the cold. Rewarm the body part by immersing it in water between 100°F and 108°F and refer the patient to a physician for follow-up evaluation and treatment.

From Kozol RA: When to Call the Surgeon: Decision Making for Primary Care Providers. FA Davis, Philadelphia, 1999, with permission.

to each other during cold exposure. Patients suffering from **hypotension** •, **hypertension** •, or other cardiovascular or cardiorespiratory diseases may experience increased blood pressure or difficulty breathing if large areas (i.e., immersion) are treated or temperatures that are too cold are used. Some recommendations advise against the application of ice treatments for acute surgical wounds.[23]

Nerve inhibition can interfere with local thermoregulation, either producing overcooling of the tissue or increased blood flow. Impaired sensory function increases the risk of cold-related injury. Decreased sensory function is often associated with conditions such as diabetes. Ice should be used with caution in these cases. Ice application is contraindicated in the presence of major nerve regeneration secondary to the possibility of ischemia and cold-induced neuropathy.[23]

Edema caused by circulatory problems such as peripheral vascular disease can be increased by cold application. Decreased blood flow to or from the treated area can cause the tissues to be overcooled.

Patients who have precautions can be treated by placing a terry cloth towel between the ice pack and the skin to prevent the temperature from becoming too cold. However, this approach can render the treatment ineffective. Adding an insulating barrier or increasing the temperature of cold immersions can prevent a negative reaction to the cold. The patient's physician should always be consulted prior to using apparently contraindicated techniques.

■ Overview of the Evidence

Researchers and clinicians generally accept the physiological efficacy of cold modalities. Most studies focus on the physiological effects, primarily tissue temperature decrease and pain reduction. Despite its widespread use, cryotherapy has not undergone randomized controlled clinical trials required to demonstrate improved outcomes, especially regulating the response to acute musculoskeletal injury.[37,73]

The Canadian Physiotherapy Association (CPA) cites postsurgical wounds as a contraindication to prolonged ice application, although "prolonged" is not defined. The rationale for this recommendation was based on reduced tissue perfusions, slowing of the healing process, and increasing the risk of infection. These effects last 1 to 2 hours post-treatment. The CPA recommends intermittent cold application only for symptom management, allowing for normal physiology between treatments.[23] Although some studies have demonstrated increased oxygen saturation in tendons following ice application[59,60] and no study has investigated the differences in healing time between those receiving ice treatment and those who do not, the implications of this recommendation on the treatment of acute injuries can be profound.

Studies have indicated that ice, compression, and elevation hasten return to athletic participation, but patient outcomes are probably strongly influenced by other treatments (e.g., compression, elevation, crutch walking) and the nature and quality of post-injury rehabilitation.[37,101] Decreased pain is a relatively consistent finding following cold application.[73]

Twenty minutes is used as the default treatment duration for ice packs (and, to a lesser extent, 15 minutes has become the "standard" for immersion and 10 minutes for ice massage), but this "one size fits all" treatment duration limits the effectiveness of cold application. With the exception of cutaneous sensory nerves that are superficial to the adipose tissue layer, the rate, depth, and magnitude of intramuscular cooling are dependent on the thickness of the adipose tissue layer. Therefore, the appropriate treatment duration is based on the thickness of this insulating layer and the depth of the target tissue.

Nerve conduction[68,69,105] and muscle function[57,68,70,90] are affected by cold. There is conflicting evidence that this interruption in normal nerve and muscle function affects proprioception. Several research articles[17,74,77,78,80,81,82,83,84] caution that proprioception is inhibited following joint or local muscle cooling, thereby possibly increasing the risk of injury. Other researchers[17,76,79,82,85,88] have concluded that there is no significant decrease in proprioception following treatment. While caution should be used in prescribing weight-bearing activity following cryotherapy, muscles and joints rapidly rewarm during exercise. In practicality, even walking should hasten the return of proprioceptive function.

The method of cold application affects treatment outcomes. Intermittent cold application results in deeper tissue cooling. Allowing some skin rewarming to occur maintains a steeper temperature gradient that allows further cooling of the underlying tissue. This is in contrast to clinical approaches that call for constant cooling, such as is often applied immediately after injury or postsurgery. The cost-effectiveness of cold compression therapy units has also been questioned.[67] The effectiveness of various methods of cold application on reducing intramuscular temperature also depends on the size (area) of the skin being treated. For example, ice massage results in a more rapid decline in intramuscular temperatures, but only when a small (4 × 4 cm) area is treated.[6]

Another common clinical practice, placing an insulating barrier between the skin and ice pack, can render the treatment ineffective by reducing the temperature gradient between the skin and the ice pack. An insulating barrier should only be used when a reusable ice pack is applied or the patient displays sensitivities or contraindications to cold treatment.

Some debate still exists about fluctuations in blood flow and other vascular reactions that occur during treatment.

Hypotension: Low blood pressure.

Hypertension: High blood pressure.

Some researchers have reported a spike in blood flow approximately 10 to 17 minutes into the treatment.[54] However, this appears to be inconsequential to most treatments. Likewise, as we will see with techniques such as contrast baths, the fact that capillaries do not change their size must be considered when determining the effectiveness of various treatment approaches.

■ Heat Modalities

Heat, the increase in molecular vibration and cellular metabolic rate, is produced by four primary methods:

1. The transfer of thermal energy
2. Chemical action associated with cell metabolism
3. Mechanical action such as is found with therapeutic ultrasound (see Chapter 7)
4. Electrical or magnetic currents such as those found in diathermy devices (see Chapter 9)

The application of therapeutic heat, **thermotherapy,** is classified as superficial or deep (Table 5-6). Superficial agents heat a larger area of tissue (the skin), but their limited depth of penetration reduces the overall volume of tissue heated (Fig. 5-7).[106] To produce therapeutic effects, superficial heating agents must be capable of increasing the skin temperature to 104°F to 113°F (40°C to 45°C). The transfer of heat to underlying tissues occurs through conduction, but superficial heating agents are limited to depths of less than 2 cm. Deep-heating agents, therapeutic ultrasound, and shortwave diathermy are capable of heating tissues located at depths greater than 2 cm. These devices are presented in the next section.

Research regarding the physiological effects of heat have not received as much attention as has cold application.[107] Heat's effects on metabolic rate, blood and fluid dynamics, and inflammation are generally opposite to those of cold (see Fig. 5-1). Both heat and cold applications decrease pain and muscle spasm by altering the threshold of nerve endings. Systemically, heating large areas results in increased body temperature, pulse rate, and respiratory rate and in decreased blood pressure. The use of heat is indicated

in the subacute and chronic inflammatory stages of injury (Table 5-7).

■ Magnitude and Duration of Temperature Increase

When therapeutic heat is applied, the temperature gradient causes the modality to lose heat and the body to gain heat. Some heat is also lost to the surrounding environment (Fig. 5-8). The larger the temperature gradient is, the faster the energy exchange occurs. Some thermal modalities, such as moist heat packs, require the use of an insulator to protect the skin from burns, thus regulating the temperature gradient within therapeutic limits.

Maximum therapeutic benefits occur when the skin temperature rapidly increases, increasing the excitability of local temperature receptors that causes an active release of vasoactive mediators.[108] If the rate of temperature increase is too slow, the associated increased blood flow will keep tissue temperatures low. If the rate of temperature increase is too great, wide dynamic range thermoreceptors will be activated, producing pain, and burns may result.

During the first 5 to 6 minutes of treatment the body absorbs heat faster than it can be dissipated. After approximately 7 to 9 minutes of exposure, the temperature gradient begins to even out and slightly decline. At this point, the body is able to counteract the energy being applied by supplying an adequate amount of blood to cool the area, stabilizing the tissue temperature. The fluctuations in skin temperature (presumably occurring as a defense mechanism to prevent burning) limit the amount of subcutaneous heating that can be obtained.[109]

When a maximal vasodilation has occurred and the intensity of the treatment stays constant (or increases), the vessels begin to constrict. This phenomenon, known as **rebound vasoconstriction,** occurs approximately 20 minutes into the treatment. This is the body's attempt to save underlying tissues by sacrificing the superficial layer. If the intensity of treatment is too great or if the duration of exposure is too long, burns will result. The likelihood of rebound vasoconstriction increases with treatments in which the temperature and intensity are kept constant, such as hot whirlpools and paraffin immersion baths. With modalities such as moist heat packs, the intensity of the treatment temperature decreases with time because the modality loses heat during the application. **Mottling** ● of the skin is a warning sign that tissue temperatures are rising to a dangerously high level. In this case, ghost-white areas and beet-red splotches mark the patient's skin. When mottling occurs, the treatment should be discontinued immediately.

Central and local mechanisms and a reflex arc attempt to maintain the core temperature at a "set point" that is monitored by the hypothalamus. The temperature of local areas

TABLE 5-6 Classification of Heating Agents	
SUPERFICIAL HEAT (< 2 CM)	DEEP HEAT (> 2 CM)
Infrared lamps [not a contemporary device]	Ultrasound (see Chapter 8)
	Shortwave diathermy (see Chapter 10)
Moist heat packs	
Paraffin baths	
Warm whirlpool and/or immersion	

Mottling: A blotchy discoloration of the skin.

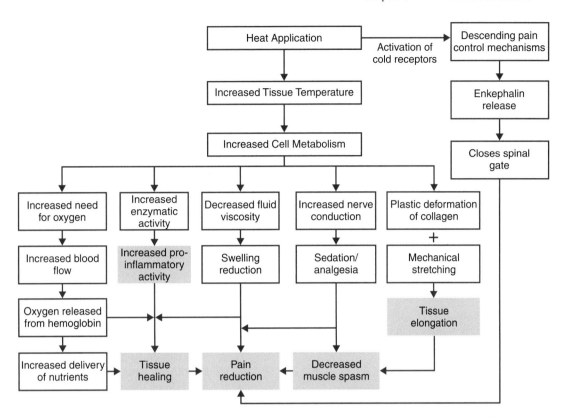

Figure 5-7. **Schematic representation of the local effects of heat application.** The primary effects are derived from increasing cell metabolism, increasing blood flow, and sedating nerve endings.

TABLE 5-7	**General Indications and Contraindications for Heat Treatments**

INDICATIONS	CONTRAINDICATIONS
Subacute or chronic inflammatory conditions	Acute injuries
	Impaired circulation
Reduction of subacute or chronic pain	Peripheral vascular disease
	Deep vein thrombosis
Subacute or chronic muscle spasm	Advanced arthritis (vigorous heating)
Decreased range of motion	Poor thermal regulation
	Anesthetic areas
Hematoma resolution	**Neoplasms** ●
Reduction of joint contractures	Thrombophlebitis
	Closed infections
	Pregnancy (avoid increasing core temperature)

Precautions

Areas of decreased sensation
Treatment around the eyes or testicles

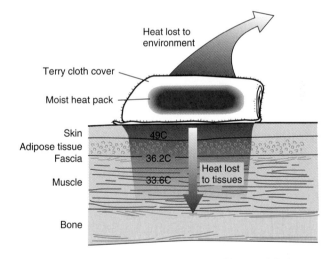

Figure 5-8. **Conductive Heating of the Skin and Subcutaneous Tissues.** When a moist heat pack is placed on the skin, the subcutaneous adipose tissue layer limits deeper penetration of the energy. The maximum treatment depth of moist heat packs is between 2 and 3 cm.

is permitted to fluctuate more than the core temperature. Blood flow is regulated to prevent excessive heat exchange, with vasodilation occurring to help cool the treated area. The body may (theoretically) decrease blood flow to prevent the increased temperature from affecting the core.[110]

Neoplasm: Abnormal tissue, such as a tumor, that grows at the expense of healthy tissue.

As we saw with cold modalities, the adipose tissue layer is also a primary limiting factor for the effective depth of heat penetration (see Box 5-1). The amount of superficial heat absorbed by the adipose tissue increases as the thickness of this layer increases, preventing temperature increase in deeper layers. The resting temperature of muscle is warmer than that of skin, decreasing the temperature gradient and slowing the exchange of heat.

Tissue Rewarming

Skin and subcutaneous adipose tissue temperatures rapidly decrease following the removal of the heating agent. Heat is lost to the surrounding air, and the increased circulation continues to deliver relatively cool blood to the treated area while the venous system removes relatively warm blood. Superficial intramuscular temperatures remain elevated for approximately 30 minutes following the conclusion of the treatment. The magnitude and duration of the latent effects of heat are less pronounced than those demonstrated with cold.

Therapeutic Temperature Benchmarks

The magnitude of heating effects is based on the temperature increase of the target tissues (Table 5-8). Increases in cell metabolism and blood flow occur soon after the application of the heating agent. Increased temperature causes blood hemoglobin to release oxygen, providing more oxygen for the healing process. At 106°F (41.1°C), the release of oxygen is approximately twice as great as at baseline temperatures (Fig. 5-9).

TABLE 5-8	Tissue Temperature Increase From Baseline Required to Achieve Therapeutic Effects*	
CLASSIFICATION OF THERMAL EFFECTS	TEMPERATURE INCREASE	USED FOR
Mild	1.8°F (1°C)	Mild inflammation Accelerates metabolic rate
Moderate	3.6°–5.4°F (2°–3°C)	Decreasing muscle spasm Decreasing pain Increasing blood flow Reducing chronic inflammation
Vigorous	5.4°–9.0°F (3°–4°C)	Tissue elongation, scar tissue reduction Inhibition of sympathetic activity

The relative temperature increase (e.g., 2°C) above resting baseline (see Controversies in Treatment for Heat Modalities).

Enzymatic activity begins to increase when temperatures approach 102°F (38.9°C) and continues to be accelerated up to 122°F (50°C). After this point, the rate of enzymatic activity rapidly decreases.

✴ Practical Evidence

A treatment duration of 20 to 25 minutes is required for a moist heat pack to increase intramuscular temperature 0.72°F (0.4°C) at a depth of 1 inch (2.54 cm).[111] This increase is not within therapeutic ranges.

Heating to 104°F to 113°F (40°C to 45°C) more easily allows for plastic deformation of collagen-rich tissues (joint capsule, ligaments, fascia, tendons). However, the structure must be physically stretched for elongation to occur.[111] Protein damage occurs and cells and tissues are destroyed when the tissue temperature is increased to greater than 113°F (45°C). Extreme heating such as that obtained by thermal lasers used to shrink capsular tissues results in a temperature increase of 140°F to 158°F (60°C to 70°C), resulting in contraction of the capsular fibers.[112]

● EFFECTS ON
The Injury Response Process

Although heat and cold produce many of the same clinical outcomes, decreased pain, for example, the timing of when to begin using heat modalities is critical. A primary effect of heat modalities is increased cell metabolism and rate of inflammation, both of which require increased oxygen. If heat is applied too soon in the injury response process, the increased cell metabolism increases the number of cells injured or destroyed because of hypoxia. Increasing the inflammatory rate could extend the acute and subacute inflammatory stages.

Cellular Response

The rate of cell metabolism increases in response to the rise in tissue temperature. For each increase of 18°F (10.0°C) in skin temperature, the cell's metabolic rate increases by a factor of two to three, the **Q10 effect**.[113,114] As the cell's metabolic rate increases, so does its demand for oxygen and nutrients. In the presence of an active inflammatory response, an increase in cell metabolism results in an increased release of inflammatory mediators and other by-products.

There is a reciprocal relationship between tissue temperature and the rate of cell metabolism. Increased temperature causes an increase in cellular metabolic rate; an increase in cell metabolism causes tissue temperature to rise. As with all heat applications, increased cellular

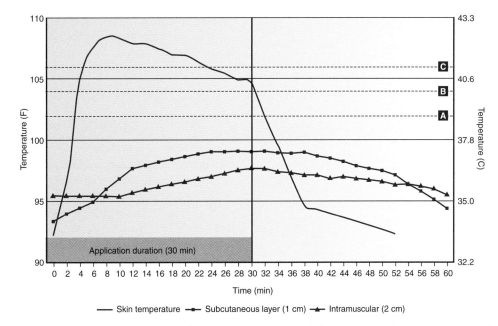

Figure 5-9. **Tissue Temperature Increase During a 30-Minute Moist Heat Pack Application.** (A) 102°F to 109°F: Enzymatic activity increases. (B) 104°F: Plastic deformation of collagen-rich tissue begins to occur. (C) 106°F: Blood hemoglobin release into tissue is twice that of baseline tissue temperature.

metabolic rate causes arteriolar dilation and increased capillary flow.

Effect on Inflammation

The local application of heat accelerates inflammation. Soft tissue repair is facilitated through an accelerated metabolic rate and increased blood supply. Blood flow must be increased to encourage the removal of cellular debris and to increase delivery of the nutrients necessary for the healing of tissues.[115] Increased oxygen delivery stimulates the breakdown and removal of tissue debris and inflammatory **metabolites** ●. Nutrients are delivered to the area to fuel the cells, and there is also an increase in the delivery of leukocytes, encouraging phagocytosis.

✱ Practical Evidence

Although subjectively a more comfortable treatment for patients with osteoarthritis or rheumatoid arthritis, increasing intra-articular temperature in these patients appears to further degrade the joint surface by activating a series of enzymatic events.[30]

Blood and Fluid Dynamics

The body responds to the rise in tissue temperature by dilating local blood vessels. Blood flow begins to increase soon after the application of the modality, increasing the delivery of oxygen, nutrients, and antibodies required for healing. Vasodilation occurs more in the superficial vessels than in the deeper vessels. Heat produces vasodilation through the combination of three mechanisms: (1) relaxing arteriole smooth muscle, (2) triggering the release of neurotransmitters and peptides, and (3) through a spinal-level reflex.

Immediately following application, vascular smooth muscle dilates (relaxes) in response to the release of substance P and calcitonin gene-related peptide, increasing the permeability of calcium channels. Shortly after this immediate response when skin temperature increases above 77°F (25°C), a sequence of events heavily reliant on the presence of calcium causes the release of nitric oxide that continues the vasodilation.[116,117]

Peak blood flow, often more than a twofold increase relative to the baseline, usually occurs during the final one-third of the treatment or within 10 minutes following the removal of the modality.[118] The viscosity of blood and other fluids decreases as the surrounding temperature increases. This elevated blood flow will continue for up to 60 minutes following the end of the treatment.[118] The presence of moisture helps to increase blood flow relative to dry heat.[117] Moist heat increases skin blood flow by 386%, while dry heat results in a 282% increase.[116]

In the presence of normal amounts of adipose tissue, this effect occurs 2 cm or less below the skin. Heat applied to muscles that are normally covered by relatively low amounts of subcutaneous adipose tissue, such as the trapezius, may experience increased blood flow up to 3 cm below the surface of the skin.[119]

Metabolite: A by-product of metabolism.

Edema Formation and Reduction

Heat application increases the volume of the treated limb, especially when the limb is placed in the gravity-dependent position such as during warm whirlpool treatment. During a 20-minute treatment, the limb volume of uninjured lower extremities increases 5 mL for every 1°F (0.6°C) rise in water temperature above 92°F (33.3°C). This increase is greater when pathology is present.[120]

The amount of edema is increased, but the capability of removing it is greater. Increased capillary pressure forces edema and harmful metabolites from the injured area. Increased lymphatic permeability aids in the reabsorption of edema and the dissolution of hematomas. These wastes can drain into the venous and lymphatic systems. However, if venous and lymphatic return is not encouraged, further edema occurs.

Nerve Conduction

The increased rate of chemical reactions and cell metabolism results in increased nerve conduction velocity. Both sensory and motor nerve function are typically enhanced through heat treatments.

Pain Control

Pain relief is obtained by decreasing mechanical pressure on nerve endings, reducing muscle spasm, resolving ischemia, and producing a counterirritant effect via a descending pain control mechanism that increases the pain threshold. Mechanical deformation or chemical irritation of nerve endings stimulates pain transmission. In acute injuries, the primary cause of pain is the mechanical damage done to the tissue in the area. In the subacute and chronic stage of injury, ischemia and irritation cause chemical pain from certain chemical mediators. Increased **catabolic** ● and **anabolic** ● activity assist in removing cellular wastes, improving the healing environment.[4]

Mechanical pain is caused by increased tissue pressure (swelling) and the tension placed on nerves by muscle spasm. Increasing circulation to the area decreases congestion, allowing oxygen to be delivered to the suffocating cells. Increased circulation (blood flow to and away from the area) assists in removing the pain-producing chemicals in the area. By decreasing the mechanical pressure on the nerves, the pain-spasm-pain cycle is reduced. By encouraging venous and lymphatic return through the use of elevation and muscle contraction, the swelling is removed, further decreasing interstitial pressure.

An increase in temperature and the tactile stimulation of the skin lead to a state of analgesia and **sedation** ● in the injured area by acting on free nerve endings.[4] Nerve fibers

are stimulated, activating areas of the thalamus and S2 region in the brain, blocking the transmission of pain with a counterirritant effect.[4] This effect appears to last only as long as the stimulus of heat is applied, and when heat is removed, the pain symptoms quickly return.[121]

■ Muscle Spasm and Function

Heat reduces muscle spasm by decreasing the sensitivity of the muscle's secondary gamma afferent nerves (that are more sensitive to tonic [constant] tension than phasic tension), which decreases muscle tone and alleviates pressure on the nerve. Increasing blood flow and reducing local muscle metabolites further alleviate spasm.[4] The most subcutaneous layer of the muscle is directly affected by superficial heating agents.

Decreased fluid viscosity, increased nerve conduction velocity, and the increased rate of Golgi tendon organ firing increase muscle function and strength, as long as the temperature is maintained within therapeutic ranges.

■ Tissue Elasticity

When collagen-rich tissue such as tendon, muscle, and fascia is heated to 104°F to 113°F (40°C to 45°C) for 5 minutes, it can be physically elongated (plastic deformation). This effect alone is not sufficient to decrease contractures or increase the elasticity of healthy tissues.[111] Tension, in the form of gentle stretching, while the tissues are still within therapeutic range is necessary to elongate muscle and capsular tissues. ROM is subsequently improved by increasing the extensibility of collagen, decreasing fluid viscosity, and plastic deformation of tissues.[122] This response is better achieved through the use of deep heating rather than superficial heat modalities.[106]

Unless an adhesion is mechanically restricting ROM, most of the ROM benefits derived from heat application are probably the result of decreasing muscle tone rather than physically elongating tissues. For example, moist heat pack application can increase short-term hamstring flexibility more than three 30-second static stretches. However, this increase is related to muscle relaxation rather than representing an increase in an elongation of the muscle.[123] Neither anterior laxity of the knee or long-term hamstring flexibility has been shown to be affected by heat modalities alone.[124,125]

■ Exercise as a Heating Agent

Increased blood flow, increased cell metabolism, and increased intramuscular temperature occur during the application of heat modalities and during active exercise. Moderate to intense exercise increases intramuscular temperatures approximately 4°F (2.2°C) at a depth of 5 cm in

---

Catabolic: A metabolic process that breaks a molecule into its component elements, thereby releasing energy.

Anabolic: The synthesis of a molecule from its component elements. Constructive metabolism.

Sedation: The result of calming nerve endings.

the involved muscles, but does not result in a temperature increase in nonexercising muscles.[126]

Although active exercise does not result in vigorous heating of the muscle, moderate heating occurs over a larger cross-sectional area and deeper into the muscle than most other forms of heat. Most important, active exercise is more functional than the use of passive heating modalities. Brief exercise produces a relatively large, short-term increase in blood flow. Heat modalities result in a smaller net increase in blood flow, but the duration of the increase lasts for a longer time.[127]

Contraindications and Precautions to Heat Application

Because the effects of heat application are essentially the opposite to those of cold, its use in the treatment of acute injuries should be avoided. Applying heat to an active inflammatory process increases the rate of cell metabolism and accelerates the amount of hypoxic injury (see Table 5-7).

Neurovascular deficits can result in overheating of the skin and consequently in burns. The patient should have normal sensory and vascular function and be able to communicate any abnormal sensations such as burning. Heating agents should not be applied to patients who are sleeping or unconscious.

High temperatures should not be used on limbs in which thrombophlebitis is present and increasing core temperature or those with deep vein thrombosis (DVT) must be avoided. The vasodilation and increased blood flow related to heat application could cause the clot to become dislodged and enter the circulatory system, potentially blocking blood supply to vital organs such as the heart or brain.[128] The application of therapeutic heat over tumors can increase the rate of tumor growth.

Heat application over areas of closed infection can result in swelling and pain. However, moist heat can be applied to open infection to promote drainage.[128]

Avoid systemic heating that increases the core temperature in patients who are pregnant, have a history of cardiac failure, or who have hypertension. Local heating agents may be used in these patients with the exception of avoiding heating the abdomen during pregnancy.

Overview of the Evidence

Research investigating the effects and outcomes of superficial heating is dwarfed by that of cold. Many of the heating methods described in the next chapter, namely fluidotherapy, paraffin treatment, and whirlpools, do not have a strong research base to support or refute their efficacy. Likewise, the reputed effects of contrast therapy have not been established in controlled studies.

The amount of temperature increase required to enhance the plastic properties of collagen-rich tissues is unclear (see Table 5-8). The temperatures of the heating ranges are based on the assumption of an initial temperature of approximately 99°F (37°C); resting muscle is typically less

than this. Increasing collagen elasticity is improved when the target tissue temperature is increased to 104°F to 113°F (40°C to 45°C). Clinically, this is different from obtaining a 5.4°F to 9.0°F (3°C to 4°C) temperature increase.[129]

The use of certain heating agents over joints affected by osteo- and rheumatoid arthritis has been questioned. Vigorous heating of arthritic joints may promote the effects of proteolytic and lysosomal enzymes, especially collagenase, which degrades articular cartilage.[30] At temperatures greater than 95F° to 97°F (35°C to 36°C) enzymatic deterioration of articular cartilage markedly increases.[27]

Contrast and Comparison of Heat and Cold Application

The effects of cold modalities penetrate deeper and are longer lasting than those of heat modalities. Heat causes a vasodilation that delivers cool blood to the area while the warmer blood is transported away. In contrast, cold application causes a vasoconstriction, resulting in a decreased amount of blood arriving to warm the area. This causes deeper tissues to be affected more by cold than by superficial heating agents (Table 5-9).

After the modality is removed from the body, the effects of cold last longer than those of heat. This is a result of the same mechanisms that account for the increased depth of the effects of cold. After a heat treatment, cool blood continues to flow to the area, decreasing the temperature. In contrast, the cool tissue temperature resulting from cold application causes the vasoconstriction of blood vessels and a decrease in the amount of blood delivered to the area, so that a longer time is needed for rewarming than for recooling.[130]

Both modalities effectively reduce pain transmission by increasing the patient's pain threshold and, through the initial stimulation of sensory nerves, activate the gate mechanism. Although patients prefer moist heat modalities, their effectiveness is short lived after the treatment.[121] Educating the patient about the potentially detrimental effects of using heat too early in the treatment program should help improve patient compliance.

The application of cold reduces the amounts of inflammatory mediators and cell by-products released into the area. These cellular wastes are insulting to the tissues and increase the amount of tissue damage and pain. When heat is applied during the proliferation stage of inflammation, the vascular response assists in removing cellular waste.

Use of Heat Versus Cold

One of the most asked questions regarding heat and cold is "How do you know when to use heat and when to use cold?" There are no clear-cut answers to this question. Many sources use definitive time frames, such as: "Use ice for the first 24 hours and heat for the next 48." One of the first points made in this text was that the body heals an injury at its own rate. Not only does this rate vary from person to person but also from injury to injury in the same person.

TABLE 5-9   Comparison of Heat and Cold Treatments

EFFECT	COLD	HEAT
Effective depth	5 cm	1–2 cm (superficial agents) 2–5 cm (deep-heating agents)
Duration of effects	Hours	Begins to dissipate after the removal of the modality
Blood flow	↓(Vasoconstriction)	↑(Vasodilation)
Rate of cell metabolism	↓	↑
Oxygen consumption	↓	↑
Cell wastes	↓	↑
Fluid viscosity	↓	↓
Capillary permeability	↓	↑
Inflammation	↓	↑
Pain	↓	↓
Muscle spasm	↓(Reduced sensitivity of muscle spindles and decreased pain)	↓(Reduced ischemia and pain)
Muscle contraction	↓(Reduced nerve conduction velocity and increased fluid viscosity)	↑(Increased nerve conduction velocity and decreased fluid viscosity)

↓= *Decrease;* ↑=*Increase.*

The patient's physical and psychological state, and the type and amount of tissue damaged factor into the time required for healing.

The transition from cold to heat modalities is based on the patient's current stage in the healing process. Cold should be used in the earlier stages; the transition to heat may be made as the patient progresses to the mid- to late proliferation stage. The amount of time for this transition varies from patient to patient and from injury to injury.

The decision-making process is similar to the steps involved when a pipe ruptures in the basement of a house. Before bailing out the water and cleaning up the mess, you have to stop the leak. Likewise, before encouraging an increase in the rate of cell metabolism in an injured area, the active process of inflammation must be reduced (Table 5-10).

A distinction should be made between using cold modalities for ROM exercises and using heat modalities before competition. Cold increases fluid viscosity and decreases the ability to perform rapid movements. During participation in a sport, athletes rely on the ability to move the extremities in a rapid, powerful manner. Heat is used for its ability to allow this type of movement. Ice is indicated after the activity to prevent reactivation of the inflammatory process. If motion is limited by pain, then cold should be used; if motion is limited by stiffness, heat would be the modality of choice.

The decision about when to use heat and cold should not be based on any predetermined time frame. This decision should be based on the desired physiological responses at any one point in time. When the desired goal is to limit

TABLE 5-10   Deciding Whether to Use Heat or Cold

Evaluate the patient to determine the answer to each of the following questions. If all of the answers to these questions are no, then heat can be safely used. As the number of yes answers increases, so does the indication to use cold:

1. Does the body area feel warm to the touch?
2. Is the injured area still sensitive to light to moderate touch?
3. Does the amount of swelling continue to increase over time?
4. Does swelling increase during activity (joint motion)?
5. Does pain limit the joint's range of motion?
6. Would you consider the acute inflammation process to still be active?
7. Does the patient continue to display improvement with the use of cold modalities?

or reduce the amount of inflammation, cold should be used. When the inflammatory response has subsided to the point at which tissue healing begins, heat is applied. When in doubt, use cold.

The patient's preference of modalities should also be considered. Some patients prefer cold modalities, but more commonly, they prefer heat. For many, the change from cold to heat is a milestone signaling that their healing process is progressing.

Chapter 6

Clinical Application of Thermal Modalities

This chapter describes common methods of applying therapeutic cold and superficial heating agents; unique physiological effects; the procedures used; and the specific indications, contraindications, and precautions in their use. The deep-heating agents, therapeutic ultrasound and shortwave diathermy, are discussed in the next section.

● Multiple methods are used to apply cryotherapy and superficial heating agents. Although the physiological effects are similar within each classification—cold or heat—each technique has its individual benefits and limitations. The stage of injury, the depth of the target tissues, the uniformity of the surface area being treated, and the patient outcomes factor into selecting the method of application. In many instances more than one technique may be appropriate. Refer to Chapter 5 for a detailed description of the physiological effects of cold and heat modalities.

The various modalities presented in this chapter generally do not require a physician's prescription or direction. However, professional responsibility dictates that clinicians become aware of state practice acts and professional standards of practice and work within those boundaries.

■ Cold Packs

Cold packs are delivered by one of four techniques: (1) plastic bags filled with cubed, crushed, or flaked ice; (2) reusable cold gel packs; (3) cold compression therapy (CCT) units; and (4) chemical (or "instant") cold packs.

The effectiveness of cold packs is based on their ability to safely decrease tissue temperatures to therapeutic levels. Superficial blood flow begins to decrease within the first minute of treatment. Subsequent cooling decreases cell metabolism and nerve conduction velocity. Maximum analgesia is obtained when skin temperature reaches 58°F (14.4°C) (see Therapeutic Temperature Benchmarks, Chapter 5).[16,40]

A layer of insulation is sometimes placed between the cold pack and the skin, often done with the well-meaning intent of patient comfort or frostbite prevention. However, with the exception of reusable cold packs, this technique limits the effects of cold to the point where the treatment yields little or no therapeutic benefits (Table 6-1).

✳ Practical Evidence

A layer of insulation is often placed between the cold pack and the patient's skin, either for comfort or convenience. In most cases this barrier layer decreases the amount of cooling to subtherapeutic temperatures.[34,133,134] An insulator should be used only when the direct placement of the cold pack on the skin is contraindicated.

The use of an insulating medium is indicated when a reusable cold pack is applied and in conditions where the patient's blood flow to the area is compromised, there is sensory deficit or cold intolerance, or the patient experiences Raynaud's phenomenon. If an insulating medium is used, extend the treatment duration beyond the normal treatment time for the target tissue to reach the desired therapeutic range. Ice applied over an elastic wrap would require a treatment duration of approximately 109 minutes to decrease the skin temperature to therapeutic ranges; when applied over a single layer of dry terry cloth toweling, a treatment duration of 151 minutes would be required.[133]

TABLE 6-1	Skin Temperatures Obtained During Cold Pack Application With Insulators Used
Insulator Between Cold Pack and Skin	**Minimum Skin Temperature Obtained (°F) (percent increase from baseline)**
No insulation (baseline)	37.8
Wet wrap	48.0 (27.0%)
Frozen wrap	51.4 (36.0%)
Tegaderm™	60.8 (60.8%)
Plaster cast	65.7 (73.8%)
Dry wrap	67.1 (77.5%)
Synthetic cast	67.5 (78.6%)
Dry towel	69.6 (84.1%)
Wool and crepe dressing	80.6 (113.2%)

Sources: Ibrahim, et al,[132] Tsang, et al,[133] and Metzman, et al.[134]

Ice Bags

Ice bags (cold packs) are the most commonly used modality in the treatment of acute injuries. They are easy, efficient, and safe to use, requiring only plastic bags and either crushed, flaked, or cubed ice. Crushed ice is preferred because it allows the pack to better conform to the body part.

Reusable Cold Packs

Reusable cold packs contain a gel consisting of **silica** ● , water, and a form of antifreeze sealed in a plastic pouch (Fig. 6-1). Although they represent a convenient method for cold application in the clinical setting, the effectiveness of reusable cold packs diminishes when they are stored in an ice chest for long periods.

When not in use, reusable packs are stored in a dedicated cooling unit or freezer at a temperature of approximately 12°F (–11.1°C) (Fig. 6-2). Most types of reusable packs must not be cooled below 0°F (17.8°C) or damage to the pack will result. Some packs are also capable of being heated in water or using a microwave oven, but do not attempt to heat those packs that are not specifically designed for this purpose.

Because reusable cold packs reach temperatures well below freezing, they carry the risk of frostbite. To prevent frostbite, an insulating medium such as one layer of wet toweling or a wet elastic wrap must be placed between the reusable cold pack and the skin. The medium helps to insulate the skin from the subfreezing temperature. Although insulation is needed with reusable cold packs, avoid overinsulating the area. One or two layers of wet toweling or a wet elastic wrap will serve as adequate protection against

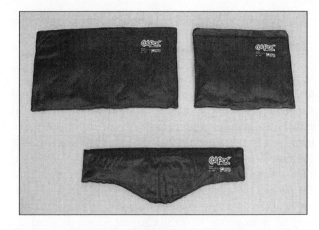

Figure 6-1. **Reusable Cold Packs.** Clockwise from upper left: Oversized (21 × 11 in.), standard size (14 × 11 in.), and cervical (23 in. long). Other sizes and shapes are also available. These packs are stored in a refrigeration unit between treatments.

Silica: A finely ground form of sand capable of holding water.

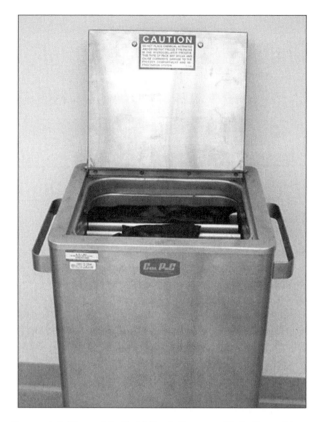

Figure 6-2. **Reusable Cold Pack Storage Unit.** Reusable cold packs are stored at a temperature of approximately 12°F (–11.1°C) when not in use. Allow an appropriate cooling period for the pack to reach its optimum treatment temperature level.

frostbite (refer to the manufacturer's recommendations). Adding too much insulation will prevent the effects of the cold from reaching the skin. Regardless of the insulating medium used, check the patient's skin regularly for signs of frostbite (see Box 5-5).

✱ Practical Evidence

Those forms of cryotherapy that undergo a change of state—that is, they melt during treatment—result in more subcutaneous cooling at 1 cm than those that do not melt.[15]

Cold Compression Therapy

Cold compression therapy (CCT) units combine constant external compression and cold application (Fig. 6-3). Individual CCT sleeves contour to specific body areas (e.g., the ankle, knee, and shoulder). The sleeves are filled with chilled water and provide up to 40 mm Hg of circumferential compression (some units allow the amount of pressure to be adjusted) that prevents the formation of swelling, may

decrease swelling, maintains deep tissue oxygen saturation, and increases the effective depth of cold penetration (also see Intermittent Compression Devices in Chapter 14.[57,135] These effects lead to decreased pain, decreased recovery time, and increased range of motion (ROM) after acute injury or surgery.[136–139] Some units have a motorized unit that eliminates the need to manually circulate chilled water into the appliance.

CCTs may not produce significant decreases in pain and joint edema formation compared to ice packs, partially because skin surface temperatures may not reach therapeutic levels.[67] Oxygen saturation in joints and tendons is improved by reducing congestion on the venule side of the capillary-venule junction.[59,60]

These units are a convenient method of applying cold and compression. Advanced CCT knee appliances are designed to prevent placing pressure on the popliteal vein. Compression of this vein can result in edema of the lower extremity.

Instant Cold Packs

Instant cold packs contain two chemicals separated from each other by a plastic barrier. Rupturing the seal allows the chemicals to mix. Cold is produced by an endothermic chemical reaction that absorbs heat from the tissues (Fig. 6-4). The relatively low decrease in skin temperature and the short duration of the reaction give instant cold packs a relatively short workable life. Instant cold packs are convenient in that they may be stored in a medical kit for emergency use. These packs can only be used once and must be properly disposed of after use.

When mixed, the chemicals contained in instant cold packs are extremely caustic to the skin. If a pack should develop a leak, discard it immediately and rinse the patient's skin with running water. For this reason, do not use instant cold packs on the face.

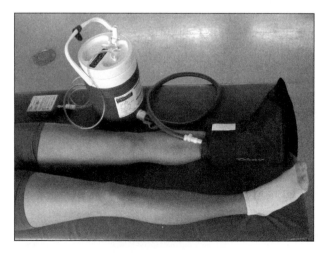

Figure 6-3. **Cold Compression Therapy Unit.** These devices deliver circumferential cold compression by a sleeve that fits around the extremity. See also Chapter 14.

At a Glance: **Cold Packs**

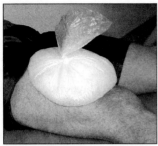

Crushed Ice Pack

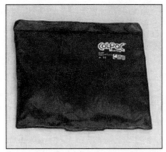

Reusable Cold Pack

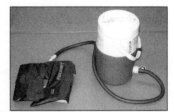

Cold Compression Therapy

Description

Cold packs include plastic bags filled with crushed, chipped, or flaked ice; **reusable cold gel packs** consist of a silica base and an anti-freeze gel; **cold compression therapy** units use chilled water to provide cold and compression; and **"instant" cold packs** use a chemical reaction to produce cold.

Indications

- Acute injury or inflammation
- Acute or chronic pain
- Prevention of swelling
- Decrease muscle spasm
- Neuralgia
- CNS spasticity

Primary Effects

ACUTE PATHOLOGY
- Decreases cell metabolism, reducing the amount of secondary hypoxic injury
- With compression and elevation, limits the formation of edema

OTHER EFFECTS
- Decreased metabolism reduces the release of inflammatory mediators and cellular by-products
- Decreases pain by slowing nerve conduction velocity and increasing the threshold of nerve endings
- Causes local vasoconstriction

Contraindications

- Uncovered open wounds
- Circulatory insufficiency
- Cold allergy and/or hypersensitivity
- Anesthetized skin
- Deep vein thrombosis
- Cardiovascular disease (see Table 5-2)

Treatment Duration

ICE BAGS, REUSABLE COLD PACKS, AND
INSTANT COLD PACKS
- The treatment duration depends on the treatment goal, target tissues, and the amount of subcutaneous adipose tissue (see Box 5.3).
- Applications should be no less than 2 hours apart.
- In the immediate care of injuries, keep the body part wrapped and elevated between treatments.
- When treating deep structures, the treatment duration should be increased as the amount of adipose tissue increases.

COLD COMPRESSION THERAPY UNITS
In addition to the preceding protocol, CCTs may be applied continuously for 24 to 72 hours after acute injury or surgery.[136,138,139] The periods used to rechill the water provide sufficient time for the body part to rewarm.[140]

Precautions

- Cardiac or respiratory involvement.
- Application of ice packs over large superficial nerves (e.g., perineal or ulnar nerves) could cause neuropathy, especially if an elastic wrap is used. If an elastic wrap is used, avoid applying too much pressure (see Clinical Techniques: Compression Wraps).
- Recheck the patient regularly for signs of nerve dysfunction, such as tingling in the distal extremity, or unwanted reaction to the treatment.
- When reusable cold packs are used or in the presence of vascular insufficiency, check the patient for frostbite.
- Application of a CCT unit over an elastic wrap can result in increased pressure being placed on the tissues.
- The content of instant cold packs can produce chemical burns if it comes into contact with the skin. Avoid use around the face, eyes, and other sensitive areas.

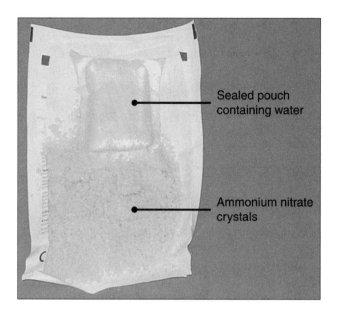

Sealed pouch containing water

Ammonium nitrate crystals

Figure 6-4. **Inside an Instant Cold Pack**. A bag containing water and ammonium nitrate crystals is sealed within a pouch. When the inner bag is ruptured, the water and crystals mix, causing a chemical reaction that produces cold (note that the chemicals may vary). Instant cold packs should not be opened. Torn packs or packs that develop a leak should be immediately discarded.

● EFFECTS ON

The Injury Response Process

The application of cold packs decreases tissue temperature, resulting in a decrease in cellular metabolic rate. All subsequent effects of cold application are related to this decreased cell metabolism. In acute injuries, the most beneficial effect of cold application is to reduce the need for oxygen. More cells are able to survive in the oxygen-starved environment because of their decreased metabolic rate. When combined with compression and elevation, the edema in the area is reduced, and compression acts to have the effects of cold affect deeper tissues.[8] These factors limit the scope of the original injury and reduce the amount of secondary injury.

Activation of cold receptors, slowing nerve depolarization and repolarization decreases the transmission rate of nerve impulses and increases the depolarization threshold, thereby decreasing pain. Decreased pain will reduce muscle spasm and help improve ROM. Inflammation is decreased as the result of reduction in the release of inflammatory mediators, decreased cell metabolism, and reduced blood flow.

Refer to Chapter 5 for a detailed description of the effects of cold.

Setup and Application

Before the application of each of the following forms of cold application, ensure that the patient is free of contraindications (see At a Glance: Cold Packs).

Ice Packs

1. Ensure the patient is free of contraindications to the application of ice packs.
2. Fill the bag with enough ice to last for the duration of the treatment but avoid overfilling. Overfilling the bag prevents it from being molded to the body part.
3. Remove excess air from the bag to allow the ice to better conform to the body part.
4. More than one bag may be required to fully cover the area.
5. In acute injuries, or when compression is desired, wet an elastic wrap and apply one layer of compression around the injured area (see Clinical Technique 1.1). A tub of cold "wet wraps" can be kept soaking in the refrigerator for this purpose.

This use of a wet compression wrap assists in increasing the effective depth of cold penetration.[8] Areas such as the acromioclavicular joint are not practical for wet wraps. In cases such as this a moist towel or thin sponge placed over the injured tissues may be substituted for the wrap. The cold packs are then held in place with dry wraps. Remember that overinsulating the ice bag will decrease the effectiveness of the treatment.

✱ Practical Evidence

To obtain maximal intramuscular temperature decrease, wrap the ice pack on using elastic wraps. Ice packs applied using elastic wraps result in more intramuscular temperature reduction than ice packs applied using flexible plastic wraps, but both techniques decreased intramuscular temperatures more than cold applied without wraps.[14]

Ice bags filled with cubed or crushed ice with a small amount of water or that is allowed to begin to melt prior to treatment (i.e., stored in a refrigerator) produce more significant skin and intramuscular cooling than cubed or crushed ice.[22]

Continuous Application

Apply the ice bags over the injured area. Secure in place with an elastic or plastic wrap using approximately 30 to 40 mm Hg of pressure (Fig. 6-5).[14] However, pressures above 50 mm Hg do not produce meaningful intramuscular temperature decrease.[141] (Note: Inflating a blood pressure cuff around your arm or leg to 30 to 40 mm Hg will give you a good estimation of the amount of pressure that should be exerted when applying the compression wrap.)

Intermittent Application

The ice pack is placed or wrapped on the skin for 10 minutes, removed for 10 minutes, and then reapplied for another 10 minutes. This process is repeated for up to 2 hours. This

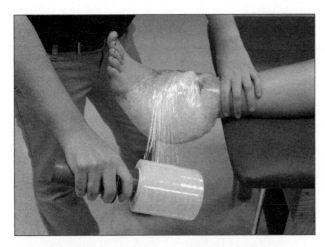

Figure 6-5. **Application of a Crushed Ice Pack.** Plastic wrapping material (that was originally used for shipping wrap) can be used to secure an ice pack in place. The plastic may help insulate the cold within the pack.

is an effective method for controlling pain, but has little effect on function or swelling.[25]

Reusable Cold Packs

1. Ensure the patient is free of contraindications for this treatment technique.
2. Select a pack large enough to cover the injured area, or use multiple packs.
3. Cover the skin overlying the treatment area with a wet towel or wet elastic wrap. Because of the risk of frostbite, a fully chilled reusable cold pack (less that 32°F [0°C]) must not contact the skin. Equally important, do not overinsulate the area. Too much insulation will decrease the heat absorption from the skin to the point where the treatment is ineffective.
4. Secure the pack in place with an elastic wrap.
5. Check the patient regularly for signs of frostbite (see Box 5-5).
6. The reusable cold pack may lose its effective treatment temperature after 20 minutes of use (refer to the manufacturer's specifications).[140]

Cold Compression Therapy Units

Refer to the instruction manual for the CCT unit being used. Following is a general overview of the setup and application of CCTs.

1. Ensure the patient is free of contraindications for this treatment technique.
2. Fill the cold cooling unit with ice as indicated. Shorter treatment times require less ice than treatments having a longer duration.
3. Add cold water to the depth of the FILL mark.
4. Allow the water to chill for approximately 5 to 10 minutes.
5. Choose the appropriate appliance for the body part and size of the treatment area.

6. Fasten the distal strap snugly, but not tight enough to cut off blood flow.
7. Fasten the proximal strap loosely enough to allow for proper venous drainage. Overtightening the proximal strap can inhibit venous and lymphatic drainage.
8. Connect the appliance to the cooler using the hose or hoses provided. If applicable, open the air vent on the top of the cooler to allow the fluid to flow into the appliance.
9. Elevate the cooler higher than the body part being treated. In manually filled CCTs the height of the cooler determines the amount of pressure within the appliance; consult your unit's user manual.
10. If applicable, remove the air-bleed cap to allow any trapped air to be forced out of the appliance.
11. Disconnect the hose or hoses from the appliance.
12. Draining the appliance or rechilling the fluid:
    (a) Reconnect the appliance to the hose or hoses.
    (b) Place the cooler at a level below the cuff.
    (c) Allow the fluid to drain from the appliance.
    (d) If the fluid is being rechilled, allow the fluid to remain in the cooler for 15 to 30 minutes; then repeat steps 7 through 10.

Instant Cold Packs

1. Ensure that the patient is free of contraindications for this treatment technique.
2. Shake the bag so that the contents are evenly distributed.
3. Squeeze or strike the bag to break the inner pouch.
4. Shake the bag to thoroughly mix the contents.
5. If indicated on the instructions of the particular brand of chemical cold pack you are using place a wet towel between the pack and the skin.
6. Secure in place with an elastic wrap.
7. If the solution within the bag leaks and makes contact with the skin, immediately remove the pack and thoroughly rinse the area with water. Monitor the patient for chemical burns. Refer to the packaging instructions for precise information on managing exposure to the pack's chemicals.
8. Properly dispose of the pack following treatment.

Treatment Duration

Historically, cold packs have been administered for 20 to 30 minutes per session. A more precise method of determining the treatment duration is to factor in the target tissues, the depth of those tissues, and—in the case of subcutaneous tissues—the amount of overlying adipose tissue. Skin numbness can occur in 10 minutes. Intramuscular cooling is related to the amount of subcutaneous adipose tissue and the depth below this layer (see Box 5-3).

✻ Practical Evidence

Muscular activity can quickly negate intramuscular cooling. The practice of wrapping an ice bag on patients and then allowing them to leave while wearing the pack prevents effective intramuscular cooling.[18,34]

▧ Ice Massage

Ice massage is used to deliver cold treatments to small, evenly shaped areas. It is most effective in cases involving muscle spasm, contusions, and other minor injuries limited to a well-localized area and to numb relatively small areas of the skin. The patient may be able to administer self-treatment either in the clinical setting or as a part of the home treatment program. When appropriate, this method of cold application is convenient, practical, and time efficient, providing cold treatments.

Ice massage produces a more rapid decline in intramuscular temperature than does an ice pack, but only when it is applied to a small treatment area (e.g., 4 × 4 cm, which is only slightly larger than the face of the ice massage cup). Although ice massage results in a quicker cooling time, following 15 minutes of ice massage and 15 minutes of ice pack application, there are no significant differences in intramuscular temperature or the duration of effects.[6]

At a Glance: **Ice Massage**

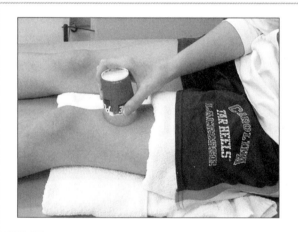

Treatment Duration

- 5 to 15 minutes (or until the ice runs out). When treating deep structures, the treatment duration should be increased as the amount of adipose tissue increases.

If the purpose of the ice massage is to produce numbness, the treatment may be discontinued when the patient's skin is insensitive to touch. These treatments may be repeated as necessary (i.e., when sensation returns).

Description

- Water frozen in a paper cup that is massaged over a small area of skin

Indications

- Subacute injury or inflammation
- Reduce muscle spasms
- Prior to ROM exercises
- Trigger point therapy
- Muscle strains
- Contusions
- Acute or chronic pain
- Rapid cooling of the skin

Primary Effects

- Decreases the sensitivity of cutaneous nerve receptors
- Decreases pain
- Breaks pain-spasm-pain cycle

Contraindications

- Cases in which pressure on the injury is contraindicated
- Suspected fractures
- Uncovered open wounds
- Circulatory insufficiency
- Cold allergy and/or hypersensitivity
- See Table 5-2

Precautions

- Anesthetized skin
- In some injuries, the pressure of the massage may be contraindicated.

● E F F E C T S   O N

The Injury Response Cycle

In addition to the general effects associated with cold application (see Chapter 5), the massaging action of this treatment assists in decreasing pain and muscle spasm. The sensation of movement stimulates large-diameter nerves and the cold temperature activates ascending pain control mechanisms. Together these effects activate the gate-control mechanism, inhibiting the transmission of pain and, in turn, causing a decrease in muscle spasm. Following treatment there is an almost immediate increase in the pain pressure threshold and decreased EMG activity, suggesting activation of descending inhibitory pathways.[105] These effects do not influence muscle torque production[98] or other muscle inflammatory markers.[2]

✳ Practical Evidence

Ice massage is effective at rapidly producing analgesia and anesthesia and decreasing intramuscular tissue temperature, but only when small treatment areas are treated (approximately 4 × 4 cm).[105,142] Although the initial decrease in temperature is greater using ice massage, there is no difference in intramuscular temperature relative to an ice pack following 15 minutes of treatment.[6]

Ice massage is not the modality of choice for acute ligament injuries because no compression is available during the treatment, potentially increasing the amount of hemorrhage and swelling, and because of the relatively small surface area that can be effectively treated with ice massage. However, when the muscle is placed on gentle stretch, ice massage is often indicated for acute strains.

Subcutaneous tissue temperatures are not reduced at the same magnitude and duration as other forms of cold application, an effect related to the decreased treatment duration and the movement of ice.[98] In the event that this is the only form of ice treatment available at the time of the injury, additional steps must be taken to limit the amount of swelling. Wrap the injured body part with an elastic bandage and elevate the body part to reduce edema after the treatment.

Setup and Application

1. Ensure that the patient is free of contraindications for this treatment technique.
2. Ice cups are made by filling paper cups three-quarters full and storing them in a freezer.

Reusable plastic cups specifically designed for ice massage are commercially available.
3. The treatment area should be no larger than two to three times the size of the ice cup. Smaller treatment areas will increase the rate of subcutaneous cooling. Large treatment areas can be ineffective because as one area cools, the previously cooled area warms.
4. Surround the treatment area with a towel to collect water runoff.
5. Slowly massage the ice over the injured area in overlapping strokes or circles.
6. Increased pressure between the ice and the skin will decrease the amount of time required to obtain skin numbness.[142]
7. The paper must be continually removed from the cup as the ice melts to prevent it from rubbing on the skin.

◼ Ice Immersion

Ice immersion (ice slush or ice bath) involves placing the body part into a mixture of ice and water having a temperature range of 50°F to 60°F (10°C to 15.6°C). This treatment is useful for injuries involving an irregular surface.

This can be an uncomfortable method of cold application. Pain is most intense during the first 3 minutes and remains high during the first 5 minutes of immersion.[143] This effect may limit patient compliance, especially when the fingers or toes are immersed.

Increased pain may be related to the increased surface area exposed to the cold. When the fingers or toes are immersed, they are exposed to cold across their circumference and at the distal end. Because their diameter is small, the effects of cold penetrate to bone level. Another factor that may account for the increased pain experienced is stimulation of the lumina in the nailbed. This is a hypersensitive area that may be overstimulated by the presence of cold. You can test this hypothesis on yourself by simply applying pressure with your thumbnail on the white crescent in your opposite thumbnail. A **Neoprene** • covering ("toe cap") can make ice immersion more tolerable when the fingers or toes are not the target of the treatment (Fig. 6-6).[46,144]

Repeated exposure to ice immersion increases the patient's tolerance to this treatment.[47] The pain and affective response to this treatment can be decreased by explaining to the patient the sensations to be expected.[45,46,143]

Despite the discomfort associated with ice immersion, this technique allows for circumferential cooling and simultaneous ROM exercise. The use of Neoprene, gradually decreasing the temperature of the immersion, and communicating with the patient can make this treatment more tolerable and maximize its therapeutic benefits.

Neoprene: A synthetic rubber material.

At a Glance: Ice Immersion

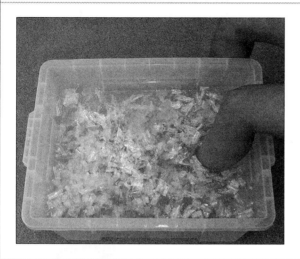

Treatment Duration

- 10 to 15 minutes. When treating deep structures, the treatment duration should be increased as the amount of adipose tissue increases.
- Lower treatment temperatures may require shorter treatment durations.
- Treatments may be repeated as needed.

Description

A tub or bucket is filled with ice and water and is used for cooling large and/or irregularly shaped areas. The body part, usually the foot and ankle or elbow, wrist, and hand is then immersed in the solution.

Indications

- Acute injury or inflammation
- Acute, chronic, or postsurgical pain
- Prior to ROM exercise

Temperature Range

- 50°F to 60°F (10°C to 15.6°C)
- The temperature should be increased as the proportion of the body area immersed increases.

Contraindications

- Cardiac or respiratory involvement
- Uncovered open wounds
- Circulatory insufficiency
- Cold allergy and/or hypersensitivity
- Absolute inability to tolerate the cold temperature
- See Table 5-2

Primary Effects

- Decreases cell metabolism, reducing the amount of secondary hypoxic injury
- Decreased metabolism reduces the release of inflammatory mediators and cellular by-products
- Decreases pain by slowing nerve conduction velocity and increasing the threshold of nerve endings
- Causes local vasoconstriction

Precautions

- Anesthetized skin
- Ice immersion is the most uncomfortable of all the cold treatments. Neoprene "toe caps" may be used to decrease discomfort.
- Avoid having the patient continually immerse and withdraw the body part from the immersion. If the limb is repeatedly removed and then reimmersed, it only increases the duration of pain.
- The limb's gravity-dependent position increases the risk of swelling.
- Care should be taken when relatively subcutaneous nerves (e.g., ulnar nerve as it crosses the elbow) are immersed. Because of the chance of cold-induced nerve palsy, slightly increase the temperature of the immersion, and check the patient regularly.

● EFFECTS ON

The Injury Response Process

The effects of ice immersion are as described in the general effects of cold application (see Chapter 5). The intensity of cold is greater with ice immersion because of the large surface area exposed. Therefore, the resulting drop in skin and subcutaneous temperature is more pronounced than with other methods of cold application.[145] Ice immersion is the most effective method to decrease sensory and motor nerve conduction velocity.[68] As long as there is a proper rewarming

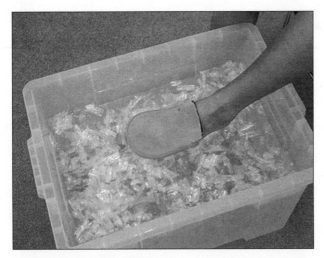

Figure 6-6. **Neoprene Toe Cap.** Covering the toes or fingers with an insulating material such as neoprene makes ice immersion treatment more tolerable.

period, ice immersion does not appear to negatively affect joint proprioception during activity.

The use of ice immersion places the limb in a dependent position, increasing the capillary **hydrostatic** • pressure within the capillaries, encouraging the leakage of fluids into the interstitial space that may cause increased swelling.[120] The use of active ROM exercises during the immersion will aid venous return (see the following sections on Whirlpools and Edema Formation and Reduction). Following treatment of acute or subacute injuries, wrap and elevate the limb to encourage venous and lymphatic drainage.

Setup and Application

1. Ensure that the patient is free of contraindications for this technique.
2. Prepare a bucket, tub, or similar container with cold water and ice. The temperature used will depend somewhat on the person's ability to tolerate the cold. Generally, patients who have had repeated exposure to this treatment can tolerate a lower temperature. Another approach is to start the patient at a tolerable temperature and to add ice as the treatment progresses.
3. The temperature of the treatment is related to the size of the body area being treated (Fig. 6-7). To prevent hypothermia during full-body immersion, as the size of the area being treated (the proportion of the total body area) is increased, the temperature of the water is increased.
4. Colder treatment temperatures may be better tolerated if the fingers or toes are insulated from the water by a Neoprene covering.
5. Avoid having the patient continually immerse and withdraw the body part from the immersion. Initially, the cold will cause a burning or aching sensation. To lessen discomfort, explain to the

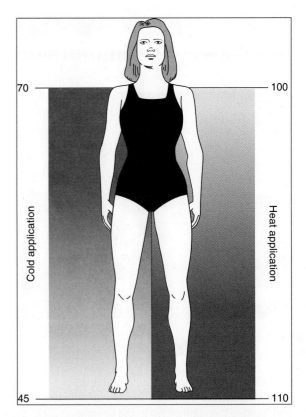

Figure 6-7. **Relationship Between Treatment Temperature and the Percentage of the Body Immersed.** During cold immersion, the temperature of the water should be increased as the percentage of the body immersed increases. During hot immersion, the temperature of the water decreases as the percentage of the body immersed increases.

patient that the treatment will be uncomfortable only for a few minutes, but numbness will soon follow. If the limb is repeatedly removed and then reimmersed, it only increases the duration of pain.
6. Continue to monitor the patient. The discomfort, sensation, and possible change in blood pressure associated with ice immersion may result in unconsciousness.
7. Following the treatment, perform active ROM exercises if they are not contraindicated.
8. Because the limb is placed in a gravity-dependent position, it should be wrapped and elevated after the treatment.

■ Cryostretch

Cryostretch combines the effects of cold application and passive stretching, leading to its alternate name, "spray and stretch." A vapocoolant spray is used to rapidly decrease skin temperature and reduce pain transmission. This is combined with simultaneous passive stretching to relieve local muscle spasm to effectively reduce the amount of pain and spasm associated with strains and trigger points (Fig. 6-8). A chart of trigger point pain patterns is presented in Appendix B.

Hydrostatic: Relating to the pressure of liquids in equilibrium or to the pressure they exert.

At a Glance: **Cryostretch**

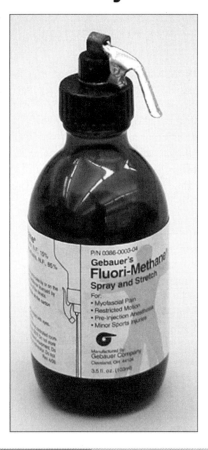

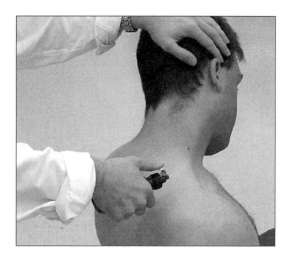

Description

A vapocoolant spray, a liquid that quickly evaporates and cools the skin, is applied to the skin while the underlying muscles and fascia are simultaneously stretched. Cryostretch is used for treating trigger points, local muscle spasm, and other myofascial conditions.

Indications

- Trigger points
- Muscle spasm
- Decreased ROM

Primary Effects

VAPOCOOLANT SPRAY
The rapid evaporation of the spray cools the skin and desensitizes nerve endings.
STRETCHING
Elongates muscle fibers and other soft tissues, breaking muscle spasm and releasing adhesions. Vapocoolant sprays are not an effective means of providing immediate treatment for acute injuries.

Contraindications

- Allergy to the spray
- Acute and/or postsurgical injury
- Open wounds
- Contraindications relating to cold applications
- Contraindications relating to passive stretching
- Use around the eyes. When treating the upper extremity, torso, or neck, protect the patient's eyes from the spray.

Treatment Duration

- The treatment proceeds through three or four sweeps, with sufficient time for the tissue to rewarm between sprays. Treatments are given once a day. When treating deep structures, the treatment duration should be increased as the amount of adipose tissue increases.
- See the text for a complete description of the procedure.

Precautions

- Cold sprays are capable of causing frostbite if improperly used.
- If ethyl chloride is used, be aware that it is extremely flammable; avoid using it around possible sources of ignition, including smoking and electrical sparks; ethyl chloride is a local anesthetic; however, if the fumes are inhaled, it very quickly becomes a general anesthetic.
- Fluoromethane contains ozone-depleting chemicals but has been granted an exception for use by the Environmental Protection Agency.

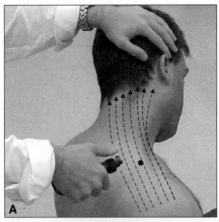

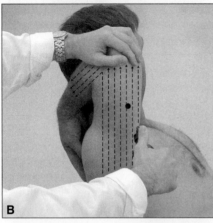

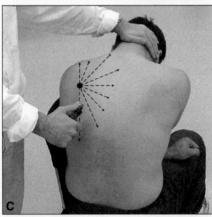

Figure 6-8. **Cryostretch Techniques**. The muscle and skin are placed on stretch and passively elongated as they are cooled (see Setup and Application). Treatment technique for the (A) upper trapezius; (B) triceps brachii; and (C) lower, middle, and upper trapezius.

Cryostretch has traditionally been performed with ethyl chloride because of its ability to evaporate quickly and cool the superficial tissue. However, ethyl chloride possesses many inherent dangers: it is highly flammable; it acts as a general anesthetic if inhaled; and because it decreases the skin temperature so drastically, there is a high potential for frostbite. Because of these risks, ethyl chloride has been replaced by fluoromethane spray, which is less volatile and has a safer cooling effect.[146] Ice massage may also be used instead of fluoromethane.

● EFFECTS ON

The Injury Response Process

The evaporation of the coolant on the skin causes stimulation of cutaneous sensory nerves and a reduction in motor neuron activity. This stimulus masks pain by reducing the intensity and speed of pain transmission. The passive stretching assists in breaking the pain-spasm-pain cycle by lengthening the muscle fibers. This combination of pain reduction and soft tissue stretching makes this a particularly effective method of trigger point therapy. The rewarming period following application is relatively brief, so the analgesic effects are less than ice packs and have a shorter duration of pain reduction.[147]

The effect of cold sprays is limited to that of a counterirritant. Vapocoolant sprays do not produce the cellular and vascular responses associated with other forms of cold application. The brief cooling of superficial nerves may impair joint position sense, but this effect is so transient that function is not hindered.[82] Vapocoolant sprays are ineffective in the treatment of acute musculoskeletal trauma. Although the evaporation of the liquid rapidly cools the skin and produces temporary pain relief, the other physiological effects of cold application do not occur.

Setup and Application

1. Ensure that the patient is free of contraindications for this treatment technique.
2. Position the patient so that the muscle group being treated may be easily stretched.
3. If the treatment is being applied to the upper extremities, cervical spine, or upper chest, position the patient's face to avoid being caught in the stream.
4. The nozzle of the bottle should be approximately 12 inches from the skin. The spray should strike the skin at a 30- to 45-degree angle. The closer to the body that the bottle is held, the warmer the coolant stream feels.
5. Spray the entire muscle length in a sweeping manner in one direction only. The speed of the sweep should allow the tissue to become covered, but not frosted because this creates the risk of frostbite.
6. Apply pressure to passively stretch the muscle group. Come to, but do not exceed, the point of pain.
7. Allow the tissue to rewarm.
8. Instruct the patient to take deep, relaxing breaths before stretching the muscle.
9. Continue for two or three more sweeps with increasing stretch on the muscle. Allow the tissue to rewarm between each sweep.
10. Repeat until the desired amount of stretch has occurred.
11. The cryostretch treatment may be followed by a moist heat treatment or massage.

Whirlpools

Whirlpools are effective for applying heat or cold to irregularly shaped areas. Large immersion tanks make it possible to perform ROM activities and exercise while also receiving the thermal benefits of the treatment by taking advantage of the physical characteristics of water. Energy is transferred to or from the body by means of convection. In a hot whirlpool, heat is transmitted to the body. In a cold whirlpool, heat is transmitted away.

A turbine is used to regulate the water flow and the amount of air introduced into the flow (aeration). Water enters through an inlet on the turbine's stem, where the motor forces it back into the tub, causing agitation of the water (the "whirlpool" effect). Air is also introduced into the stream, causing bubbles to circulate in the tank. The agitation and aeration are controlled by separate valves and can be adjusted to produce a range of effects, providing a massaging effect that produces sedation, analgesia, and increased circulation (Fig. 6-9).

For both hot and cold whirlpools, the temperature of the immersion depends on the proportion of the total body area immersed. In cold whirlpool treatments, the temperature of the water is increased as the body area being treated increases. Hypothermia can result if too large an area is cooled too rapidly for too long a duration.

During hot whirlpool treatments, the temperature of the water is decreased as the total body area immersed increases (see Fig. 6-7). When the temperature of the water is equal to or greater than the body temperature, heat loss can occur only through evaporation and respiration. If the patient's core temperature is increased too greatly, **hyperthermia** ● may result. During a full-body immersion the patient can lose heat only through the head and through breathing, increasing the risk of heat stress. Moderate to strenuous exercise while in the immersion will further increase the core temperature.

Physical Effects of Water Immersion

The physical characteristics of water, **buoyancy, resistance,** and **hydrostatic pressure,** create a good supportive medium for active ROM exercises. These benefits can be obtained by the extremities in clinical-sized whirlpools or body wide in deeper immersion tanks such as spas, exercise therapy pools, and swimming pools (Fig. 6-10). The temperature of the water is the most important property of immersion treatments.

Buoyancy describes the lifting force (thrust) provided by water and is explained by Archimedes's principle. If the body's **specific gravity** ● is equal to that of the water (1.0 for pure water), it floats just beneath the surface. If the body's specific gravity is greater than water, it sinks; if it is less, it floats. Therapeutically, buoyancy is used to reduce compressive forces on weight-bearing joints and assist in anti-gravity motions.

Resistance to movement is produced by the water's viscosity. The amount of resistance depends on the speed of the motion and the proportion of the body (or limb) that is immersed. Faster motions produce more resistance than slower motions; it is easier to walk than run through water 3 feet deep. Resistance also increases as the surface area

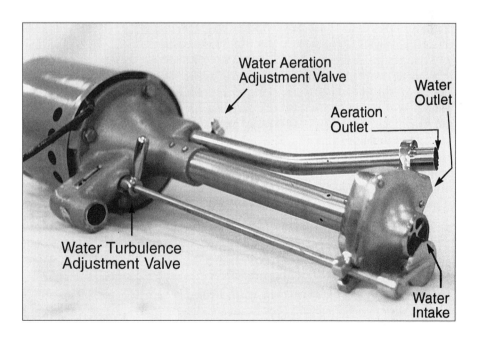

Figure 6-9. **A Whirlpool Turbine.** Note the position of the turbulence and aeration valves, and the water intake port. The water is driven through the turbine and returned to the tub under pressure. The aeration outlet is in front of the water outlet, forcing bubbles to flow in the water.

Water Aeration Adjustment Valve

Water Outlet

Aeration Outlet

Water Turbulence Adjustment Valve

Water Intake

Hyperthermia: Increased core temperature.
Specific gravity: The ratio of the density of a substance to the density of pure water taken as a standard when both densities are obtained by weighing in air.

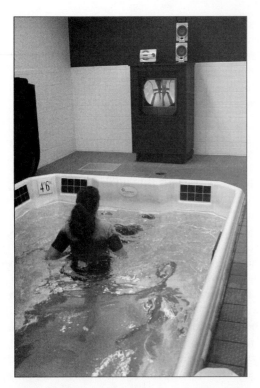

Figure 6-10. **Exercise Therapy Pool.** These water-filled tanks have a treadmill on the bottom, allowing the patient to walk or run during treatment. The water provides buoyancy and resistance during exercise.

increases; it is easier to run through ankle-deep water than through waist-deep water.

Hydrostatic pressure describes the force exerted on a body part immersed in a nonmoving fluid. As described by Pascal's law, the fluid will conform to the irregular surface area and exert an equal pressure across the circumference. The amount of pressure increases with depth, exerting 0.73 mm Hg per centimeter of immersion. When standing in an immersion, a pressure gradient is formed between the amount of pressure exerted on the skin at the surface of the water (low pressure) and the pressure exerted at the distal extremity (high pressure) (Fig. 6-11). This pressure gradient can help force fluids in the distal extremity proximally, especially when combined with walking. The combination of hydrostatic pressure and buoyancy helps provide the patient with balance and stability.

● E F F E C T S   O N

The Injury Response Process

The thermal effects of cold and heat are described in the relevant sections of Chapter 5. Hot whirlpools promote muscle relaxation, and cold whirlpools decrease muscle spasm and muscle spasticity. Cold whirlpools administered at a temperature of 50°F (10°C) for 20 minutes result in the

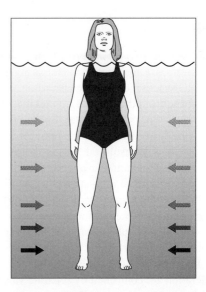

Figure 6-11. **Hydrostatic Pressure During Water Immersion.** As the depth of the body part in the water increases, the pressure exerted on the body increases by 0.73 mm Hg for each centimeter of depth. The resulting pressure gradient can encourage venous return from the lower extremity, but only when the patient is immersed at least to the mid-chest.

same amount of intramuscular cooling as found with ice packs. Because of the large treatment area, the effects of post-treatment cooling are more pronounced following a whirlpool treatment.[10] This effect is beneficial when used before rehabilitation exercises. An additional effect of the turbulence from the flowing water is the creation of a **sedative** ● and analgesic effect on sensory nerves.

Blood Flow
The increase or decrease in blood flow is proportional to the temperature of the bath. Hot whirlpool treatments above 101.5°F (38.6°C) cause a 21% increase in blood flow and a 50% increase when the temperature is increased to 108.5°F (42.5°C).[148] Although agitation of the water is thought to provide a "massaging" effect, agitation in and of itself does not significantly increase blood flow.[148]

Edema Formation and Reduction
There is a complex relationship between whirlpool baths and the formation or reduction of edema. Except for cases where the patient is supine in the tank, the limb is in a gravity-dependent position that could encourage the formation of edema.

When a patient is standing in a neutral-temperature immersion, the hydrostatic pressure gradient formed by the water pressure at the feet being greater than the water pressure at the surface will encourage venous return. Slow walking or other exercise will cause the deep venous pressure within the calf to increase to 200 mm Hg, further increasing the venous return pressure gradient, thus encouraging venous return.[48] This effect is similar to an air-filled

---

Sedative: An agent that causes sedation.

balloon in a swimming pool. The balloon will maintain its shape when it is near the surface of the water. If you grab the balloon and try to swim to the bottom of the pool with it, its shape elongates with the top being wider than the bottom.

The hydrostatic pressure exerts a force of 0.73 mm Hg per centimeter of depth. A mid-calf immersion, approximately 25 cm (10 in.) deep, would exert 18.25 mm Hg of pressure at the foot. Increasing this distance to 50 cm (20 in.) would exert 36.5 mm Hg at the feet. Normal **diastolic blood pressure** ● is approximately 80 mm Hg (see Fig. 6-11). Therefore, an immersion of approximately 110 cm (43.3 in.; 3 feet, 7 in.) is required to exceed diastolic blood pressure and prevent the formation of distal edema.

Increase in limb volume is related to the temperature of the water. As the temperature increases, so does the blood volume in the lower extremity, increasing by 44 to 64 mL.[48] The total accumulation of blood associated with hot whirlpools is based on the hydrostatic pressure and exercise acting to reduce the total accumulation. If edema formation is a concern during hot whirlpool treatments, reduce the temperature of the immersion. In moderate temperature water (approximately 86°F [30°C]), deep water immersion and moderate exercise can reduce leg edema.[149]

Cold whirlpool treatments are not recommended for the care of acute injuries where edema is still forming. If this method of acute injury management is unavoidable, the turbine should be set on "low" or not be turned on during treatment. A compression wrap should be applied and the body part should be elevated after the treatment.

Pain Control

The circulation and aeration of the water decrease pain by stimulating A-beta nerve fibers (sensory nerves), activating the gate-control mechanism. Increased blood flow, the reduction of edema, and improved ROM also assist in reducing the mechanical and chemical pain triggers. The buoyancy of the water helps to reduce compressive stresses on joint surfaces and provide short-term pain reduction or pain caused by joint loading during exercise. Temperature-dependent pain-reducing mechanisms are also activated.

Range of Motion

Increased blood flow, reduced pain, and reduced edema all contribute to increasing the joint's ROM. Gravity-assisted motion is aided by the buoyancy of the water. During dry-land exercise, the effect of gravity on the rotational movement of joints is greatest when the limb reaches parallel to the ground. When this motion is performed in water, the buoyancy of the limb helps to

counteract the force of gravity, making slow motion through the ROM possible.

✳ Practical Evidence

Lower extremity cold whirlpools (50°F, 10°C) can substantially decrease power, speed, and agility following treatment. Power is reduced for 32 minutes following treatment, while speed is decreased for 27 minutes and agility for 12 minutes.[68]

Wound Cleansing

Lavage—using water to cleanse wounds—can reach all portions of irregularly shaped surface areas and into open wounds. Water and water pressure encourage the hydration, softening, and subsequent débridement of tissues.[148] Hydrotherapy is often used in the management of open wounds, diabetic ulcers, pressure wounds, thermal burns, and **"turf burns** ● **."**

For wound cleansing, the water is heated to 96°F to 98°F (35.6°C to 36.7°C) and antibiotic agents or other chemicals are added to reduce the bacterial load of the skin.[150] In most cases, the turbine's stream should not directly strike the wound. Doing so may damage the fragile granulation tissue, force bacteria deeper into the tissue, or otherwise cause further damage to the wound.

The presence of open wounds requires that appropriate sterilization procedures be used both before and after the treatment. Tile tubs or spa-type whirlpools may harbor germs and are difficult to clean properly. Only stainless steel tubs should be used for wound cleansing or débridement.[151] The tank should be cleaned with an appropriate disinfectant before and after the treatment (see Cleaning the Whirlpool, page 149). The tank is filled with water, and a disinfectant is added. After the treatment, the tank should be drained and cleaned again. A culture kit can be used to check the whirlpool for contaminants.

Hubbard Tanks

The butterfly-shaped Hubbard tank is designed to allow a supine, partially submerged patient to abduct the arms and legs through their full ROM (Fig. 6-12). Although these devices were originally designed for orthopedic patients, their use has evolved to include the treatment of burns and spinal cord–injured patients. Because the extremities and torso are often immersed in a Hubbard tank, the standard treatment temperatures for this device are decreased to the range of 90°F to 102°F (32.2°C to 38.8°C).

Diastolic blood pressure: The lowest level of pressure in the arteries. For example, when a blood pressure reading is given as 120/80, 80 represents the diastolic value.

Turf burn: A deep abrasion caused by friction between the skin and artificial playing surfaces.

At a Glance: **Hot and Cold Whirlpools**

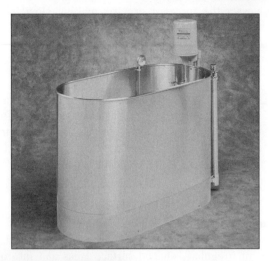

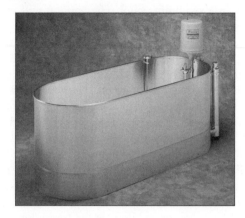

Description

A tub filled with warm or cold water. An attached turbine provides motion and aeration to the water. Left, "High Boy" whirlpool bath. The patient can immerse the extremity and perform ROM exercises. Right, "Lo Boy" whirlpool bath. The patient can sit in this tub with the legs extended.

Temperature Range

COLD WHIRLPOOL
50°F to 65°F (10°C to 16°C). Temperature is increased as the proportion of the body area treated increases.
HOT WHIRLPOOL
90°F to 110°F (32°C to 49°C). Temperature is decreased as the proportion of the body area treated increases.

Primary Effects

- Provides a supportive medium for range of motion exercises
- The water provides resistance to rapid motions
- Agitation and aeration of the water causes sedation, analgesia, and increased blood flow
- Also includes the effects of hot and cold treatments
- Cold whirlpool treatments result in longer lasting cooling of intramuscular tissues

Indications

- Decreased range of motion
- Subacute or chronic inflammatory conditions
- Promoting muscular relaxation
- Decreasing pain and muscle spasm
- Peripheral vascular disease (use a neutral temperature)
- Peripheral nerve injuries (avoid the extremes of hot and cold)

Contraindications

- Acute conditions in which water turbulence would further irritate the injured areas or in which the limb is placed in a gravity-dependent position
- Fever (in hot whirlpool)
- Patients requiring postural support during treatment
- Skin conditions in spa-type tubs. Otherwise, follow the cleaning instructions noted on page 149
- General contraindications listed for heat and cold treatments (Chapter 5)

Precautions

- The whirlpool must be connected to a ground-fault circuit interrupter (see Box 4-5).
- Instruct the patient not to turn the whirlpool motor on or off while in the water. Ideally, the switch to the motor should be out of the patient's reach.
- Patients who are receiving whirlpool treatments should be in view of a staff member at all times.
- Because of the discomfort associated with cold immersions, the treatment may be started at a comfortable, yet cool, temperature. Decrease the temperature gradually during the treatment by adding cold water.
- The combination of increased circulation and placement of the extremity in a gravity-dependent position tends to increase edema.
- Do not run the whirlpool turbine dry.
- The flowing water may nauseate some patients, especially those prone to motion sickness.[151]
- Patients who are under the influence of drugs (including alcohol) or those who have seizure disorders or heart disease are at risk of losing consciousness during treatment, especially when hot whirlpools are used.[146]
- The pressure associated with full-body immersion may impair breathing in individuals suffering from advanced respiratory disease.

Treatment Duration

- Initial whirlpool treatments are given for 5 to 10 minutes.
- The duration of treatments may be increased to 20 to 30 minutes as the program progresses. When treating deep structures, the treatment duration should be increased as the amount of adipose tissue increases.
- Treatments may be given once or twice a day.

Lo Boy and High Boy, courtesy of Whitehall Manufacturing, City of Industry, CA.

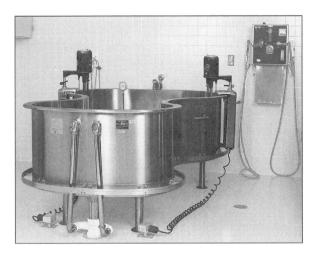

Figure 6-12. A "Hubbard Tank" Full-Body Whirlpool. These whirlpools are designed to allow the patient to lay supine and abduct the arms and legs. (Courtesy of Ferno Performance Pools, Wilmington, OH.)

Setup and Application

1. Ensure that the patient is free of contraindications to whirlpool immersion and the temperature of water used.
2. Instruct the patient not to turn the whirlpool on or off or touch any electrical connections while in the whirlpool or while the body is wet.
3. Fill the whirlpool to a depth sufficient to cover the area being treated, keeping in mind the effects of hydrostatic pressure. Be sure the amount of water is enough to run the motor safely.
4. Add a whirlpool disinfectant according to the manufacturer's directions.
5. If wounds are present on the body part being treated, add a disinfectant such as povidone, povidone-iodine, or sodium hypochlorite to the water.
6. Adjust the temperature for the type of effect desired and for the proportion of the body being treated.
7. The temperature of full-body warm whirlpool immersions should be further reduced if the patient will be performing moderate to strenuous exercise. Exercise increases the body's core temperature and would be magnified by higher water temperatures.
8. If an extremity is being treated, place the patient in a comfortable position using either a high chair or a whirlpool bench. Use rubber padding or a folded terry cloth towel to pad the limb where it contacts the tank.
9. If the entire body is being immersed, use a whirlpool stool or sling seat.
10. Turn the turbine on and adjust the turbulence. With subacute injuries, do not focus the turbulence directly on the affected area.
11. Patients receiving full-body treatments, whether hot or cold, must be monitored continuously.

Maintenance

The presence of electricity, water, and patients in the same room creates unique safety concerns. Refer to Electrical Systems and Hydrotherapy Area, in Chapter 5, regarding the safe operation of the hydrotherapy area.

Follow the manufacturer's guidelines for quarterly, 6-month, and annual maintenance requirements, including thermometer calibration by qualified personnel as a part of the annual inspection. Unplug the turbine from its power source prior to cleaning or moving the whirlpool tub.

Cleaning the Whirlpool

The whirlpool must be cleaned before and after treating a patient who has open wounds that will be exposed to the water. If no open wounds are permitted in the tub, the whirlpool should then be cleaned at the end of the workday. Spa-type whirlpools require special attention. Refer to the manufacturer's maintenance and hygiene requirements.

1. Drain the whirlpool after treatment.
2. Wear appropriate attire such as rubber gloves and a smock.
3. Refill the tub with hot (approximately 120°F [48.9°C]) water to a level sufficient to safely operate the turbine.
4. Add a commercial disinfectant, antibacterial agent, or chlorine bleach to the water, using the concentration indicated on the packaging.
5. Run the turbine for at least 1 minute to allow the cleaning agent to cycle through the internal components.
6. Drain the whirlpool and scrub the interior using a brush with a cleaner, paying close attention to the external turbine, thermometer stem, drains, welds, and other areas that could retain germs.
7. Thoroughly rinse the tub.
8. Clean the exterior surface with a stainless steel (or appropriate) cleaner. Stainless steel tubs should not be cleaned with bleach.
9. Culture kits are available to determine if bacteria are present in the tub.

Monthly or at Regular Intervals

Check the proper functioning of the ground fault circuit interrupter.

Annually

1. Have the whirlpool turbine inspected by a qualified service technician.
2. Calibrate the tub's thermometer.

■ Moist Heat Packs

A moist heat pack (MHP) is a canvas pouch filled with silica or a similar substance capable of absorbing a large number of water molecules. The pack is kept in a water-filled heating unit that is maintained at a constant temperature ranging between 160°F and 166°F (71.1°C and 74.4°C), although some packs can be heated in water on a stovetop or in a microwave oven for home use (refer to the manufacturer's instructions for at-home heating procedures).

The temperature range used for heating an MHP assists in killing any bacteria that may collect in the heating unit. Moist heat packs are a superficial heat modality, transferring energy to the patient's skin by way of conduction, with moisture assisting the transfer of energy.[7] Underlying tissue layers are heated through conduction from the overlying tissue. These packs are capable of maintaining a workable therapeutic temperature for 30 to 45 minutes after removal from the heating unit.

The layering around the hot pack (see Setup and Application) serves as insulation between the pack and the skin (Fig. 6-13). When the pack is placed on the skin, there is little compression of the protective covering, allowing air pockets to form within the layering, providing additional insulation. If the hot pack is compressed, such as when the patient is lying on it, the layering is moved together and the air is forced out. This decreases the available insulation and increases the amount of energy being transferred, increasing the possibility of the patient suffering burns. Lying on the hot pack also decreases capillary flow and energy lost to the environment, further increasing the possibility of burns occurring. For this reason patients should not lay on the MHP.

Moist heat packs are suitable for use over localized areas or on areas that normally cannot be treated by immersion in water, such as the cervical spine (Fig. 6-14). The wide array of sizes and styles of MHPs make them acceptable for use over the lumbar spine (medium or large size), the cervical spine (cervical pack), the shoulder (medium size), and the knee (medium size). The effectiveness of the MHP is diminished when used over irregular areas such as the ankle or fingers, in which case hot whirlpool or other immersion techniques should be considered.

The presence of water allows the rapid transfer of heat from the moist heat pack to the skin. Thick layers of adipose tissue insulates intramuscular tissues from this rapid heat exchange. Dry heat, such as that produced by chemical heat packs, has a lower temperature that results in a slower rate

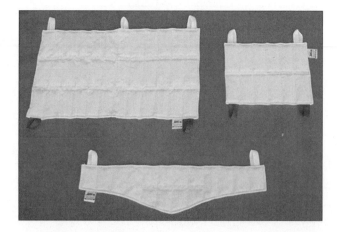

Figure 6-14. **Moist Heat Packs.** Clockwise from upper left: Oversized (15 × 24 in.), standard (10 × 12 in.), and cervical (24 in. long) packs. Other sizes and shapes are available.

of heat exchange. The lower treatment temperature allows a treatment duration of several hours. This long, slow heating is effective in increasing intramuscular temperatures beneath thick adipose tissue layers.[7]

● E F F E C T S   O N

The Injury Response Process

The specific effects of moist heat packs are the same as described for heat in general (see Chapter 5). When compared with dry heat, moist heat is considered a more comfortable method of application and may have greater benefit in reducing pain. Dry heating agents, such as chemical packs or an electrical heating pad, do not increase the skin temperature as rapidly as moist agents, allowing fresh blood to keep the tissue temperatures relatively low during normal therapeutic treatment durations. However, because electrical heating maintains a constant temperature during the treatment, over time the chance of burns increases unless temperature is controlled by a thermostat and/or timer.

✳ Practical Evidence

Moist heat packs are ineffective in increasing subcutaneous tissue temperatures in individuals who have thick adipose tissue layers. However, dry heat packs applied at a lower temperature for long treatment durations (up to 6 hours) can increase intramuscular tissue temperatures.[7] Chemical heat packs/wraps are best suited for this purpose.

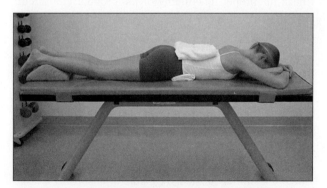

Figure 6-13. **Patient Positioning for Moist Heat Treatments of the Lumbar Spine.** Note the bolsters under the feet, abdomen, and face. This position relieves tension on the lumbar muscles.

The application of moist heat causes a rapid increase in the surface temperature of the skin. Vasodilation of the vessels produces an influx of blood to the area in an attempt to cool the tissues. Superficial muscle layers are directly

At a Glance: **Moist Heat Packs**

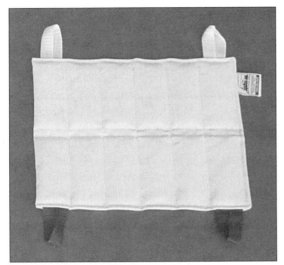

8 × 12 in. Moist Heat Pack

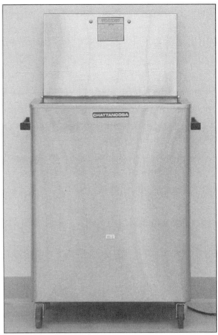

Moist Heating Unit

Description

Silica-filled packs are stored in hot water between use. The packs are then removed from the heating unit, wrapped in a terry cloth cover or towel, and used to deliver moist heat to the body. The resulting temperature increase is localized to superficial tissues.

Indications

■ Subacute or chronic inflammatory conditions
■ Reduction of subacute or chronic pain
■ Subacute or chronic muscle spasm
■ Decreased ROM
■ Hematoma resolution
■ Increasing muscle, tendon, and fascial elasticity
■ Reduction of joint contractures
■ Infection (see procedures in Setup and Application of moist heat packs)

Primary Effects

■ Increased blood flow/vasodilation
■ Increased cell metabolism
■ Muscular relaxation secondary to reducing muscle spindle sensitivity

Contraindications

■ Acute conditions: This modality will increase the inflammatory response in the area.
■ Peripheral vascular disease: The heat cannot be dissipated, thus increasing the chance of burns.
■ Impaired circulation.
■ Poor thermal regulation.

Temperature Range

■ Moist heat packs are stored in 160°F to 166°F (71.1°C to 74.4°C) water between treatments.
■ During application, insulation is added to the pack as needed to maintain a comfortable treatment.

Precautions

■ Do not allow the moist heat pack to come into direct contact with the skin because burns may result.
■ If the packs are changed during the course of the treatment, additional care must be taken to prevent burns.
■ Infected areas must be covered with sterile gauze or another type of material to collect seepage.
■ Do not allow the patient to lay on the heat pack. If this is unavoidable, add extra layers of insulation.

Treatment Duration

■ Moist heat packs are commonly used in treatment bouts of 20 to 30 minutes. When treating deep structures, the treatment duration should be increased as the amount of adipose tissue increases.
■ Treatments may be repeated as needed, but sufficient time should be allowed for the skin to cool before the next treatment is given.

heated by the heat packs, resulting in relaxation of the affected tissues. In areas with low amounts of overlying adipose tissue, blood flow can be affected up to 3 cm deep. Vasodilation and increased blood flow occur only while the hot packs are in contact with the body.[56] Using the triceps surae muscle group as a model, temperatures at 1 cm deep within the tissues are elevated by 38.5°F (±30.7°F) compared to only 17.6°F (±21.2°F) at a depth of 3 cm.[152] Thick layers of overlying adipose tissues reduce the effective depth of penetration.[152]

Relaxation of muscles or muscle layers that are more deeply situated results from soothing of the superficial motor and sensory nerves. When treating obese individuals, the clinician may find that hot packs are less effective in raising subcutaneous tissue temperature because the adipose tissue layer serves as insulation.

Setup and Application

1. Ensure that the patient is free of contraindications for this treatment technique.
2. Cover the pack with a commercial terry cloth covering, or fold a terry cloth towel so that there are five or six layers of towel between the pack and the skin (Fig. 6-15). The treatment temperature can be increased by removing towel layers or decreased by adding layers.
3. Place the pack on the patient in a comfortable manner. If having the patient lie on the pack is unavoidable, place additional toweling between the patient and the hot pack.

4. When treating an infected area, completely cover the skin with sterile gauze. After the treatment, dispose of the gauze in a biowaste container and wash the hot pack's covering using standard precautions.
5. Check the patient after the first 5 minutes for comfort and mottling. Recheck the patient regularly, and adjust the toweling if needed.
6. Some clinicians replace the hot pack every 8 to 10 minutes to maintain high treatment temperatures,[89] but properly heated packs contain sufficient energy for a 30-minute treatment.[108] If hot packs are replaced during the treatment, extra caution must be taken to check for burns arising from increased temperatures and rebound vasoconstriction.
7. After the treatment, return the moist heat pack to the heating unit and allow it to reheat for a minimum of 30 to 45 minutes before reuse.

Maintenance

Unplug the heating unit before performing any maintenance. Follow the manufacturer's guidelines for quarterly, 6-month, and annual maintenance requirements, including calibration by qualified personnel.

New Moist Heat Packs

Allow new moist heat packs to soak fully immersed in warm water for 2 hours before placing them in the heating unit.

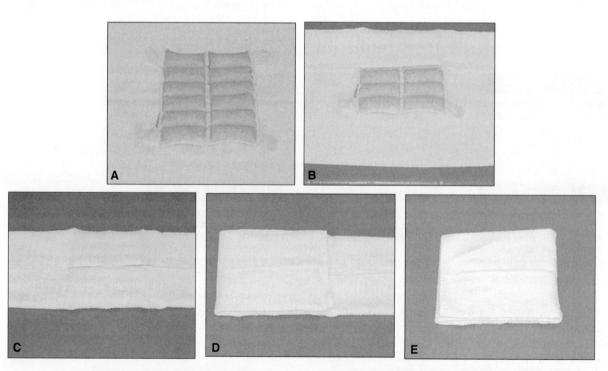

Figure 6-15. Insulating a Moist Heat Pack With a Terry Cloth Towel. (A) Center pack on a terry cloth towel. (B) and (C) Fold long edges toward the center of the pack. (D) and (E) Fold the short edges toward the center. This technique provides five layers of insulation. Additional toweling may be added to decrease the treatment intensity. Two towels may be required for larger moist heat packs.

Daily Maintenance

Ensure that the water level covers the top of the moist heating packs.

Biweekly Maintenance

1. Unplug and drain the heating unit.
2. Clean the storage unit, the racks, and the heating element with stainless steal cleanser, a vinegar and water mixture, or a mild abrasive cleanser. If the unit is made from stainless steel, DO NOT use a cleanser that contains chlorine bleach. Chlorine damages stainless steel. If local tap water has high level of chlorine, add a dechlorinator.
3. Remove sediment from the inside metal and heating coil with a firm brush or steel wool. Do not use metal objects to scrape off the sediment as this can damage the metal.
4. Fill the unit with enough water to cover the tops of the moist heat packs.
5. Scented or herbal additives should not be added to the water unless it is specifically approved by the manufacturer.

Care of the Moist Heat Packs

1. Discard any pack that may be contaminated with germs.
2. Discard any pack that is torn. The contents of the pack will leak out into the storage unit.
3. Do not allow the packs to dry out.
4. To store the packs for long periods, place wet packs in individual sealable plastic bags and store them in a freezer.

▨ Paraffin Bath

Paraffin is a superficial agent used for delivering heat to small, irregularly shaped areas, such as the hand, fingers, wrist, and foot. Although its use in sports medicine is limited, it is an effective method for delivering heat, and this form of thermotherapy may increase intra-articular temperature as much as 6.3°F (3.5°C).[28] The application of paraffin is beneficial in chronic conditions in which ROM is not an essential part of the treatment protocol, such as arthritis or chronic inflammatory conditions.

A paraffin bath contains a mixture of wax and mineral oil in a ratio of seven parts wax to one part oil (7:1). Melted paraffin is kept at a constant temperature of 118°F to 126°F (47.8°C to 52.2°C) for upper extremity treatments. Temperatures for treatments given to the lower extremity are decreased to 113°F to 121°F (45.0°C to 49.4°C) because the circulation is less efficient. Because of its low specific heat (0.5 to 0.65), paraffin can provide approximately six times the amount of heat as water. Consequently, the paraffin feels cooler and is more tolerable than water at the same temperature (see Box 5-1).

● EFFECTS ON

The Injury Response Process

In addition to the standard effects of heat application, paraffin increases perspiration in the treated area and softens and moisturizes the skin.

Setup and Application

There are several methods of paraffin application, the most common being the immersion and glove methods. Paraffin acts as both a heating agent or insulator when it is allowed to dry on the skin. With this in mind, the amount of heat delivered is adjusted by increasing or decreasing the wax layers. During immersion baths, the amount of insulation is increased with the number of layers added.

Preparation for Treatment

To avoid contaminating the paraffin, thoroughly clean and dry the body part before treatment. Remove chipped or flaking nail polish prior to treatment.

Immersion Bath

This is the best method for raising tissue temperature. However, the chance of burns is increased, so the patient must be closely monitored.

1. Ensure that the patient is free of contraindications for this treatment technique.
2. If possible, the patient should spread the fingers or toes to allow the paraffin to cover the maximum amount of surface area. The patient begins by dipping the body part into the paraffin and removing it. Allow this layer to dry (it will turn a dull shade of white).
3. Dip the extremity into the wax 6 to 12 more times to develop the amount of insulation necessary. Each dip should be slightly lower than the previous immersion. Allow the wax to dry between dips.
4. The patient then places the body part back into the paraffin for the duration of the treatment.
5. Instruct the patient to avoid touching the sides and bottom of the heating unit because burns may result.
6. Patients who are receiving an immersion treatment must not move the joints that are in the liquid. The cracking of the wax will allow fresh paraffin to touch the skin, increasing the risk of burns.
7. After the treatment, scrape off the hardened paraffin and discard it.

Pack (Glove) Method

The glove method is the safest method for delivering heat to the body with paraffin wax, but produces less heating than the immersion method. This method is recommended

At a Glance: **Paraffin Bath**

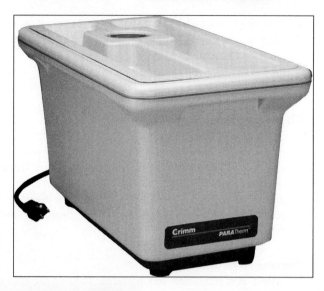

Description

A mixture of wax and mineral oil is melted in the unit. The low specific heat of the mixture allows warm temperatures to be used during treatment. Paraffin is used to deliver heat to small, irregularly shaped areas, especially when ROM exercises are not a part of the treatment, for the treatment of chronic inflammatory conditions, and softening the skin.

Primary Effects

- Increased perspiration
- Increased blood flow/vasodilation
- Increased cell metabolism

Temperature Range

118°F to 126°F (47.8°C to 52.2°C)

Treatment Duration

Paraffin treatments are given for 15 to 20 minutes and may be repeated several times daily.

Indications

- Subacute and chronic inflammatory conditions (e.g., arthritis of the fingers)
- Limitation of motion after immobilization

Contraindications

- Open wounds: Wax and oil would irritate the tissues.
- Skin infections: The warm, dark environment is excellent for breeding bacteria.
- Sensory loss.
- Peripheral vascular disease.
- See Table 5-7.

Precautions

- Do not allow the patient to touch the bottom or sides of the paraffin tank. Burns may result.
- The sensation of the paraffin is misleading as to the actual temperature of the treatment. The temperature of the paraffin is sufficient to cause burns, but its specific heat requires more time to transfer the energy.
- Avoid using paraffin with athletes who are required to catch or throw a ball (e.g., basketball players) or workers who are required to maintain a good grip (e.g., carpenters) after the treatment. The mineral oil in the paraffin mixture tends to make the hands slippery, making the task of catching a ball or holding onto a hammer difficult.

ParaTherapy, courtesy of Whitehall Manufacturing, City of Industry, CA.

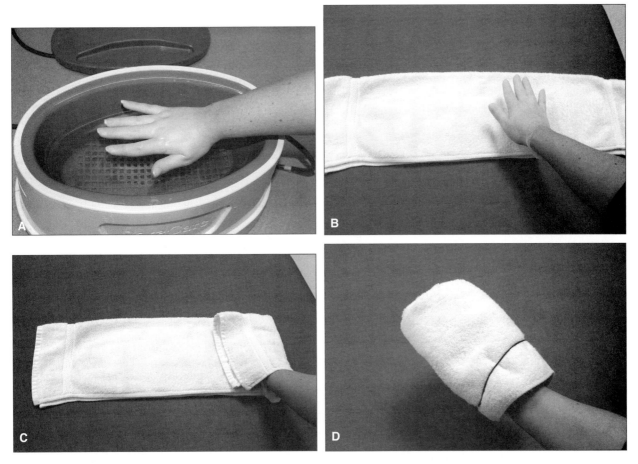

Figure 6-16. **The Glove Method of Paraffin Application.** (A) The body part, usually the hand, is dipped in the paraffin mixture 7 to 12 times. (B) and (C) After the outer layer of the wax dries, the body part is wrapped with a terry cloth towel or aluminum foil. (D) The extremity remains wrapped for the remainder of the treatment. Custom cloth mitts and boots are also sold for this purpose.

for those patients who are in the subacute stage of healing or who have a vascular or nerve condition that would predispose them to burning. The body part may also be elevated during this form of paraffin application (Fig. 6-16).

1. Ensure that the patient is free of contraindications for this treatment technique.
2. Begin the treatment by immersing the extremity in the wax so that it becomes completely covered. Remove the body part and allow the wax to dry.
3. Continue to dip and remove the body part in the wax 7 to 12 times.
4. After the final withdrawal from the wax, cover the extremity with a plastic bag, aluminum foil, or wax paper. Then wrap and secure a terry cloth towel around the area.
5. If indicated, the body part may be elevated.
6. Following the treatment, remove the towel and inner layering. Scrape off the hardened paraffin and return it to the bath for reheating, or discard it.

Maintenance

Refer to the manufacturer's maintenance requirements for the unit being used.

After Each Use

Allow any paraffin that may have dripped onto the outer surface of the heating unit to dry, and then scrape the wax off using a tongue depressor.

As Needed

The paraffin mixture should be changed when it becomes discolored or debris builds up in the bottom of the tank. Unplug the heating unit prior to performing any maintenance. Follow the manufacturer's guidelines for quarterly, 6-month, and annual maintenance requirements, including calibration by qualified personnel.

1. Unplug the unit and remove the protective grate from the bottom of the unit.
2. Allow the paraffin to harden (this may require several hours).

3. Once the paraffin has hardened, plug the unit back in and allow the paraffin to heat to the point where it dislodges from the unit.
4. Remove and discard the used paraffin.
5. Use paper toweling to remove any residual paraffin.
6. Unplug the unit and cleanse the inner tub with a mild disinfectant.

Fluidotherapy

Fluidotherapy is a convective modality that delivers dry heat to the extremities. This method of heat application is used in cases where paraffin or whirlpool application would be appropriate, but fluidotherapy results in more heat absorption in the tissues.[153] Air jets circulate heated cellulose particles that have a lower specific heat and thermal capacity than water, allowing higher treatment temperatures. Fluidotherapy applied at 118°F (47.8°C) increases the temperature of the joint capsule by 16.2°F (9°C) and superficial muscle by 9.5°F (5.3°C).[154]

The patient inserts the body part into the unit through one of the portals located on the machine. The clinician's hands can also be inserted into the unit to assist with ROM exercises or perform joint mobilization techniques.

● EFFECTS ON

The Injury Response Process

The effect and sensation of fluidotherapy is similar to that of a whirlpool, but without the benefits of buoyancy and hydrostatic pressure. The cellulose medium provides resistance to active exercise. Increasing the amount of airflow decreases resistance and vice versa.

The effects of fluidotherapy on the injury response cycle are the same as heat treatments in general. An advantage of fluidotherapy is the ability to place the limb in the nongravity-dependent position, reducing the formation of edema.

Instrumentation

Air Speed: The rate at which the medium is moved through the unit is expressed as a percentage of the total force (0 to 100). The default setting is 50. Lower force increases the viscosity of the mixture, providing more resistance to joint motion.

Preheat Timer: Used for preheating the transmitting medium. Some units are programmable, allowing the unit to automatically preheat at the start of a workday.

Pulse Time: Pulses interrupt the flow of the medium by starting and stopping the air stream. Pulses range from 1 (1 sec on/1 sec off) to 6 (6 on/6 off). Setting the pulse time to OFF provides a constant flow.

Treatment Temperature: Sets the treatment temperature from 88°F to 130°F (31.1°C to 54°C).

Treatment Time: Sets the duration of the treatment. The time remaining is displayed on the console, or the timer rotates to display the time remaining.

Setup and Application

Refer to the unit's instruction manual for precise operating instructions.

Patient Preparation
1. Ensure that the patient is free of contraindications for this treatment technique.
2. During the patient preparation period, preheat the fluidotherapy unit. If the unit is so equipped, close the heat flaps to speed preheating. Following the preheating, reopen the flaps.
3. Remove jewelry from the body part being treated.
4. Wash and dry the patient's extremity using an antimicrobial soap and then apply a hospital grade antiseptic skin cleanser.
5. To prevent the medium from entering open wounds, cover skin lesions with a nonpermeable membrane such as a plastic bag, rubber gloves, or surgical skin dressing (e.g., OpSite).

Initiating the Treatment
1. Turn the unit off.
2. Ensure that the unit contains a proper amount of the medium.
3. Secure all nonused entry portals prior to turning the unit on.
4. Select the portal appropriate for the treatment and body part. Have the patient fully insert the body part into the unit.
5. Securely fasten the appliance proximally on the body part.
6. Set thermostat to the desired temperature, usually between 100°F and 123°F (37.8°C and 50.6°C).
7. Set the treatment duration.
8. If indicated, instruct the patient to perform the appropriate ROM exercises.

Terminating the Treatment
1. Turn the unit OFF before removing the extremity being treated.
2. Loosen the appliance from the patient's extremity.
3. Before removing the body part from the tank, remove any particles that may have adhered to the patient.
4. Re-secure the entry portal used by the patient.

Maintenance

Unplug the unit before performing any maintenance. Follow the manufacturer's guidelines for quarterly, 6-month, and

At a Glance: **Fluidotherapy**

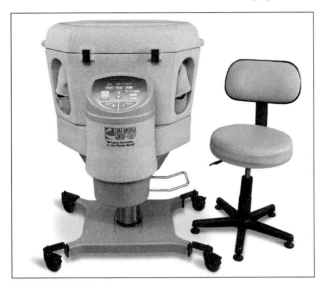

Description

Ground cellulose is heated and circulated by air to deliver dry heat to the extremity. Fluidotherapy is used for superficial heating of the extremities, especially the wrist, hand, and fingers and the ankle and toes.

Indications

- Pain reduction
- Prior to or during joint mobilization
- ROM exercises combined with heat therapy
- Nonrheumatoid arthritis

Temperature Range

110°F to 125°F (43.3°C to 51.6°C)

Contraindications

- Uncovered open wounds
- Sensory loss
- Peripheral vascular disease
- Over cancerous lesions
- General medical conditions that reduce the patient's tolerance to heat

Treatment Duration

Fluidotherapy treatments are given for 20 minutes and can be repeated multiple times per day.

Precautions

- Cover open wounds prior to treatment.
- Patients who are sensitive to allergic reactions caused by dust and pollen.

Fluido CHT, courtesy of the Chattanooga Group, Hixson, TN.

---

annual maintenance requirements, including calibration by qualified personnel.

Daily Maintenance
1. Clean air inlet filters. Remove the filter and wash with antibacterial soap and water. Allow the filter to completely dry before reinstalling it. Older filters are cleaned using a soft-bristle brush.
2. Refill medium. Refill the unit to the indicated level using the manufacturer's recommended medium.
3. Inspect sleeves. Ensure that the portal sleeves are free from rips and weak seams. Porous sleeves

will result in the spillage of the medium during treatment.

Weekly Maintenance
Launder all appliance sleeves in a mild antibacterial detergent. Refer to the operator's manual for instructions on removing the sleeves.

■ Contrast Therapy

Contrast therapy consists of alternating hot and cold treatments. Stationary water immersion, tandem whirlpools, or moist heat packs and ice packs may be used for this technique. Alternating heat and cold modalities are thought to cause a cycle of vasoconstrictions and vasodilations of the superficial blood vessels.

✱ Practical Evidence

Contrast therapy is often used as an edema reduction technique by "pumping" blood flow.[5] However there is no physiological basis or clinical evidence supporting this technique, especially in large joints such as the ankle or knee. Although there is some support for the increase in skin blood flow, the effective depth of this treatment does not penetrate the subcutaneous tissues and the lymph vessels would not be affected by any temperature changes that may occur.[155,156,157]

There is little evidence that supports the use of contrast therapy in decreasing pain thresholds, especially when compared to other therapeutic interventions.[5,156,157,158]

The most effective time ratio between hot and cold has not been determined; some protocols are based on the temperature and medium used. Commonly used ratios are 3:1 and 4:1 (i.e., 3 and 4 minutes in the hot immersion to 1 minute in the cold).[157] Other approaches use 10 minute immersion in hot water, 1 minute immersion in cold water, followed by alternating 4:1 hot/cold bouts for the duration of the treatment.[20,156]

Alternating 6-minute bouts of moist heat pack and cold pack application produces a more pronounced differential in temperatures than immersion techniques used for shorter contact times. This method keeps the temperature gradient high, resulting in a greater exchange of energy.[20]

The treatment may end after either the hot or the cold application, depending on the stage of the injury, the desired effect of the treatment, and the patient's activity plans after the treatment. When a state of vasoconstriction is desired, the treatment is terminated after cold application. If vasodilation is desired, the treatment is terminated after a warm application. In subacute conditions, it is generally beneficial to finish the treatment with following cold exposure.

● EFFECTS ON

The Injury Response Process

The exact effects on cellular responses from contrast therapy are not clear. Contrast therapy has long been used under the assumption that the influx of new blood assists in removing edema by unclogging the vasculature. The changes in tissue temperature cause fluctuations in cutaneous blood flow, but these changes do not extend into the intramuscular tissues.[5,156,157] Changes on skin blood flow are significantly decreased in patients with vascular impairment such as diabetes.[159]

The alternating bouts of vasoconstriction and vasodilation were once thought to "pump" edema from the extremity.[160] Changes in vascular diameter primarily occur in cutaneous vessels. However, lymphatic capillaries contain only epithelial cells and are unable to change sizes, that is, they are unable to vasodilate or vasoconstrict. Most importantly, as described in Chapter 1, the solid matter in edema must be removed by the lymphatic system and lymph vessels are not affected by temperature. Only gravity, muscle contractions, or external pressure moves matter through the lymph system.[5,156,159]

There is no evidence that supports the efficacy of contrast therapy in reducing edema or removing ecchymosis. If half-leg or half-arm immersion techniques where there is not sufficient hydrostatic pressure placed on the distal extremity are used to deliver contrast therapy, the limb will be placed in the gravity-dependent position, potentially increasing limb volume (see the Whirlpools section in this chapter).

Theoretically, the cellular metabolic rate increases or decreases in response to the temperature of the treatment; however, contrast therapy does not appear to significantly influence subcutaneous tissue temperatures.[20,100] There appears to be no effect on pain or pressure perception following treatment.[158]

Setup and Application

Immersion Technique

1. Ensure that the patient is free of contraindications for this treatment technique.
2. If an immersion technique is being used, position the tubs as close together as possible without touching each other. ("Tubs" refers to either immersion buckets or whirlpool tanks.) The patient should be able to remove the body part from one tub and immediately immerse it in the other.
3. Fill one tub with water in the range from 105°F to 110°F (40.6°C to 43.3°C) and the other with water between 50°F and 60°F (10°C to 15.6°C).
4. Position the patient on a chair or bench in a manner requiring a minimal amount of motion from tub to tub.

Hot/Cold Pack Technique

1. Ensure that the patient is free of contraindications for this treatment technique.
2. Position the patient so the hot and cold packs are within reach.
3. Instruct the patient on how and when to remove one pack and apply the other pack.
4. Because of cooling, the original hot pack should be replaced with a fresh, heated pack at approximately 15 minutes into the treatment.

At a Glance: **Contrast Therapy**

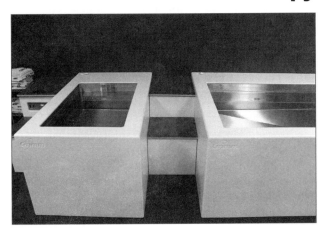

Description

Contrast baths consist of alternating bouts of heat and cold, using a hot and cold whirlpool (shown), hot and cold immersion, or moist heat packs and cold packs. Contrast therapy is used for the transition between cold and heat modalities, but there is no evidence to support this.
*The efficacy of this treatment has not been fully substantiated.

Primary Effects

Alternating periods of vasoconstriction and vasodilation of cutaneous vessels

Temperature Range

COLD IMMERSION
50°F to 60°F (10°C to 16°C). The temperature is increased as the proportion of the body area immersed increases.
HOT IMMERSION
105°F to 110°F (40.6°C to 43.3°C). Temperature is decreased as the proportion of the body area treated increases.

Treatment Duration

- 20 to 30 minutes and may be repeated as needed. When treating deep structures, the treatment duration should be increased as the amount of adipose tissue increases.
- Hot immersions are typically 3 or 4 minutes in duration.
- Cold immersions are typically 1 or 2 minutes in duration.

Indications

- Subacute or chronic inflammatory conditions
- Impaired circulation (monitor the patient closely)
- Pain reduction
- Increasing joint ROM

Contraindications

- Acute injuries
- Hypersensitivity to cold
- Contraindications relative to whirlpool use
- Contraindications relative to cold applications
- Contraindications relative to heat applications

Precautions

- If whirlpools are used, see Precautions described in At a Glance: Hot and Cold Whirlpools.
- A Neoprene toe cap may be used to decrease the discomfort associated with cold immersions.
- The combination of increased circulation and placement of the extremity in a gravity-dependent position tends to increase edema.

Common Considerations

1. A clock or watch should be available to time the treatment segments.
2. In most cases, heat treatments are given first.
3. Have the patient alternate between the treatments according to the protocol being applied.
4. As with all hot or cold treatments, the patient should be monitored.
5. The treatment ends after the hot immersion if relaxation and vasodilation are desired or after the cold immersion if vasoconstriction is desired.

End of Section

(The following discussion relates to Case Study Part 2, found on page 67 of Section 1.)

Case Study: Continuation of Case Study From Section 1

The modalities presented in Chapters 5 and 6 would benefit our patient throughout his rehabilitation program. Various forms of cold modalities can be used throughout the time frame indicated, and moist heat packs can be incorporated in the later stages of the program.

Ice Packs

Crushed ice packs would be used during the early stages of this patient's program. The patient would be placed in the supine position, with his head and neck comfortably supported to decrease the amount of electromyographic activity in the trapezius. The cold application will decrease the amount of pain by increasing the pain threshold and by decreasing the rate of the nerve conduction velocity. Muscle spasm will be decreased secondary to reducing the muscle spindle's sensitivity to stretch. Acutely, this method of cold application will also decrease the metabolic activity in the treated area, thereby decreasing the amount of secondary hypoxic injury.

As the patient's treatment progresses, active or passive range-of-motion exercises (described later) would be performed after the removal of the pack. During the more advanced stages of the rehabilitation program, ice packs would be applied after the rehabilitation session to minimize the post-exercise inflammatory response. Last, the patient would be instructed to use cold packs as a part of his home treatment program.

Ice Massage

Ice massage could be used in conjunction with stretching exercises. The patient would be in the seated position, with the cervical spine flexed and laterally bent to the left to tolerance. Once the ice massage treatment has begun and the patient reports decreased pain, the trapezius could be further stretched until discomfort is once again reported. This process would be repeated for the 10- to 15-minute duration of the treatment.

This approach relies on ice massage numbing the area and decreasing the sensitivity of the local muscle spindles. This effect, combined with the passive stretching of the muscle, helps to decrease muscle spasm and to increase range of motion.

Moist Heat Packs

When the active inflammatory process subsides, moist heat can safely be applied before therapeutic exercise and other modalities. Similar to the application of cold packs, moist heat decreases the pain and spasm associated with the injury, but other benefits are realized as well. Moist heat promotes relaxation of the cervical musculature and increases tissue extensibility, increasing the effectiveness of the patient's range-of-motion program.

Concurrent Range-of-Motion Exercises

Range-of-motion exercises for side bending and rotation (30-second hold for five repetitions) are first begun with the patient in the supine position to decrease the effects of gravity. As the patient's pain and spasm begin to subside, these exercises can be progressed to being performed in an upright position.

Case Study: Chapter Case Study

Jessica is a 16-year-old basketball player who sustained a left ankle inversion sprain while you are providing medical coverage for this event. You witnessed the incident and noted that her ankle and foot rolled onto the lateral border after landing on another player's foot after a layup. After the referee called a time out, you entered the court to assist Jessica. You noted that she was seated on the floor holding her ankle in significant pain. She reports to you that her ankle is in a lot of pain on the lateral aspect of her foot, ankle, and lower leg. After a brief injury assessment, you determine she can be assisted off the court in a non-weight-bearing mode to render treatment.

1. What is the best thermal agent to consider in this situation?

2. What are the physiological effects on the injury response cycle from the application of this thermal agent?

3. What are the clinical symptoms that you hope to address with this intervention?

4. At what other phases would this intervention philosophy apply during the injury rehabilitation process?

5. What other thermal modalities may be appropriate over the following 2 weeks for this diagnosis? Why?

● ● ●   Section 2 Quiz

1. Which of the following modalities has the greatest likelihood of frostbite?
   A. Ice immersion
   B. Reusable cold packs
   C. Ice massage
   D. Ice bag

2. Which of the following is a contraindication to the use of a paraffin bath?
   A. No range of motion
   B. Chronic conditions
   C. Pain
   D. Skin conditions

3. Which of the following devices uses convection as the method of heat transfer?
   A. Ice bag
   B. Whirlpool
   C. Moist heat packs
   D. Therapeutic ultrasound

4. Which of the following is not a local effect of cold application?
   A. Decreased rate of cell metabolism
   B. Decreased muscle spindle activity
   C. Decreased nerve conduction velocity
   D. Decreased viscosity of fluids in the area

5. Which of the following modalities has the greatest depth of penetration into the tissues?
   A. Moist heat pack
   B. Hot whirlpool
   C. Infrared lamp
   D. Ice bag

6. Heat application by itself (i.e., without stretching exercises) is sufficient to elongate collagen-rich tissues.
   A. True
   B. False

7. Which of the following is not a local effect of heat application?
   A. Increased rate of cell metabolism
   B. Increased blood flow
   C. Increased muscle tone
   D. Decreased muscle spasm

8. A ____ degree F drop in skin temperature is needed to reduce the sensitivity of muscle spindles.
   A. 5
   B. 9
   C. 13
   D. 17

9. As the size (area) of the body exposed to cold immersion increases, the temperature of the immersion should:
   A. Increase
   B. Decrease

10. The primary reason for the use of cold during the immediate treatment of an injury is:
    A. To decrease swelling
    B. To limit hemorrhage
    C. To reduce pain
    D. To decrease cell metabolism

11. The "hunting response" has been demonstrated to occur in all body parts during cold application.
    A. True
    B. False

12. Moist heat packs are stored in water having a temperature range between ____ and ____ degrees F.
    A. 140/146
    B. 150/156
    C. 160/166
    D. 170/176

13. The thermal effects obtained from a moist heat pack occur up to ___ cm beneath the skin.
    A. 1
    B. 2
    C. 3
    D. 4

14. If the goal of your treatment is to produce long-lasting cold within the quadriceps muscle prior to exercise (in the subacute or chronic stage of injury), which of the following modalities would be most appropriate?
    A. A single ice bag
    B. Vapocoolant spray
    C. Ice massage
    D. Cold whirlpool

15. A patient is standing in a warm whirlpool 100 cm deep. The water's hydrostatic pressure at the ankle is:
    A. 7.3 mm Hg
    B. 36.5 mm Hg
    C. 73.0 mm Hg
    D. 109.5 mm Hg

16. You are attempting to cool intramuscular tissue 1 cm deep with an ice pack. There is 25 mm of adipose tissue overlying the target tissues. To reach therapeutic temperatures the ice should be applied for ___ minutes.
    A. 20
    B. 25
    C. 40
    D. 60

17. Cell metabolic rate increases by a factor of two to three for each ___ degree F increase in skin temperature.
    A. 4
    B. 9
    C. 15
    D. 18

References

1. Halliday D, et al: Fundamentals of Physics, ed 6. Wiley, Hoboken, NJ, 2000, p 465.
2. Howatson G, Gaze D, van Someren KA: The efficacy of ice massage in the treatment of exercise-induced muscle damage. *Scand J Med Sci Sports.* 15:416, 2005.
3. Reid G, Flonta M: Cold current in thermoreceptive neurons. *Nature.* 413:480, 2001.
4. Nadler SF, Weingand K, Kruse RJ: The physiologic basis and clinical applications of cryotherapy and thermotherapy for the pain practitioner. *Pain Physician.* 7:395, 2004.
5. Fiscus KA, Kaminski TW, Powers ME: Changes in lower-leg blood flow during warm-, cold-, and contrast-water therapy. *Arch Phys Med Rehabil.* 86:1404, 2005.
6. Zemke JE, et al: Intramuscular temperature responses in the human leg to two forms of cryotherapy: Ice massage and ice bag. *J Orthop Sports Phys Ther.* 27:301, 1998.
7. Petrofsky J, Bains G, Prowse M, et al: Dry heat, moist heat and body fat: Are heating modalities really effective in people who are overweight? *J Med Eng Tech.* 33:361, 2009.
8. Merrick MA, et al: The effects of ice and compression wraps on intramuscular temperatures at various depths. *J Athl Train.* 28:236, 1993.
9. Myer JW, et al: Muscle temperature is affected by overlying adipose when cryotherapy is administered. *J Athl Train.* 36:32, 2001.
10. Myer JW, et al: Temperature changes in the human leg during and after two methods of cryotherapy. *J Athl Train.* 33:25, 1998.
11. Otte, JW, et al: Subcutaneous adipose tissue thickness alters cooling time during cryotherapy. *Arch Phys Med Rehabil.* 83:1501, 2002.
12. Jutte LS, Merrick MA, Ingersoll CD et al: The relationship between intramuscular temperature, skin temperature, and adipose thickness during cryotherapy and rewarming. *Arch Phys Med Rehabil.* 82:845, 2001.
13. Danielson R, et al: Differences in skin surface temperature and pressure during the application of various cold and compression devices (abstract). *J Athl Train.* 32:S34, 1997.
14. Tomchuk D, Rubley MD, Holcomb WR, et al: The magnitude of tissue cooling during cryotherapy with varied types of compression. *J Athl Train.* 45:230, 2010.
15. Merrick MA, Jutte LS, Smith ME: Cold modalities with different thermodynamic properties produce different surface and intramuscular temperatures. *J Athl Train.* 38:28, 2003.
16. Ho SS, et al: Comparison of various icing times in decreasing bone metabolism and blood flow in the knee. *Am J Sports Med.* 23:74, 1995.
17. Jameson AG, et al: Lower-extremity-joint cryotherapy does not affect vertical ground-reaction forces during landing. *J Sports Rehabil.* 10:132, 2001.
18. Myer JW, et al: Exercise after cryotherapy greatly enhances intramuscular rewarming. *J Athl Train.* 35:412, 2000.
19. Ho SW, et al: The effects of ice on blood flow and bone metabolism in knees. *Am J Sports Med.* 22:537, 1994.
20. Myer WJ, et al: Cold- and hot-pack contrast therapy: Subcutaneous and intramuscular temperature change. *J Athl Train.* 32:238, 1997.
21. Karunakara RG, et al: Changes in forearm blood flow during single and intermittent cold application. *J Orthop Sports Phys Ther.* 29:177, 1999.
22. Dykstra JH, Hill HM, Miller MG, et al: Comparisons of cubed ice, crushed ice, and wetted ice on intramuscular and surface temperature changes. *J Athl Train.* 44:136, 2009.
23. Houghton PE, Nussbaum EL, Hoens AM: Cryotherapy. *Physiother Can.* 62:55, 2010.
24. Knobloch K, Grasemann R, Spies M, et al: Intermittent KoldBlue cryotherapy of 3 x 10 min changes mid-portion Achilles tendon microcirculation. *Br J Sports Med.* 41, 2007.
25. Bleakley CM, McDonough SM, MacAuley DC: Cryotherapy for acute ankle sprains: A randomised controlled study of two different icing protocols. *Br J Sports Med.* 40:700, 2006.
26. Dahlstedt L, et al: Cryotherapy after cruciate knee surgery: Skin, subcutaneous and articular temperatures in 8 patients. *Acta Orthop Scand.* 67:255, 1996.
27. Oosterveld FG, et al: The effect of local heat and cold therapy on the intraarticular and skin surface temperature of the knee. *Arthritis Rheum.* 35:146, 1992.
28. Bocobo C, et al: The effect of ice on intraarticular temperature in the knee of the dog. *Am J Phys Med Rehabil.* 70:181, 1991.
29. Martin SS, Spindler KP, Tarter JW, et al: Cryotherapy: An effective modality for decreasing intraarticular temperature after knee arthroscopy. *Am J Sports Med.* 29:288, 2001.
30. Osbahr DC, Cawley PW, Speer KP: The effect of continuous cryotherapy on glenohumeral joint and subacromial space temperatures in the postoperative shoulder. *Arthroscopy.* 18:748, 2002.
31. Long BC, Cordova ML, Brucker JB, et al: Exercise and quadriceps muscle cooling time. *J Athl Train.* 40:260, 2005.
32. Ibrahim T, Ong SM, Saint Clair Taylor G: The effects of different dressings on the skin temperature of the knee during cryotherapy. *Knee.* 23:21, 2005.
33. Kennet J, Hardaker H, Hobbs S, et al: Cooling efficiency of 4 common cryotherapeutic agents. *J Athl Train.* 42:343, 2007.
34. Bender AL, Kramer EE, Brucker JB, et al: Local ice-bag application and triceps surae muscle temperature during treadmill walking. *J Athl Train.* 40:271, 2005.
35. Jamison CA, et al: The effects of post cryotherapy exercise on surface and capsular temperature (abstract). *J Athl Train.* 36:S91, 2001.
36. Allen JD, et al: Effect of microcurrent stimulation on delayed-onset muscle soreness: A double-blind comparison. *J Athl Train.* 34:334, 1999.
37. Bleakley C, McDonough S, MacAuley D: The use of ice in the treatment of acute soft-tissue injury: A systematic review of randomized controlled trials. *Am J Sports Med.* 32:251, 2004.

38. Halar, EM, et al: Nerve conduction velocity: Relationship of skin, subcutaneous, and intramuscular temperatures. *Arch Phys Med Rehabil.* 61:199, 1980.

39. Michalski WJ, Séguin JJ: The effects of muscle cooling and stretch on muscle spindle secondary endings in the cat. *J Physiol.* 253:341, 1975.

40. Knight KL, et al: Circulatory changes in the forearm in 1, 5, 10 and 15°C water. *Int J Sports Med.* 4:281, 1981.

41. Lievens P, Meevsen R: The use of cryotherapy in sports injuries. *Sports Med.* 3:398, 1986.

42. Greenspan JD, et al: Body site variation of cool perception thresholds, with observations on paradoxical heat. *Somatosens Mot Res.* 10:467, 1993.

43. Wilkerson GB: Inflammation in connective tissue: Etiology and management. *J Athl Train.* 20:299, 1985.

44. Ingersoll CD, Mangus BC: Sensations of cold reexamined: A study using the McGill Pain Questionnaire. *J Athl Train.* 26:240, 1991.

45. Streator S, et al: Sensory information can decrease cold-induced pain perception. *J Athl Train.* 30:293, 1995.

46. Misasi S, et al: The effect of a toe cap and bias on perceived pain during cold water immersion. *J Athl Train.* 30:49, 1995.

47. Ingersoll CD, et al: Cold induced pain: Habituation to cold immersions (abstract). *J Athl Train.* 25:126, 1990.

48. Dolan MG, et al: Effects of cold water immersion on edema formation after blunt injury to the hind limbs of rats. *J Athl Train.* 32:233, 1997.

49. Merrick MA, et al: A preliminary examination of cryotherapy and secondary injury in skeletal muscle. *Med Sci Sports Exerc.* 31:1516, 1999.

50. Merrick MA, McBrier NM: Progression of secondary injury after musculoskeletal trauma—a window of opportunity? *J Sport Rehabil.* 19:380, 2010.

51. Menth-Chiari WA, et al: Microcirculation of striated muscle in closed soft tissue injury: Effect on tissue perfusion, inflammatory cellular response and mechanisms of cryotherapy. A study in rat by means of laser Doppler flow-measurements and intravital microscopy. *Unfallchirurg.* 102:691, 1999.

52. Eston R, Peters D: Effects of cold water immersion on the symptoms of exercise-induced muscle damage. *J Sports Sci.* 17:231, 1999.

53. Thompson-Torgerson CS, Holowatz LA, Flavahan NA, et al: Cold-induced cutaneous vasoconstriction is mediated by Rho kinase in vivo in human skin. *Am J Physiol Heart Circ Physiol.* 292:H1700, 2007.

54. Taber C, et al: Measurement of reactive vasodilation during cold gel pack application to nontraumatized ankles. *Phys Ther.* 72:294, 1992.

55. Weston M, et al: Changes in local blood volume during cold gel pack application to traumatized ankles. *J Orthop Sports Phys Ther.* 19:197, 1994.

56. Baker RJ, Bell GW: The effect of therapeutic modalities on blood flow in the human calf. *J Orthop Sports Phys Ther.* 13:23, 1991.

57. Knobloch K, et al: Microcirculation of the ankle after Cryo/Cuff application in healthy volunteers. *Int J Sports Med* 27:250, 2006.

58. Curl WW, et al: The effect of contusion and cryotherapy on skeletal muscle microcirculation. *J Sports Med Phys Fitness.* 37:279, 1997.

59. Knobloch K, Grasemann R, Spies M, et al: Midportion Achilles tendon microcirculation after intermittent combined cryotherapy and compression compared with cryotherapy alone. A randomized trial. *Am J Sports Med.* 36:2128, 2008.

60. Knobloch K, Kraemer R, Lichenberg A, et al: Microcirculation of the ankle after Cryo/Cuff application in healthy volunteers. *Int J Sports Med.* 27:250, 2006.

61. Lewis T: Observations upon the reactions of the vessels of the human skin to cold. *Heart.* 15:177, 1930.

62. Daanen HA, et al: The effect of body temperature on the hunting response of the middle finger skin temperature. *Eur J Appl Physiol Occup Physiol.* 76:538, 1997.

63. Knight KL: Circulatory effects of therapeutic cold applications. In Knight KL (ed): Cryotherapy in Sports Injury Management. Human Kinetics, Champaign, IL, 1995, pp 107–125.

64. Hopkins JT, et al: The effects of cryotherapy and TENS on arthrogenic muscle inhibition of the quadriceps. *J Athl Train.* 36:S49, 2001.

65. Hopkins JT: Knee joint effusion and cryotherapy alter lower chain kinetics and muscle activity. *J Athl Train.* 41:177, 2006.

66. Smith TL, et al: New skeletal muscle model for the longitudinal study of alterations in microcirculation following contusion and cryotherapy. *Microsurgery.* 14:487, 1993.

67. Dervin GF, et al: Effects of cold and compression dressings on early postoperative outcomes for the arthroscopic anterior cruciate ligament reconstruction patient. *J Orthop Sports Phys Ther.* 27:403, 1998.

68. Herrera E, Sandoval MC, Camargo DM, et al: Motor and sensory nerve conduction are affected differently by ice pack, ice massage, and cold water immersion. *Phys Ther* 90:581, 2010.

69. Allison SC, Abraham LD: Sensitivity of qualitative and quantitative spasticity measures to clinical treatment with cryotherapy. *Int J Rehabil Res.* 24:15, 2001.

70. Algafly AA, George KP: The effect of cryotherapy on nerve conduction velocity, pain threshold and pain tolerance. *Br J Sports Med.* 41:365, 2007.

71. Brander B, et al: Evaluation of the contribution to postoperative analgesia by local cooling of the wound. *Anaesthesia.* 51:1021, 1996.

72. Knight KL, et al: The effects of cold application on nerve conduction velocity and muscle force (abstract). *J Athl Train.* 32:S5, 1997.

73. Hubbard TJ, Denegar CR: Does cryotherapy improve outcomes with soft tissue injury? *J Athl Train.* 39:278, 2004.

74. Ernst E, Fialka V: Ice freezes pain? A review of the clinical effectiveness of analgesic cold therapy. *J Pain Symptom Manage.* 9:56, 1994.

75. Tremblay F, et al: Influence of local cooling on proprioceptive acuity in the quadriceps muscle. *J Athl Train.* 36:119, 2001.

76. Thieme HA, et al: Cooling does not affect knee proprioception. *J Athl Train.* 31:8, 1996.

77. Evans TA, et al: Agility following the application of cold therapy. *J Athl Train* 31:232, 1995.

78. Berg CL, Hart JM, Palmieri-Smith R, et al: Cryotherapy does not affect peroneal reaction following sudden reaction. *J Sports Rehab.* 16:285, 2007.

79. Dover G, Powers ME: Cryotherapy does not impair joint position sense. *Arch Phys Med Rehabil.* 85:1241, 2004.

80. Wassinger CA, Myers JB, Gatti JM, et al: Proprioception and throwing accuracy in the dominant shoulder after cryotherapy. *J Athl Train.* 42:84, 2007.

81. Oliveria R, Ribeiro F, Oliveria J: Cryotherapy impairs knee joint position sense. *Int J Sports Med.* 31:198, 2010.

82. Surenkok O, Aytar A, Tüzün EH, et al: Cryotherapy impairs knee joint position sense and balance. *Isokinet Exerc Sci.* 16:69, 2008.

83. Schmid S, Moffat M, Gutierrez GM: Effect of knee joint cooling on the electromyographic activity of lower extremity muscles during a plyometric exercise. *J Electromyogr Kinesiol.* 20:1075, 2010.

84. Uchio Y, Ochi M, Fujihara A, et al: Cryotherapy influences joint laxity and position sense of the healthy knee joint. *Arch Phys Med Rehabil.* 84:131, 2003.

85. Costello JT, Donnelly AE: Cryotherapy and joint position sense in healthy participants: A systematic review. *J Athl Train.* 43:306, 2010.

86. Patterson SM, Udermann BE, Doberstein ST, et al: The effects of cold whirlpool on power, speed, agility, and range of motion. *J Sports Sci Med.* 7:378, 2008.

87. Hart JM, Leonard JL, Ingersoll CD: Single-leg landing strategy after knee-joint cryotherapy. *J Sport Rehabil.* 14:313, 2005.

88. Fore CJ, Smith BS: The effects of cryotherapy on knee joint position sense in females (abstract). *Phys Ther.* 81:A42, 2001.

89. Halvorson GA: Therapeutic heat and cold for athletic injuries. *Physician Sportsmedicine.* 18:87, 1990.

90. Denys EH: AAEM minimonograph #14: The influence of temperature in clinical neurophysiology. *Muscle Nerve.* 14:795, 1991.

91. Richendollar ML, Darby LA, Brown TM: Ice bag application, active warm-up, and 3 measures of maximal functional performance. *J Athl Train.* 41:364, 2006.

92. Ruiz DH, et al: Cryotherapy and sequential exercise bouts following cryotherapy on concentric and eccentric strength in the quadriceps. *J Athl Train.* 28:320, 1993.

93. Ferretti G, et al: Effects of temperature on the maximal instantaneous muscle power of humans. *Eur J Appl Physiol.* 64:112, 1992.

94. Thompson G, et al: Effect of cryotherapy on eccentric peak torque and endurance (abstract). *J Athl Train.* 29:180, 1994.

95. Mattacola CG, Perrin DH: Effects of cold water application on isokinetic strength of the plantar flexors. *Isokinetic Ex Sci.* 3:152, 1993.

96. Kimura IF, et al: The effect of cryotherapy on eccentric plantar flexion peak torque and endurance. *J Athl Train.* 32:124, 1997.

97. Verducci FM: Interval cryotherapy decreases fatigue during repeated weight lifting. *J Athl Train.* 35:422, 2000.

98. Borgmeyer JA, Scott BA, Mayhew JL: The effects of ice massage on maximum isokinetic-torque production. *J Sport Rehabil.* 13:1, 2004.

99. Krause A, et al: The relationship of ankle temperature during cooling and rewarming to the human soleus H reflex. *J Sports Rehabil.* 9:253, 2000.

100. Myrer JW, et al: Contrast therapy and intramuscular temperature in the human leg. *J Athl Train.* 29:318, 1994.

101. Hubbard TJ, Aronson SL, Denegar CL: Does cryotherapy hasten return to participation? A systematic review. *J Athl Train.* 39:88, 2004.

102. Perlau R, et al: The effect of elastic bandages on human knee proprioception in the uninjured population. *Am J Sports Med.* 23:251, 1995.

103. Babwah T: Common peroneal neuropathy related to cryotherapy and compression in a footballer. *Res Sports Med.* 19:66, 2011.

104. Lekakis J, et al: Cold-induced coronary Raynaud's phenomenon in patients with systemic sclerosis. *Clin Exp Rheumatol.* 16:135, 1998.

105. Anaya-Terroba L, Arroyo-Morales M, Femandez-de-las-Penas Diaz-Rodrigue L, et al: Effects of ice massage on pressure pain thresholds and electromyography activity postexercise: A randomized controlled crossover study. *J Manipulative Physiol Ther.* 33:212, 2010.

106. Robertson VJ, Ward AR, Jung P: The effect of heat on tissue extensibility: A comparison of deep and superficial heating. *Arch Phys Med Rehabil.* 86:819, 2005.

107. Martin SN, Nichols W: Does heat or cold work better for acute muscle strain? *J Fam Pract.* 57:820, 2008.

108. Tomaszewski D, et al: A comparison of skin interface temperature response between the ProHeaty instant reusable hot pack and the standard hydrocollator steam pack. *J Athl Train.* 27:355, 1992.

109. Lehmann JF, et al: Temperature distributions in the human thigh, produced by infrared, hot pack and microwave applications. *Arch Phys Med Rehabil.* 47:291, 1966.

110. Draper DO, et al: Temperature change in human muscle during and after pulsed short-wave diathermy. *J Orthop Sports Phys Ther.* 29:13, 1999.

111. Sawyer PC, Uhl TL, Mattacola CG, et al: Effects of moist heat on hamstring flexibility and muscle temperature. *J Strength Cond Res.* 17:285, 2003.

112. Perkins SA, Massie JE: Patient satisfaction after thermal shrinkage of the glenohumeral-joint capsule. *J Sport Rehabil.* 10:157, 2001.

113. Gray SR, De Vito G, Nimmo MA, et al: Skeletal muscle turnover and muscle fiber condition velocity are elevated at higher muscle temperatures during maximal power output development in humans. *Am J Physiol Regul Integr Comp Physiol.* 290:R376, 2006.

114. Rall JA, Woledge RC: Influence of temperature on mechanics and energetics of muscle contraction. *Am J Physiol.* 259(Pt 2):R197, 1990.

115. Knight KL, Londeree BR: Comparison of blood flow in the ankle of uninjured subjects during application of heat, cold, and exercise. *Med Sci Sports Exerc.* 12:76, 1980.

116. Petrofsky JS, Bains G, Raju C, et al: The effect of the moisture content of a local heat source on the blood flow response of the skin. *Arch Dermatol Res.* 301:581, 2009.

117. Petrofsky J, et al: Impact of hydrotherapy on skin blood flow: How much is due to moisture and how much is due to heat? *Physiother Theory Pract.* 26:107, 2010.

118. Abramson DI, et al: Changes in blood flow, oxygen uptake and tissue temperatures produced by the topical application of wet heat. *Arch Phys Med Rehabil.* 42:305, 1961.

119. Erasala GN, et al: The effect of topical heat treatment on trapezius muscle blood flow using power Doppler ultrasound (abstract). *Phys Ther.* 81:A5, 2001.

120. McCulloch J, Boyd VB: The effects of whirlpool and the dependent position on lower extremity volume. *J Orthop Sport Phys Ther.* 16:169, 1992.

121. Curkovic B, et al: The influence of heat and cold on the pain threshold in rheumatoid arthritis. *Z Rheumatol.* 52:289, 1993.

122. Swenson C, et al: Cryotherapy in sports medicine. *Scand J Med Sci Sports.* 6:193, 1996.

123. Funk D, et al: Efficacy of moist heat pack application over static stretching on hamstring flexibility. *J Strength Cond Res.* 15:123, 2001.

124. Benoit TG, et al: Hot and cold whirlpool treatments and knee joint laxity. *J Athl Train.* 31:242, 1996.

125. Taylor BF, et al: The effects of therapeutic application of heat or cold followed by static stretch on hamstring muscle length. *J Orthop Sports Phys Ther.* 21:283, 1995.

126. Wirth VJ, et al: Temperature changes in deep muscles of humans during upper and lower extremity exercise. *J Athl Train.* 33:211, 1998.

127. Crumley ML, et al: Do ultrasound, active warm-up, and passive motion differ on their ability to cause temperature and range of motion changes? *J Athl Train.* 36(S):S-92, 2001.

128. Houghton PE, Nussbaum EL, Hoens AM: Superficial heat. *Physiother Can.* 62:47, 2010.

129. Merrick MA. Personal communication.

130. Reed BV: Wound healing and the use of thermal agents. In Michlovitz SL (ed): Thermal Agents in Rehabilitation, ed 3. FA Davis, Philadelphia, 1990, pp 5–27.

131. De Coster D, et al: The value of cryotherapy in the management of trigeminal neuralgia. *Acta Stomatol Belg.* 90:87, 1993.

132. Bolster MB, et al: Office evaluation and treatment of Raynaud's phenomenon. *Cleve Clin J Med.* 62:51, 1995.

133. Tsang KW, et al: The effects of cryotherapy applied through various barriers. *J Sports Rehabil.* 6:345, 1997.

134. Metzman L, et al: Effectiveness of ice packs in reducing skin temperatures under casts. *Clin Orthop.* 330:217, 1996.

135. Healy WL, et al: Cold compressive dressing after total knee arthroplasty. *Clin Orthop.* 299:143, 1994.

136. Schroder D, Passler HH: Combination of cold and compression after knee surgery. A prospective randomized study. *Knee Surg Sports Traumatol Arthrosc.* 2:158, 1994.

137. Levy AS, Marmar E: The role of cold compression dressings in the postoperative treatment of total knee arthroplasty. *Clin Orthop.* 297:174, 1993.

138. Scheffler NM, et al: Use of Cryo/Cuff for the control of postoperative pain and edema. *J Foot Ankle Surg.* 31:141, 1992.

139. Whitelaw GP, et al: The use of the Cryo/Cuff versus ice and elastic wrap in the postoperative care of knee arthroscopy patients. *Am J Knee Surg.* 8:28, 1995.

140. Barr E, et al: Effect of different types of cold applications on surface and intramuscular temperature (abstract). *J Athl Train.* 32:S33, 1997.

141. Serwa J, et al: Effect of varying application pressures on skin surface and intramuscular temperatures during cryotherapy (abstract). *J Athl Train.* 36:S90, 2001.

142. Rogers JW, et al: Increased pressure of application during ice massage results in an increase in calf skin numbing. *J Athl Train.* 36:S90, 2001.

143. Rubley MD, Holcomb WR, Guadagnoli MA: Time course of habituation after repeated ice-bath immersion of the ankle. *J Sport Rehabil.* 12:323, 2003.

144. Nimchick PSR, Knight KL: Effects of wearing a toe cap or a sock on temperature and perceived pain during ice immersion. *J Athl Train.* 18:144, 1983.

145. Belitsky RB, et al: Evaluation of the effectiveness of wet ice, dry ice, and cryogen packs in reducing skin temperature. *Phys Ther.* 67:1080, 1987.

146. Newton RA: Effects of vapocoolants on passive hip flexion in healthy subjects. *Phys Ther.* 65:1034, 1985.

147. Yoon WY, Chung SP, Lee HS, et al: Analgesic pretreatment for antibiotic skin test: vapocoolant spray vs ice cube. *Am J Emerg Med.* 26:59, 2008.

148. Cohen L, et al: Effects of whirlpool bath with and without agitation on the circulation in normal and diseased extremities. *Arch Phys Med Rehabil.* 30:212, 1949.

149. Hartman S, Huch R: Response of pregnancy leg edema to a single immersion exercise session. *Acta Obstet Gynecol Scand* 84:1150, 2005.

150. Burke DT, et al: Effects of hydrotherapy on pressure ulcer healing. *Am J Phys Med Rehabil.* 77:394, 1998.

151. Press E: The health hazards of saunas and spas and how to minimize them. *Am J Public Health.* 81:1034, 1991.

152. Smith K, et al: The effect of silicate gel hot packs on human muscle temperature (abstract). *J Athl Train.* 29:S33, 1994.

153. Borrell RM, et al: Fluidotherapy: Evaluation of a new heat modality. *Arch Phys Med Rehabil.* 58:69, 1977.

154. Borrell RM, et al: Comparison of in vivo temperatures produced by hydrotherapy, paraffin wax treatment, and fluidotherapy. *Phys Ther.* 60:1273, 1980.

155. Kuligowski LA, et al: Effect of whirlpool therapy on the signs and symptoms of delayed-onset muscle soreness. *J Athl Train.* 33:222, 1998.

156. Berger Stanton DE, Lazaro R, MacDermid JC: A systematic review of the effectiveness of contrast baths. *J Hand Ther.* 22:57, 2009.

157. Higgins D, Kaminski TW: Contrast therapy does not cause fluctuations in human gastrocnemius intramuscular temperature. *J Athl Train.* 33:336, 1998.

158. Cotts BE, Knight KL, Myrer JW, et al: Contrast-bath therapy and sensation over the anterior talofibular ligament. *J Sport Rehabil.* 13:114, 2004.

159. Petrofsky J, Lohman E, Lee S, et al: Effects of contrast baths on skin blood flow on the dorsal and plantar foot in people with type 2 diabetes and age-matched controls. *Physiother Theory Pract.* 23:189, 2007.

160. Cote DJ, Prentice WE, Hooker DN, et al: Comparison of three treatment procedures for minimizing ankle sprain swelling. *Phys Ther.* 68:1072, 1988.

Deep-Heating Agents

This section describes therapeutic ultrasound, a modality that uses acoustical energy, and shortwave diathermy, an electrical modality that produces radio waves, which produce heat deep within the body's tissues. The physics, biophysical effects, and clinical application of each modality are described.

Chapter 7

Therapeutic Ultrasound

Therapeutic ultrasound is presented in this section rather than in the thermal agents section for two reasons: (1) it is an acoustical modality that uses mechanical energy rather than an electromagnetic or infrared modality and (2) it is a deep-heating agent. In addition, ultrasound is capable of producing mechanical, nonthermal effects in addition to its thermal effects. Also refer to the basic physiological responses to heat described in Chapter 5.

● Therapeutic ultrasound is a deep-penetrating agent that produces changes in tissue through thermal and nonthermal (mechanical) mechanisms. Unlike most other physical agents, ultrasound is not a part of the **electromagnetic spectrum •,** but uses acoustical energy (Box 7-1). Depending on the frequency and wavelength of the energy, ultrasound is used for diagnostic imaging (0.5 to 50 mW/cm^2), therapeutic deep tissue heating (1 to 3 W/cm^2), or tissue destruction (0.2 to 100 W/cm^2). This chapter focuses on the thermal and nonthermal effects of therapeutic ultrasound.

The human ear is capable of detecting sound waves ranging from 16,000 to 20,000 **hertz •** (Hz). Ultrasound has a frequency above this range (Box 7-2). Therapeutic ultrasound ranges from 750,000 to 3,300,000 Hz (0.75 to 3.3 **megahertz •** (MHz)). In the United States, the most frequently used ultrasound frequencies are 1 and 3 MHz (note that it is common practice to drop the .3 when reporting frequency in megahertz, so a 1-MHz frequency is actually 1,300,000 Hz or 1.3 MHz).

Traditionally, therapeutic ultrasound's deep-heating effects are used to treat musculoskeletal conditions. Depending on the output parameters, the effects of ultrasound include increased rate of tissue repair and wound healing, increased blood flow, increased tissue extensibility, reduction of calcium deposits, reduction of pain and muscle spasm by altering nerve conduction velocity, and changes in cell membrane permeability. Ultrasonic energy is also used to deliver medications to the subcutaneous tissues (phonophoresis). Another specialized form of ultrasound is used to promote fracture healing.

Electromagnetic spectrum: A continuum ordered by the wavelength or frequency of the energy produced.
Hertz (Hz): The number of cycles per second.
Megahertz (MHz): One million cycles per second.

Box 7-1. ACOUSTICAL ENERGY

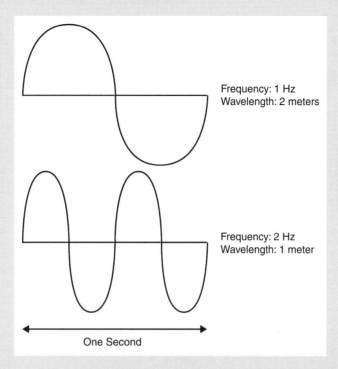

Frequency: 1 Hz
Wavelength: 2 meters

Frequency: 2 Hz
Wavelength: 1 meter

One Second

Frequency is the number of times the wave passes per second; wavelength is the distance between the start of the wave to the end of the wave (one complete cycle). As shown above, frequency and wavelength are inversely proportional: the higher the frequency, the shorter the wavelength (and vice versa). Amplitude is the maximum distance from the baseline to the peak of the wave.

Acoustical energy is transmitted differently from electromagnetic energy. Electromagnetic radiation involves the transmission of individual energy particles that do not require a transmission medium. The sun emits light particles that travel unhindered through the vacuum of space. Unlike sound waves it does not require a physical medium.

To be transmitted, acoustical energy (sound waves) requires a physical medium, such as air. Mechanical vibrations form waves in the medium that transmit acoustical energy. Therefore, the transmission of acoustical energy is impossible in the vacuum of space. If you yell at a person across the street, your voice creates waves in the air. These waves travel through the air and are received by the other person's ear.

Unlike audible sound, ultrasound's high frequency requires a medium that is denser than air to be transmitted. Water is the ideal media. The most effective ultrasound transmission media have a high water density.

In a uniform environment, sound waves travel at a constant speed. These waves have three properties: wavelength, frequency, and amplitude. Wavelength and frequency are inversely related. Referring to the above figure, the top has a longer wavelength and a lower frequency than the bottom. Frequencies are expressed in Hertz (Hz). A larger Hz number means a higher frequency. In the figure, fewer wavelengths that are 2 meters long at a frequency of 1 Hz will travel past a specific point in 1 second than sound with a wavelength of 1 meter and a frequency of 2 Hz. Amplitude is simply how loud or intense a particular sound is. As the figure shows, it does not depend on frequency or wavelength. Amplitude in the drawing is shown as the height of the waves—the higher the wave, the higher the amplitude.

Ultrasound, and its effects, is differentiated by the frequency and amplitude of the wave. Ultrasound used to produce images of the body's internal structures has a frequency of 2 to 15 MHz, but has a low amplitude. Therapeutic ultrasound has a frequency of 0.75 to 3.3 MHz and has a greater amplitude, meaning that more energy is delivered to the body per pulse.

Box 7-2. CONTRAST AND COMPARISON OF ULTRASOUND AND AUDIBLE SOUND

The way in which piezoelectric crystals produce ultrasound bears some striking similarities to the way in which an MP3 player produces audible sound. When an MP3 plays music, it detects the patterns of recorded sound impulses. These patterns are converted to electrical energy that is transferred to speakers in the headphones. Once the electrical impulses reach the speaker, it activates a magnet, causing a cone to expand and contract. The vibration of the cone produces mechanical waves that are transmitted through the air and strike our eardrums.

Ultrasound generators operate on basically the same principle. An alternating current is passed through a crystal, causing it to expand and contract. The vibration of this crystal produces mechanical waves that are passed along to the body.

The difference between the production of these two sound waves lies in the frequency at which the "speaker" vibrates. Stereos use a much lower acoustical frequency than ultrasound, so the waves can be transmitted through air and detected by the human ear. Ultrasound units use such a high frequency that the waves cannot be transmitted without the use of a dense medium and cannot be detected by the human ear.

■ Ultrasound Production

Ultrasound is produced by an **alternating current** ● flowing through a piezoelectric crystal housed in a **transducer** ● (Fig. 7-1). **Piezoelectric crystals** such as zirconate titanate produce positive and negative electrical charges when they contract or expand (Fig. 7-2). A reverse (indirect) piezoelectric effect occurs when an alternating current is passed through a piezoelectric crystal, resulting in its contraction and expansion. This mechanism, the reverse piezoelectric effect (**electropiezo effect**), is used to produce therapeutic ultrasound. The vibration of the crystal results in the mechanical production of high-frequency sound waves.

■ Transmission of Ultrasound Waves

Ultrasound produces a sinusoidal waveform that has the properties of wavelength, frequency, **amplitude** ●, and velocity (see Box 7-1). Acoustical energy is transferred by one molecule colliding with another, and in the process exchanging kinetic energy without actually displacing the molecules. Consider a leaf floating in a pond. If a pebble is dropped near it, the leaf bobs up and down as the ripples pass beneath it but does not change its position.

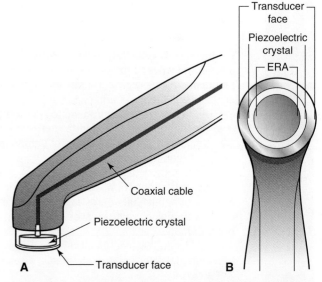

Figure 7-1. **Cross Section of an Ultrasound Transducer.** (A) Lateral view. A coaxial electrical cable delivers an alternating current that innervates the piezoelectric crystal, causing it to vibrate via the reverse piezoelectric effect and produce ultrasonic sound waves. (B) View of the transducer face. The large metallic face is the "transducer face" or "sound head." The crystal produces the ultrasonic energy, but the effective radiating area (ERA)—where the majority of the energy is produced—is smaller than the area of the crystal. In some cases the size of the transducer face may be twice the size of the ERA.[1]

Alternating current: The uninterrupted flow of electrons marked by a change in the direction and magnitude of the movement.

Transducer: A device that converts one form of energy to another.

Amplitude: The maximum departure of a wave from the baseline.

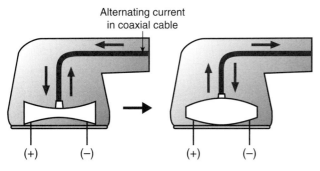

Figure 7-2. **Piezoelectric Crystals.** The reverse piezoelectric effect. The crystal expands and contracts when an electrical current is passed through it.

Because of its high frequencies, ultrasound is unable to pass through the air and requires a dense transmission medium. A coupling medium allows the ultrasonic energy to pass from the transducer to the tissues. Coupling media are discussed in Chapter 8.

Longitudinal Waves

Molecule displacement in longitudinal waves occurs parallel to the direction of the sound. A person dangling from the end of a bungee cord is an example of longitudinal waves. Longitudinal waves result in the elongation and contraction of the cord, causing the jumper to bob up and down. In this case, the energy, as represented by the jumper, is transmitted parallel to the direction of the wave.

The alternation of high and low pressure exerted by the ultrasound beam results in regions of high particle density (**compression**) and low particle density (**rarefaction**) along the path of the wave (Fig. 7-3). These pressure fluctuations transmit the energy within the tissues and, as discussed in subsequent sections, produce physiological

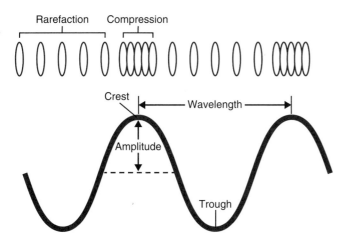

Figure 7-3. **Rarefaction and Compression of Molecules.** An ultrasound wave passing through the tissues creates alternating periods of low and high pressure. Molecules in the low-pressure areas expand (rarefaction), and molecules in the high-pressure area compress.

effects. Longitudinal waves are capable of traveling through both solid and liquid media. Ultrasound passes through soft tissue as a longitudinal wave.

Transverse (Shear) Waves

Molecules in transverse waves are displaced perpendicular to the direction of the energy. Plucking a guitar string, causing it to vibrate parallel to its length, is an example of a transverse wave (see Fig. 7-3). When the longitudinal waves of the ultrasonic beam strike bone, they become transverse waves. Transverse waves cannot pass through fluids and are found in the body only when ultrasound strikes bone.

■ Ultrasonic Energy

Low-frequency sound waves, such as those produced by human speech, diverge (spread) in all directions. The higher the frequency of the sound wave, the less the sound beam diverges. The frequencies used in therapeutic ultrasound produce relatively focused beams that have a width smaller than the diameter of the sound head. Like all sound waves, ultrasound waves are capable of reflection, refraction, penetration, and absorption (Box 7-3).

The ultrasound waves diverge as they travel through a medium, but not as much as audible sound waves. Consider the difference between a beam of light produced by a spotlight and the light produced by an ordinary light bulb. If you held the spotlight and lamp 1 foot from a wall, the spotlight would concentrate the light within an area approximately the same diameter as the lens. The light produced from the bare bulb would illuminate an area significantly larger than the bulb itself. As the distance between the lights and the wall is increased, the beams' diameters will increase, but much more so with the bare bulb than with the spotlight. Likewise, similar to the spotlight, the treatment area effectively exposed to the ultrasonic energy is limited to an area slightly larger than the diameter of the sound head.

Close to the transducer head, the pressure of the sound field is nonuniform, forming high-intensity ridges and low-intensity valleys (Fig. 7-4). This area, the **near field** or **Fresnel zone,** is the portion of the ultrasound beam used for therapeutic purposes. The pressure variations occur because the transducer head acts as if it were formed by many smaller transducers, each producing its own sound wave. Close to the transducer, these areas are individually distinguishable. As the distance from the head is increased, the waves interact to produce a more unified beam. An example of this can be found in a computer monitor. If you look very closely at the screen (a few inches away), individual colored elements are seen (hope that no one walks in the room while you are doing this). As the distance between your eye and the screen is increased, the dots lose their individuality, eventually forming a complete picture.

Box 7-3. INFLUENCES ON THE TRANSMISSION OF ENERGY

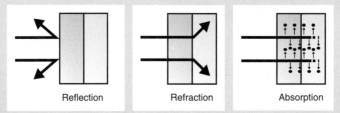

Reflection   Refraction   Absorption

Most energy prefers to travel in a straight line. However, when traveling through a medium, its course is influenced by changes in density. Energy striking the interface between two different densities may be reflected, refracted, or absorbed by the material, or continue through—penetrate—the material unaffected by the change.

Reflection occurs when the wave cannot pass through the next density. The wave strikes the object (tissues) and reverses its direction away from the material. Reflection may be complete, as when all energy is precluded from entering the next density layer, or it may be partial. An echo is an example of reflection that involves acoustical energy.

Refraction is the bending of waves as a result of a change in the speed of a wave as it enters a medium of different density. When the energy leaves a dense layer and enters a less dense layer, its speed increases. When moving from a low-density to a high-density layer, the energy decreases. A prism refracts light rays. As the light is bent within the prism each of the seven color bands becomes visible.

Absorption occurs by the tissue collecting the wave's energy and changing it into kinetic energy and then possibly into heat. The tissues may absorb part or all of the energy being delivered to the tissue. Any energy not reflected or absorbed by one tissue layer continues to pass through the tissue until it strikes another density layer. At this point, it may again be reflected, refracted, absorbed, or passed on to the next tissue layer. Each time the wave is partially reflected, refracted, or absorbed, the remaining energy available to deeper tissue is reduced, the basis for the **law of Grotthus Draper** (see Appendix A).

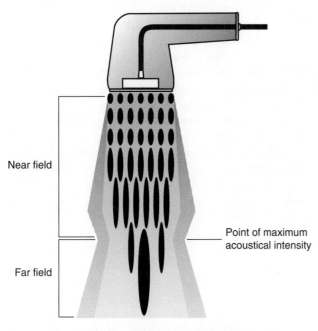

Figure 7-4. **A Schematic Representation of an Ultrasound Beam.** Note the irregular intensity of the near field and the spatial peak intensity in the far field (see Table 7-1).

Resonating: Vibrating.

Ultrasonic output is described in terms of power, the frequency of the waves, and the area that produces the power. Other measures factor in time and energy density to describe the treatment parameters (Table 7-1).

Effective Radiating Area

Ultrasound heads are available in different sizes and with different crystal **resonating** • frequencies (Fig. 7-5). The **effective radiating area** (ERA) of the ultrasound head is the proportion of the transducer's surface area that produces ultrasonic energy and is described in terms of square centimeters (cm^2). Measured 5 mm from the face of the sound head, the ERA represents all areas producing more than 5% of the maximum power output of the transducer.

The ERA is always smaller than the actual size of the transducer's face (see Fig. 7-1) and may differ from the value listed for the unit.[1] Most energy is concentrated at the center of the head, with less energy being emitted away from this point and no energy produced in the outermost part of the sound head. Large ERAs

TABLE 7-1 Ultrasound Output Parameters and Measures

PARAMETER	DESCRIPTION
Beam nonuniformity ratio (BNR)	The BNR describes the consistency (uniformity) of the ultrasound output as a ratio between the spatial peak intensity and the spatial average intensity. The lower the ratio, the more uniform the beam. A BNR greater than 8:1 is unsafe.
Duty cycle (DC)	The percentage of time that ultrasonic energy is being emitted from the sound head. A 100% duty cycle indicates a constant ultrasound output and produces primarily thermal effects within the body. A low duty cycle produces nonthermal effects.
Effective radiating area (ERA)	The area of the transducer that produces ultrasonic waves. Measured in square centimeters (cm^2). The actual ERA is usually significantly smaller than the contact area of the sound head.[1] Larger ERAs produce a more focused beam than smaller ERAs (see Fig. 7-1).[2]
Frequency	The output frequency determines the effective depth of penetration. A 1-MHz output targets tissues up to 5 cm deep; 3 MHz has a penetrating depth of at least 2 cm. These depths are influenced by tissue geometry and their relative location to bone.[3]
Intensity	The intensity describes the amount of power generated by unit.
Half layer (depth) value	Tissue depth where half of the initial output intensity has been lost.
Spatial average intensity (SAI)	The average intensity over the area of the transducer, a measure of energy density. Measured in watts per square centimeter, the SAI describes the amount of power per unit area of the sound head's ERA.
Spatial peak intensity (SPI)	The maximum output across time.
Spatial average temporal peak (SATP)	The SAI during the ON time of a pulse and is displayed as intensity on the ultrasound output meter. Meaningful only with pulsed output.
Spatial average temporal average (SATA)	Describes the SATP as calculated across the duty cycle: $1.0\ W/cm^2 \times 50\%\ DC = 0.5\ W/cm^2$ SATA. The SATA is meaningful only when delivering pulsed ultrasound.
Treatment duration	The treatment duration is determined by the output intensity and the specific goals of the treatment.

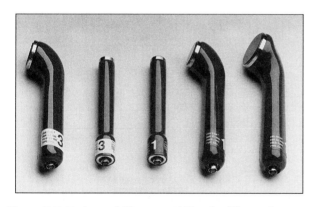

Figure 7-5. **Variety of Ultrasound Heads.** Ultrasonic transducers are available in a range of sizes and frequencies. (Courtesy of Mettler Electronics Corporation, Inc., Anaheim, CA.)

produce a **collimated** ●, focused beam. Smaller ERAs yield a more divergent beam.[2] When treating a localized area (e.g., a trigger point), use a collimated beam; when treating a larger area such as a muscle strain a divergent beam is indicated.

The ERA is used to calculate the spatial average intensity (W/cm^2) and spatial average temporal average intensities. Variation between the reported ERA and the actual ERA will affect the treatment dosage. If the ERA is smaller than indicated, then the actual spatial average intensity will be greater than the metered value and vice versa.

Frequency

Ultrasound output frequency is measured by megahertz and describes the number of waves produced in 1 second. Most commercial therapeutic ultrasound units offer 1- and/or 3-MHz outputs (a few models offer a 2-MHz option), although "longwave" ultrasound is available. Low-frequency (1 MHz) ultrasound has a beam that diverges more than high-frequency (3-MHz) ultrasound (Table 7-2).

The depth of penetration of the ultrasonic energy into the tissues is inversely related to the output frequency.[4] The lower the output frequency is, the deeper will be the penetration into the tissues. The ultrasonic energy creates molecular friction as it passes through the tissues, thereby losing energy to the tissue. Friction represents the loss of energy, thereby not **attenuating** energy left to be transmitted to the deeper tissues.[5] One-MHz ultrasound penetrates approximately 5 cm; 3-MHz ultrasound has an effective depth up to 2.5 to 3 cm.[6,7]

Collimated: Possessing a beam of parallel rays or waves that form a column of energy.

TABLE 7-2	**Comparison of 1-MHz and 3-MHz Thermal Ultrasound Application**	
	1 MHz	3 MHz
Beam profile	Relatively divergent	Relatively collimating
Depth of penetration	5 or more cm	0.8 to 3 cm
Maximum rate of heating	0.36°F (0.2°C) per minute per W/cm^2	1.1°F (0.6°C) per minute per W/cm^2
Heat latency	Retains heat twice as long as 3-MHz ultrasound	Retains heat half as long as 1-MHz ultrasound

✳ **Practical Evidence**

Although the effective depth of ultrasound penetration is often reported to be based solely on the output frequency, the output frequency is only one variable that determines the depth of heating. Over extended treatment durations (greater than 5 minutes), temperature increases are determined by heat conduction between tissues. The thermal properties, relative location to bone, and geometry influence the tissues' heating patterns.[3] While not yet definitive in humans, it appears that these factors may blur the lines between 1- and 3-MHz ultrasound.

High-frequency (3-MHz) ultrasound generators provide treatment to superficial tissues because the energy is rapidly absorbed and heats three times faster than 1-MHz ultrasound (Fig. 7-6). The 1-MHz output offers a compromise between deep penetration, adequate heating, and prevention of **unstable cavitation** ●. Because of the depth of heating, the heat produced by 1-MHz ultrasound is longer lasting than heat produced by 3-MHz ultrasound.[8]

Power and Intensity

The **power** (energy) produced by an ultrasound generator is measured in watts (W). **Intensity** describes the strength of the sound waves at a given location within the tissues being treated. There are several methods for describing the output and intensity (see Table 7-1 and Fig. 7-7).

Spatial Average Intensity

Spatial average intensity (SAI) describes the amount of energy passing through the sound head's effective radiating area (energy density). Expressed in watts per square centimeter (W/cm^2), the SAI is a measure of the power per unit area of the sound head. The SAI is calculated by dividing the power of the output (watts) by the ERA of the transducer head (square centimeters):

$$SAI = \frac{\text{Total watts (W)}}{\text{Effective radiating area (cm}^2)} = W/cm^2$$

For example, if 10 W were being delivered through a transducer head with an ERA of 5 cm^2, the SAI would be 2 W/cm^2.

Figure 7-6. **Relative Depth of Penetration of 1-MHz and 3-MHz Ultrasound.** The effects of 1-MHz ultrasound occur more deeply within the tissues than 3-MHz ultrasound, which attenuates in the superficial tissues. Note that the 1-MHz beam diverges more than the 3-MHz beam. The actual depth of penetration is based on the half-layer value of the ultrasonic energy.

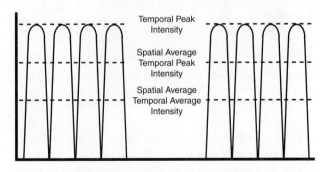

Figure 7-7. **Measures of Pulsed Ultrasound Output.** The **temporal peak intensity** represents the amplitude of a single wave. The **spatial average temporal peak intensity** is the average amount of energy delivered by a single pulse. The **spatial average temporal average intensity** is the average amount of energy delivered to the tissues during the application of pulsed ultrasound.

Unstable cavitation: The violent oscillation and subsequent rupture of bubbles during ultrasound application at too high an intensity.

Ultrasound units can display their output as either total watts or watts per square centimeter. Standard treatment doses range from 0.3 to 5 total watts (to convert this to the spatial average intensity, divide the total watts by the ERA). If the radiating area of the sound head is smaller than specified, or if a portion of the sound head is obstructed from transmitting sound (such as not being in full contact with the skin), a higher energy density is produced than that indicated on the meter.

As seen with electrical current density, altering the size of the sound head affects the power density. Passing 10 W of energy through a transducer of 10 cm^2 results in a lower density than if a head of 5 cm^2 is used (Table 7-3). Therapeutic ultrasound generators are limited to a maximum output of 3.0 W/cm^2.

Spatial Average Temporal Peak Intensity

Spatial average temporal peak (SATP) intensity describes the average intensity during the "ON" time of the pulse. The output meter on an ultrasound unit displays the SATP intensity.

Spatial Average Temporal Average Intensity

Spatial average temporal average (SATA) intensity measures the power of ultrasonic energy delivered to the tissues over a given time (total watts/time). The SATA is meaningful only for the application of pulsed ultrasound. The energy delivered to the tissues per unit of time with ultrasound operating at a 50% duty cycle is half of that delivered in a continuous mode. If we take a SAI of 2 W/cm^2 and pulse it with a 50% duty cycle, the temporal average intensity of the treatment would be 1 W/cm^2 (2 W/cm^2 × 0.5 = 1 W/cm^2).

It is important to distinguish between the SATP intensity, the average amount of power delivered during the "ON" time of the duty cycle, and the temporal peak intensity, the maximum amount of energy delivered by a single pulse. The SATP describes the total amount of energy delivered to the body during the treatment.

Ultrasound Beam Nonuniformity

The ultrasonic output consists of peaks and valleys of high and low energy that are shaped by minute imperfections in the crystal producing the sound waves. The BNR describes the variation between the peaks, the spatial peak intensity,

and valleys. This is the ratio of the highest intensity within the beam, to the average intensity reported on the output meter (Fig. 7-8):

$$BNR = \frac{\text{Spatial peak intensity}}{\text{Spatial average intensity}}$$

A perfectly uniform ultrasound beam, one that has no "peaks and valleys" would have a BNR of 1:1, but the mass manufacturing process makes producing crystals of this quality impractical. If the BNR is indicated as 3:1 and the meter displays an output of 2 W, then at some point in the beam the actual intensity is equivalent to 6 W (3 × 2 W = 6 W). The presence of high-intensity areas in the beam, "hot spots," is the primary reason for keeping the sound head moving during the treatment.

A BNR greater than 8:1 is unacceptable because the energy delivered to the body would be harmful. The U.S. Food and Drug Administration (FDA) Center for Devices and Radiological Health requires that the BNR must be indicated on the ultrasound unit.[9,10] The BNR of individual crystals do not have to be reported because the FDA allows companies to randomly sample their transducers and report the maximum BNR found.[11] The BNR of the sound head being used may be different from that indicated on the label and is indicated by "BNR < 5:1" or "6:1 Max."

Half-Layer Value

The half-layer value is the depth where 50% of the ultrasonic energy has been absorbed by the tissues. If ultrasound is applied at 1 W/cm^2 and loses 50% of its energy at a depth of 2.3 cm, the beam intensity is now 0.5 W/cm^2. At twice this depth (4.6 cm), the ultrasound intensity is reduced to 0.25 W/cm^2.[12] The effect of the half-layer value and the penetrating effects of 1- and

TABLE 7-3	Relationship of Ultrasound Radiating Area and the Total Amount of Energy Produced	
INTENSITY (W/cm^2)	EFFECTIVE RADIATING AREA (ERA) OF THE SOUND HEAD (cm^2)	TOTAL POWER PRODUCED (W)
1.5	5	7.5
1.5	6	9.0
1.5	10	15.0

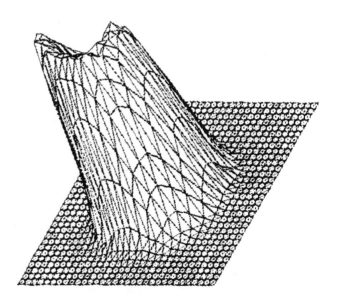

Figure 7-8. **Ultrasound Beam Profile.** This topographical map of an ultrasound beam was plotted from the intensities produced from various points on the transducer. The peak on the left side represents the beam's peak intensity. (Courtesy of IAPT. Used with permission.)

3-MHz (which has a half-layer depth of 0.8 cm) output frequencies are used to target the tissues during treatment (e.g., use 1-MHz ultrasound for deep structures).

Energy that is not reflected or absorbed is passed on to the underlying tissues (see Law of Grotthus-Draper, Appendix A). The intensity of ultrasonic energy decreases as the distance it travels through the tissues increases. This process, called **attenuation** •, occurs through the scattering and absorption of the waves within the tissues.

Duty Cycle

Each pulse has thermal and nonthermal properties. The net effects of these properties in the body are based on the duty cycle (Fig. 7-9). A continuous (100% duty cycle) output causes primarily thermal effects. A pulsed (e.g., 25% duty cycle) output produces primarily nonthermal (mechanical) effects.[13] The decision to use thermal or nonthermal ultrasound depends on the stage of healing and the treatment goals. Nonthermal ultrasound can be used during acute inflammation and thermal ultrasound is used later in the healing process.

Continuous Output

Continuous ultrasound application can effectively heat tissues located 5 (or more) cm deep, depending on the

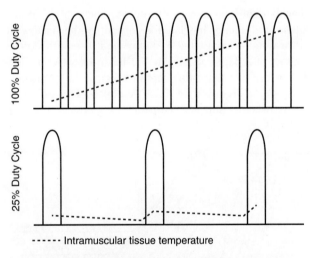

----- Intramuscular tissue temperature

Figure 7-9. **Temperature Increase per Pulse.** Each pulse produces heat and nonthermal effects. When a 100% (continuous) duty cycle is applied, the heat produced by one impulse adds to the heat produced by the prior impulse. When a pulsed output is used such as the 25% duty cycle depicted above, each wave still creates a brief increase in temperature, but the OFF cycle allows the heat to decay. Over time pulsed output still results in small increases in tissue temperature, but does not reach therapeutic ranges.

frequency used. Because the energy is produced 100% of the time, the output is measured in terms of the SATP intensity. The spatial peak intensity, as determined using the beam nonuniformity ratio (BNR), must not exceed 8 W per square centimeter (metered output × BNR).

Pulsed Output

As show in Figure 7-9, each ultrasound wave produces thermal effects. Pulsing the ultrasound output decreases the temporal average intensity, reducing the thermal effects and increasing the proportion of nonthermal effects. The duty cycle describes the percentage of time that ultrasound is being emitted from the transducer (Fig. 7-10). The ratio between the **pulse length** • and the **pulse interval** • is expressed as a percentage duty cycle:

$$\text{Duty cycle} = \frac{\text{Pulse length}}{(\text{Pulse length} + \text{Pulse interval}) \times 100}$$

The output of pulsed ultrasound is measured by the SATA intensity, but the actual amount of energy delivered to the tissue is dependent on the duty cycle. Pulsing the output reduces the temperature increase proportional to the duty cycle, but it does not entirely eliminate tissue heating.[4] The closer the duty cycle is to 100%, the greater the net thermal effects of the treatment; lower duty cycles produce greater proportions of nonthermal effects, although thermal and nonthermal effects occur at all duty cycles. With low duty cycles the heat that is formed by a pulse has time to dissipate before the next pulse.

✱ Practical Evidence

Based on the spatial average temporal average intensity, pulsed output can result in significant intramuscular temperature increases. Applying therapeutic ultrasound at 1.0 W/cm² with a 50% duty cycle will result in approximately the same amount of heating as ultrasound applied at 0.5 W/cm² and a 100% duty cycle.[14]

■ Transfer of Ultrasound Through the Tissues

Air is not dense enough to transmit ultrasonic energy. A coupling agent must be used to allow the energy to pass out of the transducer into the tissues (see Chapter 9). Ultrasound travels as pressure waves through the body. Longitudinal waves of ultrasound pass through soft tissue until it strikes bone, where some of the energy is reflected and the rest is converted into transverse waves. The propagation

---

Attenuation: The decrease in a wave's intensity resulting from the absorption, reflection, and refraction of energy.

Pulse length: The amount of time from the initial nonzero charge to the return to a zero charge, forming one complete cycle.

Pulse interval: The amount of time between ultrasonic pulses.

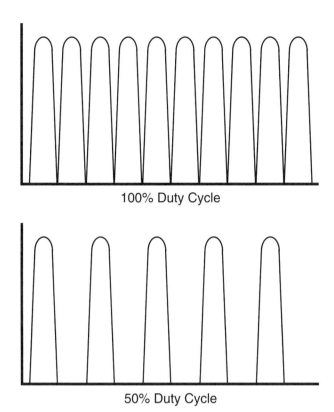

Figure 7-10. Ultrasound Duty Cycle. The amount of time that the ultrasonic energy is produced. The top figure shows a 100% duty cycle. The bottom figure shows the ultrasound that would be emitted during the same time period if a 50% duty cycle were selected.

TABLE 7-4	Percent Reflection of Ultrasonic Energy at Various Interfaces
INTERFACE	ENERGY REFLECTED (%)
Water–Soft tissue	0.2
Soft tissue–Fat	1
Soft tissue–Bone	15–40
Soft tissue–Air	99.9

high-pressure centers.[16] A high level of energy is formed in a limited amount of space, increasing the risk of tissue damage. Standing waves can be avoided by keeping the sound head moving.

Intense ultrasonic energy reflecting off of bone can produce **periosteal pain** ●. Caution is needed when applying ultrasound over bony protuberances, such as the patella or acromion process. The intensity used to treat the muscle or tendon can produce periosteal pain if applied over relatively subcutaneous bone.

Absorption of the sound waves transfers energy from the beam into the surrounding tissues through conversion of mechanical energy into thermal energy. The amount of absorption that occurs depends on the protein content of the tissues (especially collagen). Tissues that are high in water content transmit ultrasound. Protein-rich tissues such as muscles, tendon, and ligaments tend to absorb ultrasound. Ultrasound tends to reflect as it strikes bone and refract as it passes through joint spaces, potentially creating a standing wave.[15,17]

The outer portion of the skin is formed by the stratum corneum, a layer of tightly packed, dry, dead cells 10 to 15 layers thick. The low water content in this layer inhibits the transmission of ultrasound and limits the diffusion of medications used during phonophoresis treatment. Evidence suggests that hydrating the skin prior to treatment improves ultrasound transmission.[18,19]

of ultrasonic energy depends on the frequency of the sound waves and the density of the tissues. Passage of ultrasound through the body and the subsequent penetration of cell membranes cause the tissues to acquire kinetic energy, resulting in cellular vibration.

When the ultrasound beam strikes an **acoustical interface** ● such as different tissue layers, some of the energy is reflected or refracted. The amount of reflection depends on the degree of change in density at the junction between the two tissues (Table 7-4). The interface between soft tissue and bone is highly reflective. Other highly reflective interfaces include the musculotendinous junction and intermuscular interfaces. Unlike infrared energy, ultrasound is not greatly affected by adipose tissue and easily passes through it.[15]

When a reflected wave meets the incoming incident wave, a **standing wave** ● is created that increases the intensity of the energy by magnifying the high- and low-pressure areas. Free-floating gas bubbles move toward the low-pressure areas. Free-moving cells collect at the

● BIOPHYSICAL EFFECTS OF

Ultrasound Application

The physiological changes within the tissues can be grouped into two classifications, although they do not occur exclusively from one another:[20]

- Nonthermal effects: changes within the tissues resulting from the mechanical effect of ultrasonic energy

Acoustical interface: A surface where two materials of different densities meet.

Standing wave: A single-frequency wave formed by the collision of two waves of equal frequency and speed traveling in opposite directions. The energy with a standing wave cannot be transmitted from one area to another and is focused in a confined area.

Periosteal pain: A deep-seated ache resulting from overly intense application of ultrasonic energy that irritates the bone's periosteum.

- Thermal effects: changes within the tissues as a direct result of ultrasound's elevation of the tissue temperature

Nonthermal treatment is accompanied by some degree of heating, and thermal treatment is accompanied by nonthermal effects (Fig. 7-11).

These effects are limited to the treatment area, which should be no more than two to three times the sound head's ERA, but the smaller the area treated, the greater the temperature increase.[21] The proportion and magnitude of thermal and nonthermal effects are based on the duty cycle and the output intensity. The higher the duty cycle, the greater are the thermal effects; the higher the output intensity, the greater is the magnitude of the effects.

Nonthermal Effects

Nonthermal ultrasound is used when acute injuries are being treated or in other cases where tissue heating is undesirable. Nonthermal ultrasound is administered by (1) using a pulsed output (20 to 25% duty cycle) and an output intensity of 0.5 W/cm[2] or (2) using a continuous (100% duty cycle) and a low-output intensity (below 0.3 W/cm[2]).[21]

The individual pulses of ultrasonic energy cause acoustical streaming, cavitation, and microstreaming, interrelated events that produce the nonthermal effects that stimulate the healing process. Given a high duty cycle these events are also responsible for increased tissue temperatures.

Cavitation occurs as a result of the pressure changes created by the ultrasonic wave that deforms microscopic tissues. The ultrasonic peaks and troughs cause the accumulation of gas and the formation of microscopic bubbles. These bubbles then pulsate in the ultrasonic field, resulting in **stable cavitation** (see Fig. 7-3).[2,22]

Unstable cavitation (transient cavitation) involves the compression of the bubbles during the high-pressure peak, but is followed by a total collapse ("bursting of the bubble") during the trough.[21] The release of energy can destroy local tissues. In most clinical cases unstable cavitation is an unwanted, deleterious effect of ultrasound being applied at too great an intensity and can damage immobile tissue,

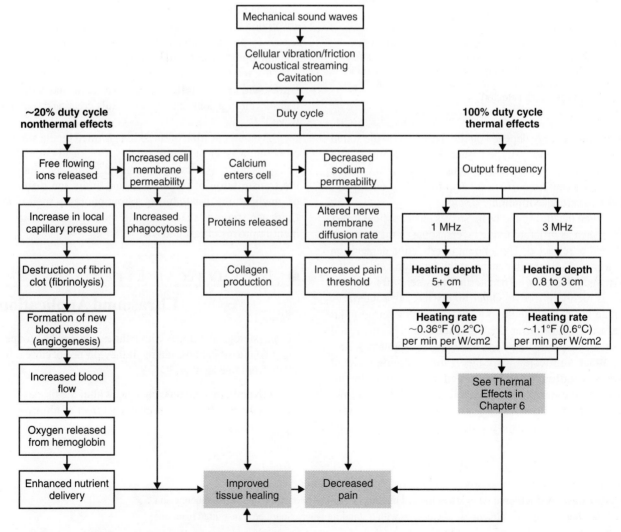

Note: Heating effects increase as the duty cycle increases.

Figure 7-11. **Schematic Diagram of the Effects of Therapeutic Ultrasound.**

free-floating blood cells, or other biological structures in the area.[4] When they are in proper working order, therapeutic ultrasound units do not have the output power or frequency required to produce transient cavitation.

Cavitation and acoustical streaming create microstreaming. Acoustical streaming is the "bulk" flow of fluids in one direction.[20] When the acoustical stream courses around gas bubbles, the cell membranes, and its **organelles** ●, **eddies** ● form.[20,23,24] The eddy current over the cell membranes causes the release of free-floating ions and small molecules, increasing cell membrane permeability that alters the diffusion rate across the cell membrane.[21,22,23] Local elevations in blood pressure, a secondary effect of cavitation and microstreaming, enhance nutrient delivery.[23]

The beneficial effects of stable cavitation, acoustical streaming, and microstreaming include early resolution of inflammation, enhancement of fibroblast recruitment, **fibrinolysis** ●, **angiogenesis** ●, increased matrix synthesis, increased tensile strength, and accelerated fracture healing.

The amount of cavitation is in direct proportion to the output intensity. Low-intensity output with a continuous output leads to more stable, prolonged cavitation than pulsed ultrasound applied at higher intensities. Low-intensity treatments are becoming the method of choice for delivering nonthermal ultrasound. Extracorporal shock wave therapy delivers low-frequency, very-high-intensity sound waves to the body to treat localized chronic inflammatory conditions.

CLINICAL TECHNIQUES: ULTRASONIC BONE GROWTH GENERATORS

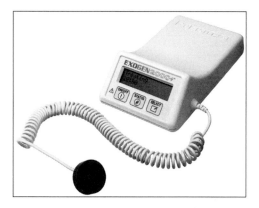

Application over unhealed fracture sites is an absolute contraindication for therapeutic ultrasound. How then can ultrasonic treatment be a promising treatment for accelerating the rate of fracture healing?

The type of ultrasound used for treating fracture sites is different from therapeutic ultrasound. Low-intensity pulsed ultrasound (LIPUS) uses output characteristics that are not available on standard therapeutic ultrasound units to produce low-level mechanical force that stimulates or accelerates bone growth.

Output Characteristics of Ultrasonic Bone Growth Generators

Parameter	Value
Output frequency	1.5 MHz
Burst width	200 microseconds
Repetition rate	1 kHz
Effective radiating area	3.88 cm^2
Temporal average power	117 milliwatts
Temporal maximum power	625 milliwatts
Spatial average temporal intensity	30 mW/cm^2 (Note: Higher intensities may inhibit healing.[19])
Treatment duration	One 20-minute treatment per day

Photograph of Exogen 2000 courtesy of Smith & Nephew, Memphis, TN.

Organelle: A specialized portion of a cell that performs a specific function, such as the mitochondria and the Golgi apparatus.

Eddy (eddies): A circular current of fluid, often moving against the main flow.

Fibrinolysis: Pathological breaking up of fibrin.

Angiogenesis: Formation of new blood vessels.

The **frequency resonance theory** explains the non-thermal effects of ultrasound using the vibration characteristics of the cellular and molecular structures. Proteins in these structures absorb the mechanical energy, altering the structure and function of individual proteins or molecules.[21] The result is stimulation of phagocytosis (assisting in the removal of inflammatory debris),[29] increase in the number of **free radicals** • in the area (increasing ionic conductance and acting on the cell membrane),[30] increased cell membrane permeability and cellular proliferation,[21] and acceleration of fibrinolysis.[21,31,32]

Increased permeability allows calcium to enter the cell, which, in turn, encourages the release of protein. Potassium, other ions, and metabolites move into and out of the cell more rapidly. Concentrations of glycosaminoglycan, the primary component needed for the proper remodeling of collagen, and hydroxyproline, one of the essential amino acids of collagen, are increased following low-dose pulsed ultrasound.[21,33] These substances result in connective tissue being stronger and more deformable, and able to withstand greater loads.

Collagen synthesis, secretion of **cytokines** •, increased uptake of calcium in fibroblasts, increased fibroblastic activity (essential for the production of functional, healthy granulation tissue and scar tissue), mast cell degranulation, and increased macrophage activity are also promoted.[16] This mild acceleration of the inflammatory stage helps the body reach the proliferation stage sooner.

Thermal Effects

The amount of temperature increase during treatment depends on the mode of application (high duty cycle), the intensity and frequency of the output, the vascularity and tissue type, and the size of the treatment area. Temperature increase is also generator dependent, with some brands producing more heating than other brands.[34] Using 1-MHz ultrasound in a treatment area two times the ERA can raise the subcutaneous tissues' temperature 6.3°F (3.5°C)[35] and 16.7°F (9.3°C) using 3-MHz ultrasound. Using the same output parameters but increasing the treatment area to six times the ERA (much larger than the recommended treatment area) results in only a 2.3°F (1.3°C) temperature increase.[8]

✳ Practical Evidence

The size of the treatment area is one of the most important factors in producing meaningful thermal effects. Given the same output intensity, frequency, treatment duration, and duty cycle, increasing the treatment area can decrease the resulting temperature increase to well below therapeutic levels if the treatment area is more than two to three times the size of the ERA.[8,35,36]

The thermal effects of ultrasound are the same as those described for heat in Chapter 5. The primary differences are that ultrasound heats deeper tissues and affects a smaller area. The physiological changes within the tissues are based on the amount of temperature increase (Table 7-5). Ultrasound applied with a 1-MHz output frequency can affect tissues located up to 5 cm deep; 3-MHz ultrasound is effective on tissues located up to 2 to 3 cm deep. Tissues heated with 1-MHz ultrasound retain heat approximately twice as long as heat generated by 3-MHz ultrasound.[8]

To achieve a therapeutic heating effect, the tissue temperature must be elevated for a minimum of 3 to 5 minutes.[16,37] Three-megahertz ultrasound heats three to four times faster than 1-MHz ultrasound, although the thermal effects of 1-MHz ultrasound last longer (see Table 7-2).[12,38] The relationship between the output intensity and treatment

---

TABLE 7-5	Temperature Increases Required to Achieve Specific Therapeutic Effects During Ultrasound Application	
CLASSIFICATION OF ULTRASOUND	TEMPERATURE INCREASE	USED FOR THERMAL EFFECTS
Mild	1°C	Mild inflammation
		Accelerating metabolic rate
Moderate	2°C–3°C	Decreasing muscle spasm
		Decreasing pain
		Increasing blood flow
		Reducing chronic inflammation
Vigorous*	3°C–4°C	Tissue elongation, scar tissue reduction
		Inhibition of sympathetic activity

Tissue temperatures must be increased to 39°C to 45°C for vigorous heating to occur. Temperatures greater than 45°C result in tissue destruction.

Free radical: A highly reactive molecule having an odd number of electrons. Free radical production plays an important role in the progression of an ischemic injury.

Cytokines: Proteins produced by white blood cells.

duration determines the amount of temperature increases. Lower output intensities require a longer treatment duration to elevate the tissue temperature to the desired level. Preheating the treatment area for 15 minutes using a moist heat pack can decrease the treatment time required to reach vigorous heating levels by 2 to 3 minutes in deep (3 cm) tissues using a 1-MHz output.[39]

Heat production is related to the amount of attenuation of the sound waves in the tissues.[40] The process involved in attenuation, absorption, and scattering creates friction between the molecules that increases temperature. Collagen-rich tissues—such as tendon, joint menisci, superficial bone, large nerve roots, intermuscular fascia, and scar tissue—are preferentially heated.[16] Tissues that are largely fluid filled, such as the fat layer and articular fluid, are relatively transparent to ultrasonic energy.[15] Because of their size and relative fluid content, muscle bellies are not well heated by ultrasound, but scar tissue and fascia within the muscle belly are.

Heating that occurs secondary to the conversion of ultrasonic energy into thermal energy is then transferred to the surrounding tissues by conduction. This effect blurs the actual effective depth of heating based on output frequency alone. The actual depth and magnitude of heating is strongly influenced by the tissues' properties and geometry (Fig. 7-12).[3]

Temperatures in poorly vascularized tissues increase by 1.4°F to 2.5°F (0.8°C to 1.4°C) per minute during the application of 3-MHz continuous ultrasound.[4,12] In highly vascularized areas like muscle, the temperature increase is not as great because incoming, cooler blood continually washes out the local warmer blood.[41] Temperature increases of up to 8.8°F (4.9°C) have been documented 2.5 cm deep within the muscle after 10 minutes of 1.5 W/cm² ultrasound application.[15]

Reflected waves also increase the amount of heating. When ultrasound waves are reflected, the energy passes through the tissues more than once (forming a standing wave), increasing the thermal effects.

● EFFECTS ON

The Injury Response Process

The effects of ultrasound application depend on the mode of application (continuous or pulsed), the frequency of the sound, the size of the area treated, and the vascularity and density of the target tissues. The deep thermal effects are

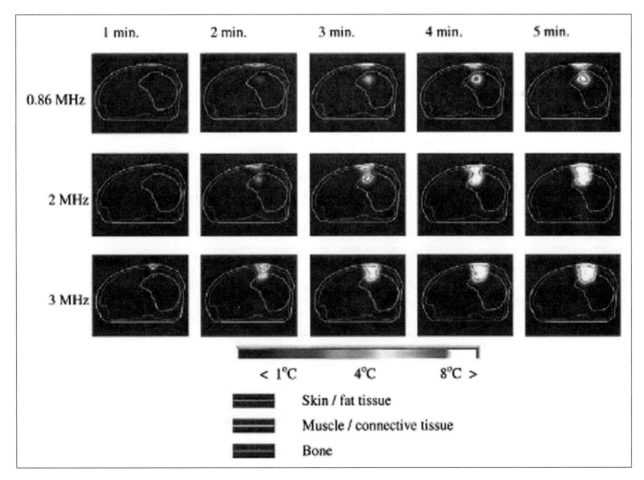

Figure 7-12. **Thermal Imaging of Ultrasonic Heating.** Cross section demonstrating the amount of heat accumulation at 1-minute increments at various output frequencies. Note that there is relatively little difference in heating depths and patterns among the three frequencies.

similar to those described in the thermotherapy section (see Chapter 6). Nonthermal effects are discussed, where relevant, in each of the following sections. A specialized form of ultrasound promotes fracture healing.

The effects of therapeutic ultrasound are not universally accepted and a great deal of discrepancy is found in the research. Refer to the Controversies in Treatment section at the end of this chapter.

Cellular Response

Acoustical streaming and cavitation increase cell membrane permeability, changing the diffusion rate across the cell membrane. Cellular responses to ultrasound include increased histamine release, increased intracellular calcium, mast cell degranulation, and increased rate of protein synthesis.[21,42,43,44] Thermal effects increase cell metabolism and accelerate the rate of inflammation.

Inflammation

In the acute stage of injury, the use of continuous ultrasound output is contraindicated because of the increased tissue temperature and the associated increased need for oxygen. Nonthermal ultrasound has been used during the acute and subacute inflammatory stages but substantial evidence does not support the use of this technique.

The acceleration of the inflammatory process results in an earlier onset of the proliferation stage of the healing process.[45] Changes in cell membrane permeability result in degranulation and the release of growth factors and platelets that stimulate fibroblast proliferation.[42] The application of continuous ultrasound has been shown to positively influence macrophage activity[43] and to increase the adhesion of leukocytes to the damaged endothelial cells.[46] When applied during the proliferation phase, ultrasound stimulates cell division.[47]

Blood and Fluid Dynamics

Continuous ultrasound can increase local blood flow for up to 45 minutes after treatment,[48] although this finding is not universally accepted.[49,50] Blood flow remains at the pretreatment level during the initial 60 to 90 seconds of treatment. After this point blood flow increases, regulating the temperature increase by carrying heat from the area.[41] Eventually a balance between the heat delivered and the heat removed by blood will reach an equilibrium and a fairly consistent temperature will be maintained.[41]

Other physiological factors may also promote increased blood flow.[51] Alteration of cell membrane permeability could result in decreased vascular tone, leading to a dilation of the vessels, and histamine released in the treated area could also cause vasodilation, further increasing blood flow.

Moist heat,[39] ice massage,[48] and cold packs[37] have been applied before ultrasound to alter blood flow during and after the treatment. The use of moist heat before ultrasound application significantly reduced the relative increase in blood flow.[39] Ice massage before ultrasound maintains the increased blood flow at the level found with ultrasound application alone. Cold pack application, long thought to increase the thermal effects of ultrasound, greatly decreases intramuscular temperature increase at a depth of 5 cm below the skin after ultrasound, 3.2°F (1.8°C) compared with a 7.2°F (4°C) rise in the temperature of tissues that were not cooled before treatment.[37]

Nerve Conduction and Pain Control

Ultrasound controls pain directly by affecting the peripheral nervous system and the result of the other tissue changes associated with ultrasound application. Ultrasound directly influences the transmission of nerve impulses by eliciting changes within the nerve fibers. Cell membrane permeability to sodium ions is affected, altering the nerve's electrical activity[20] and elevating the pain threshold.[54,55] Nerve conduction velocity is increased as a result of the thermal effects of ultrasound application.

Indirect pain reduction results from the other effects of ultrasound application. Increased blood flow and increased capillary permeability augment the delivery of oxygen to hypoxic areas, reducing the activity of **chemosensitive pain receptors** ●. Input from mechanical pain receptors is reduced because of a reduction in the amount of muscle spasm and increased muscular relaxation.[52]

✱ Practical Evidence

Ultrasound applied at 0.5 to 1.0 W/cm² for 15 minutes daily for 2 weeks can reduce the symptoms of carpal tunnel syndrome.[56]

Muscle Spasm

As described in Chapter 2, the thermal effects of ultrasound can decrease muscle spasm by reducing the mechanical and chemical triggers that continue the pain-spasm-pain cycle. Alteration of nerve conduction velocity, the counterirritant effect of increased temperature, and increased blood flow can decrease noxious stimulus. Relaxation of muscle tension by increasing blood flow, increased delivery of oxygen, and encouraging the elongation of muscle fibers can decrease the mechanical stimulus.

Tissue Elasticity

Ultrasound preferentially heats collagen-rich tissues, especially tendon, ligament, fascia, and scar tissue. To promote

---

Chemosensitive pain receptors: Nerves that are excited by the presence of certain chemical substances.

tissue elongation, the temperature of the target tissues must be elevated 7.2°F (4°C). After ultrasound application, the stretching window is short lived.[38] The thermal effects associated with vigorous heating (see Table 7-5), when applied at 3 MHz, have an effective stretching time of just over 3 minutes after the end of the treatment, although the window may be slightly longer when 1-MHz ultrasound is used.[38]

To be permanently elongated, noncontractile tissues must be heated and stretched across multiple treatments.[54] When the goal of the ultrasound treatment is to elongate tissue, place the tissues on stretch during the treatment. Any subsequent stretching or joint mobilization techniques should be performed immediately after the treatment ends. Repeated application across a number of days may be necessary to obtain the desired lengthening.[35,55]

Therapeutic ultrasound is effective only in heating a relatively small area of tissue. For this reason, it is not effective for heating a large area of muscle. Exercise or short-wave diathermy (see Chapter 9) should be used instead of ultrasound in these cases.

Muscle and Tendon Healing

Animal studies have shown that the application of continuous ultrasound increased the rate of collagen synthesis in tendon fibroblasts[47] and tendon healing,[57] and increased the tensile strength of tendons.[42,58] Tendons can transform individual ultrasound pulses into heat that causes metabolic change in the tissues. Although continuous ultrasound can produce enough acoustical pressure to damage healing fibers, pulsed ultrasound may assist in healing by increasing their tensile strength.[59]

One-megahertz, continuous output ultrasound enhances the release of preformed fibroblasts. Three-megahertz ultrasound increases the cells' ability to synthesize and secrete the building blocks of fibroblasts.[43,45,47] This response appears to be localized to areas with a high collagen content, especially tendons, and may be a more effective treatment for tendinopathies than phonophoresis.[60]

Wound Healing

Some superficial wounds have responded favorably to ultrasound application. Continuous ultrasound delivered at 1.5 W/cm² for a 5-minute treatment over a 1-week period can increase the breaking strength of incisional wounds. The same protocol, except applied at 0.5 W/cm² for a 2-week duration, produced the same results of increased breaking strength after 1 week, and facilitation of collagen deposition was demonstrated during the second week.[61] (Note: The preceding studies were performed with a 1-MHz output frequency; the results of the same protocol using a 3-MHz output have not been established.)

Pressure ulcers treated with 3-MHz, 5 cm² ERA, 20% duty cycle, at an output intensity of 0.1 to 0.5 W/cm² applied around the open wound and also treated with standard wound care techniques demonstrated accelerated healing compared with the use of standard wound care techniques (Fig. 7-13).[62] Ultrasound applied at 1 W/cm² or applied using a continuous output may have an inhibitory effect on wound healing, possibly because the necrotic tissues are unable to dissipate heat.[62]

■ Fracture Healing

Low-intensity pulsed ultrasound (LIPUS) applied in one 20-minute session per day has demonstrated an improved healing rate for acute and nonunion fractures[22,60,64,65,66,67,68] and spinal fusion.[69] The efficacy of LIPUS in the treatment of stress fractures is unclear.[70,71] This technique is not approved for skull **nonunion fractures** or with skeletally immature individuals.

Each phase of the bone-healing process, inflammation, soft callus formation, hard callus formation, and bone remodeling, may benefit from LIPUS.[65] The primary classification of cells involved in the healing process is osteoblasts, osteoclasts, macrophage, chondroblasts, and fibroblasts (see Chapter 1). Similar to soft tissue injury response, the acute fracture ruptures blood vessels leading to hematoma formation that eventually stops the bleeding, but also causes necrosis of the bone. Necrosis triggers an inflammatory action that includes the release of cytokines, osteoclasts, and macrophage to remove the debris.[23]

Angiogenesis attracts fibroblasts and osteogenic cells, forming a procallus. Fibroblasts produce a collagen bond between the fracture segments. Chondroblasts, formed from osteogenic cells, lay down fibrocartilage that forms the soft callus. Osteoblasts create a vascular network and that allows the formation of the hard callus.[72] Bone remodeling is marked by osteoclasts that remove cellular debris; osteoblasts then replace the removed debris with compact bone, forming the permanent repair (Fig. 7-14).[23]

Mechanisms proposed to assist healing are microdisplacement of the fracture segments, cavitation,[23] slight temperature increase,[22] and increased neurotransmitter activity.[73]

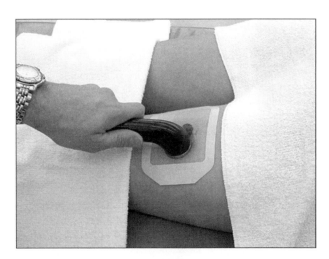

Figure 7-13. **Ultrasound Application to Promote Wound Healing.** The wound may be covered with an occlusive dressing, and MHz low-intensity, pulsed output is applied to the periphery of the wound.

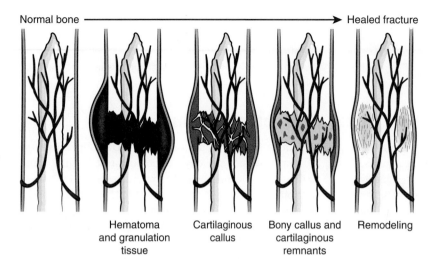

Figure 7-14. **Phases of Bone Healing.**

Although delivered at a low intensity and with a pulsed output, LIPUS still causes a slight increase in temperature, less than 1°C. Some of enzymes such as collagenase are sensitive to this subtle temperature increase, accelerating their activity.[22]

Microdisplacement assists in osteogenic cells forming fibrocartilage. When applied early in the healing stage, cavitation and acoustical streaming increase the quality and strength of the bony callus.[19,22] The production of the angiogenic factors **interleukin-8, basic fibroblast growth factor, vascular endothelial growth factor,**[74] bone-forming cell **cyclooxygenase-2,** and **messenger RNA**[68] appears to be enhanced by cavitation.[23] In particular, stimulating the proliferation of osteoblasts[72] and chondrocytes accelerates the subsequent healing events.[22] When applied toward the end of the healing process, cartilage growth is primarily stimulated.[19]

Treatment outcomes depend on the fracture site, the lapsed time to the initiation of treatment, the location of the fracture, and the stability of the fracture site.[75] In acute tibial fractures, LIPUS has been demonstrated to reduce the clinical healing time (86 days compared with 144 days for the control group) and radiographic healing time (96 days; control group equals 154 days), an outcome which was found to be both statistically significant and, perhaps most important, clinically significant.[63,64]

✱ Practical Evidence

When treatment is started soon after the injury, the preponderance of evidence indicates that LIPUS is effective in accelerating the rate of acute fractures.[63,64,76-78] Application during the inflammation and callus formation phases of healing results in a more viable, functional callus.[22,73]

LIPUS is unable to activate the healing process and therefore is less effective when applied late in the healing process.[19] This technique is not effective in accelerating the healing of tibial fractures that have been surgically reinforced using an **intramedullary rod.**[77,79] The use of medications containing calcium channel blockers, nonsteroidal anti-inflammatory medications, steroids, and, possibly, smoking decrease the probability of success of LIPUS.[80] Age is also inversely proportional to the effectiveness of LIPUS in healing nonunion fractures.[22]

CLINICAL TECHNIQUES: EXTRACORPOREAL SHOCK WAVE THERAPY

Low-frequency, high-pressure sound waves (lipsotrophy) have long been used to break down kidney stones, gall stones, and other urologic and gastric conditions. This technique has been modified to treat musculoskeletal conditions. Extracorporeal shock wave therapy (ESWT) uses focused, high-pressure sound waves that produce microtrauma to disintegrate calcific deposits, reactivate the inflammatory process, and promote healing.[2,25] The pressure wave is produced by a hydraulic, pneumatic, or electromagnetic impulse driving a piston through a cylinder. The resulting pressure wave is transmitted from a transducer into the tissues.[26] ESWT is sometimes applied under local anesthesia.

Although ESWT is used experimentally to treat a wide range of inflammatory conditions, it is currently approved by the FDA only to treat plantar fasciitis and lateral elbow tendinopathy.[27,28] In chronic calcific conditions such as calcific tendinopathy or calcaneal spurs, ESWT is proposed to degrade the calcium buildup and stimulate its reabsorption.[28] Pain reduction is thought to be the result of activation of inhibitory fibers in the brain stem and somatic pain suppression mechanisms.[26]

■ Phonophoresis

Phonophoresis describes the use of therapeutic ultrasound to assist in the diffusion of medication through the skin.[61] Proposed mechanisms of actions include ultrasonic energy causing changes in the tissues and/or changes in the medication that allow the medication to diffuse across barriers and be absorbed by the body.[81]

Although it is easy to visualize the ultrasound waves physically driving the medication through the skin, phonophoresis does not work this way. Rather, ultrasound opens pathways that allow the medication to diffuse through the skin and pass deeper into the tissues. Cavitation is believed to cause small openings in the stratum corneum and increase in pore size.[18,19] These openings allow the medication to be absorbed by superficial capillaries and thereby be absorbed subcutaneously.[19]

The advantage of introducing medications into the body through phonophoresis rather than by injection is that the medication is spread over a larger area, and phonophoresis is noninvasive.[82] Medication that enters the tissues by phonophoresis bypasses the liver, thus lessening the metabolic elimination of the substances.

Transdermally applied medications must first pass through the enzymatic barrier of the epidermis and the stratum corneum, the rate-limiting barrier to diffusion, before being absorbed by the subcutaneous tissues. The stratum corneum determines the rate and amount of medication that is transmitted to the deeper tissues. Medications that are absorbed through the skin may be stored in the subcutaneous tissues and require a longer time to diffuse into the deeper tissues.

With this in mind, the type and consistency of the skin overlying the treatment area are important elements in determining the success of the treatment. Factors such as skin composition, hydration, vascularity, and thickness combine to encourage or prohibit medication diffusion through the skin and, therefore, into the deeper tissues (Table 7-6).

Many substances such as medicated lotions or creams can be moved past the skin's barriers simply by massaging them into the skin. However, some medications have been shown to be delivered to depths of 6 cm into the tissues with the assistance of ultrasound.[83,84] The thermal and nonthermal effects associated with standard ultrasound application may increase the rate and amount of medication absorbed. The thermal effects of ultrasound increase the kinetic energy of both the local cells and the medication, dilating the points of entry (hair follicles, sweat glands, etc.), increasing circulation, increasing capillary permeability, and disordering the structured lipids in the stratum corneum.[85,86,87] Nonthermal effects enhancing diffusion across the membranes include altering the cell's resting potential, affecting the permeability of ionized and un-ionized molecules, and increasing cell membrane permeability.[86,88,89]

Preheating the treatment area with a moist hot pack to increase local blood flow and kinetic energy can further enhance delivery of the medication into the tissues. Moist heat also assists in hydrating the stratum corneum, assisting in both the transfer of ultrasound through the skin and aiding in the diffusion of medication across the skin barrier.[18]

Phonophoresis is applied using a prescription or nonprescription medication that has molecules of relatively small size and of low molecular weight (Table 7-7).[90,91] The small size and weight of the molecules is needed for the medication to diffuse through the skin. The medication is often mixed with an inert base such as ultrasound gel to help transmit the energy to the tissues. If the medication is mixed with a base, the base must be capable of transmitting ultrasonic energy (see Direct Coupling in Chapter 8).

TABLE 7-6 Skin Factors Affecting the Rate of Medication Diffusion During Phonophoresis

FACTOR	EFFECT
Hydration	The higher the water content, the more permeable the skin is to the passage of medications.
Age	Dehydration occurs as skin ages; circulation and **lipid** ● content are also decreased.
Composition	The easiest passage of medication through the skin is near hair follicles, sebaceous glands, and sweat ducts.
	Although hair follicles encourage the passage of medication through the skin, excessive hair should be shaved off the area being treated.
Vascularity	Highly vascular areas are more apt to allow for the transfer of the medication into the deep tissues. Constricted vessels localize the effects, whereas dilated vessels enhance the systemic delivery of the medication.
Thickness	Thick skin presents a much more cumbersome barrier to medication than does thinner skin. When applying phonophoresis to an area, attempt to administer it over areas of low skin density (e.g., when treating an individual suffering from plantar fasciitis, apply the medication to the medioinferior aspect of the calcaneus rather than on its plantar surface).

Lipid: A broad category of fat-like substances.

TABLE 7-7	**Medications Commonly Administered via Phonophoresis**		
CLASSIFICATION	INDICATIONS	TARGET TISSUES	EXAMPLES
Corticosteroids	Inflammatory conditions	Subcutaneous tissues	Hydrocortisone
		Nerves	Dexamethasone 0.4%
		Muscle	Diclofenac
Salicylates	Inflammatory conditions	Subdermal tissues	Myoflex*
	Pain		
Anesthetics	Pain	Nerves	Lidocaine
	Trigger points	Circulatory system	Benzydamine

Note: Does not transmit ultrasonic energy.

✱ Practical Evidence

Phonophoresis transfer may be improved by placing the medication on preheated skin and covering the area with an occlusive dressing one half-hour prior to treatment. Following the treatment, leave the dressing in place for several hours to further encourage vascular absorption and distribution of the medication.[18,86]

Do not use medication mixtures that are not specifically intended for phonophoresis. Many commonly used phonophoresis mixtures reflect most—if not all—of the ultrasonic energy. In this case the ultrasound has no effect on the treatment.[61,89]

Most thick, white, corticosteroid creams are poor ultrasound conductors. Topical gel-mixed media, such as commercially available transmission gels, are good conductors.[92] Another approach to administration of phonophoresis is the "invisible method," where the medication is first directly massaged into the skin and then followed by a traditional ultrasound application. It stands to reason that those medications that can be naturally absorbed through the skin are more effective for phonophoresis than those that are not easily absorbed.

The efficacy of phonophoresis has not been fully substantiated.[82,84,89,93,94] Many of the contradictions in the results of studies can be related to the type of coupling agent used and the concentration of the medication. For example, one study examined the subcutaneous absorption of a commercially available **salicylate** ●, Myoflex, and found no difference in the level of salicylates in the bloodstream with or without the use of ultrasound.[89] A later study revealed that Myoflex transmitted no ultrasonic energy (see Table 8.1).[92]

Still, the actual amount of medication that penetrates to the viable tissues and the effect that ultrasonic energy has on the absorption is unclear. **Hydrocortisone** ● is thought to be delivered into the subcutaneous tissues, where it slowly diffuses into the deeper tissues, but increased serum cortisol levels have not been found after treatment.[91,95] Hydrocortisone itself is a poor transmitter of acoustical energy.[92] Both pulsed and continuous ultrasound improve the transmission and subsequent absorption of **diclofenac** gel relative to topical application, resulting in a significant decrease in pain and increased function.[96]

Dexamethasone transmits 95% to 98% of ultrasonic energy and is becoming more prevalently used for phonophoresis.[97] Likewise, dexamethasone has not been proved to produce a measurable effect in the submuscular or subtendinous tissue[97] or in any amount sufficient to impair adrenal function.[98,99]

Some of the limitations found in traditional phonophoresis techniques may be circumvented through the use of low-frequency sound generators. These devices use a 20-kHz frequency (at the upper range of human hearing), 125 mW/cm^2, pulsed output to enhance the introduction of medication into the deep tissues. The lower frequency allows medications of a larger molecular size and weight, including insulin and **interferon gamma** ●, to penetrate deeper into the tissues. Initial reports on this technique indicate that low-frequency sonophoresis is capable of delivering a wide range of medications up to 1000 times more effectively than those produced with the traditional ultrasound method (Box 7-4).[90,98,100] The effect of the treatment may be enhanced by covering the treated area with a dressing following treatment to keep the area hydrated.[86]

Salicylates: A family of analgesic compounds that includes aspirin.
Hydrocortisone: An anti-inflammatory drug that closely resembles cortisol.
Interferon gamma: A group of proteins released by white blood cells and fibroblasts when devouring the unwanted tissues. The gamma classification is also referred to as "angry macrophages" because of their heightened phagocytic activity.

Box 7-4. LONGWAVE ULTRASOUND

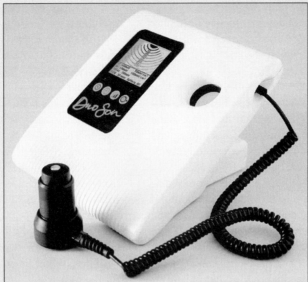

Therapeutic ultrasound traditionally has been used with an output frequency that ranges between 1.0 and 3.3 MHz. Longwave ultrasound employs a wavelength ranging between 20 and 45 **kilohertz** ● (kHz) and is used for both deep heating and for phonophoresis application. The longer wavelength is capable of effectively penetrating the body's tissues and can produce bone-depth heating in even the largest muscle mass.[101]

The longer wavelength results in greater particle displacement within the tissues and produces a more uniform beam. The increased overall power and homogeneity of the ultrasonic wave require lower output intensities to reach therapeutic levels than traditional ultrasound units. Heating can be obtained with an output intensity of 0.3 to 0.8 W/cm² and nonthermal effects occur at levels below 0.3 W/cm². Application above 0.8 W/cm² can result in tissue damage.[42]

Unlike shortwave ultrasound, longwave generators do not require the use of a transmission medium. However, a lubricant is used to assist in moving the sound head over the skin. The indications and contraindications for the use of longwave ultrasound are similar to those of traditional ultrasound.

Duoson, courtesy of Orthosonics, Devon, England.

Phonophoresis using prescription medication is regulated by most state pharmacy practice acts. Although there is variation from state to state, the law may require that the medication be specifically prescribed to the individual patient.

■ Contraindications to Therapeutic Ultrasound

In cases in which the use of ultrasound is questionable because of underlying medical conditions, consult with the patient's physician to determine if this modality should be used. Thermal ultrasound should not be applied in the presence of the general contraindications to heat application (see Table 5.7). Refer to At a Glance: Therapeutic Ultrasound in Chapter 8 for a complete list of contraindications and precautions in the use of therapeutic ultrasound.

Therapeutic ultrasound must not be applied over areas of impaired circulation, ischemic areas, or areas having sensory deficit. The lack of normal circulation reduces the body's ability to dissipate the heat and may result in burns, a risk that is increased in the absence of normal sensory function. Application over areas of active deep vein thrombosis or thrombophlebitis may cause the clot to dislodge and move elsewhere in the circulatory system. Use over sites of active infection may result in the infection spreading. Application of ultrasound over cancerous tumors can increase the tumor's mass and weight.[102]

Specific body regions are potentially hazardous targets of ultrasound, especially fluid-filled cavities. Avoid application

Kilohertz (kHz): One thousand cycles per second.

over the eyes, heart, skull, and genitals. Application over an implanted pacemaker and its leads is contraindicated because of the risk of damage to the pacemaker or causing it to malfunction. Increased bleeding may occur if ultrasound is applied over the pelvic, lower abdominal region, or lumbar area of menstruating women. Because of the risk to the fetus, do not apply therapeutic ultrasound to the abdominal, pelvic, or lumbar areas during pregnancy.

The use of therapeutic ultrasound over active fracture sites or stress fractures may cause pain and may possibly delay healing (the exception to this is ultrasonic bone growth stimulators). Application of therapeutic ultrasound over unfused epiphyses is commonly listed as a contraindication to therapeutic ultrasound, but no definitive evidence supports this claim. Metal implants are also sometimes listed as a contraindication to ultrasound application. However, metal rapidly conducts heat away from the area and this procedure should be appropriate if the sound head is kept moving. Avoid thermal application over plastic implants or areas of bone cement (e.g., joint replacements). Heating can result in pliability of the plastic or cement.

Although not a strict contraindication, use caution when applying ultrasound over the vertebral column, nerve roots, or large nerve plexus. The tissue densities in these regions may result in a rapid rate of heating. Following a **laminectomy** •, portions of the muscle and bone covering the spinal cord may retract, potentially directly exposing the spinal cord to the ultrasonic energy. See At a Glance: Therapeutic Ultrasound for a list of contraindications to therapeutic ultrasound application.

■ Overview of the Evidence

Despite the relative wealth of published research examining the effects of therapeutic ultrasound, the efficacy of this device is still being questioned. There is sufficient evidence to indicate that continuous ultrasound can significantly increase the temperature of subcutaneous tissues.[8,12,15,36,37,38,39,103-106] However, other studies suggest that the temperature increases are dependent on the ultrasound generator being used and identify variations between units of the same model.[3,11,34,41,107]

Much of the published research examining the effectiveness of ultrasound in patient care was methodologically flawed, suffered from a lack of randomized controlled trials, and was limited by an insufficient range of patient problems.[108]

In examining the biophysical effects of ultrasound, the authors concluded that there is no evidence that cavitation actually occurs during therapeutic ultrasound application and initial studies may have been misled by instrumentation errors.[20] If this is the case, then bulk streaming rather than acoustical streaming may occur in the human body. Bulk streaming has less of a biophysical effect than acoustical streaming. And if acoustical streaming does not occur, then the nonthermal effects attributed to ultrasound may not occur.[20] Subsequent research has both supported[21] and refuted[13] the potential of therapeutic ultrasound's nonthermal effects.

Despite all of the recent questions regarding the efficacy of ultrasound, sufficient evidence exists to conclude definitively that when it is applied at the proper intensity for the proper duration and the treatment area is limited to two to three times the transducer's ERA, ultrasound is capable of vigorously heating a small volume of tissue. This may be the inherent limitation to its use. Therapeutic ultrasound is probably incapable of heating a large muscle mass and improving range of motion. This deficit has, in part, given renewed interest in shortwave diathermy as a deep-heating agent.

For ultrasound to be effective, it must be used properly, an issue that has plagued this modality since entering the mainstream of health care. Common clinical errors in application include selecting the wrong output frequency, using an output intensity that is too low when attempting to produce thermal effects, treating too large an area, using inappropriate coupling media, and moving the sound head too rapidly. Therapeutic ultrasound has its place in the care of musculoskeletal injuries. However, the tool (modality) must fit the job (the treatment goals).

Continuous ultrasound has been thought to be the treatment of choice for the treatment of heterotopic ossification (myositis ossificans). Therapeutic ultrasound delivered at high treatment doses and/or long treatment durations over ectopic bone can stimulate further growth.[109]

Laminectomy: Surgical removal of the lamina from a vertebra.

Chapter 8

Clinical Application of Therapeutic Ultrasound

Ultrasound application has evolved from what was once a rote "cookbook" approach to a clinical science. Determining if ultrasound is indicated and, if appropriate, the proper output parameters requires knowledge of the type of tissues involved, the depth of the trauma, the nature and inflammatory state of the injury, and consideration of the skin and tissues overlying the treatment area.

● Although some treatment parameters have been established, patient feedback and reevaluation of the response to prior treatments form the basis for adjusting the treatment parameters. Inform the patient about the expectations and sensations that are to be expected during the treatment and inform the patient to report any uncomfortable, unusual, or unexpected sensations such as pain or burning.

To ensure safe application of therapeutic ultrasound, units must be calibrated at least once a year (many manufacturers recommend that this be done twice a year). The U.S. Food and Drug Administration (FDA) requires that the output frequency, effective radiating area (ERA), and beam type must be indicated on the generator or the transducer[10] (Fig. 8-1). The date of the last calibration must also be indicated somewhere on the unit. The reported ERA is the average for that make and model; the actual ERA may be significantly different from the reported value.[11] The size

of the transducer face may also be included if it is significantly different from the size of the ERA (see Fig. 7.1).[1]

Tissue Treatment Area

Ultrasound can only increase tissue temperatures when the treatment area is approximately two times the size of the ERA.[8] Note that the ERA is approximately half the size of the transducer face. Attempting to heat a larger area will significantly reduce the temperature increase. If the size of the target tissues is larger than three times the ERA, divide the area into two or more treatment zones (Fig. 8-2).

If more than two zones are being treated, stagger the treatment order to prevent contiguous zones from being heated consecutively. However, this method does not increase the collagen elasticity of large body areas sufficiently enough

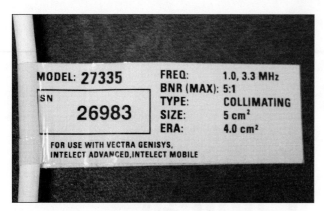

Figure 8-1. **FDA Labeling Requirements for Therapeutic Ultrasound.** The sound head pictured here is capable of producing an output frequency of 1 or 3.3 MHz and has an effective radiating area of 4.0 cm². Note that the BNR is listed as 5:1 for both outputs. The "Max." indicates that this was the maximum BNR found in a sample of sound heads.

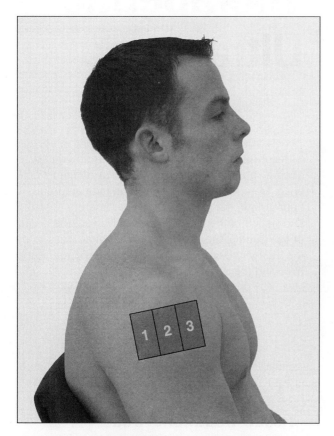

Figure 8-2. **Treatment Zones.** When treating an area more than twice the size of the sound head's ERA, divide the area into two or more "treatment zones." Use caution when treating overlapping areas. In this example treat the two outer zones and then the center zone. As one treatment zone is being heated, the prior treatment areas will cool, thus limiting the ability to effectively heat the muscle mass as a whole.

to promote their elongation. The effectiveness of thermal ultrasound treatment decreases as the area treated increases.

The size of the treatment area for nonthermal treatments may be slightly larger. However, there are no definitive guidelines for this mode of application.

Coupling Methods

Ultrasonic waves cannot pass through the air; a transmission medium is needed to transmit the energy from the transducer into the tissues. A good medium must transmit a significant percentage of the ultrasound; therefore, it should be nonreflective. The optimal medium for transmission is distilled water, which reflects only 0.2% of the energy.[110]

Attempting to pass ultrasound through a nonconductive medium can damage the crystal. Most ultrasound generators automatically shut down if application is attempted without a medium, if an unacceptable medium is used, or if sufficient contact is not made with the skin. Do not attempt to increase the output intensity without the transducer in contact with the body.

When treating large, regularly shaped body areas (such as the quadriceps muscle group), obtaining a good couple is relatively easy. However, irregularly shaped areas decrease the contact area between the transducer and the skin, causing uneven delivery of energy to the tissues, requiring modified coupling methods.

Direct Coupling

In this method of ultrasound application, the transducer is applied directly to the skin, with an approved gel used to transfer the energy between the ultrasound head and the skin. Coupling agents are made of distilled water and an inert, nonreflective material that increases the viscosity of the mixture. Coupling media that contain 1% methyl nicotinate, a superficial vasodilator may increase blood flow and help hydrate the topical skin layer and improve the transmission of energy.[106]

Not all substances efficiently transfer the ultrasonic energy from the transducer to the tissues, and many block the energy altogether (Table 8-1).

Topical counterirritants and analgesics have been used as coupling agents, but these products can decrease the

TABLE 8-1	Coupling Ability of Potential Ultrasound Media

Substance	Transmission Relative to Distilled Water (%)
Saran Wrap	98
Lidex gel, fluocinonide 0.05%	97
Thera-Gesic cream, methyl salicylate	97
Mineral oil	97
Ultrasound transmission gel	96
Ultrasound transmission lotion	90
Chempad-L	68
Hydrocortisone powder (1%) in US gel	29
Hydrocortisone powder (10%) in US gel	7
Eucerin cream	0
Myoflex cream, trolamine salicylate 10%	0
White petrolatum gel	0

US = ultrasound.

effectiveness of the treatment or altogether render the treatment ineffective. Although some analgesic creams are good conductors of ultrasonic energy (e.g., Thera-Gesic), others do not transmit ultrasonic energy (e.g., trolamine salicylate [Myoflex]) (see Table 8-1). The use of counterirritants as an ultrasound transmission agent increases the patient's perception of heat, but the actual amount of intramuscular heating may be less than that obtained from ultrasound gel.[111,112]

Application Technique

Apply the gel liberally to the area and ensure a consistent thickness and that no large air bubbles are present (Fig. 8-3). Poor conductivity can increase the spatial average intensity by decreasing the contact area between the transducer and the tissues. The effectiveness of ultrasound transmission gel or cream is decreased if the body part is hairy or irregularly shaped. The application of gel causes air bubbles to cling to hair. The greater amount of hair on the body part, the greater the reduction of ultrasound delivered to the tissues. If the body hair is excessive, consider shaving the treatment area.

Use firm, constant pressure to hold the sound head in contact with the skin.[113] Too little pressure creates an insufficient couple. Too much pressure decreases the amount of energy transferred to the tissues by scraping off

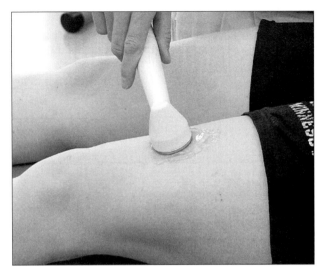

Figure 8-3. **Direct Coupling Method Using an Ultrasound Gel.** Note that the treatment area is only twice as large as the effective radiating area.

the transmission medium, and the pressure may cause the patient discomfort. Move the sound head slowly, using approximately 0.44 to 1.32 pounds of pressure.[113]

CLINICAL TECHNIQUES: SPEED LIMIT . . . SLOW DOWN WHEN MOVING THE SOUND HEAD

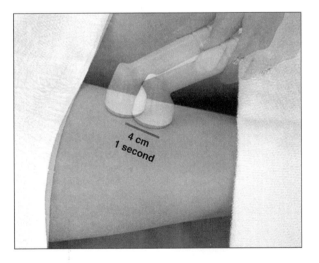

4 cm
1 second

There is a tendency to move the sound head too rapidly during treatment. When thermal ultrasound is being applied, moving the sound head too quickly can decrease the amount of temperature increase to the point of ineffectiveness. An analogy can be made between the speed that the sound head is moved and ironing a pair of pants. If the iron is moved too quickly across the pant leg, it will not be heated to the point required to remove the wrinkles. Moving the iron too slowly can scorch the cloth.

The same holds true for ultrasound. Slow, precise strokes are recommended to allow the tissues to warm, but moving the sound head too slowly can overheat the

tissues. The speed limit for moving the sound head is approximately 4 cm per second, but the slower the better.[113]

If the patient experiences discomfort from the treatment, move the head slightly faster and/or decrease the output intensity. This is related to the spatial peak intensity, creating "hot spots" in the ultrasound output. However, the patient should feel warmth if a thermal treatment is being applied.

In the **stationary head technique,** the sound head is held over the target tissue (e.g., a trigger point or area of muscle spasm). This technique is seldom used because of standing waves overheating the tissue and hot spots associated with the beam.

Heating the skin with a moist heat pack results in a more rapid increase in intramuscular temperature; the use of warm transmission gel does not. Preheating the transmission gel may be done for patient comfort. Overwarming the gel can reduce its density and decrease the efficiency of ultrasonic energy transmission.[114]

Pad (Bladder) Method

This technique originally used a balloon, condom, or plastic bag filled with water or ultrasound transmission gel that was coated with a coupling agent.[115] The bladder is able to conform to irregularly shaped areas such as the acromioclavicular or talocrural joints. The disadvantage is the formation of air pockets within the bladder that prohibit the transmission of sound waves and the difficulty holding the gel-coated bladder in place. The bladder should be made from thin plastic. Rubber products may absorb more energy as the ultrasound wave passes through the bladder on one side and then again on the other, resulting in less energy being available to be delivered to the tissues.[115]

Commercially produced gel pads have become a popular and effective alternative to the bladder method.[115] Gel pads are formed from ultrasound gel in a tight matrix that allows them to hold their shape while also conforming to the contours of the body (Fig. 8-4). Gel pads also limit the treatment area to the size selected, thus focusing the energy on an area approximately twice the size of the sound head.

Application Technique

Fill the bladder with **degassed water** • (see the Immersion Technique section) or ultrasound gel. Remove all air pockets

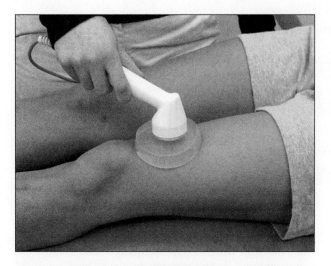

Figure 8-4. Ultrasound Application Using an Ultrasound Gel Pad. This method is used to deliver ultrasound to irregularly shaped areas when the underwater area is not practical. These pads also limit the treatment area to an appropriate size.

and large bubbles to prevent blockage of the ultrasonic energy. Apply a transmission medium to the skin and the outer surface of the bladder. The bladder is then held against the body part while the sound applicator is moved over its surface. If a gel pad is used, coat both sides with ultrasound gel to improve coupling and to ease motion of the sound head over the pad.[105]

✳ Practical Evidence

Gel pads are a convenient method of ultrasound coupling. However, 2-cm-thick gel pads transmit less energy than 1-cm-thick pads. In all cases the use of gel pads reduces the amount of heating relative to direct coupling.[104]

Immersion Technique

When treating irregularly shaped areas such as the distal extremities, a more uniform dose of ultrasound is delivered using water as the transmission medium. The body part is immersed in a tub of water (degassed water is the ideal). Water can be degassed by first boiling it for 30 to 45 minutes and then storing it in an airtight container (sterile or distilled water may be used as well).

Application Technique

A ceramic or metal tub is recommended for underwater ultrasound application.[109,110] The reflective surface creates an "echo chamber" that allows the sound waves to strike the body part from all angles. Plastic tubs are not recommended because they absorb ultrasonic energy.[109] If nondistilled water is being used, the intensity of the ultrasound can be increased by approximately 0.5 W per square centimeter to account for attenuation caused by minerals in the water. Tap water immersion, using 3-MHz ultrasound, is less effective in increasing subcutaneous tissue temperatures than the direct coupling method.[103,115]

Place the transducer in the water with the sound head approximately one-half inch away and facing the body part (Fig. 8-5). The face of the transducer should be parallel with the surface of the skin so that the energy strikes the tissues at a 90-degree angle. Angles of less than 80 degrees significantly reduce the effectiveness of the treatment (see the Cosine Law in Appendix A).[116] The operator's hand should not be continually immersed in the water. Although this is not necessarily dangerous in a single treatment, immersion could unnecessarily expose the hand to ultrasonic energy over repeated exposures.

Air bubbles tend to form along the patient's skin during the treatment, potentially interfering with the transmission of ultrasound and the energy striking the tissues. Using a tongue depressor, wisp away any bubbles that form on the

---

Degassed water: Water that has been allowed to sit undisturbed for 4 to 24 hours, allowing the gaseous bubbles to escape.

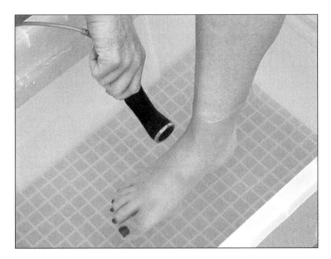

Figure 8-5. **Underwater Application of Ultrasound.** Water is used as a coupling medium to distribute the energy evenly over irregularly shaped areas. The sound head does not come into contact with the body part.

patient's skin or on the transducer face before and during the treatment.

■ Selecting the Output Parameters

The following sections describe the methodology used to select the various output parameters. This information is described in more detail in Chapter 9.

✳ Practical Evidence

Although research has identified the parameters needed to maximize the treatment, these recommendations are frequently not used clinically. Even small deviations in the treatment parameters can result in significant decreases in temperature increase. The most common errors in clinical technique are treating too large an area, using too short a treatment duration, and selecting an output intensity that is too low.[36]

Output Frequency

The effective depth of the ultrasonic energy and the rate of heating are based on the output frequency. An output frequency of 1 MHz targets tissues up to at least 5 cm deep. Three-megahertz output has traditionally been thought to target tissues up to 2 cm deep, although there is evidence that indicates that heating may occur up to 2.5 to 3 cm deep.[6,7] Table 8-2 details the differences in 1- and 3-MHz ultrasound application.

Superficial structures such as the patellar tendon, medial collateral ligament, and brachialis require a 3-MHz output. Deep structures such as the rotator cuff, vastus intermedius, and the gastrocnemius call for a 1-MHz output. Keep in mind that subcutaneous adipose tissue is relatively transparent to ultrasonic energy.

Duty Cycle

The duty cycle determines if the treatment effects will be primarily thermal or nonthermal, although the two are never truly separate. Nonthermal effects are always accompanied by thermal effects and vice versa. However, the rate and magnitude of temperature increase are markedly reduced when a low duty cycle is used. Nonthermal effects are used for acute injuries and a continuous output is used when thermal effects are desired.

The duty cycles available on most units range from 20% to 100% (continuous output) with gradations ranging from 5% to 25%. Although it is clear that a 100% duty cycle is used for thermal effects and the lowest duty cycle for the treatment of acute injuries (or when nonthermal effects are desired), it is less clear when, or even if, to use the intermediate duty cycles.

Output Intensity

The effects of the ultrasound treatment depend on the output intensity, the treatment duration, and the duty cycle. The overall amount of energy delivered to the body also depends on the BNR and the ERA.[11] When a continuous output is used, the output meter displays the spatial average temporal peak intensity in watts per square centimeter (W/cm^2) or the total output in watts (W). When the output is pulsed, the overall intensity must be thought of in terms of the spatial average temporal average (SATA) intensity, the average amount of energy per unit of time. Remember that the metered output displays only the average intensity in the near field and does not reflect the peak intensity as represented by the BNR.

TABLE 8-2	Comparison of 1-MHz and 3-MHz Thermal Ultrasound Application	
	1 MHz	3 MHz
Beam profile	Relatively divergent	Relatively collimating
Depth of penetration	5 or more cm	0.8 to 3 cm
Maximum rate of heating	0.36°F (0.2°C) per minute per W/cm2	1.1°F (0.6°C) per minute per W/cm2
Heat latency	Retains heat twice as long as 3-MHz ultrasound	Retains heat half as long as 1-MHz ultrasound

Thermal Treatments

For thermal treatments, 1-MHz ultrasound applied at 1.5 W/cm² heats at the approximate rate of 0.2°C per W/cm²; 3 MHz heats at approximately 0.2°C per W/cm² (Fig. 8-6).[12] Approximately 10 minutes of treatment time is required to heat tissues to 7.2°F (4°C) using 1-MHz output and a treatment area twice the size of the ERA and an output of 2 W/cm². For 3-MHz ultrasound, just under 4 minutes at an output intensity of 1.75 W/cm² is required (see Table 8-3). There tends to be a progressive increase in tissue temperature during the first 6 minutes of treatment, after which the rate of increase tapers out. The temperature plateau represents a balance between the energy (heat) applied and blood carrying heat away from the area.[41]

The values presented in Figure 8-6 are estimates of the treatment duration required to reach the target temperature. The body area being treated and the depth of the target tissue, the ultrasound unit's BNR, application techniques, and the coupling medium used influence the rate and degree of temperature increase. Ultimately, heat production varies between manufacturers[34] and even between identical units made by the same manufacturer.[11,41,107]

* Practical Evidence

The amount of heating depends on the output intensity, treatment duration,[117] and the duty cycle. Increasing each of these variables increases the potential for heat production.

The patient should describe "warmth" or heat during thermal treatments but not pain or burning. Discomfort could indicate that the sound head is not being moved fast enough, approximately 4 cm per second. Adjust the output intensity to the patient's tolerance and comfort. Uncalibrated units, incomplete contact of the transducer with the skin, and/or too intense a treatment dosage can result in skin burns and blistering.[118] Err on the side of caution, use shorter treatment durations and lower treatment intensities, and make subsequent adjustments based on the patient's response to the treatment. Note that the patient's report of heat may not reflect the actual temperature increase within the muscle.[112]

Nonthermal Treatments

The treatment intensity and duration for nonthermal treatments is largely based on experience and anecdotal evidence. Nonthermal effects are delivered using a low duty cycle (20% to 25%) with an intensity of 0.5 W/cm² for treatment of acute injuries.[29,119] Nonthermal effects can also be obtained using a 100% duty cycle with an output intensity less than 0.3 W/cm². Superficial skin lesions, such as pressure sores, respond well to 3-MHz ultrasound applied using a 20% duty cycle and an output intensity of 0.1 to 0.5 W/cm².[62]

Treatment Duration

The length of the treatment depends on the output frequency, output intensity, duty cycle, and the therapeutic goals of the treatment. In all circumstances, the area for any particular treatment should be no larger than two times the surface area of the sound head's ERA.[1,8]

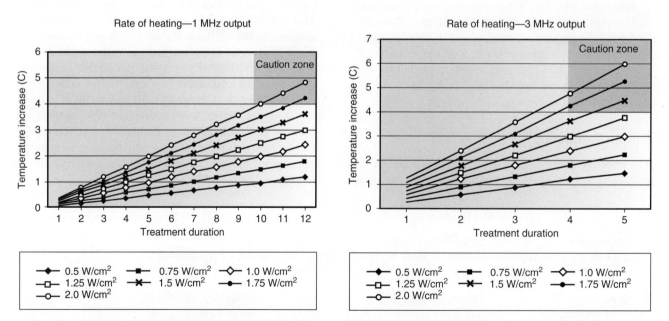

Figure 8-6. Approximate Treatment Time Based on Target Temperature Increase. Assuming a continuous output (100% duty cycle), the approximate treatment times (in minutes) required to obtain specific tissue temperatures at different output intensities. The patient should report warmth, but not pain or discomfort, during the treatment.

✳ Practical Evidence

The treatment duration ultimately determines the amount of intramuscular heating. High intensities applied for a short duration result in less heating than therapeutic ultrasound applied at a lower intensity for a longer duration.[117]

When vigorous heating effects are desired, the treatment duration should be in the range of 10 to 12 minutes for 1-MHz output and 3 to 4 minutes for 3-MHz ultrasound. Table 8-3 should be used as a guide for determining the actual treatment duration based on the frequency of the ultrasound being applied and the goals of the treatment.

Dose-Oriented Treatments

Improvements in the quality of ultrasound generators, microprocessors, and research regarding the heating effects of ultrasound have led to the development of dose-oriented treatment parameters. The desired amount of temperature increase is entered and the unit calculates the output intensity and treatment duration. The clinician may still adjust the treatment intensity, but the treatment duration would change inversely. Decreasing the intensity would increase the duration and vice versa.

■ Ultrasound and Electrical Stimulation

The combination treatment of ultrasound and electrical stimulation has been used for treatment of trigger points and other superficial painful areas, although research supporting the benefits of this combined treatment approach is lacking. In this technique, the ultrasound head serves as an electrode for an electrical stimulating current (Fig. 8-7). Theoretically, this application method would provide the benefits of ultrasound and electrical stimulation if they were applied separately, namely, improved circulation, reduction of muscle spasm, and decreased adhesion of scar tissue.

Trigger points and other stimulation points display a decreased resistance to electrical current flow (see Chapter 12).

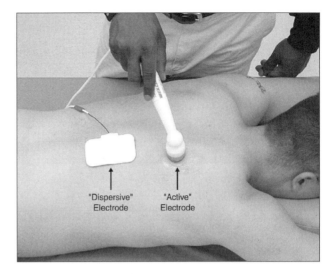

Figure 8-7. **Ultrasound and Electrical Stimulation Combination Therapy.** Using a sound/stimulation combination unit, one electrode is attached to the patient's body while the ultrasound head serves as the active "probe" electrode.

When a moderate pulse duration and moderate pulse frequency are applied at an intensity sufficient to produce a strong muscle contraction, the muscle fibers within the trigger point may fatigue to the point where they no longer have the biochemical ability to spasm. Low-amperage electrical stimulation is capable of increasing adenosine triphosphate activity within the cells, increasing their ability to repair themselves. Increased phagocytosis and increased circulation would assist in the collection and removal of cellular wastes from the treatment area.[120]

A wide range of combined ultrasound and electrical stimulation units are being marketed. The electrical stimulation part of these units delivers a monophasic, biphasic, or alternating current. Each of these parameters would affect the target tissues differently. Likewise, many ultrasound generators in this configuration, especially older ones, deliver only a 1-MHz output. In most instances, a 3-MHz output would be needed to target the stimulation points.

A slowly moving sound head is needed to produce the required amount of subcutaneous tissue temperature increase, approximately 7.2°F (4°C). Placing the target tissues on stretch during treatment could assist the reduction of trigger points and muscle spasm.[53]

■ Set-Up and Application of Therapeutic Ultrasound

Ultrasound generators are available in a wide range of makes and models. Although most models have unique features, most are capable of delivering ultrasound at different frequencies (1 and 3.3 MHz being the most common), have adjustable duty cycles, and are capable of using sound heads of different effective radiating areas. Many manufacturers produce "combo units" that are both ultrasound generators and electrical stimulators (Fig. 8-8).

TABLE 8-3	Rate of Ultrasound Heating	
Temperature Increase per Minute		
Intensity (W/cm²)	1 MHz	3 MHz
Tissue Depth	5 cm Deep	1.2 cm Deep
0.5	0.04°C	0.3°C
1.0	0.2°C	0.6°C
1.5	0.3°C	0.9°C
2.0	0.4°C	1.4°C

Applied at two to three times the effective radiating area.

At a Glance: **Therapeutic Ultrasound**

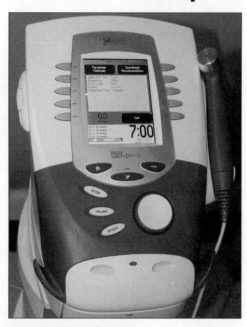

Description

- High-frequency (1 to 3.3 MHz) sound waves applied to the body to produce thermal and nonthermal effects.

Indications

- Chronic inflammatory conditions such as calcific bursitis (pulsed or continuous output)
- Acute inflammatory conditions (pulsed output)
- Pain reduction
- Joint contractures
- Muscle spasm
- Neuroma
- Scar tissue
- Sympathetic nervous system disorders
- Trigger points
- Warts
- Spasticity
- Post-acute reduction of **myositis ossificans**

Primary Effects

THERMAL
- Increased nerve conduction velocity
- Increased extensibility of collagen-rich structures
- Increased blood flow
- Increased macrophage activity

NONTHERMAL
- Increased cell membrane permeability
- Tissue regeneration
- Stimulating phagocytosis
- Synthesis of collagen

Contraindications

- Acute conditions (continuous output)
- Ischemic areas
- Areas of impaired circulation including arterial disease (continuous output)
- Over areas of active deep vein thrombosis or thrombophlebitis
- Anesthetic areas (continuous output)
- Over cancerous tumors
- Over sites of active infection or sepsis
- Exposed metal that penetrates the skin (e.g., **external fixation** devices)
- Over replaced joints using plastic or fixated bone cement.
- Areas around the eyes, heart, skull, carotid sinus, or genitals
- Over the thorax in the presence of an implanted pacemaker
- Pregnancy when used over the pelvic or lumbar areas

- Over breast implants[121]
- Over a fracture site before healing is complete
- Stress fracture sites or sites of osteoporosis
- Over the pelvic or lumbar area in menstruating female patients

Treatment Duration

- The treatment time is from 3 to 12 minutes, depending on the size of the area being treated, the intensity of the treatment, and the goal of the treatment. A minimum of 10 minutes is recommended for thermal treatments.[109]
- Ultrasound is normally given once a day for 10 to 14 days, at which time the efficacy of the treatment protocol should be evaluated.

Precautions

- Use caution when applying ultrasound around the spinal cord, especially after laminectomy. Many manufacturers list this as a contraindication to ultrasound application. The various densities provided by the spinal cord and its covering may result in a rapid temperature rise, causing trauma to the spinal cord.
- Anesthetic areas (pulsed output)
- High treatment doses over the areas of ectopic bone (e.g., heterotopic ossification, myositis ossifications) may stimulate unwanted growth.[109]
- The use of ultrasound over metal implants is not contraindicated as long as the sound head is kept moving and the treatment area has normal sensory function.
- The use of ultrasound over the **epiphyseal plates** of growing bone should be performed with caution.
- Do not apply thermal ultrasound in high doses over the spinal cord, large nerve plexus, or regenerating nerves.
- Symptoms may increase after the first two treatments because of an increase in inflammation in the area. If the symptoms do not improve after the third or fourth treatment, discontinue the use of the modality.[122]

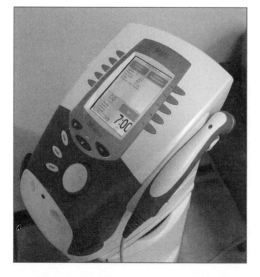

Figure 8-8. Ultrasound–Electrical Stimulation Combo Unit. These devices are electrical stimulators and ultrasound generators housed in the same unit. Electrical stimulation and ultrasound can be applied at the same time (see Ultrasound and Electrical Stimulation).

Instrumentation

Duty cycle: Adjusts between continuous and pulsed ultrasound application. Most units display the duty cycle as a percentage, with 100% representing continuous ultrasound. Low duty cycles produce primarily nonthermal effects; with a 100% duty cycle the predominant effect is thermal.

Frequency: Selects the output frequency—and therefore the depth of penetration—of the ultrasound. A 3-MHz frequency should be used for tissues 2.5 cm or less; 1 MHZ is used for greater tissue depths.[6]

Gel warmer: A heating element is used to preheat the transmission gel. This is primarily for patient comfort and has little, if any, additive effect on the treatment. Overwarming (or overcooling) the transmission medium may possibly decrease the thermal effects of ultrasound treatments.[114]

Intensity: Adjusts the intensity of the ultrasound beam. The WATT METER displays the output in either total watts (W) or watts per square centimeter (W/cm^2).

Maximum head temperature: Sets the maximum heat tolerance in the sound head in case the head is not properly coupled.

Pause: Interrupts the treatment but retains the remaining amount of treatment time when the treatment is reinstated.

Power: Allows the source current to flow into the internal components of the generator. On many units, a POWER light goes on, or the WATT METER illuminates.

Start-Stop: Initiates or terminates the production of ultrasound from the transducer.

Timer: Sets the duration of the treatment. The time remaining is displayed on the console, or the timer rotates to display the time remaining.

Watt meter: Displays the output of ultrasound in total watts or watts per square centimeter. Digital meters may require that the user manually switch between the two displays. Most **analog** • meters display the total watts on an upper scale while simultaneously displaying output in watts per square centimeter on the lower scale. These typically have a sound head with a fixed ERA.

Patient Preparation

1. Establish that no contraindications are present.
2. Determine the method and mode of ultrasound application to be used during this treatment.
3. Clean the area to be treated to remove any body oils, dirt, or grime. If necessary, shave excess body hair in the treatment area.
4. For thermal treatments, identify a treatment area that is no larger than two to three times the size of the ERA.
5. Determine the coupling method to be used.

   Direct coupling: Spread the gel over the area to be treated. Use the sound head to evenly distribute the gel.

   Gel pad: Cover both sides of the pad with ultrasound gel.[105]

   Immersion: If possible use degassed water to fill a ceramic or plastic tub deep enough to immerse the target tissue. Place the patient's extremity in the water with the sound head approximately 1 in. from the body part.

6. Explain the sensations to be expected during the treatment. During the application of continuous ultrasound, a sensation of mild to moderate warmth (but not pain or burning) should be expected. No subcutaneous sensations should be felt during the application of pulsed ultrasound. Advise the patient to inform you of any unexpected sensations.

7. For thermal treatments applied using a 1-MHz output, preheating with a moist heat pack will decrease the treatment time required to reach vigorous heating levels.[39]
8. Advise the patient to report any adverse, unusual, or painful sensations during the treatment. Improper application of therapeutic ultrasound can result in skin burns.[118]

Initiation of the Treatment

1. Reduce the INTENSITY to zero before turning on the POWER.
2. Select the appropriate mode for the output. Use CONTINUOUS output to increase the thermal effects of ultrasound application or PULSED output for nonthermal effects. The more acute the injury or the more active the inflammation process, the lower the duty cycle that is used.
3. Ensure that the WATT METER displays the appropriate output for the type of treatment.
4. Set the TIMER to the appropriate treatment duration, but treat an area no larger than two to three times the size of the unit's ERA. The actual duration of the treatment depends on the desired effects of the treatment, the output intensity, and the body area being treated. Nonthermal effects require a shorter treatment duration than thermal effects. Refer to Figure 8-6 for the approximate times required to reach various therapeutic heating levels.
5. Begin slowly moving the sound head over the medium and depress the START button to begin the treatment session. Units having low BNR may be moved at a slower rate than those with a higher BNR.
6. Slowly increase the INTENSITY to the appropriate level while keeping the sound head moving and in contact with the patient's body, immersion bath, or coupling bladder.
7. Move the sound head at a moderate pace (4 cm per second or slower) using firm, yet not strong, overlapping strokes.[113]
8. If periosteal pain is experienced (a sharp pain or ache), move the sound head at a faster rate, use a reduced duty cycle, or lower the intensity. If the pain continues, discontinue the treatment.
9. If the gel begins to wear away or if the sound head begins sticking on the skin, PAUSE the treatment and apply more gel.

Phonophoresis Application

1. Clean and, if necessary, débride and/or shave the treatment area.

Analog: A readout on a continuously variable scale. A clock with hands is a type of analog display

2. Preheating the treatment area is recommended to decrease skin resistance and increase the absorption of the medication.[83]

3. Position the extremity to encourage circulation.

4. Apply the medication directly over the target tissues and apply a liberal amount of ultrasound coupling gel over the medication. Cover the area with an occlusive dressing such as Tegaderm™. If possible, allow the mixture to pre-absorb into the skin for 30 minutes prior to applying ultrasound.[123]

5. Follow the procedures described in Initiation of the Treatment.

6. Ultrasound is delivered using a 50% or 100% duty cycle and at an output intensity ranging from 1.0 to 2.0 W/cm^2.

7. After treatment, allow the occlusive dressing to remain in place.[86]

✳ Practical Evidence

Applying an occlusive dressing over the medication 30 minutes before the treatment and allowing it to remain in place following the treatment significantly increase the subcutaneous absorption of medication during phonophoresis.[123]

Termination of the Treatment

1. Most units automatically terminate the production of ultrasound when the time expires. If the treatment is terminated prematurely, reduce the intensity before removing the transducer from the medium.

2. Immediately initiate any post-treatment stretching.

3. Remove the remaining gel or water from the patient's skin.

4. To ensure continuity of treatment sessions, record the parameters used for this treatment in the individual's file; specifically, record the output frequency, intensity, duration, and duty cycle. Keep a running count of ultrasound treatments given for this condition.

▧ Maintenance

Federal regulations require that therapeutic ultrasound units be recalibrated annually by an authorized service technician. Recalibration of the output intensity is reflected clinically by adjusting the patient's treatment intensity. For example, consider an instance where the metered output was 20% higher than the actual output intensity. The service technician would recalibrate the metered output downward by 20%. In future treatments the treatment output intensity would need to be increased by 20% to obtain the same results.[1]

Daily Maintenance

Clean ultrasound head and transducer face as recommended by the manufacturer.

Monthly Maintenance

1. Check all electrical cords for tears, fraying, or kinks.

2. Check the sound head cable for tears, fraying, or kinks.

3. Clean the transmitter face as recommended by the manufacturer.

Chapter 9

Shortwave Diathermy

Shortwave diathermy is a high-frequency electrical current that produces deep tissue heating. Similar to therapeutic ultrasound, shortwave diathermy is delivered in pulsed or continuous output modes to produce thermal and nonthermal effects. Also refer to the basic physiological responses to heat described in Chapter 5.

● Shortwave diathermy (SWD) uses oscillating high-frequency non-ionizing electromagnetic energy (similar to broadcast radio waves) to produce deep heat within the tissues. The electromagnetic energy lacks the wavelength duration needed to depolarize motor or sensory nerves. The Federal Communications Commission (FCC) has reserved the frequencies of 13.56, 27.12, and 40.68 MHz for medical use, with the 27.12-MHz (wavelength of 11 m) frequency being the most common.[124] Another type of radiofrequency deep heating modality, **microwave diathermy** (MWD), is not used clinically in the United States (Box 9-1).

The thermal effects of SWD are similar to those described in Chapter 5, but occur deeper in the tissues. Shortwave diathermy can also be applied in a nonthermal mode. The thermal and nonthermal effects are similar to therapeutic ultrasound, but SWD does not reflect from bone and is less likely to create hotspots (Table 9-1).[124] Shortwave diathermy also affects a significantly greater volume of tissue than does ultrasound, roughly the size of a cereal bowl for SWD compared with approximately the size of a ketchup packet for therapeutic ultrasound.[124]

■ Shortwave Diathermy Generation

Different forms of *diathermy,* a Greek word meaning "through heat," have been used since the late 1800s to treat a range of musculoskeletal conditions, diseases, and general medical conditions. The prevalence and popularity of shortwave and microwave diathermy (developed in the mid-1900s) has been cyclical. Leakage of the energy away from the intended target ("scatter") created concerns about patient and clinician safety that hindered the use of these devices. Diathermy also causes interference with electronic devices such as cell phones and computers.[126] Improved shielding, the ability to better focus the energy, and better control of the dosage have led to a renewed interest in SWD as a clinical treatment. Shortwave diathermy is again becoming an alternative to therapeutic ultrasound because of its ability to heat a greater volume of tissue.

Box 9-1. MICROWAVE DIATHERMY

Microwave diathermy (MWD) is a deep-heating modality that uses a magnetron to produce high-frequency electromagnetic energy that is converted into heat within the body. The FCC has reserved 915 Hz and 2450 Hz for the medical use of microwave diathermy. Although microwave diathermy is similar to SWD, there are differences between the two.

Electrical fields are predominant with microwave diathermy, in contrast to the magnetic fields that predominate in SWD. Heating occurs through a dipole response created within the cell membrane. The rotation of these molecules causes friction, resulting in heat production. Because of the spreading of the radio waves and absorption of the energy, superficial tissues tend to be heated more than deeper tissues. Although microwave diathermy produces biophysical effects similar to those of SWD, the treatment is more superficial because the microwave radiation cannot penetrate the fat layer to the same extent as shortwave radiation. Because the energy is collected by the adipose tissue, the effects occur at about one-third the depth of SWD effects, but the energy is reflected at tissue interfaces, creating standing waves that can result in unsafe increases in tissue temperatures.

The indications and contraindications for the use of microwave diathermy are similar to those for SWD. However, there can be no metal within the treatment field (4 feet from the pads, drums, or coils). This includes not only metal on the patient but implanted metal (e.g., plates, screws, **intrauterine devices** •) as well.

Microwave diathermy is not commercially available in the United States, partially because the energy tends to be reflected and scattered into the surrounding environment and has been associated with an unacceptably high incidence of miscarriages among female therapists who regularly operate these units.[125]

TABLE 9-1 Comparison of Thermal Ultrasound and Shortwave Diathermy

	ULTRASOUND	SHORTWAVE DIATHERMY
Type of Energy	Acoustical	Electromagnetic
Tissue heated	Collagen-rich	C: Adipose tissue, skin
		I: Muscle, blood vessels
Volume of tissue heated	Small (20 cm²)	Large (200 cm²)
Temperature increase	1 MHz: More than 6.3°F (3.5°C)	C: More than 7°F (3.9°C) (Adipose tissue)
	3 MHz: More than 14.9°F (8.3°C)	I: More than 18°F (10°C) (Intramuscular tissue)
Heat retention	Short (approximately 3 minutes)	Long (approximately 9 minutes)

C: capacitive method
I: inductive method

There are two types of SWD generators: (1) induction field generators and (2) capacitive field generators. The type of SWD application is generator specific. The induction field method places the patient in the **electromagnetic field** • (EMF) produced by the equipment. A capacitive field (also referred to as a "condenser field") SWD unit uses the patient's tissues in the actual electrical circuit. The tissues' resistance to the flow of energy produces heating.

The type and depth of tissues affected and the subsequent increase in temperature vary between the two types of SWD application. Induction generators produce the greatest amount of heat within the muscle layer directly beneath the coil. Capacitive generators affect tissues under each plate and selectively heat adipose tissue and bone (Fig. 9-1). Heating with capacitive SWD is highly dependent on water content and is not recommended for patients who have a thick adipose tissue layer.

Intrauterine device (IUD): A plastic or metal coil inserted within the uterus to prevent pregnancy.
Electromagnetic field: The lines of force created by positive and negative poles.

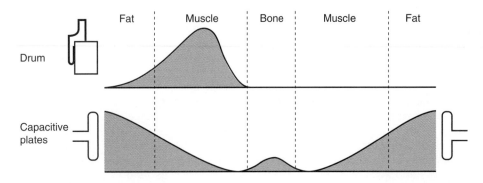

Figure 9-1. **Heat Distribution for Shortwave Diathermy, Inductive Drum, and Capacitive Plate Methods.**

Inductive SWD is not tissue-type specific and is considered to be safer.

Induction Field Diathermy

A high-frequency alternating current (see Chapter 11) flowing through a coil creates an EMF that radiates away from the cable. The patient's tissues are in the EMF but are not an actual part of the circuit. This is similar to how a microwave oven heats food. Induction field SWD, sometimes referred to as magnetic field diathermy, is delivered using either cables or via an induction drum.

Electromagnetic fields arise perpendicular from the cable, causing ions to oscillate and create **eddy currents** (Fig. 9-2). The density of eddy currents is proportional to the tissue's electrical conductivity; the friction caused by the movement of ions produces heat. Muscular tissue is selectively heated over adipose tissue.

The amount of heat produced depends on the strength of the EMF and the distance between the tissues and the source. As the distance between the source of the EMF and the tissues increases, the strength of the field decreases by the square of the distance (see the inverse square law in Appendix A).

The number of eddy currents is based on the strength of the EMF and the electrical conductivity of the tissues.

Most of the heat is produced near the source and just below the adipose tissue/muscle interface (see Fig. 9-1). Increased adipose tissue thickness will reduce the rate and magnitude of intramuscular heating.[127]

The cable method involves wrapping a conducting cable around an extremity or coiling it and placing the cable on the patient, using terry cloth toweling to buffer the cable from the patient's skin (Fig. 9-3). Because of the complexities of setup and the potential of burns if done improperly, the cable method is infrequently used.

The more common drum applicators have the cable coiled within a plastic drum. The drum is then positioned over the target tissues (Fig. 9-4). Inductive drums, approximately 200 cm^2 in size, have built-in space plates to keep the source of the energy away from the patient's skin, decreasing the risk of burns.

Capacitive Field Diathermy

In the capacitive field method of diathermy, the patient's tissues are placed between two electrodes and actually conduct the SWD's electrical energy. Two insulated plates, electrodes, are placed on either side of the site being treated. When an alternating current is applied to the circuit, the plates will always have opposite electrical charges, creating a strong electrical force between them. The flow

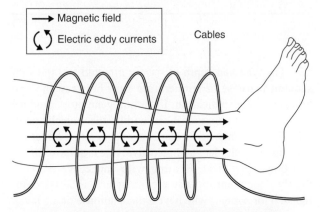

Figure 9-2. **Circular Electrical Fields—Eddy Currents— Form in the Presence of an Electromagnetic Field.** The subsequent molecular oscillation produces tissue heating.

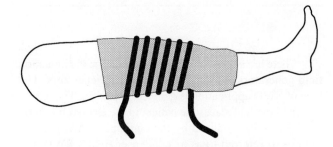

Figure 9-3. **Shortwave Diathermy Application Through an Induction Cable.** The cable is wrapped around the body part with equal spacing between the coils and an equal length leading to and from the generator. Cables that are too close together will concentrate the heat and may result in burns. Because of these risks, cables are seldom used for treatment.

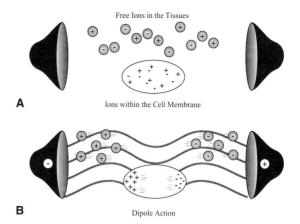

A

Ions within the Cell Membrane

B

Dipole Action

Figure 9-5. **Dipole Response to an Electromagnetic Field.** (A) Tissue ions before the application of electromagnetic energy. (B) Ionic reaction to electromagnetic energy. The ions move toward the pole having the opposite electrical charge.

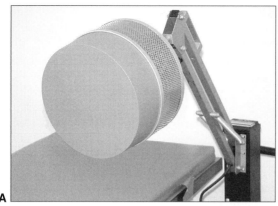

A

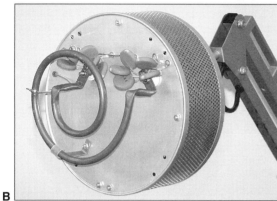

B

Figure 9-4. **Shortwave Diathermy Induction Drum.** (A) Plastic housing of the drum. (B) Drum removed to expose the coil that produces the electromagnetic field. The resulting electromagnetic field will produce a circular flow of energy similar to that of the coil. (Note: Do not remove the plastic housing.)

of electrical energy passes through the tissues as a series circuit, which acts as an electrical resistor and produces frictional heating. Those tissues that present the most electrical resistance, such as adipose tissue, produce the most heat. Unlike the inductive technique, capacitive SWD heats the body on each side.

Heat is produced by the **dipole** ● effect. Dipole molecules, molecules having no net electrical charge but having oppositely charged ends, are randomly arranged within the tissues. When exposed to the intense electrical field produced by the diathermy unit, the molecules rotate in the opposite direction of their charge. Positively charged molecules move toward the negative pole, and negatively charged molecules move toward the positive pole (Fig 9-5). The number of times the molecules rotate each second is based on the frequency of the current. The high-frequency current such as used in shortwave

diathermy produces rotation that creates kinetic energy, which is released as heat within the tissues.

The current flows along the path of least resistance, concentrating the heat in the superficial tissues and less so in the deep tissues. Adipose tissue is a poor **conductor** ● of electrical energy. The electrical resistance in the adipose tissue produces heat that is then conducted to the muscle. The capacitive method is not recommended for patients who have a large layer of adipose tissue.

The strength of the EMF is closest to the plates and weakest in the middle. The intensity near the plates causes more intense superficial heating than the induction field method, occurring at depths of 2.5 to 5 cm but the heating is uneven because of differences in the electrical resistance posed by various tissue types. Altering the distance between the plates and the skin helps keep superficial temperatures within a safe range.

Capacitive SWD is administered using pad electrodes or, in contemporary models, air space plate electrodes. To provide uniform heating, pad electrodes require even contact pressure and a uniform distance from the skin; otherwise, burns may occur. To prevent the density of energy from becoming too great, these electrodes must be spaced at least their diameter apart.

Air space electrodes are similar to induction drums in that metallic coils or plates shielded by plastic (see Fig. 9-4). An electrical charge builds on each plate until it discharges to the opposite one based on the unit's output frequency. A unit of 27.12 MHz would repeat this cycle 27,120,000 times per second.

Dipole: A pair of equal and opposite charges separated by a distance.
Conductor (electrical): A material having the ability to transmit electricity. Conductors have many free electrons and provide relatively little resistance to electrical flow. Within the body, tissues having a high water content are considered conductors.

To ensure even heating, the electrodes must be placed an equal distance from the skin on opposite sides of the body part, with the conducting plate typically about 3 cm from the skin (Fig. 9-6). A method of spacing the electrodes, usually an adjustment between the insulating cover and the electrode, helps to ensure precise placement. Uneven spacing can cause uneven heating, with more heat accumulation on the side where the electrode is closer.

■ Modes of Application

Shortwave diathermy can be delivered in either continuous or pulsed forms. Continuous SWD increases subcutaneous tissue temperature, but its use is generally limited to chronic conditions. The output may also be pulsed, allowing use with some acute and subacute conditions and preventing tissue temperatures from increasing too fast or too high.

Friction caused by the passage of energy through the tissue produces heat. The amount of heating is based on the total amount of power (measured in watts) and the ratio between the length of the "ON" pulse and the duration of the "OFF" cycle. Nonthermal effects occur when a low average intensity, short pulse duration, and low duty cycle are used. Heat is still generated

within the tissues, but the tissues are rapidly cooled by the influx of new, relatively cool blood before heat accumulates.

Pulsed shortwave diathermy (PSWD) is also referred to as pulsed electromagnetic fields (PEF), pulsed electromagnetic energy (PEME), and pulsed radiofrequency radiation (PRFR). A typical pulse duration is 20 to 400 μsec with a pulse frequency of 10 to 800 Hz. Pulsed output allows for increased treatment intensities and longer treatment durations than continuous SWD application.[128] Unlike therapeutic ultrasound, pulsed output can be used to produce thermal effects, **so do not confuse "pulsed" with "nonthermal."**

PSWD operates by interrupting the continuous output at an interval determined by the pulse frequency creating **burst trains** similar to those used in electrotherapy. Decreasing the pulse frequency decreases the time-averaged power delivered to the body. The higher the pulse frequency, the greater the amount of tissue heating that occurs.

Thermal effects are obtained when the total amount of energy delivered to the patient's body is greater than 38 watts and a high pulse frequency is used.[129] Unlike therapeutic ultrasound, the energy produced by SWD generators is not reflected by bone or other tissues and therefore does not create standing waves.

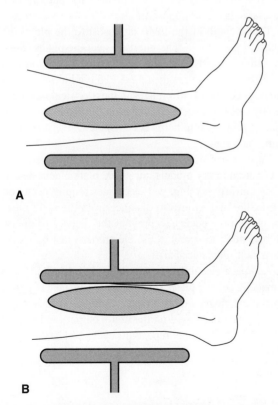

Figure 9-6. Heating Using Capacitive Pads. (A) Plates are spaced evenly from the tissue, resulting in even heating. (B) If the plates are unequally spaced (note the top electrode is closer to the skin than the bottom electrode), more heating will occur under the electrode that is closer to the skin.

● BIOPHYSICAL EFFECTS OF

Shortwave Diathermy Application

High-frequency electromagnetic energy (greater than 10 MHz) is absorbed by the patient's tissues. The **specific absorption rate** describes the rate of energy absorption per unit of area tissue. The friction caused by the movement of ions produces the heating effect. Free ions within the treatment field are attracted to the pole having the opposite charge and are repelled from the pole having the like charge. Some molecules have ions that are capable of moving only within the cell membrane, causing a dipole action in which the ions within the membrane align themselves along the charges, or creating eddy currents (see Figs. 9-4 and 9-5).[130]

The heating effects occur as a result of friction between the moving ions and the surrounding tissues, and are similar to those associated with therapeutic ultrasound (see Table 9-1). Nonthermal effects are obtained when a low output power or a low duty cycle, or both, are used (Fig. 9-7).

Nonthermal Effects

Nonthermal effects are obtained by using a low number of pulses, short pulse duration, and a low average output intensity and an output of less than 38 W. Because heat is not produced, nonthermal SWD application is advocated for the use of acute trauma and postsurgical treatment.[128,129,131]

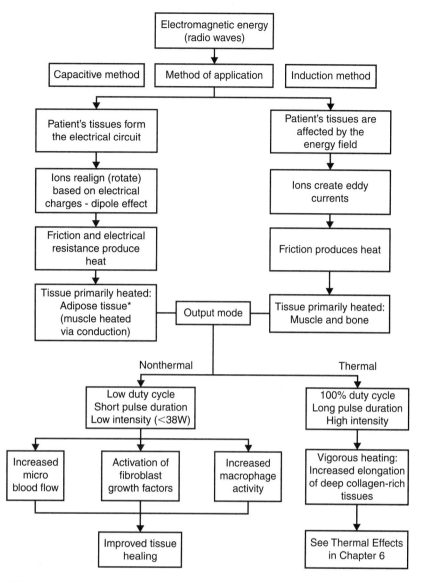

Figure 9-7. **Schematic of the Effects of Shortwave Diathermy.**

* Not recommended for patients with a thick adipose tissue layer

Nonthermal SWD changes the way that ions bind to the cell membrane, altering cellular function. The nonthermal effects of SWD include increased microvascular perfusion, activation of fibroblast growth factors, and increased macrophage activity, all of which assist in tissue healing.[132,133,134] Nonthermal SWD has been reported to promote edema reduction.

Thermal Effects

The primary advantage of shortwave diathermy is the relatively large volume and depth of tissue it can heat. Shortwave diathermy can increase intramuscular temperatures in the level of 4°C to 5°C. The heating characteristics of SWD are similar to those of ultrasound, but because of the larger amount of tissue heated, the heat is retained three times longer following the treatment than with ultrasound.[8,135] However, capacitive SWD is less effective on those persons who have a large amount of subcutaneous fat.

✱ Practical Evidence

Superficial heat modalities affect a larger area of tissue, but SWD affects a larger volume of tissue than both superficial heat modalities and thermal ultrasound. Unlike moist heat pack which loses energy during the treatment, the energy delivered by SWD remains constant, allowing for vigorous heating of intramuscular tissues.[136] Heating a larger tissue volume results in longer post-treatment effects than other heating agents.[137]

Inductive Method Heating

Induction field SWD preferentially heats tissues that are good electrical conductors, such as muscle and blood vessels. Adipose tissue is not substantially heated by induction fields because an electrical current is not passed through the tissues (see Fig. 9-1). Induction field diathermy is the most common form of shortwave used.[124]

An inductive drum heats an area approximately equal to the size of its face. Peak temperature is reached approximately 15 minutes into the treatment, increasing muscle temperature at a depth of 1.2 cm by more than 18°F (10°C).[127] A 10-minute treatment increases subcutaneous tissue temperatures 5.0°F (2.8°C).[8] The most intense heating is at the center of the drum, with slightly lower temperatures (approximately 20% less) around the periphery caused by the tissues losing heat via conduction to the surrounding tissues.[8]

Capacitive Method Heating

Capacitive field SWD preferentially heats tissues that are not good electrical conductors, such as the skin and adipose tissue. The capacitive method can increase skin temperature approximately 4.3°F (2.4°C) and intra-articular temperatures 2.5°F (1.4°C).[138] Structures with high water content, such as adipose tissue, blood, and muscle, are heated at depths of 2 to 5 cm.

Target tissue temperature may reach 107°F (41.7°C), but the adipose layer dissipates a significant portion of the energy. This leads to a secondary heating of the superficial muscle layer by heat conducted from the adipose tissue. The amount of intramuscular temperature increase compares favorably with that seen during ultrasound application, producing an increase of more than 7°F (3.9°C).[135,139]

● EFFECTS ON

The Injury Response Process

The healing properties of SWD are similar to those of other forms of heat application but occur deep within the tissues (refer to the general effects of heat in Chapter 6). The magnitude of temperature increase is based on the treatment intensity, the number of pulses per second, and the pulse duration. The biophysical effects of SWD are also similar to those of therapeutic ultrasound (see Chapter 7).

Vigorous heating occurs when the baseline tissue temperature increases 7.2°F (4.0°C) so that the intramuscular temperature is in the range of 100.4°F to 104°F (38°C to 40°C). Increasing the temperature too rapidly or beyond 104°F can cause burns and result in the breakdown of protein-rich tissues.

Inflammation

The nonthermal effects of SWD alter the rate of diffusion across the cell membrane; the thermal effects increase the rate of cell metabolism. As inductive shortwave diathermy preferentially heats muscle, it is reasonable to expect that the Q10 effect is enhanced deep within the muscle. An 18°F (10°C) increase in intramuscular temperature will approximately double the rate of cell metabolism.

✱ Practical Evidence

The treatment of osteoarthritic knees is one of the most common clinical uses of SWD.[140-148] Most studies investigating both pulsed and continuous SWD report no additive benefit in improving strength and decreasing inflammation, pain, and range of motion in the treatment of knee osteoarthritis.[140,141,142,143] Pulsed SWD also does not appear to aid in the resolution of nonspecific neck pain[144,145] or low back pain[146] relative to superficial heat, exercise, or manual therapy

Application of continuous SWD has demonstrated decreased thickness of the synovial membrane and decreased pain, indicating a reduction in arthritic-induced synovitis.[147] Also continuous SWD prior to rehabilitation exercises increases isokinetic strength and decreases pain, but at the same level as moist heat and transcutaneous electrical nerve stimulation.[148]

The cellular level effects of SWD combined with increased blood flow result in the increased delivery and concentration of white blood cells (WBC) and improved chondrocyte proliferation.[134] Increased cell membrane permeability assists in the removal of cellular debris and metabolic toxins that may have collected in the area.[131]

Nerve Conduction and Pain Control

The effects of nerve conduction velocity and pain are the same for heat in general. Primary pain relief secondary to SWD application is most often associated with decreased muscle spasm, reduction of adhesions and contractures, and increased blood flow.

Blood and Fluid Dynamics

As with all thermal modalities, the heat produced by SWD results in a vasodilation that increases blood flow, increases capillary filtration, increases capillary pressure, and increases oxygen perfusion.[149] Because of its deep-heating characteristics, increased blood flow, increased fibroblastic activity, increased collagen deposition, and new capillary growth are stimulated deeper in the tissues than superficial heating agents.[134,150] The depth of effective heating and volume of tissue affected also makes SWD useful in the resolution of hematoma.[151]

Tissue Elasticity

Shortwave diathermy is capable of reaching vigorous heating levels (7.2°F/4°C) at depths greater than 2 cm. Tissue elongation is obtained by altering the viscoelastic properties of deep, collagen-rich fibrous tissues by increasing the temperature and applying an external force to elongate the tissues.[8,136] Tissues heated by SWD retain heat for longer periods than tissues heated by therapeutic ultrasound, increasing the post-treatment stretching window.

✳ Practical Evidence

Deep heating the muscle tissue increases its extensibility more than superficial heating.[136]

Single treatment sessions of heat and stretch are not sufficient for elongating tissues.[152] Repeated sessions of combined heat and stretching are needed to obtain actual elongation of muscles and tendons,[153] but the addition of PSWD does not appear to aid in retaining the increased ROM.[154] Any increases in range of motion seen following a single treatment are most probably related to decreased muscle tone.[136]

Wound Healing

Pulsed shortwave diathermy increases WBC infiltration and increases the rate of phagocytosis, resulting in more rapid healing time and decreased need for pain medications.[131] The number and quality of mature collagen bundles are increased in the treated area, the result of increased adenosine triphosphatase (ATP) activity, and the proportion of necrosed muscle fibers decreases.[155] Superficial open wounds should not be treated because of the associated moisture.

▨ Contraindications and Precautions for Shortwave Diathermy

Technological advancements have made SWD a relatively safe and effective modality, but the electromagnetic radiation creates several contraindications and precautions to its use. The use of thermal SWD presents more contraindications than nonthermal SWD.[156] Individual manufacturing techniques may overcome some contraindications or present unique ones (refer to Chapter 11, At a Glance: Shortwave Diathermy).

The application of thermal SWD is held to the same contraindications of heat application in general, including acute inflammation, ischemia, and hemorrhage (see Table 5-7). Questions regarding the suitability of SWD for the condition being treated should be referred to the patient's physician.

The intensity for thermal treatments is based on patient feedback. Thermal SWD should not be applied over areas of sensory impairment. Extra caution is required with patients who may have diminished capacity to feel heat, interpret sensations, and/or communicate with the clinician.

Individuals who are pregnant, or may be pregnant, or who have a cardiac pacemaker or other implanted electronic device should not be permitted within 50 feet (15 m) of the unit while output is being generated.

Metal within the output field is often a contraindication to the use of SWD, including metal on clothing, jewelry, and so on (see Table 10-3).

Circular metal, such as that found with some internal fixation devices and other implants, bedsprings, and so on is always contraindicated because of the potential to create a second EMF within the metal. Metal may heat more rapidly than skin and other tissues, thus increasing the risk of burns. Certain forms of pulsed SWD may be used over some metal implants.[156,157] Refer to the manufacturer's operating instructions to determine how to handle metal in the treatment field and consult with the patient's physician prior to initiating this treatment.

The use of thermal SWD over areas of active deep vein thrombosis or thrombophlebitis may cause the clot to dislodge. Use over sites of active infection may result in the infection spreading. Heating cancerous tumors can increase the tumor's mass and weight.[102]

Thermal SWD should not be applied to areas over plastic implants or bone cement. Plastic implants contain substances that can concentrate the heat. Although it is unlikely that the intensity would not be tolerated by the patient, overheating plastic implants may cause them to become pliable.[156]

The presence of an implanted cardiac pacemaker is an absolute contraindication to the use of SWD. The EMF produced by the diathermy unit can disrupt the pacemaker's rhythm, and the implanted metal will overheat.

Shortwave diathermy applied through the skull using capacitive plates, transcerebral application, should be performed with extreme caution. The energy passing through the skull can result in headaches, dizziness, and vomiting. The eyes, frontal sinuses, and ears are particularly sensitive to SWD. Contact lenses must be removed before the application of SWD to the face or head, or both.

Application of SWD to the female pelvic region (including use of vaginal electrodes), abdomen, and lumbar spine may increase menstrual flow. Likewise, the application of SWD to these regions during pregnancy or suspected pregnancy is an absolute contraindication.

Use over unfused epiphyseal plates must be done with caution. Although there are no documented cases, repeated overheating of the growth plate can result in nonunion or malunion of the **physis** ●.

The presence of moisture in the EMF will increase the rate of heating and can cause overheating of the skin. Moist dressings, adhesive tape, and skin creams must be

---

Physis: The growth plate of bone.

removed before the treatment. If moisture collects during the treatment, pause the SWD output and dry the skin. Wet towels must not be used to attempt to provide moist heat during the treatment.

■ Overview of the Evidence

Several studies[8,126,129,136,139,147,151,154] have validated the thermal effects of SWD, although the inductive technique has been the focus of this research. There remains a limited amount of published research that investigates the efficacy of SWD in the treatment of musculoskeletal conditions. Similar to the controversies associated with therapeutic ultrasound, other published studies suffer from a lack of randomized control trials and investigated a relatively small number of patient problems.

Other than those conditions directly associated with muscular dysfunction, the current evidence does not demonstrate an additive benefit of SWD in the treatment of knee osteoarthritis,[140,141,142,143] nonspecific neck pain,[144,145] or low back pain[146] relative to other interventions. Limited research does support the use of SWD for reducing arthritic-induced synovitis and pain.[147]

Several SWD units are capable of producing a pulsed output. On some models, the pulses are used to regulate the amount of heat generated. Low-intensity treatments (either by decreasing the output power and/or using a low number of pulses) have been promoted to produce nonthermal (mechanical) effects similar to those associated with nonthermal therapeutic ultrasound. However, a review of the literature produces no studies that investigate the efficacy of nonthermal SWD.

Because electromagnetic energy is produced in relatively high quantities by SWS units, there are potential hazards associated with repeated exposure to diathermy radiation, especially for the clinician. Harm associated with exposure to microwave diathermy is well documented, and many of these effects have also been attributed to SWD. Although care should be taken to avoid repeated exposure to shortwave diathermy energy, this modality does not have the scatter and leakage of radiation found with microwave diathermy. This is especially true with newer models.

Chapter 10

Clinical Application of Shortwave Diathermy

This chapter describes the general procedures used to set up and apply shortwave diathermy. Because of the variability between units, the instruction manual for your particular brand and model must be your clinical guide for the setup and application of shortwave diathermy. The setup and application information presented here is intended to serve only as a guide.

● Shortwave diathermy (SWD) application involves placing the patient in the unit's electromagnetic field for the induction method or directly in the electrical path for the capacitive method. This energy is then converted to heat in the body's tissues.

Shortwave diathermy units are capable of producing up to 1000 watts of output energy. However, the output intensity does not reflect the amount of energy that is actually absorbed by the tissues. Unlike superficial heating agents or therapeutic ultrasound, SWD is capable of penetrating through all tissue layers. The tissues affected depend on the type of shortwave diathermy being applied (inductive or capacitive field method), the location of the tissues relative to the source of the energy, and the composition of the tissues (see Fig. 9.1).

Medical diathermy, including shortwave diathermy, is regulated under Chapter V, Subchapter C—Electronic Product Radiation Control (Sections 531 to 542) of the Federal Food, Drug, and Cosmetic Act. The Center for Devices and Radiological Health is the U.S. Food and Drug Administration (FDA) center responsible for the oversight of these devices. The exact regulations are located in Title 21, Code of Federal Regulations, Parts 1000 to 1050.

WARNING

The nuances of shortwave diathermy application are manufacturer and generator specific. The information presented in this chapter only describes the basic parameters and principles of SWD setup and application. The actual clinical delivery of this modality *must* adhere to the unit's user's manual.

Treatment Dosages

The general output parameters for pulsed SWD treatment doses are presented in Table 10-1, but dosage techniques and protocol are generator specific. The amount of heating is also based on the method of application (capacitive or inductive), the size of the electrodes or drum(s), and the distance of the source of the energy to the tissue. The output intensity for thermal treatments is based on the patient's report of heat. Parameters for vigorous heating using pulsed SWD are presented in Table 10-2.

Setup and Application of Shortwave Diathermy

Only the induction drum and capacitive plate and electrode methods of shortwave diathermy setup and application are described in this section (Fig. 10-1). Because of their relatively difficult setup procedure and potential harm, namely burns, associated with their inappropriate use, inductive shortwave cables are becoming uncommon and are not discussed in this section. Do not apply SWD in conjunction with any other device (e.g., electrical stimulation, moist heat pack).

The physical area where the SWD is applied must conform to the manufacturer's safety recommendations.[158] A minimum of 40 feet (12 m) distance from metal whirlpools, sinks, pipes, and other fixtures that have a high metal content is recommended. Refer to the manufacturer's instillation guidelines.

Instrumentation

This section presents a list of controls that are commonly found on shortwave diathermy units (Fig. 10-2). Because of the wide range of generator types and the array of manufacturers, this list serves only as an orientation. Refer to the operator's manual of the specific unit you are using for precise details. Also note that dual head shortwave diathermy units may have dual controls.

TABLE 10-2	Typical Heating Parameters—Pulsed Shortwave Diathermy
PARAMETER	SETTING
Output mode	Pulsed
Bursts per second	800
Burst duration	400 μsec
Interburst interval	850 μsec
Output intensity	RMS amplitude of 150 W RMS output of 48 W per burst

μsec = microsecond

Shortwave diathermy units that use cables, either as therapeutic electrodes to be placed on the body or as electrical leads to inductive drums or capacitive plates, require particular attention. Therapeutic cables (or their leads) will overheat and rapidly burn the patient if they cross over each other or are spaced too closely together. On some drum or capacitive plate units the leads are "hot," meaning that they can cause burns if they are placed too close together and may potentially cause an electrical short if they come into contact with each other. Consult the unit's operator's manual for specific details regarding the intricacies of the cables.

Master Power Switch: Initiates current flow to the generator as a whole. Dual head, dual control units may have individual power switches for each.

Output Intensity: Also referred to as "power" on some units. Adjusts the amount of energy delivered to the patient.

Patient Interrupt Switch (Safety Switch): A pushbutton switch held by the patient that allows immediate termination of the treatment in the event of pain, burning, or anxiety. Do not allow the Interrupt Switch to enter the shortwave diathermy treatment field. When treating the right extremity, have the patient hold the switch in the left hand and vice versa.

TABLE 10-1	Dosage Parameters Used With Pulsed Shortwave Diathermy			
DOSE	TEMPERATURE SENSATION	INDICATIONS	PULSE WIDTH	PULSE RATE
NT	No detectable warmth	Acute trauma Acute inflammation Edema reduction	65 μsec	100–200 pps
1	Mild warmth	Subacute inflammation	100 μsec-200 μsec	800 pps
2	Moderate warmth	Pain syndromes Muscle spasm Chronic inflammation To increase blood flow	200 μsec-400 μsec	800 pps
3	Vigorous heating	Stretching collagen-rich tissues	400 μsec	800 pps

NT = Nonthermal.

At a Glance: **Shortwave Diathermy**

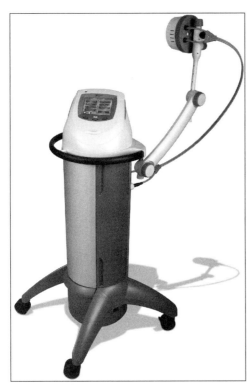

Description

High-frequency electrical currents produce deep heating to a large volume of tissue. Shortwave diathermy is often indicated in cases where thermal therapeutic ultrasound would be appropriate, but the size of the target tissues is too large. Capacitive SWD places the tissues in an electromagnetic field; inductive SWD.

Indications

- Acute and chronic pain
- Subacute and chronic inflammatory conditions in deep tissue layers
- Chronic inflammatory conditions (arthritis, bursitis, tendinitis, **myositis, osteoarthritis,** etc.)
- Range-of-motion restrictions
- Muscle spasm
- Edema reduction
- Over fracture sites
- Hematomas and contusions
- Sinusitis
- **Venous stasis ulcers**

Primary Effects

THERMAL EFFECTS
- Deep heating
- Increased blood flow
- Increased extensibility of collagen-rich tissues
- Increased cell metabolism
- Muscular relaxation
- Possible changes in some enzyme reactions

NONTHERMAL EFFECTS
- Improved tissue healing
- Edema reduction
- **Lymphedema** • reduction
- Healing of superficial, open wounds

Contraindications

In addition to the general contraindications to the use of heat (see Table 5-7):
- Cardiac pacemakers and other implanted electrode devices
- Metal implants or metals such as jewelry or body piercings: The metal collects and concentrates the energy, potentially causing burns. Pulsed SWD possibly may be used over metal implants that do not have a circular shape (consult the unit's user's manual).[157]
- Plastic implants or bone cement (thermal mode)

Lymphedema: Swelling of the lymph nodes caused by blockage of the vessels by protein-rich substances.

- Ischemic areas: The increased metabolic rate increases the need for oxygen, causing further hypoxia.
- Acute injury (thermal mode)
- Over large regenerating nerves (thermal mode)
- Peripheral vascular disease
- Over areas of active deep vein thrombosis or thrombophlebitis
- Tendency to hemorrhage, including menstruation.
- Pregnancy or the possibility of pregnancy
- Fever
- Anesthetic areas (thermal mode)
- Cancer
- Areas of particular sensitivity: Epiphyseal plates in children; genitals; open lamina; local or systemic infection; the abdomen with an implanted intrauterine device (IUD); over the heart; over carotid sinus/ anterior neck; eyes and face; application through the skull; perspiration and moist dressings: the water collects and concentrates the heat.

Treatment Duration

At moderate intensities, treatments may be given for 20 to 30 minutes and may be repeated as needed for 2 weeks. When higher treatment temperatures are used, decrease the duration of treatment to 15 minutes and apply on alternate days. Patients should not receive more than one treatment every 2 hours.

Precautions

- Anesthetic areas (nonthermal mode)
- Remove contact lenses when applying SWD around the head, face, or eyes.
- A deep, aching sensation may be a symptom of overheating the tissues.
- Individuals who are pregnant, may be pregnant, or who have *implanted electronic devices* should not be permitted within 50 feet (15 m) of the unit while output is being generated.
- It is difficult to heat only localized areas. Water pathways within the tissues dissipate heat formed in the treated area.
- Never allow the skin to come into direct contact with the heating unit or cables. Severe burns may result.
- If the cable method is used, do not allow them to touch each other. This may create a short circuit.
- If electrode pads are used, they must be spaced at least the distance of their width or diameter apart (e.g., if two 20-cm-diameter electrodes are used, they must be placed at least 20 cm apart).
- Overheating of the patient's tissues may cause tissue damage without any immediate signs. Deep tissue burning can cause destruction of muscular tissue or subcutaneous fat necrosis.
- The electromagnetic energy is not localized to the treatment area, radiating 2 to 3 feet from the source of continuous SWD and 2 feet from the source of pulsed diathermy.[159] Clinicians may be placed in the field of this scattering radiation, possibly overexposing them to diathermy. A distance of 3 feet from the source of the energy should be maintained to ensure the operator's safety. Refer to the operator's manual for generator-specific information.
- The skin exposed to the treatment should be covered by at least 0.5 inch of toweling.
- Do not allow perspiration to collect in the treatment field.
- When using capacitive electrodes, excessive amounts of adipose tissue overlying the treatment area can result in overheating the skin.

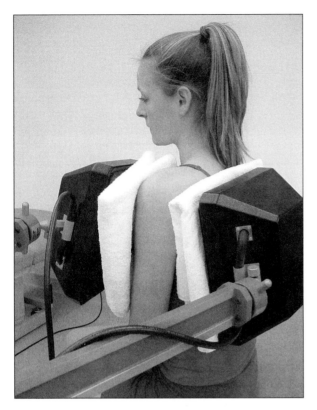

Figure 10-1. Dual Induction Drum Shortwave Diathermy. Twin drums allow for heating on both sides of the body. Note: Dual induction drums should not be confused with capacitive plates.

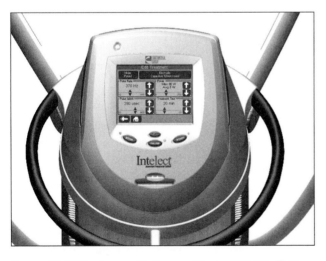

Figure 10-2. Shortwave Diathermy Control Panel. There is a significant amount of difference in the controls between makes and models.

Pause: Interrupts the treatment (while preserving the remaining treatment time) to allow repositioning of the patient, removing perspiration, or other similar situations.

Pulse Rate (Pulse Frequency): Sets the number of pulses per second (PPS) for the output. Higher PPS produce increased thermal effects.

Start/Stop: Initiates or terminates the treatment. Dual head generators may have separate "start/stop" switches for each head.

Treatment Timer: Sets the duration of the treatment. Some units may use the treatment timer to "start" the treatment: turning the timer past zero initiates the treatment.

Tuning: Adjusts the output resonance to match the patient's tissues. Tuning maximizes the energy exchange between the generator and the patient. Some units will shut off if the generator is out of tune.

Inspect Shortwave Unit

Many units require that the SWD generator be connected to a Hospital Grade Outlet.

1. Inspect the electrodes, cables, Patient Interrupt Switch, and other accessories prior to use.
2. Assure that transmission cables are not crossed.
3. Ensure that all controls are in proper working order per the manufacturer's instructions. Operating induction electrodes without a patient in the treatment field may permanently damages the electrodes.

✳ Practical Evidence

The indications and deep-heating effects of shortwave diathermy are similar to those of thermal ultrasound. The benefit of SWD is its ability to heat a much larger volume of tissue. SWD affects a volume of tissue approximately the size of a cereal bowl; therapeutic ultrasound affects tissues about the size of two ketchup packs.

Patient Preparation

1. Ensure that the patient is free of all contraindications to the use of shortwave diathermy.
2. Ensure that any implanted metals (e.g., internal fixation devices, sutures, body jewelry, hearing aids) are not contraindicated by the device (refer to the unit's operator's manual) or by the treatment protocol.
3. Remove all jewelry, coins, and other metallic items from the patient (Table 10-3).
4. The treatment tissues should not be covered by clothing. Synthetic moisture-resistant clothing, silk, and cloth that has metal implants are of particular concern because of the potential for overheating.
5. Wash the skin over the treatment area. Thoroughly dry the skin prior to treatment.
6. For personal safety, the clinician should remove any rings, watches, bracelets, and so on.
7. In many cases there must be no metal within the immediate treatment area, approximately 3 feet (1 m) for continuous output and 1.5 ft (0.5 m) for a pulsed output.[124,156] Other medical equipment should be at least 40 feet (12 m) from the SWD

TABLE 10-3 **Precautions Against Metal Within the Field of Shortwave Diathermy**

IN THE ENVIRONMENT	NEAR OR ON THE PATIENT	IN THE PATIENT
Beds	Jewelry	Orthodontic braces
Treatment tables	Body piercings	Dental fillings
Chairs	Earrings	Implanted fixation devices
Wheelchairs	Watches	External fixation devices
Metal stools	Metal in pockets (keys, etc.)	Metal heart valves
CPM units	Belt buckles	Artificial joints
Splints	Zippers	Metal IUDs
Braces	Metal underwire bras	Body piercings
Medical instruments	Hearing aids	Cardiac pacemakers
Electrical modalities		Implanted bone growth generators
		Phrenic pacers

CPM = continuous passive motion; IUDs = intrauterine devices.
  NOTE: *Each shortwave diathermy model has individual thresholds and tolerances to the presence of metal in and around the treatment field. Refer to the operator's manual for definitive information.*

---

unit. The presence of metal will collect and concentrate the energy from the treatment in the same manner that an antenna collects radio waves.[160] Some manufacturers build metal-free tables for use with shortwave diathermy.

8. Keep the patient out of reach of any metal objects that can serve as a ground (e.g., outlets, pipes).
9. Clean and dry the body part. Water, skin oils, or cosmetics can increase superficial heat production.
10. Position the patient in the most appropriate manner for the body area being treated and assure that the patient is comfortable prior to initiating the treatment.
11. The patient must not come into contact with objects that are connected directly to the ground such as whirlpools, pipes, or electrical outlets (see At a Glance: Shortwave Diathermy).
12. To encourage venous return, elevate the extremity being treated if possible.
13. Cover the body part with a *dry* terry cloth towel. This provides spacing between the source of the shortwave diathermy and absorbs perspiration, both of which decrease the risk of burns. A portion of the treatment area must remain visible to check for burns during the treatment. Avoid any moisture buildup during the treatment because water tends to collect heat. The intensity must be turned to zero or the treatment PAUSED before drying the area. Moisture does not affect pulsed SWD applied using a mean power less than 30 W.[156]
14. For thermal treatments, explain to the patient that a mild to moderate warmth should be felt. Instruct the patient to inform you if any unusual sensations are experienced.

Patient/Generator Tuning

"Tuning" refers to the resonance between the generator's output and the body's ability to absorb this energy. If more than half of the available power is used to pass the energy through the patient's tissue, the setup is out of tune, requiring calibration. Older units require that the clinician manually tune the unit. Newer units are capable of automatically tuning their output to the patient's resonance.

The following section provides an overview for the method used to manually tune a SWD unit. Refer to the user's manual and follow the manufacturer's instructions for the specific model being used.

1. Position the electrodes over the patient.
2. Increase the output intensity to approximately 40% of the maximum.
3. Adjust (increase or decrease) the TUNING control until the output meter reaches its peak, then decrease the TUNING control to the patient's comfort.
4. A unit is in tune when less than half of the maximum output is used. Some units automatically shut off if more than 50% of the maximum output is used. If this occurs, the unit must be tuned again.

Application (General Setup)

1. Turn the unit on; allow it to warm up if necessary.
2. Some units must be tuned to allow for maximal energy transfer (see Patient/Generator Tuning).

Inductive Drum

1. If indicated by the manufacturer's instructions, place a folded layer between the body part and the drum.
2. Select the appropriate drum style (Fig. 10-3).

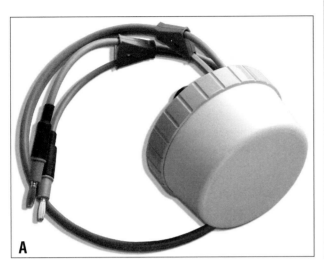
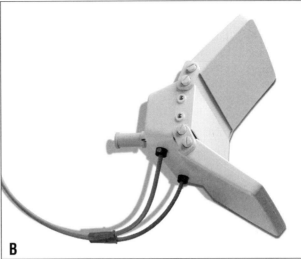

Figure 10-3. **Types of Inductive Drums.** (A) **Monode drum:** Used to treat medium to large areas such as the quadriceps. (B) **Diplode drum:** The hinged surfaces allow three sides of the body part to be treated simultaneously such as the shoulder or back.

3. Position the drum approximately 0.5 to 1 inch above the toweling. There is a direct relationship between the distance of the drum from the patient and the intensity of energy required for the treatment.
4. The surface of the drum must be parallel to the skin surface being treated, otherwise the skin closest to the drum will be overheated, the cosine law (see Appendix A).
5. If appropriate, select the appropriate PULSE RATE.

Capacitive Plate Setup
1. If indicated by the unit, cover the area to be treated with a towel.
2. Adjust the plates so that they are parallel to the body part, approximately 3 cm from the skin.
3. To heat superficial tissues place the electrodes close to the skin; to heat deeper tissues increase the distance from the skin. Increased space is needed to heat intramuscular tissue in patients who have a thick adipose tissue layer.
4. Place both plates at an equal distance above the tissue. If a spacer is used for this purpose it must be removed before the treatment is started.

Electrode Application
1. Connect the electrode cables into the generator and electrodes.
2. Choose the appropriate spacers and affix them to the electrodes (Fig. 10-4).
3. Position the electrodes on the patient's skin.
4. Assure that no part of the electrode comes into contact with the patient's skin.
5. Secure the electrodes in place using rubber straps or sandbags.

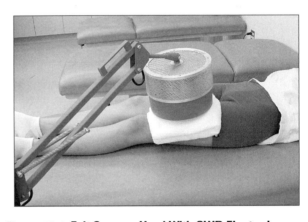

Figure 10-4. **Felt Spacers Used With SWD Electrode Application.**

All Methods
1. Assure that the movement arms and/or the generator's wheels are securely locked prior to initiating the treatment.
2. Instruct the patient not to move until the machine is shut off.
3. Set the TIMER to the desired treatment duration.
4. Increase the intensity until the patient feels mild warmth.
5. If the electrodes must be moved or if it becomes necessary to dry the area, return the INTENSITY to zero before making any adjustments.
6. Do not leave the patient unattended. Observe the skin regularly for signs of burns, and inquire as to any unusual sensations. Adjust the INTENSITY, PULSE RATE, or electrode placement as necessary.

Terminating the Treatment

1. After the treatment, return the intensity dial to zero and shut off the unit.
2. Inspect the skin for signs of burns or other abnormal treatment outcomes.
3. Record the treatment parameters in the patient's file.

Maintenance

The production of electromagnetic energy may require additional health and safety precautions because of worker exposure to radiation.

After Each Use

Unplug the unit and clean the face of the drum or cables using a cleaning agent recommended by the manufacturer. In general, the use of abrasive cleansers is not recommended. Do not re-energize the unit if moisture is still present on the cables, drums, or electrodes.

At Regular Intervals

Inspect electrical cords for kinks, cuts, and frays.

Annually

The unit must be serviced and calibrated by a qualified service technician.

End of Section

Chapter Case Study

Carlos is a 32-year-old man with marked muscle spasms of his lumbar musculature. He has had progressive symptoms for the past 10 years, but recently he has had significant pain with forward flexion. He also has a lot of difficulty standing up after a prolonged period of a flexed posture, such as with digging or shoveling. He has a 4 × 3 inch gash as a result being hit with a pipe on the job in the small of his back. Evaluation findings show marked spasm throughout his lumbar paraspinals and 25% to 50% limitation in trunk range of motion.

1. What are the best thermal agents to consider for this patient?

2. What are the physiological effects on the injury response cycle from the application of this thermal agent?
3. Why are heat packs, ice, and ultrasound less than optimum choices for this patient?
4. What are the clinical symptoms that you hope to address with this intervention?
5. Name three indications and three precautions for this modality.

Continuation of Case Study From Section 1

(The following discussion relates to Case Study 2 in Section 1)

Pulsed ultrasound (20% duty cycle) could be incorporated into our patient's program to reduce pain and promote tissue extensibility. Alterations in the cell membrane permeability bring about changes in the nerves' electrical activity, reportedly increasing the pain threshold, and assist in the healing process.

When applied with a continuous output (100% duty cycle), ultrasound preferentially heats collagen-rich tissues and assists in reducing muscle spasm. When vigorously heated (3°C to 5°C increase), tissue extensibility can be increased. To obtain the maximal benefits of tissue elongation, the trapezius must be placed on stretch during the treatment and any flexibility exercises must be performed within 3 minutes after the conclusion of the treatment.

The treatment area would be limited to an area two to three times the size of the sound head; the output frequency would depend on the depth of our patient's trauma. The intensity and duration of the treatment would be sufficient to produce a vigorous heating effect. Recall that use of ultrasound is a precaution to ultrasound application, so extra care must be taken when applying these treatments.

● ● ● Section 3 Quiz

1. When applying ultrasound with metered output of 4 W and an indicated beam nonuniformity ratio (BNR) of 4, the highest intensity in the beam is:
   A. 4 W
   B. 8 W
   C. 16 W
   D. 32 W

2. Which of the following is not an indication for the use of ultrasound?
   A. Ischemic conditions
   B. Pain reduction
   C. Trigger points
   D. Joint contractures

3. Spreading of ultrasonic energy is termed:
   A. Attenuation
   B. Collimation
   C. Thermal synthesis
   D. Divergence

4. A metered reading of 2 W per square centimeter passing through a sound head having an effective radiating area of 10 cm^2 produces an output of ___ total watts.
   A. 5 W
   B. 10 W
   C. 15 W
   D. 20 W

5. The least amount of reflection of ultrasonic energy occurs between:
   A. Water and soft tissue
   B. Soft tissue and fat
   C. Soft tissue and bone
   D. Soft tissue and air

6. All of the following are nonthermal (mechanical) effects of ultrasound *except:*
   A. Increased blood flow
   B. Increased extensibility of collagen-rich structures
   C. Synthesis of protein
   D. Increased cell membrane permeability

7. When treating the quadriceps tendon with ultrasound, what output frequency should be used?
   A. 1 MHz
   B. 2 MHz
   C. 3 MHz
   D. It does not matter.

8. When cells are exposed to high-pressure ridges, their size:
   A. Increases
   B. Decreases

9. Ultrasound that is pulsed so that it flows for 0.5 seconds and does not flow for 1 second is operating at a _____ percent duty cycle.
   A. 33
   B. 50
   C. 66
   D. 133

10. Determining the treatment duration for thermal US application is most closely dependent on what other output characteristic?
    A. Duty cycle
    B. Output intensity
    C. Coupling method
    D. Output frequency

11. To promote extensibility, the tissues must be stretched within how many minutes after the conclusion of the treatment?
    A. 1
    B. 3
    C. 10
    D. 30

12. Standard (clinical) therapeutic ultrasound generators can be employed to assist in the healing of fractures.
    A. True
    B. False

13. Which of the following substances transmits the highest percentage of ultrasonic energy relative to water?
    A. White petrolatum gel
    B. Eucerin cream
    C. Ultrasound transmission gel
    D. Hydrocortisone powder (1%) in US gel

14. During shortwave diathermy application, high-frequency electromagnetic energy is changed to heat by the process of:
    A. Convection
    B. Conduction
    C. Conversion
    D. Collection

15. Which of the following types of shortwave diathermy application places the athlete's tissues within the generator's physical circuit?
    A. Capacitive method
    B. Inductive method

16. When using a shortwave diathermy induction drum, the drum should be positioned ___ from the patient's skin.
    A. 1 in.
    B. 2 in.
    C. 4 in.
    D. 8 in.

17. The energy from a shortwave diathermy unit may scatter as much as _____ from the source.
    A. 1 ft
    B. 3 ft
    C. 6 ft
    D. 9 ft

18. Which form of shortwave diathermy should NOT be used over large areas of adipose tissue?
    A. Capacitive method
    B. Inductive method

19. What four factors determine a medication's ability to diffuse through the tissues?
    A.
    B.
    C.
    D.

20. Complete the following table comparing and contrasting therapeutic ultrasound and shortwave diathermy:

	ULTRASOUND	SHORTWAVE DIATHERMY
Type of energy	_____	_____
Tissue heated	_____	_____
Volume of tissue heated	_____	_____
Temperature increase	_____	_____
Heat retention	_____	_____

References

1. Johns LD, Straub SJ, Howard SM: Variability in effective radiating area and output power of new ultrasound transducers at 3 MHz. *J Athl Train.* 42:22, 2007.

2. Speed CA: Therapeutic ultrasound in soft tissue lesions. *Br J Rheumatol.* 40:1331, 2001.

3. Demmink JH, Helders PJM, Hobaek H, et al: The variation of heating depth with therapeutic ultrasound frequency in physiotherapy. *Ultrasound Med Biol.* 29:113, 2003.

4. Ter Haar G: Basic physics of therapeutic ultrasound. *Physiother.* 73:110, 1987.

5. Kitchen SS, Partridge CJ: A review of therapeutic ultrasound: I. Background, physiological effects and hazards. *Physiother.* 76:593, 1990.

6. Hayes BT, Merrick MA, Sandrey MA, et al: Three-MHz ultrasound heats deeper into the tissues than originally theorized. *J Athl Train.* 39:230, 2004.

7. Schneider NC, et al: 3 MHz continuous ultrasound can elevate tissue temperature at 3-cm depths (abstract). *Phys Ther.* 81:A8, 2001.

8. Garrett CL, et al: Heat distribution in the lower leg from pulsed short-wave diathermy and ultrasound treatments. *J Athl Train.* 35:50, 2000.

9. Ferguson BH: A Practitioner's Guide to the Ultrasonic Therapy Equipment Standard. U.S. Department of Health and Human Services, Public Health Service, Food and Drug Administration, Rockville, MD, 1985.

10. U.S. Department of Health and Human Services, Public Health Service: Guide for preparing product reports for ultrasonic therapy products. Food and Drug Administration, Center for Devices and Radiological Health, Rockville, MD, 1996. http://www.fda.gov/downloads/AboutFDA/ReportsManualsForms/Forms/UCM081645.pdf.

11. Straub SJ, Johns LD, Howard SM: Variability in effective radiating area at 1 MHz affects ultrasound treatment intensity. *Phys Ther.* 88:50, 2008.

12. Draper DO, et al: Rate of temperature increase in human muscle during 1 MHz and 3 MHz continuous ultrasound. *J Orthop Sports Phys Ther.* 22:142, 1995.

13. Tiidus PM, et al: Ultrasound treatment and recovery from eccentric-exercise-induced muscle damage. *J Sport Rehabil.* 11:305, 2002.

14. Gallo JA, Draper DO, Brody LT, et al: A comparison of human muscle temperature increases during 3-MHz continuous and pulsed ultrasound with equivalent temporal average intensities. *J Orthop Sports Phys Ther.* 34:395, 2004.

15. Draper DO, Sunderland S: Examination of the law of Grotthus-Draper: Does ultrasound penetrate subcutaneous fat in humans? *J Athl Train.* 38:246, 1993.

16. Dyson M: Mechanisms involved in therapeutic ultrasound. *Physiother.* 73:116, 1987.

17. White D, Evans JA, Truscott JG, et al: Modelling the propagation of ultrasound in the joint space of a human knee. *Ultrasound Med Biol.* 36:1736, 2010.

18. Ting WW, Vist CD, Sontheimer RD: Review of traditional and novel modalities that enhance the permeability of local therapeutics across the stratum corneum. *Int J Dermatol.* 43:538, 2004.

19. ter Haar G: Therapeutic applications of ultrasound. *Prog Biophys Mol Biol.* 93:111, 2007.

20. Baker KG, et al: A review of therapeutic ultrasound: Biophysical effects. *Phys Ther.* 81:1351, 2001.

21. Johns LD: Nonthermal effects of therapeutic ultrasound: The frequency resonance hypothesis. *J Athl Train.* 37:293, 2002.

22. Dijkman BG, Sprague S, Bhandari M: Low-intensity pulsed ultrasound: Nonunions. *Indian J Orthop.* 43:141, 2009.

23. Mundi R, Petis S, Kaloty R, et al: Low-intensity pulsed ultrasound: Fracture healing. *Indian J Orthop.* 43:132, 2009.

24. VanBavel E: Effects of shear stress on endothelial cells: Possible relevance for ultrasound applications. *Prog Biophys Mol Biol.* 93:374, 2007.

25. Rompe JD, Bürger R, Hopf C, et al: Shoulder function after extracorporal shock wave therapy for calcific tendinitis. *J Shoulder Elbow Surg.* 7:505, 1998.

26. Hammer DS, Rupp S, Esslin S, et al: Extracorporal shock wave therapy in patients with tennis elbow and painful heel. *Arch Orthop Trauma Surg.* 120:304, 2000.

27. Metzner G, Dohnalek C, Aigner E: High-energy extracorporeal shock-wave therapy (ESWT) for the treatment of chronic plantar fasciitis. *Foot Ank Int.* 31:790, 2010.

28. Rasmussen S, Christensen M, Mathiesen I, et al: Shockwave therapy for chronic Achilles tendinopathy. A double-blind, randomized clinical trial of efficacy. *Acta Orthop.* 79:249, 2008.

29. De Deyne P, Kirsch-Volders M: In vitro effects of therapeutic ultrasound on the nucleus of human fibroblasts. *Phys Ther.* 72:629, 1995.

30. Adinno MA, et al: Effect of free radical scavengers on changes in ion conductance during exposure to therapeutic ultrasound. *Membr Biochem.* 10:237, 1993.

31. Blinc A, et al: Characterization of ultrasound-potentiated fibrinolysis in vitro. *Blood.* 81:2636, 1993.

32. Francis CW, et al: Enhancement of fibrinolysis in vitro by ultrasound. *J Clin Invest.* 90:2063, 1992.

33. Byl NN, et al: Low-dose ultrasound effects on wound healing: A controlled study with Yucatan pigs. *Arch Phys Med Rehabil.* 73:656, 1992.

34. Holcomb W, Joyce C: A comparison of temperature increases produced by two commonly used therapeutic ultrasound units. *J Athl Train.* 38:24, 2003.

35. Chan AK, et al: Temperature changes in human patellar tendon in response to therapeutic ultrasound. *J Athl Train.* 33:130, 1998.

36. Demchak TJ, Stone MB: Effectiveness of clinical ultrasound parameters on changing intramuscular temperature. *J Sport Rehabil.* 17:220, 2008.

37. Draper DO, et al: Temperature changes in deep muscle of humans during ice and ultrasound therapies: An in vivo study. *J Orthop Sports Phys Ther.* 21:153, 1995.

38. Draper DO, Ricard MD: Rate of temperature decay in human muscle following 3 MHz ultrasound: The stretching window revealed. *J Athl Train.* 30:304, 1995.

39. Draper DO, et al: Hot-pack and 1-MHz ultrasound treatments have an additive effect on muscle temperature increase. *J Athl Train.* 33:21, 1998.

40. Weinberger A, Lev A: Temperature elevation of connective tissue by physical modalities. *Crit Rev Phys Rehabil Med.* 3:121, 1991.

41. Demchak TJ, Straub SJ, Johns LD: Ultrasound heating is curvilinear in nature and varies between transducers from the same manufacturer. *J Sport Rehabil.* 16:122, 2007.

42. Dyson M, et al: Longwave ultrasound. *Physiotherapy.* 81:40, 1999.

43. Young SR, Dyson M: Macrophage responsiveness to therapeutic ultrasound. *Ultrasound Med Biol.* 16:809, 1990.

44. Pires Oliveria DAA, De Oliveria RF, Magini M, et al: Assessment of cytoskeletan and endoplasmic reticulum of fibroblast cells subjected to low-level laser therapy and low-intensity pulsed ultrasound. *Photomed Laser Surg.* 27:461, 2009.

45. Kitchen SS, Partridge CJ: A review of therapeutic ultrasound: II. The efficacy of ultrasound. *Physiotherapy.* 76:595, 1990.

46. Maxwell L, et al: The augmentation of leukocyte adhesion to endothelium by therapeutic ultrasound. *Ultrasound Med Biol*. 20:383, 1994.

47. Ramirez A, et al: The effect of ultrasound on collagen synthesis and fibroblast proliferation in vitro. *Med Sci Sports Exerc*. 29:326, 1997.

48. Baker RJ, Bell GW: The effect of therapeutic modalities on blood flow in the human calf. *J Orthop Sports Phys Ther*. 13:23, 1991.

49. Robinson SE, Buono MJ: Effect of continuous-wave ultrasound on blood flow in skeletal muscle. *Phys Ther*. 75:147, 1993.

50. Plaskett C, et al: Ultrasound treatment does not affect postexercise muscle strength recovery or soreness. *J Sport Rehabil*. 8:1, 1999.

51. Fabrizio PA, et al: Acute effects of therapeutic ultrasound delivered at varying parameters on the blood flow velocity in a muscular distribution artery. *J Orthop Sports Phys Ther*. 24:294, 1996.

52. Downing DS, Weinstein A: Ultrasound therapy of subacromial bursitis. A double blind trial. *Phys Ther*. 66:194, 1986.

53. Srbely JZ, Dickey JP: Randomized controlled study of the antinoceptive effect of ultrasound on trigger point sensitivity: Novel applications in myofascial therapy? *Clin Rehabil*. 21:411, 2007.

54. Lehmann JF, et al: Effect of therapeutic temperatures on tendon extensibility. *Arch Phys Med Rehabil*. 51:481, 1970.

55. Reed BV, et al: Effects of ultrasound and stretch on knee ligament extensibility. *J Orthop Sports Phys Ther*. 30:341, 2000.

56. Michlovitz SL: Is there a role for ultrasound and electrical stimulation following injury to tendon and nerve? *J Hand Ther*. 18:292, 2005.

57. Jackson BA, et al: Effect of ultrasound therapy on the repair of Achilles tendon injuries in rats. *Med Sci Sports Exerc*. 23:171, 1991.

58. Enwemeka CS: The effect of therapeutic ultrasound on tendon healing: A biomechanical study. *Am J Phys Med Rehabil*. 68:283, 1989.

59. Koeke PU, Parizotto NA, Carrinho PM, Salate ACB: Comparative study of the efficacy of the topical application of hydrocortisone, therapeutic ultrasound and phonophoresis on the tissue repair process in rat tendons. *Ultrasound Med Biol*. 31:345, 2005.

60. Hoppenrath T, Ciccone CD: Evidence in practice. *Phys Ther*. 86:136, 2006.

61. Henley EJ: Transcutaneous drug delivery: Iontophoresis, phonophoresis. *Phys Rehabil Med*. 2:139, 1991.

62. Nussbaum EL, et al: Comparison of ultrasound/ultraviolet-c and laser for treatment of pressure ulcers in patients with spinal cord injury. *Phys Ther*. 74:812, 1994.

63. Heckman JD, et al: Acceleration of tibial fracture-healing by non-invasive, low-intensity pulsed ultrasound. *J Bone Joint Surg Am*. 76:26, 1994.

64. Cook SD, et al: Acceleration of tibia and distal radius fracture healing in patients who smoke. *Clin Orthop*. 337:198, 1997.

65. Azuma Y, et al: Low-intensity pulsed ultrasound accelerates rat femoral fracture healing by acting on the various cellular reactions in the fracture callus. *J Bone Miner Res*. 16:671, 2001.

66. Hadjiargyrou M, et al: Enhancement of fracture healing by low intensity ultrasound. *Clin Orthop*. 333(S):S216, 1998.

67. Tsunoda M, et al: Low-intensity pulsed ultrasound initiates bone healing in rat nonunion fracture model. *J Ultrasound Med*. 20:197, 2001.

68. Wark JD, et al: Low-intensity pulsed ultrasound stimulates bone-forming responses in UMR-106 cells. *Biochem Biophys Res Commun*. 288:443, 2001.

69. Eck JC, et al: Techniques for stimulating spinal fusion: Efficacy of electricity, ultrasound, and biologic factors in achieving fusion. *Am J Orthop*. 30:535, 2001.

70. Jensen JE: Stress fracture in the world class athlete: A case study. *Med Sci Sports Exerc*. 30:783, 1998.

71. Needle AR, Kaminski TW: Effectiveness of low-intensity pulsed ultrasound, capacitively coupled fields, or extracorporeal shockwave therapy in accelerating stress fracture healing. *Athletic Training & Sports Health Care*. 1:133, 2009.

72. Olkku A, Leskinen JJ, Lammi MJ, et al: Ultrasound-induced activation of Wnt signaling in human MG-63 osteoblastic cells. *Bone*. 47:320, 2010.

73. John PS, Poulose CS, George B: Therapeutic ultrasound in fracture healing: The mechanism of osteoinduction. *Indian J Orthop*. 42:444, 2008.

74. Reher P, et al: Effect of ultrasound on the production of IL-8, basic FGF, and VEGF. *Cytokine*. 11:416, 1999.

75. Zorlu U, et al: Comparative study of the effect of ultrasound and electrostimulation on bone healing in rats. *Am J Phys Med Rehabil*. 77:427, 1998.

76. Walker NA, Denegar CR, Preische J: Low-intensity pulsed ultrasound and pulsed electromagnetic field in the treatment of tibial fractures: A systematic review. *J Athl Train*. 42:530, 2007.

77. Busse JW, Bhandari M, Kulkarni AV, et al: The effect of low-intensity pulsed ultrasound therapy on time to fracture healing: A meta-analysis. *CMAJ*. 166:437, 2002.

78. Dell Rocca GJ: The science of ultrasound therapy for fracture healing. *Indian J Orthop*. 43:121, 2009.

79. Emami A, et al: No effect of low-intensity ultrasound on healing time of intramedullary fixed tibial fractures. *J Orthop Trauma*. 13:252, 1999.

80. Mayr E, et al: Ultrasound: An alternative healing method for nonunions? *Arch Orthop Trauma Surg*. 120:1, 2000.

81. Ferrara KW: Driving delivery vehicles with ultrasound. *Adv Drug Deliv Rev*. 60:1097, 2008.

82. Davick JP, et al: Distribution and deposition of tritiated cortisol using phonophoresis. *Phys Ther*. 68:1672, 1988.

83. Quillen WS: Phonophoresis: A review of the literature and technique. *J Athl Train*. 15:109, 1980.

84. Ciccone CD, et al: Effects of ultrasound and trolamine salicylate phonophoresis on delayed-onset muscle soreness. *Phys Ther*. 71:666, 1991.

85. Meidan VM, et al: Phonophoresis of hydrocortisone with enhancers: An acoustically defined model. *Int J Pharmacol*. 170:157, 1998.

86. Byl NN: The use of ultrasound as an enhancer for transcutaneous drug delivery: Phonophoresis. *Phys Ther*. 75:539, 1995.

87. McElnay JC, et al: Phonophoresis of methyl nicotinate: A preliminary study to elucidate the mechanism of action. *Pharmacol Res*. 10:1726, 1993.

88. Machluf M, Kost J: Ultrasonically enhanced transdermal drug delivery. Experimental approaches to elucidate the mechanism. *J Biomater Sci Polym Ed*. 5:147, 1993.

89. Oziomek RS, et al: Effect of phonophoresis on serum salicylate levels. *Med Sci Sports Exerc*. 23:397, 1991.

90. Mitragotri S, et al: Transdermal drug delivery using low-frequency sonophoresis. *Pharmacol Res*. 13:411, 1996.

91. Kuntz AR, Griffiths CM, Rankin JM, et al: Cortisol concentrations in human skeletal muscle after phonophoresis with 10% hydrocortisone gel. *J Athl Train*. 41:321, 2006.

92. Cameron MH, Monroe LG: Relative transmission of ultrasound by media customarily used for phonophoresis. *Phys Ther*. 72:142, 1992.

93. Bensen HAE, et al: Use of ultrasound to enhance percutaneous absorption of benzydamine. *Phys Ther.* 69:113, 1989.

94. Nagrale AV, Herd CR, Ganvir S, et al: Cyriax physiotherapy versus phonophoresis with supervised exercise in subjects with lateral epicondylagia: A randomized clinical trial. *J Man Manip Ther.* 17:171, 2009.

95. Bare AC, et al: Phonophoretic delivery of 10% hydrocortisone through the epidermis of humans as determined by serum cortisol concentrations. *Phys Ther.* 76:738, 1996.

96. Deniz S, et al. Comparison of the effectiveness of pulsed and continuous diclofenac phonophoresis in treatment of knee osteoarthritis. *J Phys Ther Sci.* 21:331, 2009.

97. Byl NN, et al: The effects of phonophoresis with corticosteroids: A controlled pilot study. *J Orthop Sports Phys Ther.* 18:590, 1993.

98. Franklin ME, et al: Effect of phonophoresis with dexamethasone on adrenal function. *J Orthop Sports Phys Ther.* 22:103, 1995.

99. Darrow H, et al: Serum dexamethasone levels after decadron phonophoresis. *J Athl Train.* 34:338, 1999.

100. Mitragotri S, et al: Ultrasound-mediated transdermal protein delivery. *Science.* 269:850, 1995.

101. Meakins A, Watson T: Longwave ultrasound and conductive heating increase functional ankle mobility in asymptomatic subjects. *Phys Ther Sport.* 7:74, 2006.

102. Sicard-Rosenbaum L, et al: Effects of continuous therapeutic ultrasound on growth and metastasis of subcutaneous murine tumors. *Phys Ther.* 75:3, 1995.

103. Draper DO, et al: A comparison of temperature rise in human calf muscles following applications of underwater and topical gel ultrasound. *J Orthop Sports Phys Ther.* 17:247, 1993.

104. Draper DO, Edvalson CG, Knight KL, et al. Temperature increases in the human Achilles tendon during ultrasound treatments with commercial ultrasound gel and full-thickness and half-thickness gel pads. *J Athl Train.* 45:333, 2010.

105. Bishop S, Draper DO, Knight KL, et al: Human tissue-temperature rise during ultrasound treatments with the Aquaflex gel pad. *J Athl Train.* 39:126, 2004.

106. Gulick DT, Ingram N, Krammes T, et al: Comparison of tissue heating using 3 MHz ultrasound with T-Prep® versus Aquasonic® gel. *Phys Ther Sport.* 6:131, 2005.

107. Merrick M, Benard K, Devor S, et al: Identical three-MHz ultrasound treatments with different devices produce different intramuscular temperatures. *J Orthop Sports Phys Ther.* 33:379, 2003.

108. Romano CL, Romano D, Logoluso N: Low-intensity pulsed ultrasound for the treatment of bone delayed union or nonunion: A review. *Ultrasound Med Biol.* 35:529, 2009.

109. Houghton PE, Nussbaum EL, Hoens AM: Continuous and pulsed ultrasound. *Physiother Can.* 62:13, 2010.

110. Williams R: Production and transmission of ultrasound. *Physiotherapy.* 73:113, 1987.

111. Ashton DF, et al: Temperature rise in human muscle during ultrasound treatments using Flex-All as a coupling agent. *J Athl Train.* 33:136, 1998.

112. Myrer JW, et al: Intramuscular temperature rises with topical analgesics used as coupling agents during therapeutic ultrasound. *J Athl Train.* 36:20, 2001.

113. Klucinec B, et al: The transducer pressure variable: Its influence on acoustic energy transmission. *J Sport Rehabil.* 6:47, 1997.

114. Oshikoya CA, et al: Effect of coupling medium temperature on rate of intramuscular temperature rise using continuous ultrasound. *J Athl Train.* 35:417, 2000.

115. Klucinec B, et al: Transmissivity of coupling agents used to deliver ultrasound through indirect methods. *J Orthop Sports Phys Ther.* 30:263, 2000.

116. Kimura IF, et al: Effects of two ultrasound devices and angles of application on the temperature of tissue phantom. *J Orthop Sports Phys Ther.* 27:27, 1998.

117. Burr PO, Demchak TJ, Cordova ML, et al: Effects of alternating intensity during 1-MHz ultrasound treatment on increasing triceps surae temperature. *J Sport Rehabil.* 13:275, 2004.

118. Frye JL, Johns LD, Tom JA, et al: Blisters on the anterior shin in 3 research subjects after a 1-MHz, 1.5-W/cm^2, continuous ultrasound treatment: A case series. *J Athl Train.* 42:425, 2007.

119. Byl NN, et al: Incisional wound healing: A controlled study of low and high dose ultrasound. *J Orthop Sports Phys Ther.* 18:619, 1993.

120. Cheng N, et al: The effects of electric currents on ATP generation, protein synthesis, and membrane transport in rat skin. *Clin Orthop.* 171:264, 1982.

121. Rand SE, Goerlich C, Marchand K, et al: The physical therapy prescription. *Am Fam Physician.* 76:1661, 2007.

122. McDiarmid T, Burns PN: Clinical application of therapeutic ultrasound. *Physiotherapy.* 73:155, 1987.

123. Saliba S, Mistry DJ, Perrin DH, et al: Phonophoresis and the absorption of dexamethasone in the presence of an occlusive dressing. *J Athl Train.* 42:349, 2007.

124. Merrick MA: Do You Diathermy? *Athletic Ther Today.* 6:55, 2001.

125. Ouellet-Hellstron R, Stewart WF: Miscarriages among female physical therapists who report using radio- and microwave-frequency electromagnetic radiation. *Am J Epidemiol.* 138:775, 1993.

126. Draper DO, et al: Temperature change in human muscle during and after pulsed short-wave diathermy. *J Orthop Sports Phys Ther.* 29:13, 1999.

127. Lehmann JF, et al: Selective muscle heating by shortwave diathermy with a helical coil. *Arch Phys Med Rehabil.* 50:117, 1969.

128. Trock DH, et al: A double-blind trial of the clinical effects of pulsed electromagnetic fields in osteoarthritis. *J Rheumatol.* 20:456, 1993.

129. Murray CC, Kitchen S: Effect of pulse repetition rate on the perception of thermal sensation with pulsed shortwave diathermy. *Physiother Res Int.* 5:73, 2000.

130. Kloth LC, Ziskin MC: Diathermy and pulsed electromagnetic fields. In Michlovitz SL (ed): Thermal Agents in Rehabilitation, ed 3. FA Davis, Philadelphia, 1996, pp 213–284.

131. Santiesteban AJ, Grant C: Post-surgical effect of pulsed shortwave diathermy. *J Am Podiatr Med Assoc.* 75:306, 1985.

132. Markov MS: Electric current electromagnetic field effects on soft tissue: Implications for wound healing. *Wounds.* 7:94, 1995.

133. Pilla AA, Markov MS: Bioeffects of weak electromagnetic fields. *Rev Environ Health.* 10:155, 1994.

134. Wang J, Cheng H, Huang C, et al.: Short waves-induced enhancement of proliferation of human chondrocytes: Involvement of extracellular signal-regulated map-kinase (ERK). *Clin Exp Pharmacol Physiol.* 34:581, 2007.

135. Draper DO, et al: Temperature rise in human muscle during pulsed short wave diathermy: Does this modality parallel ultrasound (abstract)? *J Athl Train.* 32:S35, 1997.

136. Robertson VJ, Ward AR, Jung P: The effect of heat on tissue extensibility: A comparison of deep and superficial heating. *Arch Phys Med Rehabil.* 86:819, 2005.

137. Mitchell SM, Trowbridge CA, Fincher AL, et al: Effect of diathermy on muscle temperature, electromyography, and mechanomyography. *Muscle Nerve*. 39:992, 2008.

138. Oosterveld FG, et al: The effect of local heat and cold therapy on the intraarticular and skin surface temperature of the knee. *Arthritis Rheum*. 35:146, 1992.

139. Castel JC, et al: Rate of temperature decay in human muscle after treatments of pulsed short wave diathermy. *J Athl Train*. 32:S34, 1997.

140. Laufer Y, Porat RZ, Nahir AM: Effect of pulsed short-wave diathermy on pain and function of subjects with osteoarthritis of the knee: A placebo-controlled double-blind clinical trial. *Clin Rehabil*. 19:255, 2005.

141. McCarthy CJ, Callaghan MJ, Oldham JA: Pulsed electro-magnetic energy treatment offers no clinical benefit in reducing the pain of knee osteoarthritis: A systematic review. *BMC Musculoskelet Disord*. 7:51, 2006.

142. Callaghan MJ, Whittaker PE, Grimes S, et al: An evaluation of pulsed shortwave on knee osteoarthritis using radioleu-coscintigraphy: A randomised, double blind, controlled trial. *Joint Bone Spine*. 72:150, 2005.

143. Rattanachaiyanont M, Kuptniratsaikul V: No additional benefit of shortwave diathermy over exercise program for knee osteoarthritis in peri-/post-menopausal women: An equivalence trial. *Osteoarthritis Cartilage*. 16:823, 2008.

144. Dziedzic K, Hill J, Lewis M, et al: Effectiveness of manual therapy or pulsed shortwave diathermy in addition to advice and exercise for neck disorders: A pragmatic randomized controlled trial in physical therapy clinics. *Arthritis Rheum*. 53:214, 2005.

145. Lewis M, James M, Stokes E, et al: An economic evaluation of three physiotherapy treatments for non-specific neck disorders alongside a randomized trial. *Rheumatology*. 46:1701, 2007.

146. Chou R, Huffman LH: Nonpharmacologic therapies for acute and chronic low back pain: A review of the evidence for an American Pain Society/American College of Physicians clinical practice guidelines. *Ann Intern Med*. 147:492, 2007.

147. Jan M, Chai H, Wang C, et al: Effects of repetitive short-wave diathermy for reducing synovitis in patients with knee osteoarthritis: An ultrasonographic study. *Phys Ther*. 86:236, 2006.

148. Cetin N, Aytar A, Ataly A, et al: Comparing hot pack, short-wave diathermy, ultrasound, and TENS on isokinetic strength, pain, and functional status of women with osteoarthritic knees. A single-blind, randomized, controlled trial. *Am J Phys Med Rehabil*. 87:443, 2008.

149. McCray RE, Patton NJ: Pain relief at trigger points: A comparison of moist heat and shortwave diathermy. *J Orthop Sports Phys Ther*. 5:175, 1984.

150. Brown M, Baker RD: Effect of pulsed shortwave diathermy on skeletal muscle injury in rabbits. *Phys Ther*. 67:208, 1987.

151. Schurman DJ, et al: Shortwave diathermy and fracture healing in rabbit fibula model: Preliminary report (abstract). Transactions of the 26th Annual Meeting Orthopedic Research Society, Atlanta, GA, 1980.

152. Draper DO, et al: The carry-over effects of diathermy and stretching in developing hamstring flexibility. *J Athl Train*. 37:37, 2002.

153. Peres SE, et al: Pulsed shortwave diathermy and prolonged long-duration stretching increase dorsiflexion range of motion more than identical stretching without diathermy. *J Athl Train*. 37:43, 2002.

154. Brucker JB, Knight KL, Rubley MD, et al: An 18-day stretching regimen, with or without pulsed, shortwave diathermy, and ankle dorsiflexion after 3 weeks. *J Athl Train*. 40:276, 2005.

155. Bansal PS, et al: Histomorphochemical effects of shortwave diathermy on healing of experimental muscular injury in dogs. *Indian J Exp Biol*. 28:776, 1990.

156. Houghton PE, Nussbaum EL, Hoens AM: Short-wave therapy. *Physiother Can*. 62:63, 2010.

157. Draper DO, Castel JC, Castel D: Low-watt pulsed short-wave diathermy and metal-plate fixation of the elbow. *Athl Ther Today*. 9:28, 2004.

158. Sarwar SG, Farrow A: Investigation of practices and proce-dures in the use of therapeutic diathermy: A study from the physiotherapists' health and safety perspective. *Physiother Res Int*. 12:228, 2007.

159. Martin CJ, McCallum HM, Heaton B: An evaluation of the radiofrequency exposure from therapeutic diathermy equipment in light of current recommendations. *Clin Phys Physiol Meas*. 11:53, 1990.

160. Scott DG, Wallbank WA: Electrode burns during local hyperthermia. *Br J Anaesth*. 70:370, 1993.

Electrical Stimulation

This section is divided into three chapters concerning the basic electrical principles, concepts, and terms; the effect that an electrical current has on the body and subsequent treatment objectives; and the effects of various electrical stimulation units.

Chapter 11

Principles of Electrical Stimulation

This chapter describes the different types of currents used for therapeutic electrical stimulation. The basic physics and principles of electricity are also presented to build a solid foundation on which to build a good understanding of electrical stimulation goals and techniques.

● The effects of electricity on the body can be difficult to comprehend, and the thought of actually sending 500 volts through a person's body can be intimidating. In this chapter, it will become apparent that electrotherapy, when used properly and appropriately, is a safe and effective form of therapy. Just as important, you will also see that electrical stimulation is an adjunct to other therapeutic modalities and rehabilitation exercises. However, electrical stimulation is not always an appropriate treatment approach.

Electricity is the force created by an imbalance in the number of negatively charged **electrons** • between two points, referred to as "poles." This force, known as **electromagnetic force, potential difference,** or **voltage,** creates a situation in which electrons flow in an attempt to equalize the difference in charges, creating an electrical current. In its simplest form, an electrical current takes the path of least resistance from the negative pole **(cathode),** an area of high electron concentration, and flows to the positive pole **(anode),** an area of low electron concentration.

For electron flow to occur there must be a complete pathway, a **closed circuit.** An incomplete path, **open circuit,** prevents the electrons from flowing. When you walk into a room and flip a switch to turn on the light, you are closing a circuit that allows the electricity to flow from its source, through the light, and back to its source. Likewise, a closed circuit is created between your patient and an electrical stimulator by attaching opposite electrodes to the body. The electrons flow from the generator, through the patient's body in the form of ions, and then back to the generator via electrons.

■ Electrical Stimulating Currents

Generally, electrical currents are classified as either being a **direct current** (DC) or an **alternating current** (AC), depending on how the electrons flow. A third classification, **pulsed current,** represents a type of current that has been modified to produce specific biophysical effects (Box 11-1).

Electron: A negatively charged atomic particle.

Box 11-1. CLASSIFICATION OF ELECTRICAL STIMULATING CURRENTS

Current Classification	Sample Waveform	Uses
Direct Current Uninterrupted, unidirectional flow of electrons.	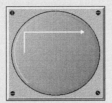	DC can produce polarity-based changes in the tissue, resulting in ions being moved to and from the area. Long duration can directly affect muscle fibers and can alter local pH. ***Common Generators/Techniques:*** Iontophoresis: Medication delivery Low voltage stimulation: Eliciting contractions from **denervated** ● muscle.
Alternating Current Uninterrupted, bidirectional flow of electrons.	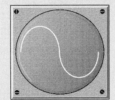	High frequency of the AC decreases skin resistance, leading to a more comfortable current. ***Common Generators/Techniques:*** Interferential Stimulation: Pain control; muscle contractions Premodulated currents; Neuromuscular Stimulation: Muscle contractions
Pulsed Current *Monophasic* Unidirectional flow of electrons marked by periods of non-current flow.	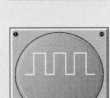	Like a direct current, monophasic currents are applied to the body with a known charge under each electrode. The resulting current can depolarize sensory and motor nerves. ***Common Generators/Techniques:*** High Voltage Pulsed Stimulation: Muscle contractions, pain control

Biphasic
Bidirectional flow of electrons marked by periods of non-current flow.

Symmetrical Each phase is a mirror image of the other.	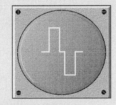	The electrode carries equal positive and negative charges. The effects are equal for both the positive and negative flow and there is no net residual electrical charge. **Common Generators/Techniques:** Neuromuscular electrical stimulation

Asymmetrical
The two phases do not mirror each other.

Balanced The two phases carry equal electrical charges.	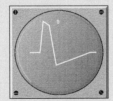	The shape of the pulse allows for greater positive (anodal) or negative (cathodal) effects, but over time the net electrical charge is 0. **Common Generators/Techniques:** Transcutaneous Electrical Nerve Stimulation: Pain control.
Unbalanced The two phases do not carry equal electrical charges.	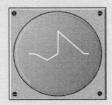	The shape of the pulse allows for greater positive (anodal) or negative (cathodal) effects. Over time there is a net electrical charge. **Common Generators/Techniques:** Neuromuscular Electrical Nerve Stimulation

Denervation (Denervated): Lack of the proper nerve supply or nerve function to, for example, an area or muscle group.

The terms "alternating" and "direct" describe the uninterrupted flow of electrons; "pulsed" indicates that the electron flow is interrupted by discrete periods of no electron flow. Pulsed currents may flow in one direction, similar to a DC, or may have bidirectional movement, as in an AC.[1] Polyphasic currents are hybrids that contain multiple current types.[2]

The primary properties of electrical current are amplitude (intensity) and pulse/phase duration. The **amplitude** is the maximum distance that the pulse rises above or drops below the baseline **(isoelectric point),** the point where the electrical potential between the two poles is equal and no current flow occurs. The horizontal distance required to complete one full cycle of the pulse represents the **pulse duration.** The term "pulse width" is often incorrectly substituted for pulse duration.[3] The total area within this waveform represents the amount of current the pulse contains, the **pulse charge.**

Direct Currents

Direct currents are the uninterrupted, one-directional flow of electrons. The basic pattern is recognized by continuous current flow on only one side of the baseline as the electrons travel from the cathode (negative pole) to the anode (positive pole) (Fig. 11-1). Despite any fluctuations in voltage or amperage, the current flow remains in one direction and stays on one side of the baseline. In medical applications, the term "galvanic" is used to describe direct currents. Iontophoresis, a technique that uses electrical stimulation to introduce medication into the body, is an example of a DC used therapeutically.

Perhaps a flashlight is the simplest example of a DC. The battery possesses a positive pole, which lacks electrons,

and a negative pole that has an excess of electrons. Electrons leave the negative pole of the battery and flow through a wire to the bulb. After leaving the bulb, the electrons return to the positive pole of the battery (Fig. 11-2). When the number of electrons at the negative pole equals the number at the positive pole, no further potential for current flow exists. The battery is dead.

Alternating Currents

In an AC, the direction of flow cyclically changes from positive to negative, although the magnitude of change may not be equal in both directions. Unlike DC, an AC possesses no true positive or negative pole. Rather than constantly moving in one direction, electrons shuffle back and forth between the two electrodes as each take turns being the "positive" and "negative" poles. Household electricity uses AC.

Consider the flashlight example used to describe DC flow (see Fig. 11-2). If a battery were placed on a device that allowed it to rotate between the two wires, we could more or less duplicate an AC. Electrons would flow away from terminal when the cathode is in line with it. When the anode aligns with terminal, electrons would flow toward it (Fig. 11-3). The basic pattern of an AC is the sine wave (Fig. 11-4). Interferential stimulators use multiple ACs.

The amplitude, or **peak value,** of an AC is the maximum distance that the wave rises above or drops below the baseline. In the case of the pure sine wave shown in Figure 11-4, the peak value is the same on both sides of the baseline. The **peak-to-peak** amplitude is the distance from the peak on the positive side of the baseline to the peak on the negative side (Fig. 11-5).

The cycle duration of an AC is measured from the originating point on the baseline to its terminating point and represents the amount of time required to complete one full cycle. The number of times that the current reverses direction in 1 second is the current's number of cycles per second (frequency) and is expressed in hertz (Hz) (Fig. 11-6). A current of 100 Hz would change its direction of flow 100 times during 1 second. A current of

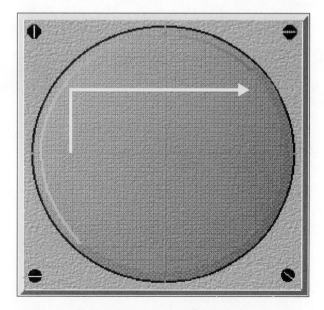

Figure 11-1. **Direct Current.** Characterized by the constant flow of electrons in one direction, a direct current remains uninterrupted (does not return to the baseline) until the circuit is opened, thus stopping the flow of electrons.

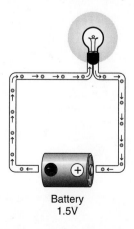

Battery
1.5V

Figure 11-2. **Example of a Direct Current.** Electrons exit the battery through the cathode (negative pole), flow through the wire and bulb, and return to the anode (positive pole).

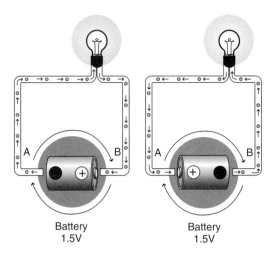

Figure 11-3. **Example of an Alternating Current.** Alternating currents possess no true positive or negative poles. In this type of current, electrons flow back and forth between poles.

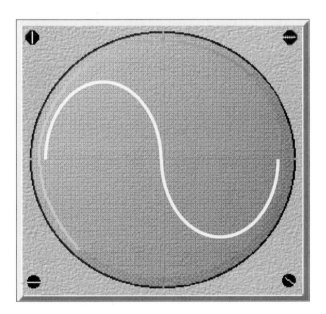

Figure 11-4. **The Sine Wave.** One cycle of an alternating current.

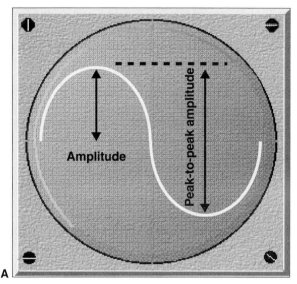

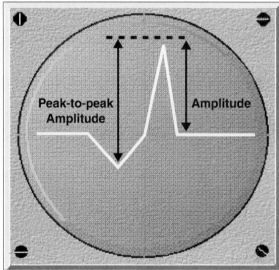

Figure 11-5. **Measures of Amplitude.** Peak amplitude and peak-to-peak values for (A) symmetrical and (B) asymmetrical pulses.

1 megahertz (MHz) would change its direction 1 million times a second. Frequency and cycle duration are inversely related. Because ACs are measured in cycles per second, as the duration of the cycles increases, fewer cycles can occur per second.

Although amplitude is often used to describe the magnitude of an electrical current, it does not describe the actual amount of time that the current is flowing. This applies to both alternating and pulsed currents. Box 11-2 presents measures that take into consideration the cycle's duration.

Pulsed Currents

Pulsed currents are the unidirectional **(monophasic)** or bidirectional **(biphasic)** flow of electrons that are interrupted by discrete periods of noncurrent flow (see Box 11-1). Using the flashlight analogy from the DC section, turning the switch on and off rapidly (about 3000 times per second) is an example

of a monophasic current (it is a monophasic current because the electrons are flowing only in one direction). The current is flowing for only microseconds (1/1,000,000 of a second, μsec) or milliseconds (1/1000 of a second, msec).

Phases are the building blocks of pulses, the individual section of a pulse that rises above or drops below the baseline for a measurable period of time. The number and type of phases then classify the pulse as being monophasic or biphasic.

Monophasic Currents

Monophasic pulses have only one phase per pulse, and the current flows in only one direction. Notice in Figure 11-7 that each pulse consists of only one component part, the phase. Despite the different shapes involved, there is only one phase, and it remains on one side of the baseline. Monophasic currents have a known polarity under each electrode. With this type of current one electrode is the cathode (negative electrode), and the opposite electrode is the

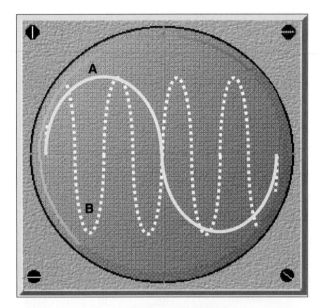

Figure 11-6. **Frequency of an Alternating Current.** Each complete wave is termed a cycle. The frequency, hertz (Hz), describes the number of cycles per second. If the oscilloscope represents 1 second, waveform (A—solid line) has a frequency of 1 Hz and waveform (B—dashed line) has a frequency of 4 Hz.

anode (positive electrode). High-voltage pulsed stimulation uses a monophasic current.

In a monophasic current, **amplitude** is the maximum distance that the pulse rises above the baseline. The **pulse duration** is the horizontal distance required to complete one full waveform (Fig. 11-8). The horizontal baseline is labeled as "time," so the distance a pulse travels represents the duration that the pulse is flowing. With monophasic currents, the terms "pulse," "phase," and "waveform" are synonymous.

Biphasic Currents

Biphasic currents consist of two phases, each on opposite sides of the baseline (Fig. 11-9). The lead phase of the pulse is the first area rising above or below the baseline, and the terminating phase occurs in the opposite direction.

The pulse represented in Figure 11-10A is **symmetrical** because the two phases are mirror images of each other. In this case, each phase has equal, but opposite, electrical balance. Figure 11-10B and C represent **asymmetrical** pulses because each phase has a different shape. When asymmetrical pulses are used, the characteristics of each phase should be considered separately. If the charges (area) of both phases are equal, the pulse is electrically **balanced;** otherwise, it is

Box 11-2. MEASURES OF A CURRENT'S ELECTRICAL POWER

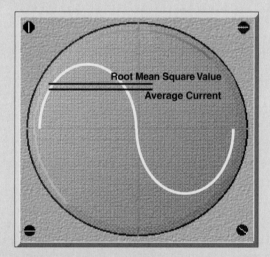

The **average current** of a wave is one-half of its complete cycle and takes into account the amount of time the current is flowing. To calculate the average value of a wave, the sine values of all angles up to 180° are added together and divided by the number of measurements. In the case of a perfect sine wave, this value is about 0.637 (63.7% of the peak current). This figure is then multiplied by the peak value to obtain the average value:

$$\text{Average value} = \text{Mean of sines} \times \text{peak value}$$
$$\text{Average value} = 0.637 \times 100 \text{ V}$$
$$\text{Average value} = 63.7 \text{ V}$$

The **root-mean-square** (RMS) value takes into account the current's amplitude and duration. It describes the total amount of charge delivered by a single cycle and is useful when asymmetrical biphasic currents are used. The RMS is important because it translates the power delivered by a biphasic current into the equivalent amount of power that would be needed by a direct current to produce the same amount of heat. In the case of a pure sine wave, the RMS value is calculated by multiplying the peak value by 0.707.

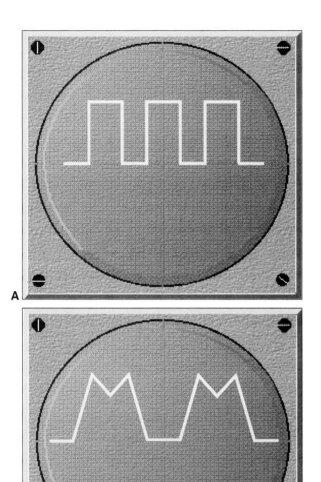

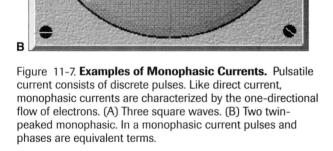

Figure 11-7. **Examples of Monophasic Currents.** Pulsatile current consists of discrete pulses. Like direct current, monophasic currents are characterized by the one-directional flow of electrons. (A) Three square waves. (B) Two twin-peaked monophasic. In a monophasic current pulses and phases are equivalent terms.

unbalanced. The phases in a symmetrical pulse or balanced asymmetrical pulse cause the physiological effects of positive and negative current flow to cancel each other out over time. Unbalanced asymmetrical pulses may lead to residual physiological changes based on imbalances in charges. Symmetrical biphasic waveforms tend to be the most comfortable because they deliver relatively lower charges per phase.[4] Neuromuscular stimulation units often deliver a symmetrical biphasic current; transcutaneous electrical nerve stimulators use a balanced asymmetrical current.

Pulse Attributes

The charge produced by an electrical generator depends on the duration and amplitude of the pulse. The relationship

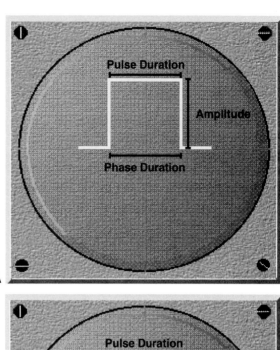

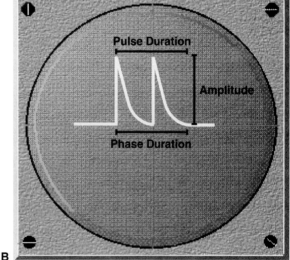

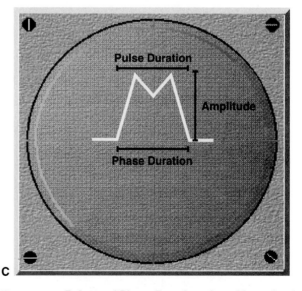

Figure 11-8. **Pulse and Phase Durations for a Monophasic Current.** Monophasic currents have phases and pulses of equal duration. (A) Square wave; (B) sawtooth wave; (C) twin-peaked wave.

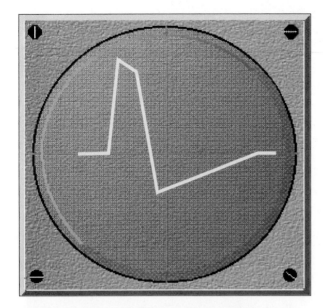

Figure 11-9. **Biphasic Pulse.** An example of biphasic pulsed current commonly used with transcutaneous electrical nerve stimulation (TENS). In the above pulse the lead phase rises above the baseline; the terminating phase drops below the baseline.

between intensity and duration of a single pulse determines the total charge delivered to the body. Increasing the amplitude or duration, or both, increases the total charge of the pulse. Time-dependent pulse characteristics are presented in Table 11-1.

Pulse and Phase Duration

As we've seen, the baseline (horizontal axis) represents time. The distance that a pulse covers on the horizontal axis represents the pulse duration: the elapsed time from the beginning of the initial phase to the conclusion of the final phase, including the intrapulse interval.[1] The duration of biphasic pulses is described by the time required for each phase to complete its shape: the phase duration (see Figs. 11-8 and 11-10).

In a monophasic current, "pulse duration" and "phase duration" are equivalent terms. In biphasic currents, the pulse duration is the sum total of the two phase durations plus the intrapulse interval (if present).

The phase duration, and its associated electrical power (charge), is the most important factor in determining what type of tissues will be stimulated.[5] If the phase duration is

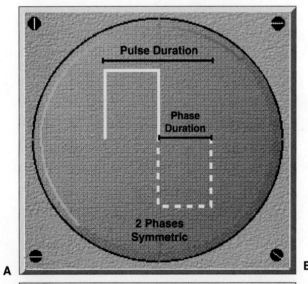

A

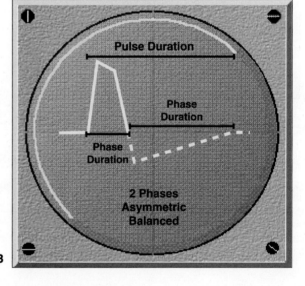

B

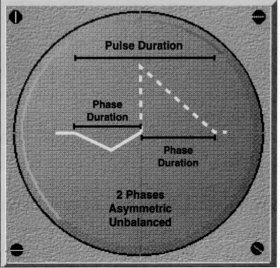

C

Figure 11-10. **Pulse and Phase Durations for a Biphasic Current.** Pulse and phase durations for (A) symmetrical biphasic, (B) balanced asymmetrical biphasic, and (C) unbalanced asymmetrical pulses. The balanced pulses, A and B, have an equal area on each side of the baseline, yielding an equal net charge (the difference between the positive and negative charges) during the treatment. Pulse C has unequal areas within each phase. This waveform would yield a net positive charge because the charge of the positive (second) phase is larger than the negative (first) phase. (The lead phase is shown using a solid line. The terminating phase uses a dashed line.)

TABLE 11-1	Time-Dependent Pulse Characteristics

Phase duration
Pulse duration (phase duration + intrapulse interval + phase duration)
Intrapulse interval
Interpulse interval
Pulse period (Pulse duration + Interpulse interval)

too short, the current will not be able to overcome the capacitive resistance of the nerve membrane and no action potential will be elicited. As the phase duration is increased, different tissues are depolarized by the electrical current.

Interpulse Interval, Intrapulse Interval, and Pulse Period

Pulsed currents have periods during which electrons are not flowing. The **interpulse interval** is the time between the end of one pulse and the start of the next pulse. A single pulse or phase may be interrupted by an **intrapulse interval** (also referred to as the "interphase interval"); the duration of the intrapulse interval cannot exceed the duration of the interpulse interval (Fig. 11-11).[1] The intrapulse interval allows time for certain metabolic events, such as repolarization of cell membranes to occur. The interpulse interval provides time for mechanical events and chemical recharging to occur. The pulse duration and the interpulse interval and, if present, the intrapulse interval form the **pulse period,** the elapsed time between the initiation of one pulse and the start of the subsequent pulse.

By definition, uninterrupted currents (alternating and direct currents) do not possess pulses. Therefore, pulse duration and pulse periods do not exist for these types of currents.

Pulse Charge

The pulse charge is the number of electrons contained within a pulse and is expressed in coulombs. A coulomb is too large a unit to use when describing the charge produced by electrical stimulation units. Most electrotherapeutic modalities produce charges measured in microcoulombs (the charge produced by 10^{-6} electrons).

The pulse charge is a function of the amount of area within the waveform. Increasing or decreasing the amplitude or duration alters the charge of the pulse accordingly. The shape of the wave may also be altered to deliver more or less charge to the tissues per pulse.

Each phase also carries its own charge, the **phase charge.** With biphasic currents, the phase charge is important when trying to evoke a strong muscle contraction. The higher the phase charge, the stronger the contraction will be.[2]

Pulse Frequency

Any waveform or pulse that repeats at regular intervals may be described in terms of its frequency or the number of events per second.[6] When a pulsed current is being used, the frequency is measured by the number of pulses per second (pps). The cycle frequency of an AC is measured by

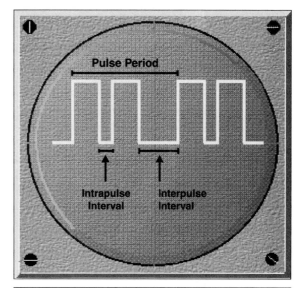

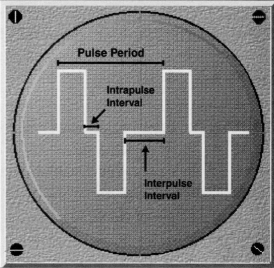

Figure 11-11. **Calculation of Time-Dependent Pulse Characteristics**. (A) Monophasic currents. (B) Biphasic currents. The Pulse Period is the time (horizontal axis) from the start of one pulse to the start of the subsequent pulse. The Interpulse Interval separates two pulses. The Intrapulse Interval interrupts a single pulse.

the number of cycles per second (cps) or Hertz (Hz) (see Fig. 11-6).

The use of the term "frequency" can be confusing because it is used to describe where the current falls on the electromagnetic spectrum, such as identifying shortwave and microwave diathermy (see Chapter 9). In electrotherapy frequency is also used to describe the number of electrical pulses (or cycles) delivered to the tissues. Electrical stimulation units are grouped by their carrier frequency. Low-frequency currents, less than 1000 cycles or pulses per second, are used for their biological effects; medium-frequency currents range from 1000 to 100,000 cps and high-frequency currents, greater than 100,000 cps, are used for their heating effects, as seen with diathermy. To help alleviate this confusion within this text, the term "pulse frequency" is used to describe an adjustable output parameter. "Stimulation frequency" is used to denote device-specific current frequencies. In each case, the actual numerical value of the frequency is the preferred nomenclature rather than "low," "medium," and "high."

There is an inverse relationship between the frequency of an electrical current and the capacitive resistance offered by the tissues. A current having 10 pps encounters more tissue resistance than a 1000 pps current and would require an increased intensity to overcome the resistance.

Pulse frequencies over 100 pps have little additive effect on nerve depolarization. As the pulse frequency increases above 100 pps, the current flow begins to occur during the absolute and relative refractory periods. In most cases, the current intensity is insufficient to cause another depolarization during the relative refractory period. A nerve cannot be depolarized during its absolute refractory period.

Pulse Rise Time and Pulse Decay Time

Pulse rise is the amount of time needed for the pulse to reach its peak value and is usually measured in **nanoseconds** • Rapidly rising pulses cause nerve depolarization. If the rise is slow, the nerve accommodates to the stimulus and an action potential is not elicited. The counterpart of pulse rise time is the pulse decay time, the amount of time required for the pulse to go from its peak back to zero (Fig. 11-12).

Pulse Trains (Bursts)

Pulse trains, or bursts, are currents that are regularly interrupted by periods of noncurrent flow. These linked patterns repeat at regular intervals (Fig. 11-13). Bursts are regulated based on their duration and frequency, and the interburst interval, the length of time between bursts. Each burst results in the nerve(s) depolarizing multiple times.[7]

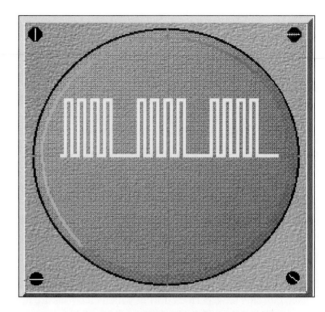

Figure 11-13. **An Example of a Pulse Train (Burst).** A pattern of electrical pulses repeating at regular intervals. In the example presented, each group of four monophasic pulses, the burst, is followed by an interburst interval of noncurrent flow.

The gradual increase in the amplitude of a pulse train is the **amplitude ramp** (ramp) (Fig. 11-14). The ramp causes a gradual increase in the output intensity and the force of muscle contractions. As the intensity of the ramp continues to increase, more and more motor units are recruited into the contraction as the amplitude increases.[8] The resulting contraction more closely resembles a voluntary muscle contraction than if no ramp were

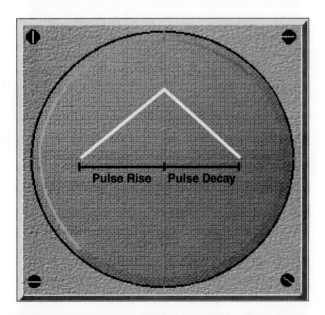

Figure 11-12. **Pulse Rise and Decay Time for a Monophasic Current.**

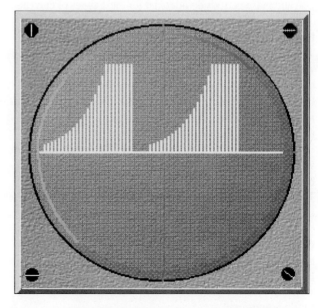

Figure 11-14. **Amplitude Ramp.** The gradual increase in the intensity (amplitude) of a current, allowing for more comfortable muscle contractions.

Nanosecond: One billionth (10^{-9}) of a second.

used. The patient appreciates a slow rise time because the intensity is gradually increased, reducing the sensation of "shock."

Measures of Electrical Current Flow

The strength of an electrical current is expressed in amperes and is related to the voltage of the current and the resistance it meets. This relationship, **Ohm's law,** is the fundamental principle governing electrical current flow (Box 11-3). The following sections describe the factors affecting the strength of an electrical current passing through the human body and relevant terminology (Table 11-2).

Electrical Charge

Electrical current results from the flow of electrons. The number of electrons required for electrical current flow is so great that it is impractical to count each one. Just as we may describe 12 objects as a dozen, or a dozen dozens as a gross, a large number of electrons can be described as a single unit. A coulomb ("Q") is used to describe the charge produced by 6.25×10^{-18} electrons (negative charge) or protons (positive charge).

Coulomb's law describes the relationship between like and unlike electrical charges: opposite charges attract and like charges repel. The strength of the attractive or repulsive forces may be amplified by increasing the magnitude of the charges or by decreasing the distance between the two objects.

Voltage

Voltage, the potential difference between two poles, measures the tendency for current flow to occur. Electrons placed within an electrical field move to the opposite pole, thus creating the potential for work to occur (Work = Force × Distance). The volt is the unit of potential difference and represents the amount of work required to move 1 coulomb of charge. The energy required to move this coulomb is termed a joule. The symbol used to represent voltage is "E" or "V."

The flow of electrons is not the simple movement of particles through a medium. Rather, the flow consists of the passing of electrons between atoms in a manner similar to a bucket brigade. Picture a line of people passing buckets of water. In this analogy, the people represent atoms and the buckets of water are electrons. The first person hands the bucket to the next person. This person then passes the bucket to the next person and the process

---

Box 11-3. OHM'S LAW

Ohm's law describes the relationship between amperage, voltage, and resistance. Generally stated, current (I) is directly proportional to voltage (V) and inversely proportional to resistance (R):

$$I = V/R$$

By using derivations of Ohm's law, the amperage, voltage, or resistance in a circuit can be calculated if two of the three variables are known. In a circuit where the potential is 120 V with 10 ohms of resistance, the amperage would be calculated as 120 V/10 ohms, or 12 A. Circuits having a very high voltage can still have a very small current flow if the resistance is high. For example, applying 1000 V to a circuit with a resistance of 1,000,000 ohms would produce only 0.001 A. Likewise, low voltages can give rise to a very high current flow. Consider a 10-V circuit with 0.01 ohms of resistance. The resultant current would be 1000 A.

To determine the effect that current (I) and resistance (R) have on voltage (V), we may transpose Ohm's law to give:

$$V = IR$$

For current to flow through a resistance, the voltage applied must be equal to or greater than the product of the amperage times the resistance. To produce a current of 12 A flowing through a circuit of 10 ohms, 120 V (12 A × 10 ohms) would be required.

The resistance (R) found in a circuit may be calculated by again transposing the formula so that we divide the voltage (V) by the resistance (I):

$$R = V/I$$

Therefore, if we are using a device that requires 120 V and 12 A, we can calculate the amount of resistance by dividing 120 V by 12 A to give 10 ohms.

You will notice that in all of our equations, current is equal to 10 A, voltage is equal to 120 V, and resistance is equal to 10 ohms. This illustrates the interrelationship between the variables. If we were to reduce the current to 5 A and increase the voltage to 200 V, the resistance would then be 40 ohms. In any case, the voltage applied to the circuit must be greater than the resistance, or no current will flow.

TABLE 11-2   Electrical Terminology

Amperage (I):	The rate at which an electrical current flows. One ampere is equal to the rate of flow of 1 coulomb per second. It is analogous to the rate of flow of water through a pipe. $I = V/R$.
Charge:	See Coulomb.
Coulomb (Q):	The basic unit of charge is the coulomb, the net positive or negative electrical charge produced by 6.25×10^{18} electrons or protons.
Coulomb's law:	Like charges repel and unlike (opposite) charges attract each other.
Joule (J):	Basic unit of work in the International System of Units. Representing the work done by moving 1 coulomb, 1 J equals 0.74 foot-pounds of work. The conversion equation is $J = QV$.
Ohm (V):	Unit of electrical resistance (R). $R = V/I$.
Ohm's law:	Current is directly proportional to voltage and inversely proportional to resistance. $I = V/R$.
Voltage (V):	The potential for electron flow to occur. Analogous to the height of a waterfall, it indicates how much energy is available in the system. The greater the height of a waterfall, the more energy it can impart to a mill below. $V = I/R$.
Watt (W):	Unit of electrical power (P). May be calculated from the relation Watts = Volts × Amperage ($P = VI$). Watts measure the ability to perform work.

repeats. The flow of electrons is similar; rather than a single electron passing through a wire, electrons are passed from atom to atom.

Current

Amperage is the rate at which the electrical current (measured in coulombs) flows. More specifically, 1 ampere (A) is the current when 1 coulomb passes a single point in 1 second. Conceptually, we may make the analogy to the number of people passing through a turnstile at any given time. If 1 coulomb passes a point in 1 second, the rate of flow is 1 A. If 20 coulombs pass a point in 1 second, the rate of flow is 20 A.

The symbol for current flow is "I" or "A." Most electrical therapeutic modalities have current flow measured in **milliamperes** (mA), 1/1000 of an ampere, or **microamperes** (μA), 1/1,000,000 of an ampere.

Resistance

All materials present some degree of opposition to the flow of electrical current. Those materials allowing current to pass with relative ease are labeled conductors and those that tend to oppose current flow, resistors. A material's resistance to the movement of electrons is measured in ohms. One ohm is the amount of resistance needed to develop 0.24 calories of heat when 1 A of current is applied for 1 second. The symbol for resistance is "R," and for ohms, Ω (omega). The skin is the primary biological resistor to therapeutic electrical current flow.

Conductance is a measure of the ease with which current is allowed to pass. Conductance is the mathematical reciprocal of resistance and is measured by the unit **mho**—ohm spelled backward.

The amount of electrical resistance is a function of the type, length, cross-sectional area, and the temperature of the conductor (Box 11-4). As we have already discussed, the potential difference at each end of the circuit must be great enough to overcome the resistance, or no current will flow.

Impedance

In an AC, two additional properties, inductance and capacitance, resist current flow. Collectively known as impedance, this form of resistance is also measured in ohms, but uses the symbol "Z."

Inductance, the ability to store electrical energy by means of an electromagnetic field, is measured by the **henry** ●. Variation in the magnitude and direction of electrical current creates a **flux** ● that induces voltage. Inductors tend to oppose electrical current flow. A transformer used to convert household current into a lower voltage DC is an example of an inductor. Inductance is negligible in biological systems.[1]

Capacitance is the ability to store energy by means of an **electrostatic field** ● that provides frequency-dependent resistance to electric current flow. Cell membranes act as capacitors that separate positive and negative charges between the inside and outside of the cell. The lipid membrane layer is an electrical insulator between the conducting plates, in this case, the intracellular and extracellular fluids (Fig. 11-15).

Capacitance is a factor in determining the effects of current flow in the body. Higher frequency currents meet less capacitive skin resistance than lower frequency currents. The output of capacitors is measured in farads (F),

---

Henry: A measure of inductance (H). One henry induces an electromagnetic force of 1 V when the current changes at a rate of 1 A per second.

Flux: A residual electromagnetic field created by two unlike charges.

Electrostatic field: A field created by static electricity.

Box 11-4. FACTORS DETERMINING THE RESISTANCE OF AN ELECTRICAL CIRCUIT

	Material of the Circuit	Length of the Circuit	Cross-Sectional Area of the Circuit	Temperature of the Circuit
Concept	Materials are classified as resistors or conductors based on the number of free electrons in the **valence shell** •.	There is a proportional relationship between the length of a circuit and the resistance to electron flow.	The resistance of an electrical circuit (path) is inversely proportional to its cross-sectional diameter.	Increased temperature increases the random movement of free electrons.
Relationship	The more free electrons a material has, the better conductor of current it becomes.	The shorter the distance an electron has to travel, the less resistance there will be to electrical current flow.	The greater the cross-sectional area of a path, the less resistance there will be to current flow.	Increasing the temperature of a circuit decreases the resistance to current flow.
Applicability	Not all of the body's tissues conduct an electrical current as well as others.	The distance between an electrical stimulator's two leads affects the output intensity needed to evoke the desired response.	Nerves having a large diameter are depolarized before nerves having smaller diameters.	Preheating the treatment area may increase the comfort of the treatment by decreasing the resistance and the need for higher output intensities.
Example	Blood and nerves have more free electrons than do skin or bone, so the current prefers to travel along this path.	Effects are seen at a lower output intensity if the electrodes are placed closer together rather than farther apart. Superficial tissues are stimulated before deeper tissues.	This, in part, explains how an electrical current selectively stimulates nerves. Sensory nerves tend to be stimulated before motor nerves because sensory nerves have a larger diameter.	The clinical efficacy of body temperature and decreased electrical flow has not been substantiated.

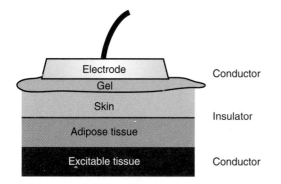

Figure 11-15. **Tissues as Capacitors.** Charge-carrying conductors, the electrode and excitable tissues, are separated by insulators, the skin and adipose tissue.

microfarads (mF, 10^{-6} F), or picofarads (pF, 10^{-10} F). A farad stores a charge of 1 coulomb when 1 V is applied. As we saw when frequency was discussed, the lower the capacitance of a circuit, the higher the frequency of an AC it allows and vice versa.[9]

Wattage

The relationship between voltage and amperage is expressed in units of wattage (W) and is used to designate the power of a current. Power (P) describes the amount of work performed in a unit of time. The voltage describes amount of work being done by the current; amperage defines the time unit. One watt is the power produced by 1 A of current

Valence shell: An imaginary shell in which the electrons responsible for chemical reactivity orbit around the nucleus of an atom.

flowing with the force of 1 V. With this in mind, wattage is describe as

$$W = VI$$

Using the variables from Box 11-3, we can calculate the power used by a device requiring 12 A from a 120-V source to be 1440 W.

The change in wattage of an electrical circuit reflects the change in amperage, voltage, or both. If either amperage or voltage is increased or decreased, the wattage changes accordingly. However, if one variable is increased and the other decreased, the wattage increases or decreases depending on the relative magnitude of the changes in voltage and amperage.

■ Circuit Types

An electrical current introduced into a conductive medium may flow along one set route (series circuit), through many different pathways (parallel circuit), or through a combination of each. Consider an old-fashioned string of Christmas tree lights. If the string is wired as a series circuit, when one bulb burns out, all the other lights go out as well because the current has no other path to take (Fig. 11-16)

In a string of lights wired in a parallel circuit, a burned-out bulb does not affect the other lights because the current still has other routes by which to reach them. Electricity operates under different constraints when traveling through series and parallel circuits, and each type of circuit has unique properties.

Series Circuit

Electrons in a series circuit have only one pathway available for travel. Connecting a wire between the two poles of a battery forms a simple series circuit (see Fig. 11-2). In more complex series circuits, resistors such as light bulbs are aligned "end to end" so that the current leaving one resistor will enter the next. In a series circuit, the current remains the same in all components along the circuit and the total resistance is equal to the sum of the individual resistors (see Appendix E).

Parallel Circuit

Electrons in a parallel circuit have multiple paths that they can follow, and tend to take the path of least electrical resistance. Each path has its own amperage and the voltage remains constant. The flow in each of these pathways is inversely proportional to the resistance provided. In a parallel circuit, the amperage is varied among the paths, but the voltage remains constant. Refer to Appendix E for the calculations of Ohm's law within a parallel circuit.

■ Characteristics of Electrical Generators

Electrical modalities are driven by either standard household current (120-V AC) or by batteries (1.5-V to 9-V DC). Before this current is delivered to the body, it is modified to the desired stimulation parameters.

In a simplified view, the current passes through a transformer that produces the desired type of current (AC to DC, or DC to AC). Another component, generically known as a generator, shapes the current (waveform) used by the modality. Other components within the generator control the characteristics of the electrical pulses.

Each element of the waveform has an effect on the tissues' reaction to the current flow. The following sections discuss each generator characteristic and relate how each affects the treatment.

Current Attributes

The current's attributes affect its ability to depolarize excitable tissue. The intensity of the current, the amount of current per unit of body area, the duty cycle, and the amount of time the current is ON relative to the time the current is OFF influence the therapeutic effects of the treatment.

Average Current

Average current describes the absolute value of current per unit of time and is only meaningful for monophasic currents and unbalanced biphasic currents. The physiochemical changes in the tissues are based on the average current.[10]

Increasing the number of pulses per second or increasing the pulse duration increases the average current and the perception of the stimulus. There is more current per unit of time in high-frequency generators than with other types. Long pulse durations combined with a high average current result in an increased sensation of discomfort.

The average current found in most electrical stimulation units is measured in milliamperes. This measure is

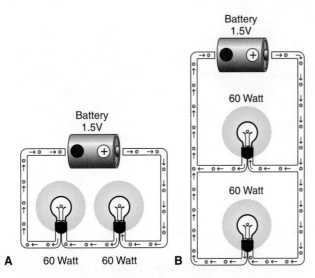

Figure 11-16. **Series and Parallel Circuits.** (A) In a series circuit there is only one pathway for the electrical current to follow. (B) In a parallel circuit the current can take one of several paths.

not meaningful for a balanced symmetrical current because the phase charges for this type of current are equal and the average current is zero. Because the net charge for balanced biphasic currents and ACs is zero, the root-mean-square value should be used for these currents (see Box 11-2).

Current Density
The physiological effects of electrical stimulation are related to the current density, the amount of current per unit area. The current density is inversely proportional to the size of the electrode. For example, if you are passing 300 V through a 10-square-inch electrode, the resulting current density would be 30 V/in^2. Reducing the electrode's surface area by half, 300 V is now passing through an electrode of 5 square inches, with a current density of 60 V/in^2. If the electrode's surface area is again reduced to 1 square inch, the result is a current density of 300 V/in^2.

As the current density increases, so does the perception of the stimulus. If the stimulus was comfortable to the patient in our first example, it would be much more uncomfortable in the last example because the same amount of current is being delivered through one-tenth of the initial surface area.

Duty Cycle
The duty cycle describes the amount of time the current is flowing (ON) relative to the time the current is not flowing (OFF). Expressed as a percentage, duty cycles are calculated by dividing the time the current is flowing by the total cycle time (the time the current is flowing plus the time it is not). For example, to calculate the duty cycle of a generator producing 10 seconds of stimulation, followed by 10 seconds without current flow, use the following equation:

$$\text{Duty cycle (percentage)} =$$
$$\text{Time current is ON/Total cycle time} \times 100$$
$$= 10 \text{ s (ON)}/10 \text{ s (ON)} + 10 \text{ s (OFF)} \times 100$$
$$= 10 \text{ s}/20 \text{ s (Total cycle time)} \times 100 = 0.5 \times 100$$
$$= 50\% \text{ duty cycle}$$

This relationship may also be expressed as a ratio. Using the parameters from the previous examples:

$$\text{Duty cycle (ratio)} = 10 \text{ s (ON)}{:}20 \text{ s (OFF)} = 1{:}2$$

Muscular stimulation is started with a 25% duty cycle and is progressively increased as the condition improves.[11] Providing longer rest intervals (e.g., 2 minutes) between repetitions reduces the amount of fatigue during the course of the treatment.[12]

Electrical Stimulation Techniques

This chapter describes the therapeutic objectives, methods, and effects of a therapeutic electrical current applied to the human body.

● The primary effects of electrotherapy are the result of the depolarization of sensory, motor, or pain nerves. Other effects are caused by electrochemical changes in the tissue and any resulting muscle contraction. Chapter 12 describes the different electrical parameters that can be applied and modified, each type of current producing unique effects within the tissues and causing a wide range of therapeutic responses (Table 12-1).

The type of current, the current's parameters (intensity, phase duration, and pulse frequency), and the electrode size and arrangement can produce specific physiological events and target specific tissues. Electrical stimulation has little, if any, direct effect on the cellular-level inflammation response, but this does not imply that it does not have a useful role in injury management.

■ The Body Circuit

The human body is a mass of tissues and fluids, each having varying ability to conduct an electrical current based on its water content. As the percentage of the water in tissue increases, its ability to transmit electricity increases.

Tissues are either excitable or nonexcitable. **Excitable tissues** such as nerves, muscle fibers, and cell membranes are influenced directly by the electrical current. **Nonexcitable tissues** such as bone, cartilage, tendons, adipose tissue, and ligaments do not directly respond to current flow but may be indirectly influenced by the electrical fields caused by the current (Fig. 12-1).

The outer layer of the skin has a low water content, making it an electrical resistor. Bone, tendons, fascia, and adipose tissue are also poor conductors of electrical currents because of their low water content (20% to 30%). Cell membranes have the greatest resistance to current flow. Muscle, nerve, and blood have a high water content (70% to 75%) and are good conductors of electrical currents. The internal organs, especially the heart, have a low resistance to electrical current flow (Box 12-1).

The current enters the body through a parallel circuit. Although the composition and texture of skin is relatively consistent, there are areas of varying resistance. **Stimulation points** are areas of skin that have decreased electrical resistance (see Box 12-3). Because of increased fluid and ion concentration, inflamed tissues have decreased electrical resistance relative to healthy tissues.[13] Once the current enters the tissues, it may take many different paths, forming a parallel circuit, with the current preferring to follow the path of least resistance, such as those formed by muscle, nerves, effusion, and blood.

TABLE 12-1	**Therapeutic Uses of Electrical Currents**

Controlling acute and chronic pain
Reducing edema
Reducing muscle spasm
Reducing joint contractures
Inhibiting muscle spasm
Minimizing disuse atrophy
Facilitating tissue healing
Facilitating muscle reeducation
Facilitating fracture healing
Strengthening muscle
Effecting orthotic substitution (Electrical stimulation
can be used to force contractions of specific muscles
during gait.)

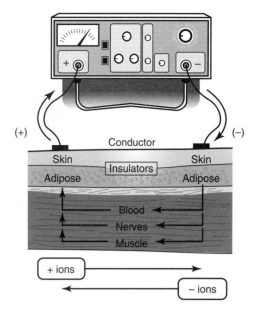

Figure 12-1. **Flow of Therapeutic Electrical Current.** At the skin-electrode interface the flow of electrons is exchanged for the flow of ions within the body. Within the tissues, the current has multiple paths from which to choose. Positively charged ions move toward the cathode (–) and away from the anode (+). Negatively charged ions move toward the anode (+) and away from the cathode (–).

The passage of current through living tissues produces varying biophysical effects, including physiochemical effects and physiological reactions. At therapeutic intensities clinical electrical stimulation causes negligible thermal changes in the tissues, primarily as the result of muscle contractions.[10] High-frequency electrical currents, such as those

Box 12-1. THE PATH OF LEAST RESISTANCE

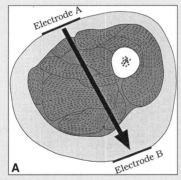

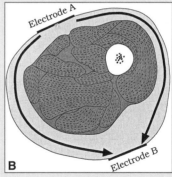

Recall that electrons follow the path of least resistance and that the amperage and voltage must be sufficient to overcome the total resistance imposed by the circuit. Consider a situation in which electrodes are placed on the anterior and posterior surfaces of the thigh. We may think that the current will flow directly through the tissues from one electrode to another as presented in A, above. Most therapeutic treatment dosages lack the electrical power required to overcome the sum of the resistance formed by the cross section of the tissues. In most cases, the current travels around the periphery by flowing through superficial blood vessels and nerves (B, above). The deeper tissues are affected by stimulation of superficial nerves.

Transthoracic and transcranial stimulation is often contraindicated, but not necessarily out of fear of sending a current through the heart or brain. Appropriately placed electrodes can affect the functions of these organs secondary to stimulation of superficial nerves. Many stimulation techniques, such as those for temporomandibular joint dysfunction and auriculotherapy, involve application of electricity to the head. However, at these intensities the current stays within the tissues that are immediately subcutaneous.

Exercise caution when applying an electrical current anywhere on the upper torso, neck, or head. In these areas the path of least resistance may involve nerves that regulate heart rate, blood pressure, and other involuntary life functions.

used with medical diathermy, do produce thermal effects (see Chapter 9).

Electrode Leads

Electrode leads connect the electrodes to the generator. Electrodes then transfer the current to and from the patient's tissues. A minimum of two leads is required to complete the electrical path, with each lead representing a pole of the circuit. Individual leads can be **bifurcated,** allowing multiple pairs of electrodes to be attached to each of the leads (Fig. 12-2).

The U.S. Food and Drug Administration (FDA) Performance Standard for Electrode Lead Wires and Patient Cables (Code of Federal Regulations, Chapter 21, Part 898) requires that electrode lead wires have jacks (plugs) that prevent unintended contact between the patient and an electrical power source (Fig. 12-3). There have been cases where electrode leads were plugged directly into electrical wall outlets (not a recommended form of treatment). The new jack design prevents this from happening. Older units must be retrofitted with these jacks (Fig. 12-4).

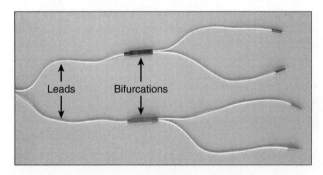

Figure 12-2. **Bifurcated Electrode Lead.** A single lead can be split, or bifurcated, to allow two electrodes to be attached.

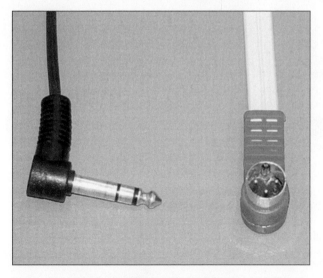

Figure 12-3. **Electrode Leads.** The lead on the left is noncompliant with FDA standards because the current-carrying surfaces are exposed. The lead on the right is compliant because the conductors are shielded.

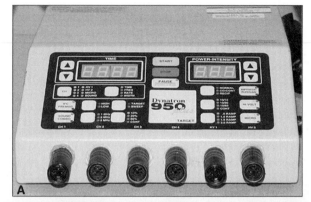

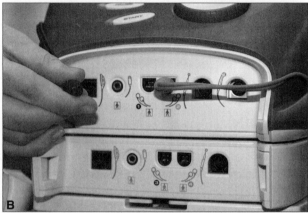

Figure 12-4. **Complying with the FDA Performance Standard for Electrode Lead Wires and Patient Cables.** (A) An older, previously noncompliant generator retrofitted with new jacks to bring the unit into compliance with the standard. (B) A new unit having compliant leads (note the face electrode lead wires in the bottom right).

Electrodes

Formed of metal, or carbon-impregnated silicon rubber, electrodes introduce the current to the body from the stimulator via the electrode leads, forming a closed circuit (Fig. 12-5). When the electrons reach the electrode, they move toward its periphery.[14] The site where the electrodes touch the skin is the point where the flow of electrons used by the stimulator changes to the flow of ions in the body's tissues (Box 12-2). Ion flow consists of positively charged sodium and potassium ions moving toward the negative pole and negative ions, primarily chlorides, moving toward the positive pole.[6] The interface between the electrode and the skin is also the primary source of resistance to current flow.

To form a closed circuit between the generator and the body's tissues, at least one electrode from each of the generator's two leads (poles) must be in firm contact with the skin. Properly prepared and positioned electrodes increase the efficiency of the electrical current by reducing the skin/electrode resistance, thereby improving patient comfort (Table 12-2). If the current is not evenly distributed across the electrode, increased current density will cause "hot spots" that may cause discomfort.

The skin presents both capacitive and parallel resistance to current flow. The stratum corneum creates a

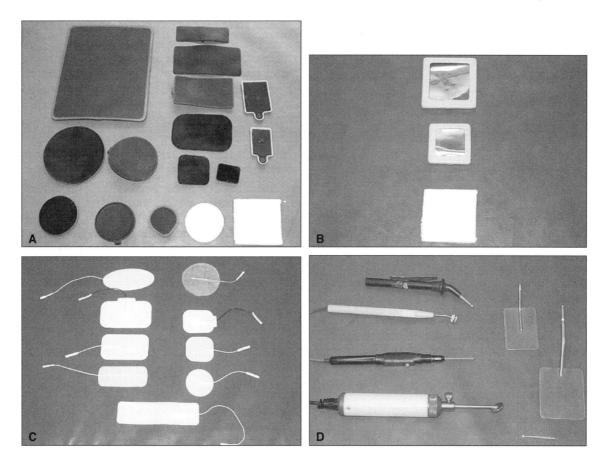

Figure 12-5. **Electrical Stimulation Electrodes.** (A) Carbon-impregnated silicon rubber electrodes. A sponge or other conducting medium is required. (B) Metal electrodes. A moistened sponge (bottom) is needed to conduct the current. (C) Self-adhesive polymer electrodes. (D) Probes (point stimulators) and paddles.

Box 12-2. IONIC CHANGES

In its normal state, an atom has a number of electrons equal to the number of protons. Because the charges of the electrons (negative) and protons (positive) are equal, the atom has a zero (neutral) charge. Atoms that no longer have a zero net charge are known as ions. When an atom loses one or more electrons, it becomes a positive ion (cation) because the number of protons is greater than the number of electrons. Likewise, atoms that gain electrons become negatively charged ions (anions) because the number of electrons is greater than the number of protons.

Ions behave differently from their neutrally charged relatives. Because they possess an electrical charge, they are subject to electromagnetic and **electro-osmotic** ● influences. When placed in the path of a direct current, positively charged ions migrate toward the negative pole and vice versa.

---

capacitor between the electrode and the underlying excitable tissues (see Fig. 12-15). As the thickness of the stratum corneum decreases, the capacitive resistance decreases. Parallel resistance is formed as the ions pass through portals in the skin, such as glands and pores, to the underlying tissues. As the number of parallel paths increases, the overall parallel resistance decreases. Water, gel, or self-adhesive electrodes more efficiently transmit the current by conforming to the small contours of the skin.

Electro-osmotic: Pertaining to the movement of ions as a result of electrical charges. Positive ions move away from the positive pole toward the negative pole; negative ions move away from the negative pole toward the positive pole.

TABLE 12-2 Methods of Reducing Skin-Electrode Resistance

Moisten electrodes with water or conductive gel (sponge or rubber electrodes).

Remove dirt, oil, or flaky skin by washing with soap and water, alcohol, or acetone.

Warm area with a moist heat pack.

Gently scrub area with fine emery paper.

Remove excess hair.

Saturate sponges with commercial saline solution rather than tap water.

Use silver electrodes.

The type of electrode and the conductive medium used affect the efficiency and comfort of electrical stimulation. Of the standard electrode types, **carbon-rubber electrodes** deliver the most current at the lowest skin impedance, about 200 ohms, allowing for more comfortable stimulation. Silver electrodes (most commonly used with iontophoresis, microcurrent stimulators, and electrodiagnostic units) provide about 20 ohms of resistance, so less energy is required to pass the current through them.[15,16] However, silver electrodes are expensive.

Self-adhesive electrodes are commonly used during clinical electrotherapy. With this type of electrode, the conducting gel is a part of the electrode. Although self-adhesive electrodes are convenient and easy to use, they produce the most resistance to electrical current flow.[14,16] Self-adhesive electrodes are more uncomfortable during the treatment, with an increased burning sensation occurring under the electrode's metal connector.[16] Self-adhesive electrodes have a finite life span and are relatively expensive because they have to be replaced. Discard them when they begin to dry out, become dirty or worn, or reach their recommended expiration date.

Metal electrodes use moistened sponges to complete the electrical connection with the skin. Carbon-rubber electrodes may also use moist sponges or a conducting gel. Although tap water is often used to moisten the sponges, the quality and high mineral content of tap water can increase electrical resistance. Usually, this is not a problem, but patients who are sensitive to electrical currents may be more comfortable if the sponge is saturated with a commercially available saline solution. Carbon-rubber electrodes lose their conductivity over time. Discard the electrode if it becomes cracked or worn, or if the electrode face loses its sheen.

Carbon-rubber and metal electrodes require a conducting medium to improve the contact between the skin and electrode, improve current distribution, and decrease the resistance formed by the skin.[14] Conducting gels are salt-free coupling agents that minimize skin-electrode resistance. The gel contains water with a thickening agent, a bactericide or fungicide, and ionic salts. The salt's ions increase the gel's conductivity, allowing diffusion into the skin, decreasing the skin's capacitive resistance. The ionic salts can, however, result in skin irritation. Their chemical properties allow long-term use with little breakdown associated with current flow or evaporation, and because of the gel's high water content and low mineral content, skin irritation and allergic reactions are minimized.

Before placing nonadhesive rubberized electrode on the patient's skin, spread a liberal amount of gel over the entire area of the conducting surface. After positioning the electrode on the skin, slightly rotated and slide it to ensure that the gel has been evenly distributed. Nonadhesive electrodes used during short-term treatments are generally held in place by elastic straps. In the case of long-term treatments, the electrodes must be secured through the use of adhesive patches. Gel, rather than water, should be used for this type of treatment. Generally, these types of electrodes and their adhesives are very durable and water resistant.

Electrode Size

The size of the electrode is inversely related to the current density; as the size of the electrode increases, the current density decreases. Consider, for example, a current passing through two electrodes, one having a surface area of 10 square inches and the other 5 square inches. The smaller electrode (5 square inches) would have twice as much current passing through it per square inch than the larger one (Fig. 12-6).

The electrode's contact with the skin also influences the stimulation parameters (current density), comfort, and muscular tension associated with electrical stimulation.[17] As the electrode surface area increases, there is a greater current flow at any given voltage.[1] **Most electrodes have a maximum current density that must not be exceeded.** This value (e.g., 0.1 watts/cm^2) is included with the electrode's packaging information.

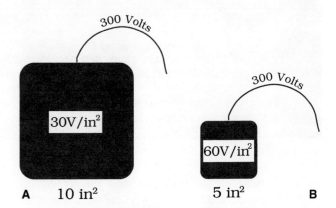

Figure 12-6. **Current Density.** Electrodes must transmit the entire voltage flowing through the circuit. In this case the large electrode, electrode A, has 300 volts flowing through it. Electrode B is half the size of A, yet 300 volts must pass through it as well. In this example, electrode A has a current density of 30 volts per square inch (in^2); electrode B has 60 volts per square inch. The stimulation would be more intense under electrode B because of the increased current density.

The relative sizes of the electrodes alter the various physiological responses. Smaller electrodes require less current to stimulate tissues than do larger electrodes because of the high current density. The size of the electrode to be used is determined by the size of the body area being treated, the treatment goal, and/or the other electrodes being used. As we will see in the next section, the size of an electrode to be used is relative to the other electrode(s) being used and the body part being treated.

✳ Practical Evidence

Small electrodes (approximately 0.8 cm²) yield a more comfortable treatment when superficial nerves are targeted or the patient has a thin (< 0.25 cm) adipose tissue layer. Large electrodes (approximately 4.1 cm²) are more comfortable when recruiting deeper nerves and/or the patient has an adipose tissue layer of more than 2 cm.[18]

The resistance to current flow (impedance) offered by the skin decreases as the size of the electrode increases. Larger electrodes are thought to produce stronger contractions without causing pain, but the stimulation of the tissues is less specific because the current is distributed over a larger area.[16,17] Large electrodes are also thought to yield a more comfortable treatment. In practice the comfort level relative to electrode size varies from patient to patient and is different in the same patient on different days.[5,13]

Electrode Placement

The size of the treatment area, current intensity, and tissue type being stimulated are determined by a combination of electrode size, electrodes' relative location on the body, and the current parameters. Certain areas of the skin are more conducive to electrical stimulation than other areas. These sites, collectively referred to as **stimulation points,** consist of motor points, trigger points, and acupuncture points (Box 12-3). Anatomically, the three types of stimulation points tend to be located close to each other, so one electrode often stimulates multiple points. Likewise, the patient's perceived intensity and the intensity of muscle contractions are dependent on the number of nerve fibers that are stimulated.

The proximity of the electrodes to each other influences the tissues that are stimulated, the depth of the stimulation, and the number of parallel circuits that are formed. When electrodes are close together the current flows superficially, forming a relatively small number of parallel paths. As the distance between electrodes is increased, the current can reach deeper into the tissues. If the distance between the two electrodes is too great, so many parallel

circuits are formed that the specificity of the stimulation decreases (Fig. 12-7). Muscle fibers are four times more conductive when the current flows with the direction of the fibers than when it flows across them.[6]

Although each electrical circuit must have two leads from the generator, more than one electrode can be connected to a single lead. Through **bifurcation,** two or more electrodes can originate from a single lead (see Fig. 12-2). It is common for both leads to possess two electrodes each, or for one lead to have two electrodes and the other lead to have only one. The relationship between the total current density of one electrode (or set of electrodes) to the other electrode determines the electrode configuration, which may be classified as monopolar, bipolar, or quadripolar.

The terms "bipolar" and "monopolar" are often confused with "biphasic" and "monophasic." This is primarily done to confuse students. Remember that *electrodes* represent electrical poles (mono**polar** technique) and electrical *currents* are built out of phases (mono**phasic** current).

Bipolar Technique

Bipolar application involves the use of electrodes having equal or near-equal size (Fig. 12-8). Both electrodes are usually located in the target treatment area. Because the current densities are equal, an equal amount of stimulation should occur under each electrode or set of electrodes. Other factors may affect the quality and equality of stimulation under each electrode. If electrode A is placed over a motor point or other hypersensitive stimulation point (see Box 12-3) and electrode B is not, the effects of the treatment will be weighted toward electrode A. This scenario would be appropriate if a single point, such as a trigger point, were being targeted during the treatment. In this case, a monopolar configuration (described in the next section) would be preferable because a single, well-localized area is being targeted. However, if the treatment goal is to elicit a muscle contraction, electrodes A and B both should be placed over motor points within the same muscle or muscle group.

Monopolar Technique

Monopolar application involves the use of two classifications of electrodes: (1) one or more **active electrodes** placed over the target tissues and (2) **a dispersive electrode** used to complete the circuit (Fig. 12-9). The surface area of the dispersive electrode is significantly larger, at least 2.5 times the total area of the active electrodes. Because of the relatively low current density no physiological effects, including sensation, should occur under the dispersive electrode although current is still flowing through it. The dispersive electrode is often incorrectly referred to as the "ground."

The active electrode is placed on or near the target tissue, and the dispersive electrode is fastened elsewhere on the body (e.g., opposing muscle group, opposite limb, low back). The high current density focuses the treatment effects

Box 12-3. STIMULATION POINTS

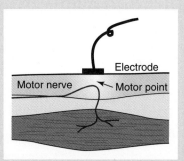

Certain areas of the skin conduct electricity better than other areas. These locations, collectively known as stimulation points, represent areas that require less current to produce muscle contractions, sensation, or pain. Many therapeutic techniques are designed to specifically stimulate one or more of these stimulation points. The proximity of these areas to each other results in a single electrode stimulating all three points.

Motor Points

Each muscle has one or more skin surface areas that are hypersensitive to electrical current flow. These points, known as motor points, are discrete areas above the location where motor nerves and blood vessels enter the muscle mass. Because of their low electrical resistance, stimulation of these points elicits a stronger contraction at lower intensities than the surrounding tissues. Motor points associated with an injured area show an increased sensitivity to current flow and palpation.

Although there is a degree of consistency in the location of motor points, there is some variation between individuals and, depending on the pathology involved, can vary within the same person over time. The thickness of the overlying adipose tissue layer influences the current intensity required to depolarize the motor nerve; increased adipose tissue requires increased intensity.[19] Appendix D presents commonly accepted motor points and is presented for reference purposes. These points must be located on each patient by finding the point at which the strongest contraction results from the lowest intensity of stimulation.

Trigger Points

Trigger points are pathological, localized areas of pain that are hypersensitive to stimulation. Stimulation of these areas "triggers" radiating or referred pain. Unlike motor points, trigger points may be found not only in muscle but also in other soft tissues, such as ligament, tendon, and fascia (see Appendix B).

Acupuncture Points

Acupuncture points are specific sites on the skin possessing a decreased electrical skin resistance and increased electrical conductivity. Acupuncturists propose that these points are connected by meridians through which blood and energy flow.[20,21,22,23,24,25] Superficial **master points** ●, consisting of 12 main channels, 8 secondary channels, and a network of subchannels, connect areas of the skin to deeper channels and allow systemic regulation of many body functions. These master points are often effective in alleviating pain along the entire meridian and are thought to result in the release of endogenous opioids.[23] Although acupuncture has been successfully used for many centuries, its theoretical basis has never been fully substantiated.

under the smaller active electrode. As the distance between the active and dispersive electrodes increases, more parallel electrical paths are formed, resulting in less specific stimulation of deeper motor nerves.

If sensation is experienced under the dispersive electrode, move it to a different site, rewet it, or use a larger electrode. Sensation under the dispersive electrode does not negate the effects of the treatment, but it is unnecessary. Motor nerve stimulation under this electrode indicates that the current

densities of the electrodes are too similar. In this case, use a larger dispersive electrode or a smaller active electrode.

Quadripolar Technique

Quadripolar application involves the use of two sets of electrodes, each originating from its own electrical **channel** ●; it is the concurrent application of two bipolar circuits. The currents from each of the two channels intersect, intensifying and localizing the treatment effects. The most common

---

Master points: Points that, according to the theory of acupuncture, connect skin areas to deeper energy channels. Stimulating master points results in systemic changes.

Channel (electrical): An electrical circuit consisting of two poles that operate independently of other circuits.

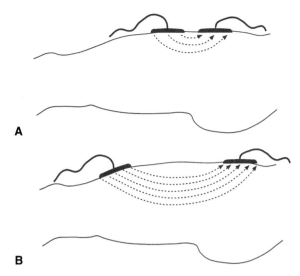

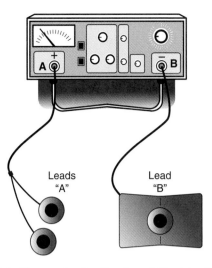

Figure 12-7. **Electrode Proximity.** (A) When electrodes are placed in close proximity to each other, the current flow forms relatively few parallel paths and does not penetrate as deeply into the tissues. (B) As the distance between the electrodes is increased, the number of parallel paths increases and the current tends to flow more deeply within the tissues. However, along with this the focus of the stimulation becomes less defined because the current meets more resistance and more parallel pathways are formed.

Figure 12-9. **Monopolar Application of Electrical Stimulation.** The total area of the active electrodes is significantly less than the area of the dispersive electrode. The imbalance in current density focuses the stimulation to the area under the active electrodes.

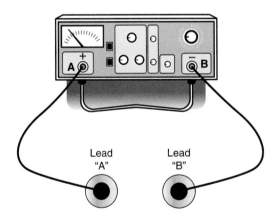

Figure 12-8. **Bipolar Application of Electrical Stimulation.** The surface area of the electrodes originating from each lead is equal. This creates an equal current density, and the effects of the stimulation occur equally under each electrode. Each lead may be split to accommodate two electrodes. As long as the electrodes are of equal size and the resulting current density is equal, the application is classified as bipolar.

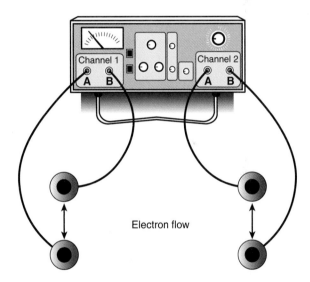

Figure 12-10. **Quadripolar Application of Electrical Stimulation.** Two sets of electrodes operating with two independent channels.

example of this is interferential stimulation. Other quadripolar configurations include parallel placements, as are found in certain transcutaneous electrical nerve stimulation techniques, or agonist-antagonist placements used in neuromuscular electrical stimulation techniques (Fig. 12-10).

Movement of Electrical Currents Through the Body

Most forms of clinical electrical stimulation are applied transcutaneously. When a current is passed through the

skin, it has the potential to upset the resting potential of nerves and other excitable tissues, resulting in depolarization (Box 12-4).

Once a therapeutic electrical current enters the body, the movement of ions replaces the flow of electrons (see Fig. 12-1). Ions move away from the pole having the same charge and migrate toward the pole having the opposite charge (Coulomb's law). When an AC or pulsed biphasic current is used, the ions move back and forth between the electrodes based on the number of cycles per second (see Figure 12-6). When a DC or pulsed monophasic current is used, this migration occurs in one direction only.

Box 12-4. EXCITING EXCITABLE TISSUES

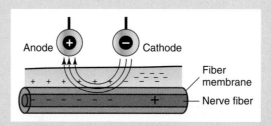

When an excitable tissue (nerves, muscle fibers, cell membranes, etc.) remains undisturbed, its resting potential stays constant. The resulting potential acts as a stored energy source to be used in the transmission of impulses; the energy is stored as separated electrical charges on the inside and outside of the cell membrane. In this sense, the membrane serves as a capacitor.

A decrease **(depolarization)** or increase **(hyperpolarization)** in the cell membrane's electrical charge is required before an action potential can take place. **Rheobase** is the minimum amount of voltage, under the negative pole, required to produce a stimulated response when a direct current is used. Unless specifically noted otherwise, the term "depolarization" will be used to denote the triggering of an action potential by either depolarization or hyperpolarization.

At a sufficient magnitude any stimulus, be it electrical, mechanical, chemical, thermal, or hormonal, can cause depolarization by changing cell permeability, resulting in an action potential. A membrane requires approximately 0.5 msec to recover its excitability after an action potential. This "down time" is the absolute refractory period. The membrane will not discharge during this period. After the absolute refractory period, there is a relative refractory period, during which another depolarization can occur if the magnitude of the stimulus is increased (see Box 1–2).

Under the cathode, the membrane potential is reduced, resulting in depolarization. Negative charges are repelled from the cathode and migrate to the relatively positively charged outer side of the nerve membrane, increasing the negative charge outside the cell and reducing the electrical potential between the inside and outside of the membrane. The resting potential shifts toward the positive and—given sufficient electrical potential—triggers an action potential.

Excitable tissues under the anode are hyperpolarized. Negative ions migrate from the nerve membrane toward the anode, creating an increased net positive charge outside of the membrane. The relative increase in the negative charge within the membrane triggers an action potential.

To trigger an action potential, the stimulus must be greater than the nerve's threshold potential. Cathodal stimulation, or the negative phase of a biphasic or alternating current, tends to more easily trigger an action potential.[14]

Nerve Type	Diameter	Conduction Velocity	Stimulus Level for Depolarization
A-beta	12 to 20 μm	30 to 70 m/s	Low
A-delta	1 to 4 μm	6 to 30 m/s	High
C-fibers	< 1 μm	0.5 to 2 m/s	High

Selective Stimulation of Nerves

The different nerve types are depolarized in an orderly, predictable manner. A nerve's response to electrical stimulation is based on three factors: (1) the diameter of the nerve, (2) the depth of the nerve relative to the electrode, and (3) the phase duration of the current.[5] Sensory nerves are stimulated first, followed by motor nerves and then pain fibers. Only after these structures have reached their depolarization threshold (or if these nerves are incapable of depolarizing) can the electrical current directly affect muscle fibers.

Large-diameter nerves are depolarized before smaller diameter nerves. The amplitude necessary to stimulate a nerve is inversely proportional to the nerve's diameter. Because the larger cross-sectional area of the nerve provides less capacitive membrane resistance, less current is required (Box 12-5).

Stimulation Levels

Stimulation intensities are described with reference to the type of nerve depolarized:

Subsensory-level: Stimulation occurs between the point at which the output intensity rises from zero to the point where the patient first receives a discrete electrical sensation. This type of stimulation does not appear to cause therapeutic benefits.

Box 12-5. THE LAW OF DUBOIS REYMOND

Causing a nerve to depolarize is a relatively easy task; simply apply enough voltage with sufficient amperage and depolarization is bound to occur. However, this type of stimulation is rarely therapeutic or selective.

According to the law of Dubois Reymond, the variation in current density, rather than the absolute current density, causes the depolarization of nerves or muscle tissue.[26] Variations in current density overcome the cell membrane's resistance at a lower intensity than at unchanging densities. To depolarize excitable tissues in an orderly and sequential manner, the following criteria must be met[27]:

- The intensity of the current must be intense enough to depolarize the cell membrane.
- The rate of rise of the leading edge of the pulse must be rapid enough to prevent accommodation.
- The current must flow long enough in one direction (phase duration) to cause the nerve to depolarize. Smaller-diameter nerves require a longer phase duration to depolarize than larger-diameter nerves.
- Sufficient time must be allotted to allow the membrane to repolarize.

Sensory-level: Stimulation depolarizes only sensory nerves. This level is found by increasing the output to the point at which a slight muscle twitch is seen or felt and then decreasing the output intensity by approximately 10%.

Motor-level: Stimulation is an intensity that produces a visible muscle contraction without causing pain.

Noxious-level: Stimulation is current applied at an intensity that stimulates pain fibers.

Muscle fiber-level: Stimulation is applied with a long phase duration and output intensity that directly causes muscle fibers to depolarize.

There is a cumulative effect as the intensity of the stimulation is increased. As the output passes through the sensory level and reaches the motor level, sensory nerves are still being depolarized; as the output intensity is increased to the noxious level, sensory and motor nerves are still being depolarized.

Superficial sensory nerves receive more stimulation than the more deeply located motor nerves. To activate a deep motor nerve, the current must first pass through the superficial tissues, including adipose tissue.[19] Pain fibers are more superficial than motor nerves, but they also tend to have a smaller diameter. Their resistance to current flow is so great that motor nerves reach threshold first, allowing muscle contractions to be elicited before pain is felt. Sine waves (alternating currents) penetrate deeper into the tissues than pulsed currents.[5]

Superficial pain fibers may, however, be stimulated before the deeper motor nerves. Surface stimulation of the skin always results in the activation of sensory receptors before motor or pain nerves.[28]

✱ Practical Evidence

With the exception of wound healing, bone growth stimulators, and iontophoresis, the benefits of clinical electrical stimulation are derived from the depolarization of sensory nerves (e.g., pain control), motor nerves (e.g., muscle reeducation), or pain fibers (e.g., pain control). Electrical stimulation has little, if any, direct effect on the inflammatory process.

Short phase durations allow the greatest range in stimulation intensity for depolarization of the three nerve types. As the phase duration is increased, two events occur. First, less amplitude is required to stimulate each nerve type. Second, the difference in the intensity required to reach the depolarization threshold between each type of nerve is decreased.[5,29] Figure 12-11 depicts a typical strength-duration curve between phase duration and the threshold of excitation for the nerve types indicated. Theoretically, if the phase duration were continued out along the baseline, there would be a point at which each type of nerve would be stimulated almost simultaneously and at a very low intensity.

Various electrical stimulation protocols require that the stimulation parameters be sufficient to produce a comfortable muscle contraction, edema "milking" or muscle reeducation for example. Clinical electrical stimulators produce a muscle contraction by depolarizing motor nerves, not by directly depolarizing muscle fibers. Since motor nerves have a larger diameter than muscle fiber they present decreased electrical resistance relative to muscle fibers, so they are prone to depolarize first.

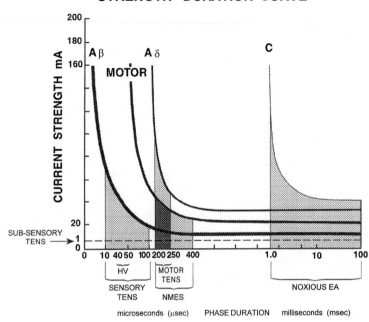

STRENGTH - DURATION CURVE

Figure 12-11. **Strength-Duration Curve.** Because of the capacitive resistance formed by the cell membranes, short pulse or phase durations are more selective in the nerve fibers stimulated than pulses having a longer duration. Shorter-duration currents require increasing amounts of current to stimulate the same type of nerve fiber than currents having a longer duration. (Courtesy of IAPT. Used with permission.)

Another reason for this lies in the resting potential of nerves and muscle fibers. On average, nerves have a resting potential of -75 mV and the resting potential of muscle fibers is -90 mV. Therefore, more electrical charge is needed to cause muscle fibers to depolarize.

Electrical stimulators that have a long phase duration and sufficient amplitude can cause muscle fibers to depolarize and contract. However, referring to the selective stimulation of nerves, these parameters would also cause pain fibers to depolarize. Direct muscle fiber depolarization is sometimes used to produce muscle contractions in patients who are suffering from paralysis, enabling them to partially regain use of their limbs.

Central and Peripheral Nervous System Interference

When a stimulus sufficient to cause depolarization of a cell membrane remains unchanged, the resting potential of the membrane rises to above its prestimulus level. This peripheral nervous system (PNS) response, **accommodation,** occurs when the nerve's rate of depolarization decreases while the depolarization stimulus, in this case an electrical current, remains unchanged. Nerves undergoing accommodation require increasingly intense stimulus throughout the treatment to reach the depolarization threshold (Fig. 12-12).

The threshold for the initiation of an action potential varies based on the stimulation applied. Slowly rising pulses require a greater amount of amplitude to initiate an action potential. Nerves accommodate quickly; thus, an abrupt pulse rise is needed. Muscle fibers accommodate more slowly than nerve fibers, so a gradual pulse rise is used.[10] The pulse rise is preset by the generator and is not changeable by the user.

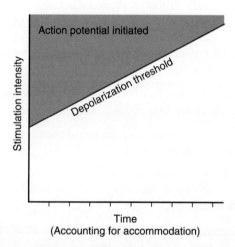

Figure 12-12. **Changes in Depolarization Threshold During Accommodation.** When excitable tissues are exposed to an unchanging stimulus, the cell membrane adapts to the stimuli, requiring an increased level of stimulation to trigger an action potential. This figure illustrates how the level of stimulation, over time, would have to be increased to cause depolarization of the cell membrane. The onset of accommodation can be combated when using electrical stimulation by adjusting the output parameters such as intensity, frequency, and duration at random intervals. These modulation parameters are built into many electrical stimulators.

The central nervous system (CNS) may also play a role in decreasing the long-term sensory stimulation associated with electrical stimulation. **Habituation** is the CNS process of filtering out a continuous, nonmeaningful stimulus.[30,31] This is experienced in everyday life: you sit down to study in the kitchen. Your roommates have gone out for the evening, so the apartment is quiet except for the humming of the refrigerator. After you begin studying, the sound of the refrigerator gets pushed further and further into the background of your consciousness. Eventually, you no longer realize that the sound is there. Although you still hear it, the stimulus stays in your mental "background" until the refrigerator stops humming. At this point, you are struck by the roaring silence of the room.

Accommodation and habituation occur during the application of an electrical modality. Increase the intensity of an electrical modality to the point at which the patient expresses slight displeasure in the comfort of the stimulus. Allow the person to experience the current flow for about 5 minutes, and then ask if the intensity can be increased. More times than not, the patient will say yes. This ability to increase the intensity represents accommodation of the involved nerves. People become accommodated to an electrical current and are able to tolerate increased intensity as their number of treatment sessions increases.[32] Habituation is the tolerance to the stimulus developed across multiple treatments.

Many electrotherapeutic modalities have **modulation parameters** to combat the effects of accommodation. The generator can randomly alter the pulse intensity, frequency, and/or duration to prevent the body from receiving a constant, unchanging stimulus (Table 12-3, and see Fig. 13.3).

Medical Galvanism

Galvanic stimulation is the application of a low-voltage direct current to the body. Since DC is used, there is a known polarity under each electrode. By controlling the polarity of the electrodes, certain cellular and biochemical responses may be elicited. The **pH** ● of tissues under the cathode (negative pole) becomes basic (the alkalinity of the tissues is increased), increasing the risk of chemical burns. Acids collect under the anode that can cause coagulation of proteins and hardening of the tissue. Direct current stimulation can elicit a muscle contraction from denervated muscle, but the phase duration is so long that C fibers are also stimulated, making the contraction painful.

TABLE 12-3 **Modulation Parameters to Delay Physiological Accommodation to an Electrical Current**

Amplitude
Phase/pulse duration
Frequency
Ramp
Surge
Burst
Multiple (the combination of two or more of the above parameters)

Through an electro-osmotic process, ions are attracted to the pole having the opposite charge and repelled from the pole with the same charge. Positively charged sodium ions (Na^+) move toward the cathode (negative pole), where they gain an electron and form an uncharged sodium atom. Through the reaction of sodium with water, proteins are liquefied, causing a general softening of the tissues in the area and a decrease in nerve irritability.[33] Physiological events under the anode are essentially opposite those occurring at the cathode. Here, tissues are thought to harden because chemical mediators force a coagulation of protein.

These effects are not as pronounced when monophasic, biphasic, or alternating currents are used. The short pulse duration and long interpulse interval reduce the chemical effects of monophasic currents.[34] Symmetrical or balanced asymmetrical biphasic currents or ACs result in no galvanic changes because both phases have an equal but opposite charge. An unbalanced asymmetrical current can result in residual chemical changes if the duration of the current is sufficient.

■ Clinical Electrical Stimulation

This section presents common goals of electrical stimulation and techniques on how to achieve them. The next chapter relates these goals to the different types of electrical stimulation units commonly used in the treatment of orthopedic and some neurological conditions. With the most notable exceptions of wound and fracture healing, the effects of electrical stimulation are the result of depolarizing sensory, motor, or pain nerve fibers (Fig. 12-13).

Motor-Level Stimulation

If applied at a sufficient intensity, almost any type of electrical stimulator can elicit a contraction in normal, healthy muscle. But not every electrical stimulator is appropriate for each type of motor-level treatment (Table 12-4). Through different types of electrical currents, different electrical stimulators allow for more efficient, intense, and comfortable contractions. The combination of the pulse rise, phase duration, and current amplitude determines the quality and quantity of the contraction. The pulse duration and intensity factor together to increase the recruitment of motor nerves **(spatial summation)**. The pulse frequency increases the rate of muscle contractions per unit of time **(temporal summation)**.[35]

Electrical stimulation is used to create tension in the muscle to prevent (or delay) atrophy, reestablish neurological pathways, restore the strength of inhibited muscle, or increase muscular strength. Clinically, the basis of these theories is that maintaining a safe load on muscle creates tension relative to total immobilization. Since there is less

---

pH (potential of hydrogen): A measure of acidity or alkalinity (bases). A neutral solution has a pH of 7. Acids have a pH of less than 7; bases have a pH greater than 7.

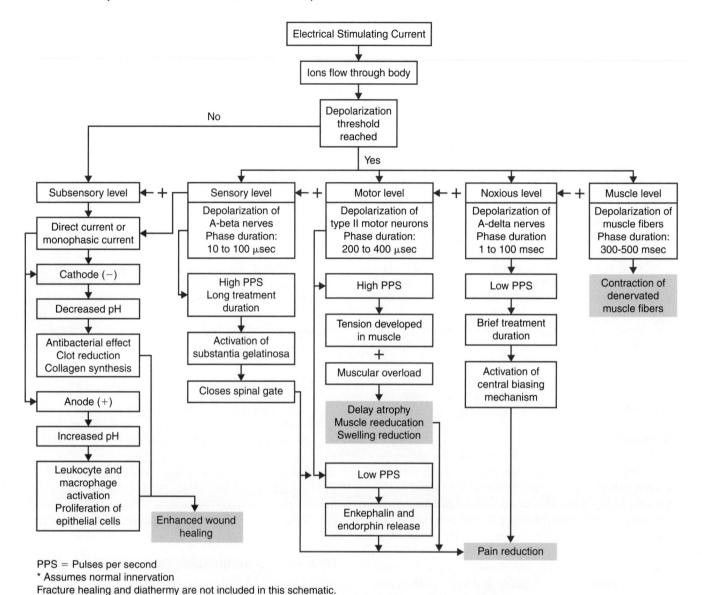

Figure 12-13. **Schematic of the effects of electrical stimulation.** There is an additive effect as the depolarization threshold increases from the subsensory level to the muscle fiber level. For example, motor-level stimulation also activates sensory nerves.

atrophy, there is less function lost.[36] The more tension safely developed in the muscle, the greater the benefits will be:

No contraction < Electrically induced contractions < Voluntary contractions < Voluntary contractions + electrical stimulation

NO TENSION   MAXIMUM TENSION

The torque produced by electrical stimulation is dose dependent and is limited by discomfort.[7,29] Generators that are intended for neuromuscular stimulation should produce a strong, comfortable contraction.[32,37]

Electrical stimulation of **innervated** ● muscle activates the motor nerve rather than the muscle fibers directly. Because the capacitance of motor nerves is less than that of muscular tissue, the current overcomes the resistance of the nerve first (Table 12-5). When the magnitude of the stimulation is sufficient, an action potential is initiated, sending a signal to the motor unit that results in contraction of the muscle. For this reason, the electrodes should be placed over the muscle's motor points (see Appendix D). These contractions may be used to retard the effects of atrophy, reeducate muscle, reduce edema, or augment the force-generating capacity of healthy muscle.

Innervate (inervated): Normal and sufficient nerve supply to a muscle, body area, and so on.

TABLE 12-4 Common Uses of Motor-Level Stimulation Protocol by Generator Type

Generator/Current Type	Clinical Usage/Limitations
High Volt Pulsed Stimulation *Monophasic*	Neuromuscular reeducation Motor-level pain control Motor-level edema reduction Some units do not have a duty cycle control Lacks total current needed for maximum force production
Transcutaneous Electrical Nerve Stimulation *Biphasic*	Motor-level pain control No duty cycle control Low total current limits force production
Interferential Stimulation *Alternating*	Motor-level pain control Motor-level edema reduction No duty cycle control Premodulated parameters target current to motor nerves
Neuromuscular Electrical Stimulation *Monophasic, biphasic, alternating*	Neuromuscular reeducation Strength augmentation

TABLE 12-5 Comparison of Physiologically Versus Electrically Induced Muscle Contractions

Physiologically Induced Contractions	Electrically Induced Contractions
• Small-diameter, slow-twitch muscle fibers are recruited first. • Contractions and recruitment are asynchronous to decrease muscle fatigue. • Golgi's tendon organs protect muscles from too much force production. Slow onset of fatigue	• Large-diameter, fast-twitch muscle fibers are recruited first (reversal of the voluntary recruitment order). • Contractions and recruitment are synchronous, based on the number of pulses per second. • Golgi's tendon organs cannot override the developing tension within the musculotendinous unit. Faster onset of fatigue

During voluntary contractions, small type I fibers (alpha motoneurons) are the first to depolarize. The strength of the contraction is based on the number of motor units recruited and the firing frequency of the motor units. Electrically induced muscle contractions cause type II fibers to be activated before type I fibers. With electrically induced contractions, all of the involved motor units fire at the same time. Tension is increased based on the pulse frequency of the motor units. Electrical stimulation causes muscle fatigue more rapidly than voluntary contractions.[7]

Motor nerves are recruited into the contraction based on the diameter of their axons and their proximity to the electrodes.[38] Large-diameter motor neurons are recruited before smaller ones, and nerves in proximity to the electrode respond before those more distant. During voluntary muscle contractions, type I motor fibers are recruited before type II fibers. During motor-level electrical stimulation, type II fibers are recruited first.

Current Attributes Influencing the Contraction

The quality, efficiency, and comfort of electrically induced muscle contractions are contingent on the type of current and the pulse characteristics. Alternating or pulsed currents are capable of yielding contractions, but the relative comfort is variable. The primary pulse characteristics that determine the quality of the contraction are the amplitude (intensity), phase duration, and pulse frequency.

✱ Practical Evidence

Clinically, each type of current except direct current is used to produce a muscle contraction. The perceived comfort of each is often patient dependent.[39] In general, there is no difference in the amount of muscle torque that can be produced by different current types, but a sine wave has been demonstrated to yield a stronger contraction with less discomfort than other current types.[40] Biphasic currents have a longer onset to muscle fatigue than an alternating current (e.g., Russian simulation), potentially maximizing the treatment benefits.[7]

Pulse Amplitude (Intensity)

The force generated by the muscle contraction is linearly correlated to the amount of current introduced into the tissues. The strength of the contraction increases as the amplitude (intensity) of the current increases.[35,41,42] The depth of penetration of the current increases as the peak current increases, thus recruiting more nerve fibers. To depolarize deeper motor nerves the current must first pass through the adipose tissue layer. Individuals with more adipose tissue overlying the target motor nerves require a greater output intensity to evoke a strong muscle contraction than those with thinner layers.[19]

The patient's tolerance to the current is often the limiting factor in the strength of the contraction produced.[29] The maximum comfortable intensity tends to be less than 30% of the maximum voluntary isometric contraction (MVIC).[43] Prior exposure to electrical stimulation and an understanding of the treatment and the expected sensations may lead to increased muscular tension.[44]

Cold treatments are often used for their anesthetic effects. Research on the ability of cold application before or during electrical stimulation to improve patient comfort has produced mixed results.[45,46,47] The pain experienced during high-amplitude electrical stimulation is caused by stimulation of the cutaneous pain receptors and nociceptors located deep within the muscle.[48] Cold application prior to treatment increases the maximum output tolerated by the patient, but does not translate into increased torque production.[47]

Phase Duration

The phase charge, the amount of current delivered by each phase, determines the quality and quantity of the muscle contraction. A phase duration of 200 to 400 microseconds (μsec) specifically recruits motor nerves.[10,49] Short phase durations require greater amplitude to evoke an action potential than phases of longer durations.[50] Phase durations of less than 1 millisecond (msec) will not be able to stimulate denervated muscle, regardless of the current's amplitude.[8,9,51] Phase durations longer than 400 microseconds begin to recruit pain fibers.[29]

Pain fibers have a small diameter relative to motor nerves and are normally only stimulated at higher intensities and with longer phase durations, allowing for muscle recruitment without a disproportional amount of discomfort. However, the pain associated with the intensity of the stimulation and the sensation of muscle tension often prevents maximum contractions from being achieved.

Pulse Frequency

When the stimulation is applied at a pulse rate of less than 15 pulses per second (pps) (or in the case of AC, Hz), there are distinguishable muscle contractions for each electrical pulse. At this pulse rate, there is sufficient time for the mechanical process required for the muscle fibers to return to their original length before the next pulse begins. Each of these individual contractions is referred to as a twitch contraction (Table 12-6).

Because of **summation,** individual contractions become less and less distinguishable between 15 and 25 pps. In this case, the pulses occur in such rapid succession that the muscle fibers do not have the time to return to their original position before the next pulse begins (Fig. 12-14). As the pulse frequency increases, the amount of summation increases as a result of the greater overlap in the mechanical process of muscle contraction.[10]

Summation continues until the muscle reaches the **critical fusion frequency,** the point at which **tetany** ● is obtained. At this point, the muscle enters a **tonic contraction** ●. The critical fusion frequency is slightly different from person to person and between muscle groups, but it usually occurs between 30 to 40 pps.[52] Postural muscles (type I muscle fibers) reach tetany before nonpostural muscles.[9]

Increasing the frequency of the stimulation will do little to further increase muscle tone. Pulse frequencies above 60 pps cause an increased rate of muscle fatigue if used for a sufficient duration.

A strong tetanic contraction is required to delay atrophy or enhance strength. Moderate pulse frequency stimulation (20 pps) reduces fatigue, but the muscle develops 45% less force than it could at higher pulse frequencies.[3] Higher frequencies reach tetany more comfortably than lower frequencies. Medium-frequency biphasic currents selectively fatigue type II muscle fibers, resulting in decreased torque production as the treatment progresses.[53]

TABLE 12-6   Pulse Frequency Ranges Commonly Used in Electrotherapy

Descriptor	Pulses per Second (pps)	Neuromuscular Effects
Low (Twitch)	<15	Individual muscle contractions
Medium (Summation)	15–40	Blending of individual contractions resulting in increased muscle tone
High (Tonic)	>40	Steady or constant contraction

Note: The above ranges will differ depending on the individual and muscle group.

Tetany: Total contraction of a muscle achieved through the recruitment and contraction of all motor units.

Tonic contraction: Prolonged contraction of a muscle.

1 pps   20 pps   40 pps

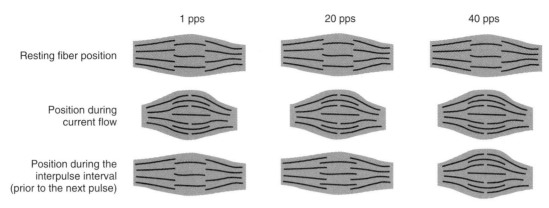

Figure 12-14. **Muscle Fiber's Reaction to Pulse Frequency.** The tone of a muscle undergoing electrically induced contractions varies with the pulse frequency. At less than approximately 15 pps, the muscle fibers have the time to return to their original starting position. As the pulse frequency increases, the duration of the interpulse interval decreases, prohibiting the muscle fibers from returning to their original starting position before the next pulse.

Force decay across the treatment can be counteracted by increasing the amount of rest between treatment cycles or decreasing the pulse frequency during treatment.

Denervated Muscle

Motor nerves that have been denervated for less than 3 weeks are still capable of depolarization. In this case, motor nerves can continue to produce a muscle contraction via electrical stimulation until **wallerian degeneration** • sets in.[10] Prior to this point motor nerves can be depolarized by a pulse that has a short duration and a slowly rising waveform.

When a muscle is fully denervated, the muscle fibers can no longer communicate with the motor nerve, or the motor nerve cannot receive signals from the spinal cord, so the muscle fibers must be directly stimulated to evoke a contraction.[51] The phase duration produced by most clinical electrical stimulators is too short to directly depolarize muscle fibers. The current must flow for a longer time in one direction to depolarize muscle fiber membranes. A galvanic (direct) or monophasic current with a long phase duration (low voltage stimulation) must be used. In cases in which the patient has suffered a spinal cord injury but the peripheral nerves are still intact, such as an **upper motor neuron lesion** •, muscle contractions can still be obtained through the use of a pulsed current.[10,35]

Neuromuscular Reeducation

Neuromuscular reeducation involves the "teaching" of a muscle how to contract again. Edema, pain, immobilization and disuse atrophy, and/or nerve damage can interfere with the neurological loop between the muscle, peripheral nerve, spinal cord, and brain.[32] Electrical stimulation can reestablish neural pathways to restore voluntary contractions.[36] Neuromuscular reeducation differs from strength augmentation, which is electrical stimulation applied to healthy muscle.

Generators that are capable of producing a duty cycle and ramping the current maximize the neuromuscular benefits.[54] A low duty cycle allows the muscle to relax and recover between contractions.[32] Ramping the current allows for a natural increase in tension. The pulse frequency must be sufficient to produce a tetanic contraction, with 60 pps being commonly used. For neuromuscular reeducation programs, the force generated should be at least 10% of the MVIC of the uninvolved extremity.[55]

The patient may experience **delayed-onset muscle soreness** • following the treatment. As with any exercise program, the intensity should be adjusted to find a proper balance between therapeutic benefits and patient comfort.[44] Neuromuscular reeducation protocols should not be administered when the tendinous attachment is not secure, the muscle cannot tolerate the tension, or joint motion is contraindicated.

✴ Practical Evidence

To maximize the early effects of neuromuscular reeducation, use long rest periods (approximately 2 minutes) between sets of electrical stimulation. This rest time decreases the decline in force production over time.[12]

Wallerian degeneration: Gradual physiological breakdown of a nerve axon that has been severed from its body.

Upper motor neuron lesion: A spinal cord lesion resulting in paralysis, loss of voluntary movement, spasticity, sensory loss, and pathological reflexes.

Delayed-onset muscle soreness: Residual muscle soreness, caused secondary to damage of the muscle cells, which appears within 24 hours after heavy muscular activity, particularly with eccentric muscle actions.

Similar to voluntary muscle contractions, electrical stimulation strengthening protocols may affect the muscle group in the opposite extremity, increasing strength by as much as 10%. These strength gains can be attributed to a neurological crossover effect, motor learning, or subconscious contraction of the nontreated muscle.[32,56] When the patient is unable to contract a muscle, secondary either to disuse or immobilization (i.e., splint or cast), strengthening the uninvolved limb by voluntary or electrically induced contractions can delay atrophy or assist in the reeducation of the involved limb.[36]

Strength Augmentation

When the goal is to increase the muscle's strength, electrically induced muscle contractions can supplement but should not substitute for voluntary contractions. Electrical stimulation is less effective in increasing quadriceps torque than is biofeedback (see Chapter 18).[57] Strength gains obtained by electrical stimulation follow the same parameters of specificity as any other form of exercise; that is, isometric training improves only isometric strength and does not carry over to **isotonic** ● or **isokinetic** ● strength.[58]

Strength gains realized through the use of electrical stimulation are attributed to two factors[59]:

1. Muscular overload
2. Reversal of type I and type II motor nerves

Strength gains are a response to placement of an increased functional load on the muscle. For strength gains to occur through electrical stimulation, the functional load placed on the muscle must be equal to at least 30 to 60% of MVIC.[2,43] You may recognize this factor as being, in part, the basis of the **overload principle** ●. To produce overload, the muscle must exceed the minimum electrically evoked torque (EET) production threshold, the point at which the contraction produces measurable and meaningful tension on the muscle. As the strength of the muscle increases, the EET also increases.[60]

The increased functional load produced by electrical stimulation is supplemented by the increased recruitment of type II muscle fibers, the second factor in strength augmentation. Because electrical current depolarizes larger diameter nerves first, type II fibers are brought into the contraction sooner and fatigue first.[38,53,61] Type II fiber recruitment and increased functional load work together so that muscle strengthening through electrical stimulation may occur at levels producing 30% of the tension found in the MVIC.[3,59]

Several variables must be considered when attempting to increase muscle strength through electrical stimulation. If the duty cycle is too high, premature fatigue can occur because of increased use of the **phosphocreatine system** ●. Also, the protective function of Golgi tendon organs is overridden during electrical stimulation. Precautions must be taken to damper the terminal ends of the patient's range of motion. For these reasons, the patient should always be given a safety switch that, when depressed, shuts off the stimulation unit if the intensity or muscle tension becomes too intense for the patient.

Prehabilitation

Prehabilitation, the process of increasing muscle strength, power, endurance, and proprioception, is used to improve functional outcomes following surgery. Inflammatory-related muscle deficits are more related to neurological inhibition than atrophy of the muscle, especially in arthritic conditions.[62] The use of electrical stimulation to strengthen muscle prior to surgery results in improved postsurgical recovery, especially in the quadriceps.[63]

Pain Control

Electrical currents are used to reduce the amount of pain experienced by either assisting in the healing process or affecting the transmission and perception of pain. Lessening the mechanical pressure placed on nerve endings or decreasing the degree of muscle spasm or edema eliminates the mechanical and chemical events that stimulate pain transmission. In specific pain-control approaches, electrical stimulation simply masks the pain or encourages the body to release pain-controlling endogenous opiates (Table 12-7).

High-pulse-frequency, short-phase-duration, sensory-level currents activate the gate mechanism of pain modulation. Stimulating sensory nerves closes the gate to the transmission of pain. Low-pulse-frequency, moderate-pulse-duration, high-intensity stimulation and noxious-level stimulation also activate the spinal gait, but have the additive effect of stimulating the release of the body's natural opiates—β-endorphins from the anterior pituitary gland and enkephalins from the spinal cord (Table 12-8). High-pulse-frequency (more than 80 pps) motor-level stimulation triggers the release of enkephalins.[64]

In the initial phases of pain control, electrical currents stimulate the dorsal horn of the spinal cord. Activation of types I, II, III, and IV neurons may cause the dorsal horn to transmit less noxious information to the supraspinal levels.[65] Decreased nerve conduction of small, pain-carrying nerves reduces the amount and rate of noxious impulses transmitted up the spinal cord. In large motor nerves, decreased nerve conduction decreases

---

Isotonic (contractions): Muscle contraction through a range of motion against a constant resistance.

Isokinetic (contraction): A muscle contraction against a variable resistance where limb moves throughout the range of motion at a constant speed.

Overload principle: For strength gains to occur, the body must be subjected to more stress than it is accustomed to. This is accomplished by increasing the load, frequency, or duration of the exercise.

Phosphocreatine system: A compound that is important in muscle metabolism.

TABLE 12-7	**Spinal Levels of Pain Control**		
SPINAL LEVEL	THEORY	ACTIVATING STIMULI	PHYSIOLOGICAL EVENTS
I	Presynaptic inhibition (Ascending)	Sensory stimulation of A-beta fibers Phase duration 75 μsec	Enkephalin interneurons block the transmission of impulses traveling along small C fibers within the dorsal horn T cell.
II	Descending inhibition (Descending)	Intense (high-frequency) stimulation of C fibers Phase duration 1000 μsec	Central biasing mechanisms in the periaqueductal gray matter and the raphe nucleus activate descending influences along the dorsolateral tract of the spinal cord.
III	β-Endorphin modulation (Descending)	Noxious, low-frequency, motor stimulation (A-delta) Phase duration 200–400 μsec	Activates the tract cell and reticular formation, resulting in the release of β-endorphin from the anterior pituitary gland, causing the degeneration of prostaglandin and dorsal horn inhibition.

TABLE 12-8	**Electrical Parameters Used in Pain Control Approaches**			
APPROACH	TARGET NERVES	PHASE DURATION	PULSE FREQUENCY	INTENSITY
Sensory level	A-beta	<100 μsec	60–100 pps	Submotor
Motor level	Motor nerves	200–400 μsec	2–4 pps 80–120 pps	Strong contraction Moderate to strong contraction
Noxious level	A-delta C fibers	1–100 msec	Variable	As painful as can be tolerated

the amount of pain-producing muscle spasm in the treated area.[66] Peripheral stimulation could relieve chronic pain if applied to the site of pain or to an area serviced by the involved peripheral nerve.

✱ Practical Evidence

The placebo effect of electrotherapeutic modalities contributes to the success in pain reduction (see Chapter 2).[67] Many studies exploring the effects of electrical stimulation (and other modalities and medications as well) on pain perception report that patients receiving sham treatments described a decrease in the amount of pain experienced, supporting the theory that cognitive processes are involved in pain modulation.[67,68,69,70,71,72,73]

Blood Flow

Muscle contractions are needed for electrical stimulation to increase blood flow in muscle.[74] Electrically induced contractions increase local blood flow approximately the same amount as voluntary contractions, but heart rate, systemic blood pressure, and cutaneous blood flow are not affected.[74,75] The increased blood flow may be caused by the release of endothelial relaxing factors that cause vasodilation and the associated oxygen demand of muscle contractions.[75] Sensory-level stimulation does not evoke changes in muscle or skin blood flow.[76]

Wound Healing

The use of a low-intensity DC or HVPS may reduce the time needed for superficial wound healing to 1.5 to 2.5 times that needed for wounds not receiving such treatment.[77,78,79,80] The electrical current acts by directly killing the invading organisms, producing antimicrobial factors, and by attracting antimicrobial factors to the wound.[52] Most of the evidence supporting the use of electrical stimulation in wound healing in humans has involved chronic conditions, with the majority of the cases being **dermal ulcers** ● or surgical incisions. Specialized or advanced training is recommended for advanced wound care using electrical stimulation.

Dermal ulcer: A slow-healing or nonhealing break in the skin.

Explanations for the effectiveness of tissue repair include increased circulation, antibacterial effects, influences on migration of cells, and the presence of an **injury potential** • in damaged tissues.[80] In healthy tissue the outer skin surface is negatively charged relative to the deeper skin layers. When tissues are damaged, the electrical charges are reversed.[81,82] This injury potential is theorized to electrically control tissue repair.

✳ Practical Evidence

Regardless of the applied polarity, direct current increases the healing rate of skin wounds. A positive polarity on the wound during the first 3 days and a negative polarity during the remaining treatment duration (usually 12 days) result in the best outcomes. With this method both the time to healing and the strength of the repair is maximized.[80]

The anode may enhance the formation of clots.[78] Negative polarity has demonstrated the ability to break down and absorb blood clots and other hemorrhagic by-products (Table 12-9).[80] Leukocytes migrate toward the anode, resulting in increased blood clotting in the area.[78] Depending on the polarity of the electrode, certain inflammatory mediators, including neutrophils, macrophages, epidermal cells, and fibroblasts, are attracted or repelled from the area.[78,83] Low-intensity DC encourages hydration, increases the number of growth factor receptors, increases the rate of collagen formation,[84] stimulates the growth of fibroblasts and granulation tissues,[85] reduces the number of mast cells in the injured area,[86] and destroys bacteria and other microbes.[87]

TABLE 12-9	Wound Healing Effects Under the Anode and Cathode
ANODE (POSITIVE POLE)	**CATHODE (NEGATIVE POLE)**
Increased pH (acidic → basic)	Decreased pH (basic → acidic)
Blood clotting	Antibacterial effects
Leukocyte migration to the area	Removal of necrotic tissues
Macrophage migration to the area	Decreasing skin edema
Extermination of microorganisims	Fibroblast proliferation
Proliferation of epithelial cells	Increased collagen synthesis

In healthy skin the current tends to flow directly from one electrode to the other. Skin wounds create several parallel pathways, with the area around the wound having decreased resistance. During the treatment of superficial wounds with moderate inflammation the current flows around the margins of the wound and through the center of the wound. In cases where there is profound inflammation, the current may flow entirely around the wound, rendering the treatment ineffective.[13]

Using animal models, DCs have also shown efficacy in promoting healing of the medial collateral ligament. Traumatized ligaments treated with electrical stimulation demonstrated an increased rupture force, increased amount of energy absorption, and decreased stiffness and laxity compared with nonstimulated ligaments.[88] When applied to healing tendons, DC appeared to suppress the proliferation of adhesion-causing cells compared with untreated tendons.[89]

Control and Reduction of Edema

Electrical stimulation is often used to control or reduce the amount of edema formed following orthopedic trauma, surgery, certain diseases, and burns. Sensory-level stimulation is theorized to inhibit edema formation by preventing the fluids, plasma proteins, and other solids from escaping into surrounding tissues. If edema has already formed, motor-level stimulation assists the venous and lymphatic systems in returning the edema back to the torso, where it can be filtered and removed from the body.

Sensory-Level Stimulation for Edema Control

In acute trauma, sensory-level HVPS applied to, or directly around, the injury site has been found to limit the volume of edema formed in laboratory animals. The central concept of this theory is to limit the formation of edema rather than to remove existing edema. In fact, attempting these techniques when swelling has already formed may inhibit edema reduction. A possible mechanism for this response is reduced capillary pressure and capillary permeability, which discourages plasma proteins from entering the extracellular tissues.[90] Pulsed monophasic current may cause a vascular spasm that prevents fluids from leaking out of the vessels.[91]

The output parameters result in decreased permeability of the microvascular structures in the target tissues. Decreased permeability blocks the passage of plasma proteins and helps to maintain the osmotic gradient that is lost during the acute inflammatory response and prevents fluids from escaping into the interstitial space.[54] Negatively charged blood cells and plasma proteins are—theoretically—repelled from the cathode, creating a concentration gradient that encourages local reabsorption of fluids.[55]

The permeability of the local microvessels must be decreased before gross edema forms. If the stimulation is

---

Injury potential: Disruption of a tissue's normal electrical balance as a result of injury.

applied too late in the injury response process, decreased vascular permeability may inhibit reabsorption of the edematous proteins and fluids back into the venous and lymphatic system, virtually trapping them within the extracellular tissues and preventing edema reduction.[92]

When applied immediately after trauma, this protocol, delivered in four 30-minute treatments interspersed with 60-minute rest periods, suppressed edema formation for 17 hours. A single 30-minute treatment curbed edema formation for 4 hours but did not significantly decrease long-term edema formation.[90,93,94,95,96] The pulse frequency also influences the effectiveness of sensory-level edema control. A low pulse frequency (e.g., 1 pps) does not significantly limit edema formation.[94,97,98] Most of these findings have involved animal studies and have not been substantiated in humans.

The clinical application of sensory-level edema control, described in the section High-Voltage Pulsed Stimulation in the next chapter, is not supported by current research.

Motor-Level Stimulation for Swelling Reduction

The role of the motor-level response in reducing edema formation is less controversial and has demonstrated more clinical efficacy than the sensory-level approach. Muscular contractions encourage venous and lymphatic return by squeezing the vessels, moving the fluids proximally, and "milking" the fluids out of the area. Many types of electrical stimulation devices can be used to produce an involuntary muscle contraction that forces the fluids out of the area, but the output must be configured so that the current develops a tetanic contraction that forces the fluids proximally along the extremity and then is followed by a relaxation period (e.g., duty cycle). This technique is also referred to as "muscle milking" or the "muscle pump."

Electrodes are arranged on the involved extremity so that they follow the course of the primary vein exiting the swollen area. If the generator does not allow for a duty cycle, a low pulse frequency, usually 1 pps, is used to allow enough time for the contents of the venous and lymphatic system to move between muscle contractions. If a duty cycle is available, increase the number of pulses per second so that a tonic contraction is achieved. A 50% duty cycle is then used to obtain the desired off-and-on contractions.

The output intensity is adjusted so that the contraction is within the patient's tolerance, and contraindicated joint movement is avoided. Although electrically induced muscle contractions do increase the rate of venous return, the volume of flow is less than that which occurs with voluntary contractions. If the individual is capable of producing strong contractions, this method should be preferred over electrically induced contractions.

✳ Practical Evidence

Motor-level swelling reduction appears to be less effective in the acute inflammatory phase of injury response than in later stages.[99]

As would be expected from what we know of the venous and lymphatic return mechanisms (see Chapter 1), the efficiency of this technique is improved when the limb is elevated so that gravity may assist in the fluid flow. In addition, the use of an elastic wrap or tubular compressive stockings applied to the extremity assists in edema reduction.

Fracture Healing

Implantation of electrodes into acutely fractured bones and the subsequent introduction of a direct current to the healing structure have shown an increased bending rigidity and bone mineral density in animal models.[100] Normally, fractures heal through the process of **osteogenesis** ●. If the fracture fails to heal properly, further repair must occur through endochondral bone formation, the process by which the soft tissue callus transforms itself into bone.[101] Historically, nonunion fractures required the surgical grafting of bone into the fracture site to assist the healing process.

The use of electrical stimulation to aid in the healing of bone is based on the theory that bone cannot differentiate between the body's innate charges needed for normal bone remodeling (see Wolff's law in Chapter 1) and those derived from outside sources, such as electrical generators. The natural sources of these intrinsic stresses are piezoelectric charges (electrical charges produced by mechanical stress) caused by the deformation of the bone's collagen matrix.[102] These piezoelectric charges require an intermittent stress to be delivered to the bone. Static or constant stresses do not produce an electric charge.

Collectively known as bone growth generators, these units attempt to produce electromagnetic fields that mimic the normal electrical signals produced by bone or to activate the bone's piezoelectric properties. Each approach encourages the deposition of calcium through increased osteoblastic activity, regardless of the technique used to introduce the current (Table 12-10). Generally, those generators applied transcutaneously use ACs, whereas those having electrodes implanted in the body use DCs.[103] The cathode is placed near the fracture site when the electrodes are implanted into the tissues because new bone callus is electropositive.[104,105] Implanted electrodes are then surgically removed once successful healing has been obtained.

Osteogenesis: Healing of fracture sites through the formation of callus, followed by the deposition of collagen and bone salts.

TABLE 12-10	Types of Electrical Bone Growth Stimulators
CURRENT TYPE	USE
Direct current	Invasive: Electrodes are implanted in the fracture site. Semi-invasive: Electrodes are placed subcutaneously.
Inductive Coupling	Two or four electrodes introduce a pulsed electromagnetic field through the skin. Treatments are given 30 minutes daily.
Capacitive coupling	An electromagnetic field similar to shortwave diathermy (see Chapter 9) affects the fracture site or sites of osteoporosis.

Adapted from Driban, 2004.

Capacitive coupling generators with external electrodes are similar to diathermy units (see Chapter 9) in that their electrodes produce strong electromagnetic fields. These fields then create piezoelectric currents at the fracture site.

The usefulness of electrical bone growth generators is debatable and is less effective than ultrasonic bone growth stimulators.[101,103,104,106] Evidence exists that electrical bone growth generators may actually delay fracture healing, with stress fractures perhaps being the most negatively impacted or deriving no benefit from the treatment.[100,107] This negative effect may be, at least in part, a result of the fact that many generators use a current "orders of magnitude" more powerful than that required for healing.[102]

Electrical bone growth generators are prescribed only in extraordinary circumstances such as certain nonunion fractures and require long-term treatments (6 months or more). However, the success rates of electrical stimulation in resolving nonunion fractures are the same of that for surgical procedures alone. Because it appears that the currently proposed protocol for treating acute fractures involves implanting electrodes into the damaged bone, the risks and time delays of the associated surgery may limit use of this device to cases in which the patient is at risk for a nonunion or **malunion fracture** ●. However, clinicians should be familiar with the functions, benefits, and limitations of this device. As this technology grows and the efficacy of this modality is established, its possibilities for use in the treatment of acute fractures increase. A specialized form of ultrasound is also used to improve fracture healing.

■ Contraindications and Precautions

The general contraindications and precautions in electrical stimulation are presented in Table 12-11. Contraindications particular to specific electrical stimulators are presented in the appropriate sections of the next chapter.

The primary precautions and contraindications to the use of electrical stimulation are rooted in the placement of the electrodes. The intensity (total current) of the treatment also determines if a treatment can be safely applied in the presence of a potential contraindication.

The patient must be able to provide immediate and understandable feedback regarding the treatment. Patients who do not have cognitive function or who do not have the ability to communicate require special attention should the need to use electrical stimulation present itself. Impaired sensory function prevents the patient from providing feedback regarding the intensity of the treatment or other abnormal effects such as burning.

Avoid current flow through the heart, **carotid sinus** ●, and pharynx because of the potential disruption in normal cardiovascular function. Most therapeutic currents do not directly affect the heart and other deeply lying tissues (see Box 12-1). However, current flow can affect the heart's superficial stimulation points (e.g., the carotid sinus). Implanted cardiac pacemakers may be affected by stimulation of the thorax, lumbar region, or upper extremity. Because of the unknown and unpredictable effects, electricity is not normally applied over sites of infection.

Motor-level stimulation is contraindicated in the presence of active deep vein thrombosis (DVT). The muscle contractions and associated muscle pump can dislodge the clot and release it into the venous system. Electrical stimulation can, however, be used to prevent DVT.[108,109]

Avascular areas, areas of infection, and hemorrhagic conditions present precautions and contraindications. Areas with decreased circulation may benefit from electrical stimulation secondary to increased blood flow as the result of muscle contractions. If the area is too ischemic electrical stimulation can worsen the condition and cause severe pain. Infection may become compartmentalized and in areas prone to hemorrhage, bleeding may increase.

The application of electrical stimulation to a pregnant patient presents a range of contraindications and precautions, primarily because of the unknown effects of electrical stimulation on fetal development. Although transcutaneous electrical nerve stimulation (TENS) has been used to reduce pain prior to and during labor, other types of electrical stimulation over the abdomen, lumbar spine, and pelvis are generally contraindicated. Motor-level stimulation of large

---

Malunion fracture: The faulty or incorrect healing of bone.

Carotid sinus: An enlargement of the carotid artery near the branch of the internal carotid artery, located distal to the inferior arch of the mandible. Baroreceptors at this site monitor and assist in the regulation of blood pressure.

TABLE 12-11 General Contraindications and Precautions for Electrotherapy

CONTRAINDICATIONS

Cardiac disability	Stimulation of the thorax or neck may result in disruption of normal respiratory or cardiac function.
Demand-type pacemakers	Electrode placement over areas where current flow may interfere with pacemaker's function. If the patient has a pacemaker, consult the patient's physician to determine the safety of the intervention.
Arterial disease	May result in pain and/or exacerbate ischemia
Uncontrolled hemorrhage	Application of electrical stimulation to areas of hemorrhage may increase the amount of blood lost.
Sites of infection	Infection, including osteomyelitis, can be spread from the treatment, including contaminating equipment. The exceptions to this are protocols specifically designed for wound care.
Blood clots	Do not apply electrical stimulation to any point on the body when the patient has active DVT and/or thrombophlebitis. Electrical stimulation can be used in cases of controlled DVT.
Pregnancy	Stimulation of the abdominal, lumbar, or pelvic region may have an adverse effect on the developing fetus. Specific guidelines, however, have been developed to decrease pain for pregnant women, but these protocols must be closely monitored by a physician. Electrical stimulation has also been used during delivery, although the current may interfere with fetal monitoring machines.
Cancerous lesions	Electrical current may possibly result in a growth or spread of the tumor.
Exposed metal implants	Contact of a metal fixation rod to a grounded object can result in severe electric shock. Application over staple sutures increases subcutaneous current flow.
History of seizures	Application of electrical stimulation to the head or neck may trigger a seizure. Patients with epilepsy require additional precautions including advice from the patient's physician and increased monitoring of the patient is required.
Sensory or mental impairment	The patient is unable to provide feedback regarding tolerance to the stimulation, potentially resulting in burns or muscle trauma.
Unstable fractures	Motor-level stimulation can place unwanted stress on the healing tissues.

Precautions

Menstruation	Stimulation of the abdominal, lumbar, or pelvic region may increase hemorrhage.
Areas of nerve sensitivity	Caution must be used when applying electrical stimulation to: • The carotid sinus • The esophagus • The larynx • The pharynx • On or around the eyes • The upper thorax • The temporal region
Unfused epiphyseal plates	
Communication impairments	The inability to provide meaningful feedback regarding the patient's response to the treatment can result in electrical stimulation being applied at unsafe intensities.
Severe obesity	Adipose tissue may provide insulation against effective stimulation, increasing the risk of skin irritation from the gel, adhesive, or current flow in individuals who wear electrodes for extended periods. Altering the position of the electrodes reduces irritation.
Electronic monitoring equipment	Concurrent use of electrical stimulators may cause the equipment (e.g., ECG monitors, ECG alarms) not to operate properly.

DVT = deep vein thrombosis

muscle groups and stimulation of acupuncture points are contraindicated.[110]

Electrical stimulation is contraindicated over cancerous sites because of the possibility of accelerating the growth of the tumor or causing the cancer to spread. Electrical

stimulation is sometimes used to help control pain in terminal cancer patients. At this point, the treatment approach no longer focuses on controlling the spread of the cancer but rather focuses entirely on patient comfort. Sensory-level pain control such as TENS can reduce the reliance on narcotic medications to the point where the patient may remain **lucid** • and relatively pain free.

■ Overview of the Evidence

Electrical stimulation is an effective modality for stimulating sensory, motor, and pain nerves and, given the proper phase duration, muscle fiber. Although there is not universal agreement in the parameters,[8,42,111] the use of electrical stimulation to control pain[21,65,112] and reeducate muscle has been substantiated,[113,114] but conflicting results can be found in the literature.[115,116] Wound healing, stimulation of bone healing, and changes in tissue pH following various forms of electrical stimulation have yet to be conclusively demonstrated.

The theoretical basis for cathodal sensory-level edema control has been substantiated in the laboratory using an animal model.[68,90,96] However, there still remains a lack of evidence conclusively demonstrating the clinical effectiveness of this approach.

No evidence exists that suggests that electrical stimulation has an effect on cellular level function. This leads to errors in clinical application of various forms of electrical stimulation. There is no evidence that suggests that subsensory or sensory-level electrical stimulation affects cellular function or affects inflammation.

Electrodes are often placed over the edematous area under the guise that the current will "drive" the edema out of this area. This effect has not been demonstrated to occur with any type of current or any type of treatment protocol.[117]

Lucid: Of clear and rational mind.

Chapter 13

Clinical Application of Electrical Agents

This chapter describes the typical setup and clinical application of electrical stimulators based on the type of current delivered. Although each stimulation method is presented as a distinct modality, many generators are capable of producing multiple forms of electrical current. The information presented in the Biophysical Effects section for each modality should be supplemented with the information presented in Chapter 12. The setup and application protocol are described in generalized terms. Always familiarize yourself with the operator's manual of the specific equipment used.

● The diverse array of electrical stimulation units, techniques, and theories can make understanding the application of electrical stimulation difficult and can be further complicated by individual manufacturers creating their own terminology. A common question is "When do I use each type of stimulator or current?" In some cases, there is one obviously correct answer; in other cases, there may be more than one correct option; and in other cases electrical stimulation may not be appropriate.

It is important to remember that most effects of electrical stimulation are the direct result of the depolarization of sensory nerves, motor nerves, pain nerves, **and, rarely, muscle fibers directly** (see Fig. 12-13). The depolarization thresholds are sequential and cumulative; for example, motor nerves cannot be depolarized without also depolarizing sensory nerves.

Some electrical stimulators deliver only one type of current. **Multimodalities** are capable of generating many different types of therapeutic currents and may also include therapeutic ultrasound (Box 13-1). Some multimodalities allow for two patients to be treated simultaneously.

Some state practice acts may require that electrical stimulation devices be applied only under a physician's order. Clinicians must be aware of state practice acts governing their

Box 13-1. MULTIMODALITIES

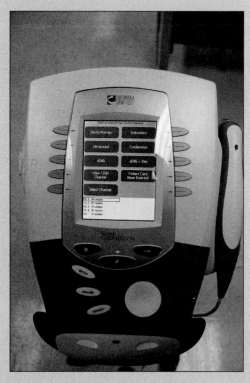

The development of microprocessors, advanced circuitry, and improved battery supplies has led to an evolution in the design and function of electrical stimulators. Once, each type of electrical stimulating current described in this chapter required a specific generator. Now a single microprocessor-based multimodality is capable of producing all of the current types described in Chapter 12 and may include other therapeutic agents, such as ultrasound.

Many multimodalities' output is based on the treatment goal, pain control or muscle reeducation, for example, rather than the type of current. In this case a menu function will display the current being used for the treatment.

The user simply selects the type of output desired, usually described by the type of current, and selects a preprogrammed treatment regimen (e.g., motor-level edema reduction, sensory-level pain control). The instrumentation and output controls are unique to each unit. Because of the differences among multimodalities, their use is not described in this text.

profession's use of these devices as well as the policies and procedures for use at their institution. Likewise, an appropriately credentialed individual should supervise use of these devices.

■ Basic Guidelines for the Setup and Application of Electrotherapy

This section describes the general steps used to prepare the generator, the electrodes, and the patient for electrotherapy. The steps involved in using the generator are described in further detail in their individual sections.

Electrical stimulators may operate from either household current or batteries. Clinical units that are driven by household (120 V) current require less output intensity to reach therapeutic goals than do portable, battery-driven stimulators.[2] Portable units may be powered by standard or rechargeable batteries (1.5 V to 9 V).

Larger portable units may also have the option of working from a transformer.

Preparation of the Generator

1. If a portable or battery-operated unit is being used, make sure the batteries are fully charged. If a clinical model is being used, make sure it is properly plugged into an appropriately grounded wall socket. If the treatment involves water immersion, plug the unit into a ground-fault interrupter circuit. Do not use extension cords.

2. Make sure the electrode leads are not tangled. Regularly inspect the leads for frays, broken insulation, and loose connections. Repair or replace frayed leads before they are used.

3. Ensure that all controls are in their zero (OFF) position.

Preparation of the Electrodes

1. Clean the electrodes to remove any residual gels or skin oils. Clean rubber electrodes with alcohol; gel-based, self-adhesive electrodes should be cleaned with soap and water as recommended by the manufacturer. Dispose of these electrodes when they become worn, dry out, or reach their recommended expiration date. Using the same self-adhesive electrodes between multiple patients is not recommended.
2. Carbon-impregnated rubber electrodes should be used only with a wet medium, such as a sponge. Do not use gels unless specifically recommended by the manufacturer.
3. If conductive sponges are used, moisten them with water. If sponges are not required, apply an even coat of conductive gel to the electrodes.
4. Connect the leads to the unit and to the electrodes.
5. In all cases, read and follow the manufacturer's recommendations for the electrodes being used.

Preparation of the Patient

1. Ensure that the patient has no contraindications to the treatment.
2. If indicated, conduct a sensory test of the area to be treated, checking both light and intense stimuli (or cold and heat). Light stimulation and cold sensation are transmitted along the dorsal column of the spinal cord. Heat and pain are transmitted along the spinothalamic tract.
3. If the goal of the intervention is pain control, question the patient regarding caffeine intake such as coffee, energy drinks, soft drinks, or medications containing caffeine. More than 200 mg of caffeine can reduce the effectiveness of electrical stimulation pain control techniques.
4. If this is the patient's first exposure to electrical stimulation, explain the sensations to be expected (e.g., "tingly sensation" or "muscle twitch"). Be aware that some individuals are apprehensive about electrotherapeutic treatments. The patient should be advised against any unnecessary movements because this may break the circuit between the electrodes.

   If the patient has had previous electrical stimulation for the current condition, question the patient about the outcomes of the prior treatment.
5. Determine the electrode placement technique.
6. Clean the skin with alcohol to remove any body oils, lotions, dirt, and grime. Keep in mind that body hair increases resistance to electrical current flow. Decreasing skin resistance increases patient comfort. When possible, place the electrode over areas of low hair density or shave the area where the electrodes will be placed (see Table 12-2).
7. If a monopolar technique is used, attach the dispersive electrode to a large body mass, such as the thigh or lower back. If the dispersive electrode is placed on the lower back, place the electrode so that it lies on one side of the spine and not across it. The indentation formed by the erector muscles causes incomplete contact with the dispersive electrode and may result in sensation under this electrode. Avoid placing the dispersive electrode over the abdomen or torso.
8. If the electrodes are not self-adhesive, use rubber and Velcro straps, elastic wraps, or sandbags to secure them in place.

Termination of the Treatment

1. Most units automatically stop the current flow when the treatment time has expired. If this is not the case with your unit, or if the treatment is being terminated prematurely, gradually decrease the INTENSITY and/or depress the STOP button.
2. Remove the electrodes from the body, and wipe away any residual water or gel.
3. Check the treatment area for burns or skin irritation.
4. Interview the patient immediately following the treatment to determine the effectiveness of the parameters used. The treatment parameters and results should be noted in the patient's file. Future modifications of the treatment protocol should be indicated. Interview the patient again before the start of the next treatment.

Maintenance

Adhere to the manufacturer's required maintenance protocol. Failure to follow these recommendations may void the manufacturer's warranty.

Daily Maintenance

1. Clean the exterior housing of the unit using a mild household cleanser.
2. Keep the electrical power cord and electrode leads neatly stored.
3. Sponges used with carbon-rubber electrodes are a haven for germs. These should be regularly cleaned using an approved solution. Soaking a sponge in water and placing the container in a microwave oven for 2 minutes is also effective in killing bacteria. Replace sponges as needed.

Monthly Maintenance

1. Check lead wires for fraying, cut or torn insulation, or loose connections.
2. Check power cord and plug for fraying, kinks, or cuts.
3. Check carbon-rubber electrodes for cracks, wearing, or dulling of the electrode surface. Replace as necessary.

Annual Maintenance

The unit must be recalibrated by an authorized technician.

■ High-Voltage Pulsed Stimulation (Monophasic Current)

High-voltage pulsed stimulation (HVPS) delivers monophasic current, so the polarity of each electrode is known (Box 13-2). HVPS is a versatile form of electrical stimulation and has a wide variety of uses, including muscle reeducation, nerve stimulation, reduction of edema, and pain control.[54]

A typical HVPS generator produces a twin-peaked waveform or a train of two single pulses having a short phase duration and a long interpulse interval. The low pulse charge requires an output voltage of approximately 150 V or more to stimulate motor and sensory nerves.[3] The short phase duration allows for the activation of sensory and type II motor nerves at a low output intensity (voltage) without stimulating pain fibers.

The interpulse interval is much longer than the pulse duration. Consider a current consisting of pulses having a duration of 140 μsec and a frequency of 125 pps. In 1 second, the current is actually flowing for 0.0175 second (0.00014 × 125 = 0.0175). Because of the short total time the current is flowing, there is time for the ions attracted to each electrode to return to their original position. As a result, the amount of physiochemical reaction beneath the electrodes is limited,

---

At a Glance: High-Voltage Pulsed Stimulation

Parameters

CURRENT TYPE:	Monophasic
AMPLITUDE:	0–500 mA RMS
VOLTAGE:	0–500 V
PULSE FREQUENCY:	1–120 pps
PULSE FURATION:	13–100 μsec
PHASE FURATION:	13–100 μsec

Waveforms

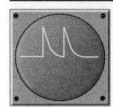 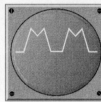 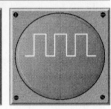

Saw tooth (1 pulse)   M-wave (2 pulses)   Square wave (3 pulses)

Output Modulation

Duty cycle
Electrode alternating rate
Electrode balance
Intensity
Polarity
Probe electrode
Surge/ramp

Treatment Duration

The typical duration of HVPS treatments is 15–30 minutes, and the treatments may be repeated as many times a day as needed.

Indications

- Reeducation of peripheral nerves
- Delay of denervation and disuse atrophy by stimulating muscle contractions
- Reduction of post-traumatic edema
- Increase in local blood circulation (unsubstantiated)
- Restoring range of motion
- Reduction of muscle spasm
- Inhibition of spasticity
- Reeducation of partially denervated muscle
- Facilitation of voluntary motor function

Precautions

- Stimulation of muscles can cause unwanted tension to be placed on the muscle fibers, the tendons, or the bony insertion.
- Muscle fatigue can rapidly develop if the duty cycle is too high.
- Improper use can cause electrode burns or irritation.
- Intense or prolonged stimulation may result in muscle spasm and/or muscle soreness.

Note: See Table 12-11 for a list of contraindications to the use of electrical modalities.

Box 13-2. WHAT'S IN A NAME? (PART I)

The term "high-voltage pulsed galvanic stimulation" is an oxymoron similar to "jumbo shrimp." The contradiction arises from the use of the terms "pulsed" and "galvanic" in describing the flow of the same current. As you will recall from the discussion on direct current flow, "galvanic" refers to "a continuous, waveless, unidirectional current."[118] Therefore, a galvanic current cannot be pulsed. The confusion stems from the constant use of this term in the literature and in manufacturers' descriptions.

and no skin significant pH changes occur under the cathode.[119] The fact that galvanic changes do not seem to occur within the tissues indicates that many of the effects attributed to polarity during HVPS may be the result of some other mechanism.

Electrode Configuration

HVPS is applied using either a monopolar or bipolar technique. Monopolar application is used when the focus of the treatment is over a wide area, such as in sensory-level pain control, and finite areas when point stimulation probes are used. A bipolar technique is often used when attempting to evoke a contraction from a specific muscle or in motor-level pain control.

● EFFECTS ON

The Injury Response Process

Neuromuscular Stimulation

The short phase duration allows a moderately high-intensity muscle contraction with relatively little patient discomfort. The strength of the contraction is less than that of neuromuscular electrical nerve stimulators or interferential stimulators.[54] Unlike muscle contractions produced by other electrical modalities, the pulse frequencies above 30 pps seem to have little effect on the maximum tension produced in a muscle being stimulated by HVPS.[32,113]

These contraction do not appear to translate into increased muscular strength. The short-term benefits derived from HVPS neuromuscular stimulation are unclear, with study results ranging from significant increases in isometric strength to significant decreases in strength relative to a nonexercising control group.[120]

The most important role for HVPS in neuromuscular stimulation is to "teach," or reeducate, a muscle how to contract after periods of immobilization or transient denervation. Other types of currents, such as biphasic or alternating, that provide for a duty cycle (as found on neuromuscular stimulators) should be used when the treatment goal is strength augmentation.

Pain Control

HVPS may be used as an adjunct treatment in controlling acute and chronic pain through both sensory-level (gate control) and/or motor-level (opiate release) stimulation. The

Treatment Strategies
Neuromuscular Stimulation Using High-Voltage Pulsed Stimulation

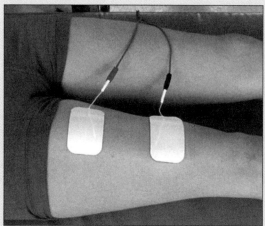

Parameter	Setting
Output intensity	Strong, intense, comfortable contractions.
Pulse frequency	If duty cycle cannot be adjusted: low for individual muscle contractions (<15 pps). If adjustable duty cycle available: tonic contractions (> 50 pps).
Polarity	Negative over primary motor point if monopolar arrangement is used. (Note that bipolar is pictured above.)
Electrode placement	**Bipolar:** Proximal and distal to the muscle (or muscle group) to be stimulated. This method offers the most direct method of stimulating specific areas. **Monopolar:** Over motor points or muscle belly.
Duty cycle	Initial treatments should begin with a low (e.g., 20%) duty cycle and be increased as the muscle responds.

These parameters are modified to meet the goals of the specific treatment regimen being used.

gate control mechanism of pain modulation is activated through the application of sensory-level currents at 100 to 150 pps. The unchanging series of pulses allows the body to accommodate to the stimulation, decreasing the effectiveness of long-term pain control techniques.[31] Because of the relative lack of portability of some high-voltage generators, HVPS is not the modality of choice for pain control treatments that require long-term stimulation.

HVPS can also stimulate the release of opiates. Although the phase duration associated with HVPS does not easily activate A-beta fibers, the high output intensity (voltage) can stimulate these fibers.[121] A monopolar electrode configuration should be used, with the active electrodes being only as large as the area being stimulated. A handheld probe is often used for this method of application (Fig. 13-1). Pain reduction can also be obtained through the brief-intense stimulation protocol.

The polarity of the active electrode (monopolar techniques) or the electrode placed over the target tissue (bipolar) influences the treatment effectiveness.[118] Acute pain is associated with an acid reaction that may be repelled by the positive pole. In the case of chronic pain, the negative pole is used for its potential liquefying and vasodilative properties.

In practicality, long-term pain relief derived from HVPS application most probably stems from the other biophysical effects described in the following sections. Swelling reduction, decreased muscle spasm, muscle reeducation, and increased blood flow assist in decreasing the mechanical and chemical factors triggering the nociceptors. These factors are usually not sufficient, however, to decrease pain caused by delayed-onset muscle soreness.[122,123]

Treatment Strategies
Pain Control Using High-Voltage Pulsed Stimulation via the Opiate Release Mechanism

Parameter	Setting
Output intensity	Motor level
Pulse frequency	2–4 pps
Polarity	Acute: positive
	Chronic: negative
Mode	Continuous
Electrode arrangement	Monopolar or bipolar
Electrode placement	Directly over painful site, distal to the spinal nerve root origin, trigger points, or acupuncture points.
Duty cycle	Continuous

These parameters are modified to meet the goals of the specific treatment regimen used.

Treatment Strategies
Pain Control Using High-Voltage Pulsed Stimulation via the Gate Control Mechanism

Parameter	Setting
Output intensity	Sensory level
Pulse frequency	60–100 pps
Mode	Continuous
Electrode arrangement	Monopolar or bipolar
Polarity	Acute: positive
	Chronic: negative
Electrode placement	Directly over the painful site

These parameters are modified to meet the goals of the specific treatment regimen used.

Treatment Strategies
Pain Control Using High-Voltage Stimulation via the Brief-Intense Protocol

Parameter	Setting
Output intensity	Noxious
Pulse frequency	>120 pps
Polarity	Acute: positive
	Chronic: negative
Mode	Continuous
Electrode arrangement	Probe (monopolar)
Electrode placement	15–60 sec at each site Gridding technique, stimulating hypersensitive areas, working distal from the painful area to proximal to it.
Duty cycle	Continuous

These parameters are modified to meet the goals of the specific treatment regimen being used.

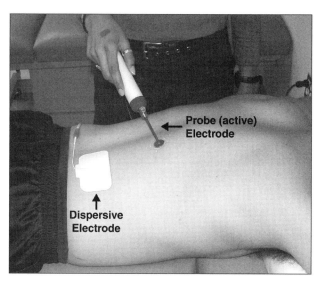

Figure 13-1. Use of an Electrode Probe With High-Voltage Pulsed Stimulation. This form of electrical stimulation is used to target stimulation points. Because of the current density under the probe, this type of stimulation is monopolar.

Control and Reduction of Edema

Motor-level stimulation is used to reduce the amount of swelling that has formed in the traumatized tissues during the subacute or chronic stages of inflammation. Sensory-level HVPS has been theorized to limit the formation of acute edema after trauma.

Sensory-Level Edema Control

In acute injuries in which HVPS is intended to prevent or limit the amount of swelling, the polarity, the time of intervention after the onset of the injury, the pulse frequency used, and the sequencing of the treatments are critical in obtaining positive treatment outcomes. The treatment parameters are configured to keep the current flowing as long as possible and to focus the cathode (negative electrode) over the target tissues.

✱ Practical Evidence

Although animal studies demonstrate the ability of cathodal HVPS to limit the formation of edema following soft tissue injury,[90,93,94,95,96] these results have not been replicated clinically on humans following lateral ankle sprains.[124,125,126]

Treatment guidelines involve cathodal stimulation applied at 10% below the motor threshold with a frequency of 120 pps using the immersion method.[91] For sensory-level edema control to be effective, the treatment must be initiated as soon as possible after injury, preferably within 6 hours.[91] To preserve the benefits associated with the recommended treatment protocol, care must be taken to limit edema formation between treatment sessions and treatment bouts. The injured limb should be elevated or a compression wrap applied to discourage fluids from leaking into the interstitial space while encouraging venous and lymphatic return.

Blood clot formation was once thought to be enhanced under the positive electrode, and the use of anodal stimulation to control acute edema has been suggested. However, this treatment approach has not been substantiated.[91,118]

High sensory-level stimulation (just below the threshold of visible muscle contractions) of HVPS significantly increases the lymphatic uptake of protein associated with edema but does not reduce limb volume.[124,127] This technique, combined with elevation, sequential compression (see Chapter 14), or muscle contractions, may assist in reducing limb volume.

Motor-Level Swelling Reduction

Chapter 1 described how muscle contractions assist in venous and lymphatic return by manually forcing ("milking") the contents of these vessels out of the extremity. Motor-level edema reduction attempts to replicate this effect by eliciting the required muscle contractions. Milking is used during the subacute or chronic stage of injury because the force of muscle contraction or the associated joint motion may either limit the effectiveness of this technique or may be contraindicated.

Treatment Strategies

Motor-Level Reduction of Edema Using High-Voltage Pulsed Stimulation via the Muscle-Milking Technique

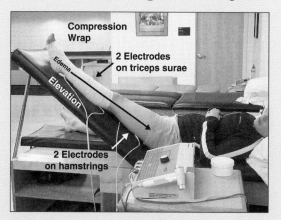

Parameter	Setting
Output intensity	Strong, yet comfortable muscle contraction. Avoid joint movement that may be contraindicated.
Electrode placement	**Bipolar:** Proximal and distal ends of the major muscle (or muscle group) proximal to the edematous area.

Continued

Parameter	Setting
	Monopolar: Active electrodes follow the course of the venous return system. If the unit has electrode alternating, place one set of electrodes on the belly of the calf and the other over the hamstrings.
Mode	Alternating preferred
Pulse frequency	Non-alternating electrodes: Low. Alternating electrodes: High
Polarity	Positive or negative.
Duty cycle	100%
Comment	Ice may be applied to the injured area, but this could impede venous return by increasing the viscosity of fluids in the area (see Chapter 5).

These parameters are modified to meet the goals of the specific treatment regimen being used.

The key to muscle milking is eliciting strong, intermittent muscle contractions. If the generator has alternating electrode output, place one set of electrodes over the calf and the other over the hamstrings. A high pulse frequency (greater than 100 pps) and sufficient output will create a tetanic contraction. As the current switches between the calf and hamstring the contractions will mimic the natural venous return mechanism. If electrode alternating is not available, a low pulse frequency is used.

In either case place the electrodes over the motor points of the major muscle groups through which the vessels course, following the path from the swollen area proximally to the torso. Elevating the limb, allowing gravity to assist in the venous return process, enhances the effectiveness of this treatment. As with all edema reduction techniques, provide the patient with home-care instruction to keep the limb elevated and wrapped between treatment sessions.

Blood Flow

It is unclear if HVPS significantly increases local blood flow. Any influence would depend on the output intensity and pulse frequency. Motor-level stimulation increases metabolism of the affected tissues, increasing their need for oxygen. If the oxygen demand exceeds the oxygen supply, the deficit is met by increasing the amount of blood delivered to the area. The number of pulses per second may also influence the increase in blood flow, although this relationship is not understood.

Isometric contractions producing muscular tension between 10 and 30% of the maximal voluntary contraction produce a slight increase in local blood flow, but at a level significantly less than that associated with voluntary contractions.[128] Increasing the output intensity is positively correlated with increased blood flow.[129] However, strong muscle contractions, joint motion, and the associated stresses placed on the involved tissues are often contraindicated.

✳ Practical Evidence

Pulse frequencies of 10, 20, and 50 pps significantly increased blood flow, although not all studies support these conclusions.[130] Pulse frequencies of 2 and 128 pps have also produced a significant increase in blood flow, but no significant increase has been demonstrated at 32 pps.[129,130]

If the treatment goal is to increase blood flow, other techniques should be considered before HVPS. Ideally, voluntary muscle contractions using therapeutic exercise should be used to meet this goal, providing that the patient is able. If not, the use of moist heat or 3-MHz ultrasound (for superficial blood flow) or 1-MHz ultrasound (deep blood flow) should be considered.

Wound Healing

The use of HVPS to facilitate wound healing stems from the results seen with the application of low-intensity direct currents (DCs). HVPS is similar to DC in that there is a positive (anode) and negative (cathode) electrode. HVPS uses short phase durations that do not cause responses equal to those of a low-intensity DC. HVPS, however, has been used to promote healing of decubitus ulcers and surgical incisions.[87]

An antimicrobial effect is obtained during HVPS application that persists after the treatment is discontinued.[87] Depending on the polarity of the treatment electrode, leukocytes, epidermal cells, and fibroblasts are attracted to the area,[83] and the level of collagenase is increased.[131] High-voltage pulsed current has also been shown to inhibit the growth of certain bacteria in infected wounds.[132] No changes in tissue pH or temperature that could affect wound healing occur during a 30-minute HVPS treatment.[87]

Negative polarity encourages blood clots to dissolve and increases the inflammatory/hemorrhagic by-products, promoting the healing of necrotic tissues.[78] Clot formation around the margin of the wound and in granulation tissue is promoted by a positive polarity.[78]

Because most of the biophysical effects of electricity on wound healing are polarity specific, the application protocol should reflect the desired outcomes of the treatment. To account for the effects of polarity during the treatment of cutaneous wounds, the application of 20 minutes of negative polarity followed by 40 minutes of positive polarity stimulation has been recommended.[133]

Instrumentation

Power: In the ON position, the current flows to the internal components of the generator.

Reset: This safety feature ensures that the voltage is reduced to zero before the treatment is started.

Timer: This control sets the duration of the treatment and subsequently displays the remaining time.

Start-stop: When this button is depressed to start the treatment, the circuit is closed, allowing the current to flow to the patient's tissues. When it is depressed again, the circuit is opened, interrupting (or pausing) the current flow.

Intensity (voltage): This knob adjusts the amplitude of the pulse from zero (OFF) to the maximal value of the unit (500 V). The applied output is displayed on the OUTPUT meter.

Pulse frequency: This parameter controls the number of pulses (or pulse trains) per second. Increasing the number of pulses per second decreases the interpulse interval and vice versa.

Low numbers of pulses per second stimulate endorphin release for pain control, moderate levels produce tetanic contractions, and the upper levels are useful in activating the gate mechanism of pain control.

Polarity: This switch determines the polarity (positive or negative) of the ACTIVE electrode or electrodes. Depending on the manufacturer of the product, the polarity may be changed during the course of the treatment without first decreasing the voltage. Other units require that the voltage be reduced before changing polarity.

Mode: When this switch is set to CONTINUOUS, the current is always flowing to each of the active electrodes. Switching to the ALTERNATING modes causes the current to be routed to only one set of active electrodes at a time. Many units also have a PROBE selection that activates the handheld electrode.

Alternating rate: This switch sets the amount of time the current is routed to each active electrode. For example, selecting an electrode alternating rate of 2.5 seconds routes the current to one set of electrodes for 2.5 seconds, then the other set for the same amount of time. This function is meaningful only when the MODE is set to ALTERNATING and two sets of active electrodes are attached to the "ACTIVE" electrode jack.

Alternating the electrodes is useful for reciprocal stimulation of agonist-antagonist muscle groups. Another use is to stimulate different muscle groups to produce a milking action to reduce edema.

Balance: During the course of a treatment, the greater sensation may be experienced under one set of active electrodes than the other. This situation may be corrected through the BALANCE adjustment. When this dial is in its midposition, an equal amount of current is routed to both sets of electrodes. If this dial is moved in one direction, toward the "B" electrodes for example, a greater amount of current flows to the "B" electrodes and less to the "A" electrodes.

The imbalance in stimulation under the electrodes can be the result of many factors. These may include improper preparation of the electrodes, the location of the electrodes, and loose connections between the electrodes and the generator or between the electrodes and the patient's body. If adjusting the BALANCE dial does not equalize the sensation, discontinue the treatment, reapply the electrodes, and start again.

Duty cycle: Not available on all HVPS units. Adjusts the ON/OFF time of current flow.

Setup and Application

Refer to manufacturer's operating instructions for the procedures specific to the unit being used.

Initiation of the Treatment

1. Turn the unit on: Activate the POWER switch.
2. Reset output parameters: Fully reduce the INTENSITY control and depress the RESET button.
3. Select output parameters: Based on the goal of the treatment, adjust the POLARITY, DURATION (width), FREQUENCY, and electrode ALTERNATING rates.
4. Set treatment duration: Indicate the duration of the treatment by adjusting the TIMER.
5. Begin treatment: Press the START button to close the circuit between the generator and the patient's tissues.
6. Increase intensity: Slowly increase the INTENSITY control until the appropriate current level is obtained.
7. Adjust electrode balance: If necessary or applicable, adjust the BALANCE control to maximize comfort.

Alternate Methods of Application

Water Immersion

HVPS may be combined with water immersion to treat irregularly shaped areas, such as the hand or foot (Fig. 13-2). In this method of application the water touching the skin serves as the active electrode. Even using a large dispersive electrode, the size of the contact area between the patient's skin and the water creates a current density equal to or less than the dispersive electrode. In many cases, the change in current density causes the treatment configuration to become bipolar.

For safety, use rubber electrodes for the immersion with the insulated (rubber-coated) side facing toward the body part. Intense stimulation would occur if the patient were to contact one of the electrodes. The dispersive electrode is placed on the closest large body mass. When treating the foot or ankle, the thigh is a logical site. The application of the current is similar to that in all other forms of HVPS. It is important to instruct the person not

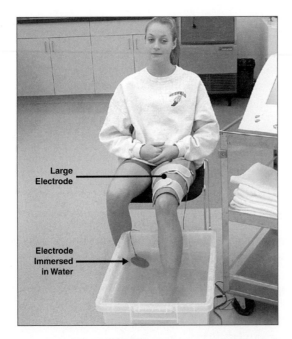

Figure 13-2. **Immersion Method of Electrical Stimulation.** The water serves as the contact point between the electrical current and the patient's skin. This method is useful when irregularly shaped areas such as the foot or hands are being treated at the sensory level.

to remove the treated body part from the water; if the intensity of the treatment is too strong, a greater proportion of the body part should be immersed or the output intensity decreased (see Current Density).

Treatment of acute injuries with water immersion raises the same concerns about edema management as ice immersion. Because the limb is placed in a gravity-dependent position, the hydrostatic pressure within the capillaries is increased and the formation of edema is encouraged rather than discouraged. After treatment, the treated limb should be wrapped and elevated to encourage venous return.

Probe

A probe electrode is used to specifically stimulate trigger points or other localized areas. The probe serves as a very small active electrode in a monopolar configuration that causes a high current density being placed on a limited group of tissues. A dispersive electrode is required to complete the circuit. A typical probe consists of a handle with a metal tip that is designed to hold a conductive medium (see Fig. 13-1).

The handle contains an INTENSITY control knob and an INTERRUPT button. The probe is activated by setting the electrode alternating switch to PROBE or by plugging the probe into a separate jack on the generator. In either case, the INTENSITY adjustment on the probe overrides the adjustment on the generator. This allows the operator to remotely adjust the intensity of the treatment. The INTERRUPT button allows the operator to open and close the circuit. When the button is depressed, the circuit is closed and the patient's tissues are stimulated.

■ Transcutaneous Electrical Nerve Stimulation (Balanced Biphasic Current)

Although all electrical modalities described in this chapter deliver their current transcutaneously, the term "transcutaneous electrical nerve stimulation" (TENS) has evolved to describe a specific electrotherapeutic approach to pain control. TENS describes the process of altering the perception of pain through the use of a biphasic electrical current (Box 13-3). Depending on the parameters used during treatment, electrical stimulation may reduce pain through activation of the gate control mechanism or centrally through the release of **endogenous opiates** ●. The primary benefit of TENS in pain control is that the treatment effects are frequency dependent. Lower pulse frequencies require more output intensity to cause the targeted nerve— based on the phase duration—to reach the depolarization threshold.[135]

The use of TENS in the treatment of pain is a spin-off of the work conducted by Melzack and Wall during their gate control pain modulation experiments (see Chapter 2).[136] This technique is effective in the management of acute or chronic musculoskeletal pain but has little effect on reducing visceral or **psychogenic** ● pain. TENS addresses only the transmission of pain, not the actual cause of the pain.

The effectiveness of TENS is as varied as its application techniques. The treatment depends on the nature of the pain, the individual's pain threshold, electrode placement, the intensity of the stimulation, and the electrical characteristics of the stimulus.[115] Traditionally, TENS units incorporate an asymmetrical biphasic pulsed current. However, some manufacturers use variants of this pulsed current including a symmetrical biphasic or monophasic waveform. When this treatment is given for extended periods, the waveform should be designed so that there is no net physiochemical effect on tissues.

● EFFECTS ON

The Injury Response Process

Pain Control

The primary purpose of TENS is to control pain by depolarizing sensory, motor, or nociceptive nerves. The patient's perception of pain is reduced by decreasing the conductivity

---

Endogenous opiates: Pain-inhibiting substances produced in the brain. These include endorphins and enkephalins.
Psychogenic: Pain of mental rather than physical origin.

At a Glance: Transcutaneous Electrical Nerve Stimulation (TENS)

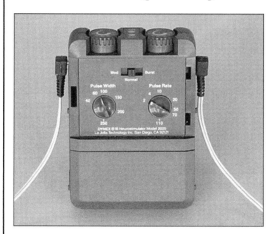

Parameters

CURRENT TYPE: Asymmetrical balanced biphasic
TOTAL CURRENT FLOW: 0–100 mA
PULSE FREQUENCY: 1–~150 pps
PHASE DURATION: 5–250 μsec
PULSE DURATION: 10–500 μsec

Waveform

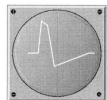

Output Modulation

Intensity — Pulse/phase duration
Mode (output modulation) — Pulse frequency

Treatment Duration

- Conventional high-frequency TENS may be used as needed, but should be used with caution when the patient is sleeping. The use of a TENS device during athletic competition has been attempted; however, because of the potential of TENS to mask pain, its use should be discouraged. An alternate approach would be to keep the electrodes affixed to the athlete and apply stimulation while the athlete is on the sideline.
- Low-frequency TENS may be given as needed in treatment bouts not exceeding 30 minutes.
- Brief-intense–type TENS application should be performed only once a day, in treatment bouts not exceeding 30 minutes.

Indications

- Control of acute or chronic pain
- Management of postsurgical pain
- Reduction of post-traumatic acute pain

Contraindications

In addition to the contraindications presented in Table 12-11:
- Pain of central origin
- Pain of unknown origin

Precautions

- Transcutaneous electrical nerve stimulation is a symptomatic treatment that can mask underlying pain and other conditions.
- Improper use can result in electrode burns or skin irritation.
- Intense or prolonged stimulation may result in muscle spasm and/or muscle soreness.
- Intake of 200 mg or more of caffeine may reduce the effectiveness of TENS.[133]
- Narcotic use decreases the effectiveness of TENS.

Box 13-3. WHAT'S IN A NAME? (Part II)

Transcutaneous electrical nerve stimulation, or TENS, is the term used to describe an electrotherapeutic modality used in pain control. In reality, each of the electrical modalities described in this chapter could be termed TENS. "Transcutaneous" means "through the skin," and "nerve stimulation" implies that the current has sufficient intensity to cause the depolarization of sensory, motor, or pain nerves. Therefore, whenever electrodes are attached to the body, an electrical current is passed through them, and the patient first reports a tingling sensation, TENS is being performed.

The names given to electrotherapeutic modalities most probably arise from, and are reinforced by, the marketing of the product. As multimodalities become more prevalent, names such as "TENS" and "HVPS" will most likely be replaced by more accurate descriptors of the current being used (e.g., low-voltage biphasic, high-voltage monophasic). Transcutaneous electrical stimulation is also sometimes used in the literature to describe any electrical stimulation procedure administered through the skin. When conducting a literature review, always check the PROCEDURES section to identify the characteristics of the electrical current being used.

and transmission of noxious impulses from the small pain fibers to the central nervous system. By affecting the large motor fibers, TENS may interfere with the normal guarding pattern of the muscle (muscle spasm), further reducing painful stimuli.[66,137] The pulse frequency and phase duration, combined with the current intensity, activate responses at different pain-modulating levels (Table 13-1).[138] The combination of output parameters, rather than a single setting, is more important in obtaining the desired outcome than any single parameter.[137]

Pain reduction associated with TENS application occurs primarily through changes in the nervous system. The number of treatments required to resolve the pain is proportional to the duration of pain: the longer the patient has been experiencing pain, the more treatments that are required.[67] Although patients are more satisfied with sensory-level TENS application than those in a sham group, over time there is no difference in the pain intensity between the two groups. In both cases, verbal suggestions that the treatment will reduce pain resulted in significantly decreased pain ratings when both actual TENS and sham TENS were applied.[67]

Neither sensory-level nor moderate motor-level TENS application significantly increases blood flow in the treated area. Indeed, evidence supports the concept that TENS application may activate the preganglionic and postganglionic neurons and produce a mild vasoconstriction.[139] Most prolonged TENS applications can modulate the activity of dorsal horn neurons secondary to stimulation of peripheral nerves and chemical stimulation of visceral organs by the release of endogenous opiates.[65] Last, pain relief obtained through the various forms of TENS application may occur through psychological factors either exclusively from, or in addition to, the neurophysiological effects.[140,141]

The patient's consumption of moderate levels of caffeine (200 mg, approximately equal to two or three cups of coffee) can decrease the effectiveness of TENS.[132] Caffeine and opioid medications compete with adenosine, a primary mediator of TENS-induced pain reduction, for its receptor sites.[142] Because caffeine binds to these sites, adenosine is prohibited from filling its receptors, causing a decreased effectiveness in TENS pain reduction. In addition to coffee, many soft drinks and over-the-counter medications (e.g., Midol™) contain significant amounts of caffeine.

Note that although the following techniques decrease the individual's perception of pain, the treatment has little effect on the underlying pathology. This modality should be

---

TABLE 13-1	Protocol for Various Methods of Transcutaneous Electrical Nerve Stimulation Application		
PARAMETER	HIGH TENS	LOW TENS	BRIEF-INTENSE TENS
Intensity	Sensory	Motor	Noxious
Pulse frequency	60–100 pps	2–4 pps	Variable
Pulse duration*	60–100 μsec	150–250 μsec	300–1000 μsec
Mode	Modulated rate	Modulated burst	Modulated amplitude
Treatment duration	As needed	30 min	15–30 min
Onset of relief	<10 min	20–40 min	<15 min
Duration of relief	Minutes to hours	Hours	<30 min

The sum of the two phases forming the pulse.

Source: Adapted from Bechtel and Fan, p 41.

used in conjunction with other therapies that attempt to treat the source of the pain.[143]

✳ Practical Evidence

Although TENS is often no more effective than sham treatments in reducing pain,[31,144] the effectiveness of TENS treatment is greatest during the first 6 weeks of use.[143] In all cases TENS should be used to increase patient compliance with therapeutic exercise programs.[145,146]

High-Frequency TENS (Sensory Level)

Conventional TENS treatment, applied with a high pulse frequency (60 to 100 pps), short pulse duration (less than 100 μsec, yielding a phase duration of approximately 50 μsec), and sensory-level intensity that stimulates A-beta fibers, activates the pain-modulating gate at the spinal cord level.[31] Painful impulses are transmitted along slow-transmitting, unmyelinated, small-diameter nerves. Nonpainful sensory information travels at a faster rate along neurons of larger diameter.

The short phase duration and high pulse frequency used with high-frequency TENS selectively target large-diameter A-beta fiber sensory nerves.[31,147,148] Activation of A-beta nerves causes presynaptic inhibition of A-delta and C fibers within the substantia gelatinosa, blocking transmission of painful impulses to the T cells. In other words, the gate is closed to pain transmission and opened to the transmission of sensory information. The result is segmental analgesia within the dermatome(s) treated.[24,31]

High-frequency, low-intensity stimulation decreases the activity of spontaneously firing nerves, decreases the activity in noxiously evoked dorsal horn neurons, and decreases nerve activity compared with the low-frequency TENS, high-intensity TENS protocol (described in the following section).[65] Patients who are seeking pain reduction subjectively prefer the high-frequency TENS protocol.[149]

The benefits of sensory-level pain control are short lived. Touch sensation returns to the pre-treatment level within 30 minutes after the TENS was discontinued, although thermal thresholds may remain elevated.[148]

Accommodation and habituation are concerns when high-frequency TENS is used for an extended time. If the stimulation parameters are kept constant, the nervous system will adapt to the unchanging stimulus. Most TENS generators have current modulation parameters designed to diminish these effects. The generator should be adjusted so that the output is modulated to decrease accommodation, with burst and frequency modulation being the most preferred by patients.[150,151] Even so, the current intensity is normally increased during the course of the treatment.

High-frequency TENS is effective in the treatment of acute soft tissue injury, but care must be taken to avoid unwanted muscle contractions. Other indications for high-frequency TENS include treatment of pain associated with musculoskeletal disorders, post-operative pain, inflammatory conditions, and myofascial pain.

Low-Frequency TENS (Motor Level)

Low-frequency TENS (low TENS) is applied with a low pulse frequency (2 to 4 pps), long phase duration (150 to 250 μsec, yielding a phase duration of approximately 75 to 125 μsec), and a strong, but nonpainful motor-level intensity in treatment bouts lasting a minimum of 45 minutes. These stimulation parameters activate small-diameter motor nerve fibers and possibly C fibers.[24] This protocol also activates A-beta fibers.

The sensory information travels along the muscle spindle's afferent nerves, which activate descending pain suppression mechanisms. Pain relief obtained through this method is thought to occur by the release of β-endorphin, which results in narcotic-like pain reduction.[140] Low-frequency TENS is sometimes referred to as "acupuncture-like TENS," but this is based on the nerves targeted rather than the stimulation of acupuncture points.[31,152]

During the treatment, the pituitary gland releases ACTH and β-lipotropin into the bloodstream. Once present, these two mediators trigger the release of β-endorphin that binds to the receptor sites of A-beta and C fibers, blocking the transmission of pain. Pain decrease is most prominent in the myotome supplied by the motor nerve(s).[24]

Some studies have concluded that there is no difference in pain reduction between sensory and motor-level TENS.[21,115] Motor-level TENS significantly increases the mechanical pain threshold relative to sensory-level TENS.[153,154] In cases where pain is the result of mechanical pressure, such as swelling, muscle spasm, or trigger points, the patient may gain more benefit from motor-level TENS.

Actual relief of pain may not be experienced for some time after the treatment has been completed, but the effects last much longer than with high-frequency TENS.[20,34,155] Suggested uses for low-frequency TENS include the treatment of chronic pain, pain caused by damage to deep tissues, myofascial pain, and pain caused by muscle spasm. Because this method of TENS application involves muscle contractions, care must be taken to avoid any joint movement that may be contraindicated.

Brief-Intense TENS (Noxious Level)

This method of TENS application is delivered at a high pulse frequency (greater than 100 pps), long pulse duration (300 to 1000 μsec, yielding a phase duration of approximately 150 to 500 μsec), and a motor-level intensity in treatment bouts lasting a few seconds to a few minutes. Pain relief is achieved by activating mechanisms in the brain stem that dampen or amplify pain impulses. Although this application protocol is sometimes referred to as noxious-level TENS, true noxious-level stimulation is not actually obtained because the limited phase duration found on TENS generators is too short to activate C fibers.

Pain relief is obtained in this TENS protocol by the formation of a negative feedback loop within the central nervous system. The intense stimulation activates ascending neural mechanisms that, on reaching the brain, make the person conscious of the pain caused by the stimulation. During the impulse's passage through the midbrain, a "short circuit" occurs, stimulating the release of endogenous opiates in the raphe nuclei. A descending pain suppression system is activated that loops efferent impulses down the spinal cord.[140] Here, the opiates inhibit the release of substance P, a neurotransmitter of noxious impulses, thus blocking the transmission of pain.[156]

A high level of analgesia is achieved through this application protocol, but the effects are more transitory than those derived from high- and low-frequency TENS. Because of the short duration of pain relief, this technique is recommended for pain reduction before rehabilitation exercises.[20]

Other Biophysical Effects of TENS

Range of motion and muscle strength may be improved secondary to pain reduction. The use of low-frequency TENS may be more effective at improving range of motion than the high-frequency TENS protocol.[112,156] During the early stages of rehabilitation, patients using TENS have demonstrated the ability to reduce the need for pain medication and a more rapid return to active exercise relative to patients not using TENS.[70]

Electrode Placement

The placement of TENS electrodes for optimal treatment has not been established, but the process is made easier if a consistent decision-making process is followed. Placement techniques are described by the electrodes' location relative to the painful area: direct placement, contiguous placement, stimulation points, dermatome placement, and placement at the level of the involved spinal nerve root (Box 13-4).[157]

High-frequency TENS most commonly uses direct, contiguous, dermatome, or nerve root–level electrode placement. Low-frequency TENS and brief-intense TENS treatments target the stimulation points. The parameters can be mixed and matched to obtain the best treatment results.

Most TENS units use four electrodes, two originating from each of two channels used. However, some units may have as few as two electrodes (one channel) or as many as eight (four channels). When two or more channels are used, electrode placement is further defined by one channel's electrode placement relative to the other possible placements.

The effects of TENS can be maximized if the nerve or nerves involved in the transmission of pain are targeted. For example, the reduction of pain associated with an injured thumb is facilitated if the radial nerve, or portions of its path, is stimulated, rather than the median or ulnar nerve.[148]

Instrumentation

Intensity: On most units there is one intensity dial for each channel. Although the intensity of each channel is individually controlled, the other current parameters (pulse duration and pulse frequency) regulate the activity in all channels.

Pulse duration: Usually labeled "PULSE WIDTH" on the unit, this adjustment should be set according to the treatment method being used. Lower durations are used for sensory-level approaches, moderate durations are used for motor-level technique, and long durations for noxious stimulation.

Pulse frequency: Also labeled "PULSE RATE," this adjustment sets the number of pulses per second used during the treatment. Increasing the pulse frequency decreases the interpulse interval.

Modulation Mode: Modes are used to alter the current in an attempt to reduce the amount of accommodation that occurs (Fig. 13-3). The various modes that are commonly selectable are:

Constant: Current flow occurs at a constant amplitude, rate, and pulse duration. This mode is best described as unmodulated, to avoid confusion with uninterrupted current. This mode is used when the treatment is not required for an extended length of time and accommodation is not a concern.

Burst modulation: In the burst mode, pulse frequencies are interrupted at regular intervals. Bursts allow "OFF" time from stimulation and assist in reducing muscle fatigue in low-frequency TENS treatments.

Frequency modulation: This setting alters, at a preset percentage, the frequency at which the stimulus is delivered. For example, if the pulse rate were adjusted to 100 pps, the unit would alternate the rate between 90 and 110 pps. Modulating the frequency has been found effective in the treatment of chronic musculoskeletal pain.[20]

Amplitude modulation: The pulse amplitude is increased and decreased by a preset percentage. Modulating the amplitude has been shown to provide short-term analgesia in the area.

Multiple modulation (random): Intensity, frequency, and pulse duration are alternately modulated in such a way that there is delivery of a steady amount of current to the body, but the body has a varying sensory perception of the treatment. This mode decreases the effects of accommodation during prolonged TENS application.

Setup and Application

Refer to manufacturer's operating instructions for the procedures specific to the unit being used.

Initiation of the Treatment

1. Adjust output parameters: Depending on the method of TENS application used (see Table 13-1), set the pulse duration (WIDTH) and pulse frequency (RATE) dials to the midrange of the recommended parameters.
2. Select the electrodes: High-frequency TENS should be applied with larger electrodes. Low-frequency TENS and brief-intense TENS should use progressively smaller electrodes.

Box 13-4. TENS ELECTRODE PLACEMENT

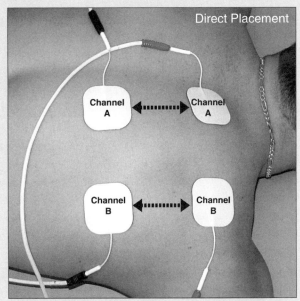

Direct Placement

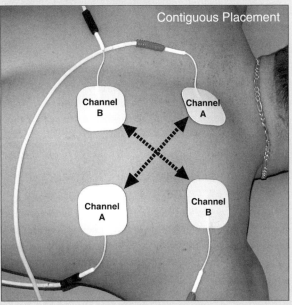

Contiguous Placement

Direct Placement

Electrodes are placed directly on the painful site. The electrical channels run parallel to each other.

Stimulation Point Placement

Motor, trigger, and/or acupuncture points are targeted (see Box 11.3). Because of the close location of these areas, a single TENS electrode may stimulate all three points at once.

Spinal Cord–Level Placement

The spinal cord nerve roots associated with the pain are targeted. The electrodes are placed between the spinous process parallel to the spinal column.

Contiguous Placement

Used when direct placement is contraindicated. Electrodes are placed around the painful tissues. Electrical channels can run parallel to each other or their currents can cross over the target tissue.

Dermatome Placement

One electrode is placed at the corresponding spinal cord nerve root and the other at the distal end of the dermatome. When pain is distributed across one or more dermatomes, place the electrodes within the affected dermatome and the contralateral dermatome.[148]

Contralateral Placement

Based on the concept of bilateral transfer, electrodes are placed on the opposite side of the body, approximating the location from which the pain is arising on the injured side.

3. Set the output mode: Select the appropriate MODE for the method and duration of the TENS application.
4. Make sure the unit is off: Make sure that the output intensity is reset to zero, and turn the unit on. Note that many TENS units have the power switch built into the intensity knobs. In this case, the intensity level of zero is equal to "OFF."
5. Increase the output intensity (channel 1): Slowly turn up the INTENSITY of channel 1. If this treatment involves sensory-level stimulation, continue increasing the intensity until a slight muscle contraction is visible, then reduce the intensity by approximately 10%. (Monitor the

patient for comfort while increasing the intensity.)
6. Increase the output intensity (channel 2): If more than one channel is used, increase the intensity of the remaining channels.
7. Balance the channels: Adjust the intensity of the channels so that an equal amount of stimulation occurs under each set of electrodes.
8. Fine-tune the output: When "fine-tuning" the treatment parameters, most manufacturers recommend first adjusting the intensity, then the pulse duration, and finally the pulse frequency.
9. Provide home-care instructions: If the patient is being sent home or to class while wearing this unit,

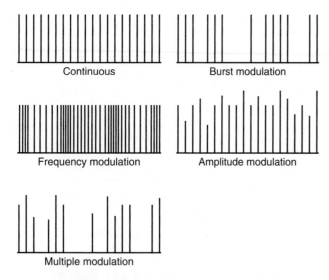

Figure 13-3. **Output Modulation.** To prevent accommodation and habituation the generator can randomly alter several output parameters.

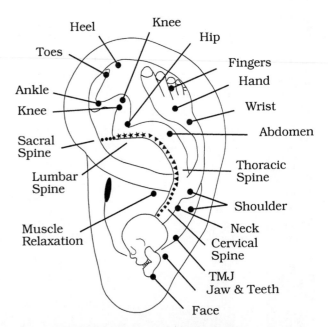

Figure 13-4. **Auriculotherapy Points.** These acupuncture points are arranged on each ear, roughly in the shape of an inverted fetus. Stimulation of these points reportedly decreases pain in the corresponding body area.

instruction should be provided on how to adjust the intensity. If indicated, provide instructions on how to disconnect the unit before taking a shower or retiring for the night, and during recharging.

Alternate Forms of Application

Point Stimulators

Devices such as the Neuroprobe™ are modified TENS devices designed to locate and stimulate trigger and acupuncture points by measuring skin resistance. Neuroprobes and galvanic stimulators are the only types of current that directly cause activation of C fibers. Point stimulators can decrease the conduction velocity of superficial nerves.[158]

Auriculotherapy

Auriculotherapy describes TENS stimulation of acupuncture points on the ear.[69,159] This method is based on the premise that an injured or diseased body reflects pain or tenderness to specific points on the ear. These points, arranged in the form of an inverted fetus, are said to represent the point at which all the acupuncture channels meet and respond to stimulation by decreasing the perception of pain in the corresponding area of the body (Fig. 13-4). Although not conclusively supported by research, this form of electrostimulation has been found effective in reducing pain caused by musculoskeletal trauma.[159]

■ Neuromuscular Electrical Stimulation (Monophasic, Biphasic, or Alternating [Premodulated] Current)

Neuromuscular electrical stimulation (NMES) is used for muscle reeducation, reduction of spasticity, delaying atrophy, and muscle strengthening. The use of electrical stimulation reverses the order in which muscle fibers are recruited into the contraction. During voluntary muscle contractions, small-diameter type I motor nerves are the first to contract. Type I fibers do not generate much force but are able to sustain the contraction for a prolonged period. Electrical stimulation causes large-diameter type II motor nerves to evoke a contraction before type I fibers. Because type II fibers are capable of producing more force, the strength of the contraction is increased.

This reversal in the order of motor nerve recruitment is a result of the relative sizes of the nerves and their depths below the surface of the skin. Electrical stimulation first causes a depolarization of large-diameter type II nerves because their cross-sectional area provides less resistance to current flow. In addition, type II motor nerves, being more superficial, receive greater stimulation than the deeper type I nerves.

The amount of muscle torque produced is directly related to the amount of current introduced into the motor nerve.[41] The strength of the contraction can be further altered through manipulation of the electrode placement. Generators for NMES use a wide range of waveforms, but the majority of the units currently on the market use a biphasic wave, but alternating currents (see Russian stimulation in the Instrumentation section) penetrate deeper into the muscle.[5]

A review of the literature indicates that no one waveform is universally "comfortable." Perceived comfort is based on individual patient preference. Symmetrical pulses tend to be less painful over a large muscle mass because there is an equal amount of stimulation under both electrodes.[49] To decrease treatment discomfort both ice and TENS have been applied at the same time as NMES. Both of these strategies were unsuccessful in increasing the patient's tolerance to the treatment.[37]

Neuromuscular stimulation is a frequency-dependent modality. The current must be strong enough to overcome the

At a Glance: **Neuromuscular Electrical Stimulation**

Parameters

CURRENT TYPE:	Biphasic or premodulated
TOTAL CURRENT FLOW:	0–200 mA
PULSE FREQUENCY:	1–200 pps
PHASE DURATION:	20–300 µsec
INTRAPULSE INTERVAL:	Appx. 100 µsec

Wave forms

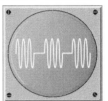

Balanced biphasic   Premodulated

Output Modulation

Intensity   Pulses per second
Duty cycle   Reciprocal rate
Ramp

Treatment Duration

Treatments used for muscular reeducation may be given daily, but as with any muscle-building program, the patient should be monitored for undue pain. Treatment to delay atrophy is given throughout the day with the use of a portable stimulator.

Indications

- Maintaining range of motion
- Prevention of joint contractures
- Increasing local blood flow
- Muscle reeducation
- Prevention of disuse atrophy
- Decreasing muscle spasm

Contraindications

In addition to the contraindications presented in Table 12-11, contraindications to the use of NMES include:
- Musculotendinous lesions, in which the tension produced by the contraction will further damage the muscle or tendon fibers
- Cases in which there is not a secure bony attachment of the muscle

Precautions

- Improper use may result in electrode burns or skin irritation.
- Intense or prolonged stimulation may result in muscle spasm and/or muscle soreness.
- An electrically induced contraction can generate too much tension within the muscle (the function of the Golgi tendon organs is overridden).

---

capacitive resistance of the tissues before the motor nerves can be stimulated. The capacitive tissue resistance is inversely proportional to the frequency of the current. Therefore, the relatively low frequencies used by NMES generators must produce a greater current to overcome this resistance.

● EFFECTS ON

The Injury Response Process

Neuromuscular Stimulation

Because of the large amplitude and long phase duration, NMES provides stronger stimulation than other forms of electrical stimulation. The increased phase duration and amperage, however, tend to result in decreased comfort. Increasing the duration of the pulses results in increased stimulation of pain nerve fibers. When the aim of the treatment session is to increase muscular strength, the output of the treatment should be as high as the patient will allow; if the aim is muscle reeducation, a mild tonic contraction for "cueing" is all that is required.[3]

NMES is capable of improving isometric muscle strength, which occurs as a result of increasing the functional stress placed on the muscle and as a result of the reversal of motor nerve recruitment.[59] NMES can produce torque equal to 90% of the maximal voluntary contraction.[42]

✳ **Practical Evidence**

Long phase durations are needed to elicit quality electrically induced muscle contractions.[50] Stronger, more comfortable treatments are obtained when the shortest phase duration required to obtain a muscle contraction at the lowest intensity is used. Increasing the output intensity will produce a stronger, more comfortable contraction than when a longer phase duration is used (thereby recruiting pain fibers as intensity is increased).[35]

Patients who reeducate muscle with NMES can significantly increase strength as opposed to patients who are not exercising. Patients using NMES applied with a 60% duty cycle demonstrated significantly higher strength gains than patients who used only isometric exercise.[160,161] After ACL reconstruction, high-intensity NMES may increase the strength of the involved quadriceps muscle to 70%, compared with 57% for voluntary contractions and 51% for low-intensity NMES.[162]

Muscle contractions obtained through NMES can increase peripheral blood flow to the treated extremity. This occurs as a result of the increased metabolic rate associated with the contractions. During treatment, blood flow increases during the first minute, whereas it reaches a steady state for the remainder of the treatment.[109] This response is independent of the stimulation intensity. Sympathetic changes in blood flow may also occur in the opposite side of the body.[163]

Table 13-2 presents several different types of benefits and effects reported to be associated with NMES and various protocols.

Swelling Reduction

NMES is similar to other forms of electrotherapy for motor-level edema reduction. The protocol described for motor-level reduction of edema using HVPS can be used with this current. Venous and lymphatic return is enhanced through the milking of these vessels by muscle contractions. Because the aim of this method is to produce individual muscle contractions, a low (1 to 10 pps) pulse frequency or a high frequency (100 or more pps) and a 50% duty cycle is used. The intensity of the current should produce a visible contraction but should not cause unwanted movement of the joint. As with other methods of edema reduction, the benefits of this treatment are enhanced if the limb is elevated.

Electrode Placement

Bipolar electrode placement is commonly employed in NMES treatments. The electrodes are placed over the proximal and distal ends of the muscle or muscle group. Because large electrodes lie over several muscles or motor points, a more generalized contraction is obtained. The use of small electrodes will elicit a more specific contraction by directly stimulating a muscle's motor point. As the electrodes are brought closer together, the effect of the stimulation becomes more superficial, and the relative intensity of the contraction decreases.

Quadripolar application requires the use of two separate channels, with each channel having at least two electrodes. This method of application is used when stimulating agonist-antagonist muscle groups.

A monopolar technique may be employed through the use of one small and one large electrode or through the use of a handheld applicator. This method of electrode placement is useful when a specific muscle, or a small muscle group, is the target of the treatment.

The size of the electrodes should be only as large as is required to stimulate the desired tissues. Electrodes that are too small result in a very high current density, whereas electrodes that are larger than needed may stimulate unwanted nerves.

Instrumentation

Power: When this switch is in its ON position, the current is allowed to flow to the internal components of the generator.

TABLE 13-2   **Effects Associated With Neuromuscular Electrical Stimulation**

Electrically induced isometric quadriceps contractions can significantly increase strength in certain joint positions:
- Knee joint positions ranged from 30°–90° of flexion.
- The amount of hip flexion can influence the strength of the contractions, possibly secondary to providing the muscle group with a mechanical advantage.
- Strength gains summarized ranged from 7%–48%.
- Electrical stimulation can increase isokinetic strength at certain speeds.
- Speeds of 65° per second showed the most substantial increases.
- No significant strength increases have been reported at speeds greater than 120° per second.
- No statistically significant strength increases have been demonstrated to occur between strength gains obtained via ES, voluntary contractions, and a combination of ES and voluntary contractions.
- Most of the literature reviewed indicated greater strength gains in voluntary contractions than in electrically induced contractions.
- Although the differences in strength gains obtained from voluntary contractions compared with those obtained from ES were not statistically significant, the results may be clinically significant. Strength increases obtained from ES were on average 10% greater than those derived from voluntary contractions.

Reset: This safety feature ensures that the output is reduced to zero before the treatment is started.

Timer: This control sets the duration of the treatment and subsequently displays the remaining time.

Intensity: This knob adjusts the amplitude of the pulses.

Pulse rate: This parameter determines the type of muscle contraction to be elicited. Depending on the muscle or muscle group being stimulated, a pulse rate of less than 15 pps causes a distinct contraction for each impulse. Between 15 and 25 pps, the muscle begins to contract smoothly, eventually leading to a tonic contraction at approximately 35 to 50 pps.

Mode: This switch allows the user to select the type of waveform used in the treatment.

Duty cycle: This feature allows the user to set the duty cycle for the treatment. Neuromuscular stimulation units have separate dials to adjust independently the number of seconds that the current is flowing and the number of seconds it is not. Other units have preset duty cycles that the user cannot alter. A CONSTANT mode (100% duty cycle) may be provided. This is useful for adjusting the other treatment parameters (intensity, pulse duration, etc.) without waiting for the duty cycle to switch to its ON mode.

External trigger: A handheld device that allows the user to manually control the ON-OFF time of the stimulation. When the trigger is depressed, current is allowed to flow to the tissues.

Reciprocal rate: When two channels are being used, this feature selects the duration of time that the current is flowing to each channel.

Ramp: The RAMP parameter allows the user to determine the amplitude rise time until the peak current is obtained. Often the RAMP represents the percentage of the ON duty cycle time required to reach the maximum intensity. For example, a 20% RAMP with an ON duty cycle time of 5 seconds would require 1 second to reach the maximum intensity.

Interrupt switch: This device is held by the patient and is used to terminate the treatment if the intensity becomes too great or too painful.

Setup and Application

Refer to manufacturer's operating instructions for the procedures specific to the unit being used.

Initiation of the Treatment
1. Prepare the generator: Reduce the output intensity to zero and turn the unit on. If applicable, press the **RESET** button.
2. Prepare electrodes: Connect the leads to the unit and to the electrodes and secure the electrodes to the patient.

3. Make the interrupt switch available: Give the patient the INTERRUPT SWITCH and provide instruction on its purpose and use.
4. Set pulse variables: Set the phase duration (WIDTH) and pulse frequency (RATE) to the midrange of the parameters to be used.
5. Set current variables: If the RAMP and ON-OFF parameters are manually adjustable on the unit, increase the RAMP to a rapid rise and adjust the ON-OFF controls to a 100% duty cycle. This configuration allows the INTENSITY to be increased without waiting for the generator to run through its duty cycle. If these parameters cannot be changed during the course of the treatment, adjust them to the desired settings now. (Certain generators may be designed to allow the intensity to be increased without adjusting these parameters.)
6. Adjust frequency: Adjust the output FREQUENCY to the appropriate level for this treatment (see step 11 below).
7. Set treatment duration: Set the TIMER for this session.
8. Initiate treatment: Press the START button to activate the unit.
9. Increase intensity: Begin the treatment by slowly increasing the INTENSITY until the desired tension is developed in the muscle.
10. Adjust ramp for treatment goals: If applicable, reset the RAMP time to match the treatment goals and patient needs.
11. Adjust the DUTY CYCLE to match the treatment goals: The following protocol may be used as an example: 127.
12. Muscle strengthening: ON = 10 seconds, OFF = 50 seconds.
13. Muscle endurance: ON and OFF have approximately equal durations (4 to 15 seconds). FREQUENCY equals 50 to 200 Hz.

▮ Interferential Stimulation (Alternating Currents)

Interferential stimulation (IFS) units generate two ACs on two separate channels. One channel produces a constant high-frequency sine wave (4000 to 5000 Hz), and the other channel produces a sine wave with a variable frequency. The two currents meet in the body to produce an interference wave having a frequency of 1 to 299 Hz. The medium-frequency carrier currents penetrate the tissues with very little resistance. The resulting interference currents are in a range that allows effective stimulation of deeper tissues than other forms of electrical stimulation with relatively little patient discomfort.[31,164]

Interferential generators combine constructive and destructive interference patterns to form a continuous interference pattern (Box 13-5). These circuits are superimposed in the tissues using a quadripolar technique, two independent electrical currents. **Premodulated currents**

At a Glance: **Interferential Stimulation**

Parameters

CURRENT TYPE:	Two alternating currents forming a single interference current. Premodulated output is based on a single alternating current.
CURRENT FLOW (AMPLITUDE):	1–100 mA
CURRENT FLOW (RMS):	0–50 mA
VOLTAGE:	0 to 200 V
CARRIER FREQUENCY:	Fixed at: 2500 to 5000 Hz
BEAT FREQUENCY:	0–299 Hz
SWEEP FREQUENCY:	10–500 μsec

Waveform

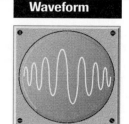

Output Modulation

Beat frequency—Analogous to the number of cycles or pulses per second
Burst duty cycle—Bursts separated by periods of no stimulation (interburst interval)
Intensity
Interburst interval—Duration of time between bursts
Premodulation (e.g., Russian stimulation)
Ramp
Sweep—Variation in the beat frequency; set with a low value and a high value
Vector/Scan—Variation in current intensity

Treatment Duration

■ Interferential stimulation may be applied once or twice daily in treatment bouts normally ranging from 15 to 30 minutes.
■ Premodulated neuromuscular stimulation bouts are normally applied three times a week in 30-minute bouts (see Neuromuscular electrical stimulation).

Indications

■ Acute pain
■ Chronic pain
■ Muscle spasm

Contraindications

In addition to the contraindications presented in Table 12-11, the use of INF is contraindicated in:
■ Pain of central origin
■ Pain of unknown origin

Precautions

■ Improper use can result in electrode burns or skin irritation.
■ Intense or prolonged stimulation may result in muscle spasm and/or muscle soreness.

are mixed within the generator and use a single channel (bipolar technique).[135,165]

The rate at which the interference waveform changes its amplitude is the **beat pattern,** the difference in frequency between the two circuits.[31] One channel has a fixed frequency (e.g., 5000 Hz), and the second channel has a variable frequency. By selecting a beat frequency of 1 Hz, the second channel produces a current with a frequency of 5001 Hz. Selecting a beat frequency of 100 Hz increases the frequency of the second channel to 5100 Hz. The beat produced by IFS elicits responses similar to the waveforms produced by TENS units but is capable of delivering a greater total current to the tissues (70 to 100 mA).[166]

Capacitive skin resistance is inversely proportional to the frequency of the current. An AC of 50 Hz encounters approximately 3000 ohms of resistance per 100 cm² of skin. Increasing the frequency to 4000 Hz reduces capacitive skin resistance to approximately 40 ohms.

Box 13-5. ELECTRICAL INTERFERENCE

Constructive Interference

When two electrical currents are in perfect phase—that is, the wavelengths are equal and the phases cross the baseline at the same point—the amplitude of the combined wave is equal to the sum of its two parts.

Destructive Interference

Two currents are perfectly out of phase. The positive peak of the first waveform occurs at the same point on the horizontal baseline as the negative peak of the second wave. When these two waves meet, the amplitudes cancel each other out, resulting in a wave intensity of zero.

Continuous Interference

When two currents have slightly different frequencies (e.g., plus or minus 1 Hz), the resulting wave alternates between constructive and destructive interference.

Consequently, IFS encounters less skin resistance than other low-frequency forms of stimulation. Inside the tissues, the interference between the two waves reduces the frequency to a level that has biological effects on the tissues.

● EFFECTS ON

The Injury Response Process

Interferential stimulation has been used to control pain and elicit muscle contractions to increase venous return. A variation of IFS, with a superimposed duty cycle, is used to reeducate muscle and to increase muscular strength.

Pain Control

Mechanisms of pain control are similar to those found with TENS. High beat frequencies, about 100 Hz, when accompanied by sensory-level stimulation, activate the spinal gate, inhibiting the transmission of noxious impulses. Low beat frequencies of 2 to 10 Hz, applied at the motor level, should initiate the release of opiates and result in a narcotic-like pain reduction. Although both high- and low-frequency IFS result in decreased pain perception, the mechanism is probably associated with the gate mechanism or occurs secondary to the placebo effect. Serum cortisol levels, an important marker associated with the release of β-endorphin, are not increased following treatment.[64]

Stimulation of acupuncture points with a frequency of 2 Hz or 100 Hz results in pain mediation at specific receptor sites. A 30-Hz frequency affects the widest range of receptors, but the amount of pain reduction is less.[167]

Treatment Strategies
Pain Control via Gate Mechanism Using Interferential Stimulation

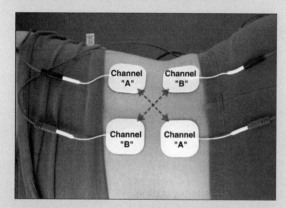

Parameter	Setting
Carrier frequency	Based on patient comfort
Burst frequency	80 to 150 Hz
Sweep	Fast
Electrode arrangement	Quadripolar
Electrode placement	Place around the periphery of the target area
Output intensity	Strong sensory level
Treatment duration	20 to 30 minutes

Treatment Strategies
Pain Control via Opiate Release Using Interferential Stimulation

Parameter	Setting
Carrier frequency	Based on patient comfort
Burst frequency	1–10 Hz (endorphins)
	80–120 Hz (enkephalin)

Parameter	Setting
Sweep	Slow
Electrode arrangement	Quadripolar
Electrode placement	Place around the periphery of the target area
Output intensity	Moderate to strong sensory level
Treatment duration	20–30 minutes

Neuromuscular Stimulation
Medium beat frequencies of approximately 15 Hz may be used to reduce edema. Venous and lymphatic return can be increased by motor-level stimulation. The IFS does not appear to significantly increase blood flow in the injured area.[108]

Treatment Strategies
Motor-Level Stimulation Using a Premodulated Current

Parameter	Setting
Carrier frequency	2500 Hz
Burst frequency	30–60 bursts per second
Burst duty cycle	10%
Cycle duration	400 μsec
On/off duty cycle	10:50 sec
Ramp	2 sec
Electrode placement	Bipolar: Proximal and distal ends of the muscle (or muscle group)
Output intensity	Strong muscle contraction. Discomfort (as opposed to pain) may be experienced.
Treatment duration	10 cycles or until fatigue occurs

Premodulated Currents
A premodulated current is the result of alternating currents being mixed within the generator (rather than the body), producing a sine or biphasic square wave with varying amplitude.[31,135,168] The output is interrupted to produce 1 to 100 bursts per second that are capable of producing strong muscle contractions with relatively little discomfort, although it is difficult to balance the parameters required to produce a strong muscle contraction and those that produce

pain.[44,168] Premodulated currents use two electrodes on a single channel and are indicated when the use of four electrodes is impractical because of the size of the treatment area (e.g., the vastus medialis oblique).

Long interburst intervals reduce the root mean square amperage of the applied current but allow for increased intensity per burst, increasing the intensity of the contraction. The interburst interval is not long enough to allow for muscle relaxation but improves the comfort of the current.[44,168] Russian stimulation is one of the most well-known premodulated currents (Box 13-6).

Edema Reduction

Chronic post-traumatic edema can be reduced by the use of IFS.[170] This effect is attributable to milking of the venous and lymphatic return systems through electrically evoked muscle contractions. Avoid unwanted joint motion that could produce further injury of the involved structures.

✱ Practical Evidence

With both true IFS and premodulated alternating current, the appropriate carrier frequency depends on the treatment goal. Maximum treatment benefits are obtained when a high carrier frequency is used for sensory-level treatments and low carrier frequencies for motor-level treatments. The patient's comfort is also influenced by the electrode size.[171]

Electrode Placement

True IFS requires the use of a quadripolar electrode arrangement. Premodulated output may use either bipolar or quadripolar arrangements. When an alternating current is used the electrodes should be no more than 5.9 inches (15 cm) apart.[5]

Box 13-6. "RUSSIAN" STIMULATION

After the 1972 Summer Olympics, much attention was given to an electrical strength-training regimen used by Russian athletes. A Soviet physician, Dr. Yakov Kots, reported that athletes training under this technique demonstrated a 30–40% strength improvement over those training with isometric exercise alone. Other reported benefits of this technique included increased muscular endurance and changes in the velocity of muscular contractions. These results, owing in part to Dr. Kots's failure to specify the parameters used by these athletes, have never been duplicated in the United States.[3,41,45,46,53,59,169,170] This method of application has gained the name "Russian" stimulation based on its country of origin.

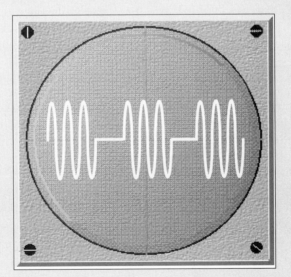

Classic Russian stimulation involves the use of a 2500-Hz carrier sine wave with burst modulation. The theory behind Russian stimulation, as with IFS, is that the higher frequencies would decrease the amount of capacitive skin resistance and allow more current to reach the motor nerve at lower intensities.[3] The 2500-Hz carrier frequency is also thought to "block" superficial sensory nerves while stimulating deeper motor fibers.[5,44] Although the strength-gain benefits have not been duplicated, this form of electrical stimulation is an excellent method to decrease muscular atrophy.

Quadripolar Technique

The four electrodes are positioned around the painful area so that each channel runs perpendicular to the other and the current crosses at the midpoint (Fig. 13-5). The interference effects branch off at 45-degree angles from the center of the treatment, in the shape of a four-leaf clover. Tissues within this area receive the maximal treatment effect; however, the distribution of the current is inconsistent, potentially leading to discomfort and decreased treatment effecitveness.[135] When the electrodes are properly positioned, the stimulation should be felt only between the electrodes, not under the electrodes.

Referring to Figure 13-5, notice that the interference effect covers only part of the area between the electrodes. If the patient has a very discrete area of pain, the interference pattern should be able to encompass the appropriate tissues. However, in cases in which the pain is diffuse, maximal pain reduction may not occur. This problem can be reduced through rotating the interference effect area. By slightly unbalancing the currents, the interference pattern "rotates" or "scans" 45 degrees back and forth between the electrodes, resulting in treatment of a larger area (Fig. 13-6).

✳ Practical Evidence

Avoid using small electrodes with interferential and premodulated currents. The high current density combined with the high power (amplitude) of the current may increase the risk of electrical burns of the skin. This risk may be increased if cold packs are applied concurrently.[172,173]

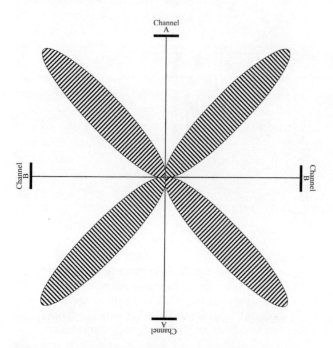

Figure 13-5. **Interference Pattern.** Maximal benefit from interferential stimulation occurs at 45-degree angles from the intersection of the channels.

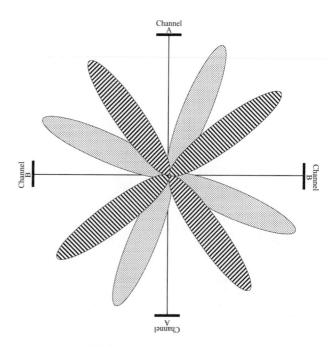

Figure 13-6. **Dynamic Interference Vectoring.** The normal vector pattern is rotated throughout the treatment to stimulate a broader tissue area.

Bipolar Electrode Placement

When IFS is applied using a bipolar technique, the mixing of the two channels occurs within the generator rather than in the tissues. Two channels are used within the generator, with a single output channel applied to the tissues. Although bipolar IFS does not penetrate the tissues as deeply as quadripolar application, the result is a more precise mixing and distribution of the current.[135]

When muscle contractions are the goal of the treatment session, either through IFS or Russian stimulation, bipolar electrode placements are used. When the effects are targeted for one specific muscle or muscle group, only one channel is used. Four electrodes are incorporated into a dual channel, agonist-antagonist treatment regimen.

Instrumentation

Power: When the switch is in its ON position, the current is allowed to flow to the internal components of the generator.

Reset: This safety feature ensures that the intensity is reduced to zero before the treatment is started.

Timer: This control sets the duration of the treatment and subsequently displays the remaining time. On some units, the TIMER serves as the master power switch.

Start-stop: This switch is used to initiate and terminate the treatment.

Intensity: This control adjusts the amplitude of the pulse and is displayed in milliamperes (mA). When quadripolar stimulation is used, the intensity control regulates both channels simultaneously or each channel may be individually adjustable.

Mode: This switch allows the user to choose between true interferential therapy and bipolar stimulation. The interferential mode allows the current to stimulate deep tissue. In the bipolar mode, only one channel is used, and the resultant current flow stimulates relatively subcutaneous nerves.

Premodulated/Russian stimulation: This mode changes the output from amplitude-modulated to burst-modulated for evoking strong muscle contractions. This technique may use one or both channels. This is an option on many IFS units, and other units provide Russian stimulation as well.

Beat frequency: The "beat" is the result of the fixed rate of the carrier wave and the variable rate of the second channel causing changes in the amplitude of the applied current.

On-off control (duty cycle): When Russian-type stimulation has been selected from the MODE control, this adjusts the duty cycle by determining the amount of time the current is ON versus OFF.

Ramp: Allows the user to determine the amplitude rise time until the peak current is obtained. Often the RAMP represents the percentage of the ON duty cycle time required to reach the maximum intensity.

Balance: This dial allows the user to control the balance of electrical current under each set of electrodes and to equalize the sensory stimulation. It may only be meaningful during quadripolar stimulation.

Setup and Application

Refer to manufacturer's operating instructions for the procedures specific to the unit being used.

Initiation of the Treatment
1. Turn on the unit by activating the POWER switch.
2. Reset parameters: Fully reduce the INTENSITY control and depress the RESET button.
3. Select application mode: Determine the MODE of application: quadripolar, bipolar, or Russian stimulation.
4. Adjust beat frequency: Select the appropriate BEAT frequencies based on the goals of the treatment.
5. Adjust sweep frequency: Use the appropriate SWEEP frequency for this treatment protocol.
6. Adjust treatment duration: Set the duration of the treatment by adjusting the TIMER.
7. Begin treatment: Press the START button to close the circuit between the generator and the patient's tissues.
8. Increase output intensity: Slowly increase the INTENSITY control until the appropriate current level is obtained.
9. Adjust balance: If necessary, adjust the BALANCE control to obtain maximal treatment comfort.

■ Iontophoresis (Direct Current)

Iontophoresis is the introduction of ionized medications into the subcutaneous tissues using a low-voltage DC. The amount of medication entering the tissues is based on the current density and the duration of the treatment. By adapting to fluctuations in tissue resistance, iontophoresis generators (iontophoresors) produce a constant voltage output by adjusting the amperage. The medication types most commonly used for iontophoresis include anesthetics, analgesics, and anti-inflammatory agents. Experimental work has begun that explores the use of iontophoresis as a substitute for certain types of **dialysis** ● and repeated injections, such as insulin.

Based on the ionic reaction between the positive and negative poles of the generator, ionized medication molecules travel along the lines of force created by the current. At the positive electrode, positive ions are driven through the skin; negative ions are introduced through the skin using the negative pole. Iontophoresis has been shown to deliver the medication to depths of 6 to 20 mm below the skin.[175,176]

Iontophoresis requires the use of custom electrodes that are designed to store medication or a buffer. Electrode sizes are expressed by the amount of medication required to saturate them. For instance, a 3.0-mL electrode will hold 3 mL of medication.

The transdermal introduction of medication has advantages over oral ingestion or injection of medication. An advantage over oral medication includes bypassing the liver, thus reducing the metabolic breakdown of the medication. The medication can also be concentrated in a localized area rather than be absorbed in the gastrointestinal tract, providing local rather than systemic delivery of the drug.[174] Most of these advantages also hold true with injected medication, but iontophoresis is less traumatic and less painful than injected medication. In addition, the injection of medication can result in a high concentration of medication in a localized area, resulting in tissue damage.[175,176]

Iontophoresis also has its disadvantages. Unreliable results are obtained with certain medications, and the amount of medication that is actually introduced into the tissues is unknown.[33] Areas of thick skin, such as the plantar aspect

---

Dialysis: The process performed by an external device that is used to assist or replace the kidney's function of filtering blood.

At a Glance: **Iontophoresis**

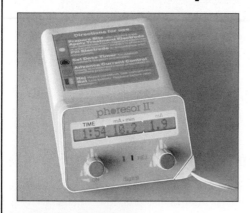

Parameters

CURRENT TYPE:	Direct current
TOTAL CURRENT FLOW:	Up to 5 mA
VOLTAGE:	80 V
PULSE FREQUENCY:	Not applicable
PULSE DURATION:	Not applicable
PHASE DURATION:	Not applicable
DOSAGE:	0–80 mA/min

Waveform

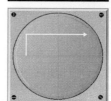

Output Modulation

Amperage
Dosage
Duration
Polarity (medication delivery electrode)

Treatment Duration

The duration of an individual treatment is based on the intensity of the treatment and the desired treatment dose (see Medication Dosage). Treatments are usually given every other day for up to 3 weeks. Consult the patient's prescription for the exact treatment regimen.

Indications

- Acute inflammation
- Chronic inflammation
- Arthritis
- Myositis ossificans
- Myofascial pain syndromes
- As a vehicle for delivering local anesthetics before injection or other minor invasive procedures[174]
- Hyperhidrosis

Contraindications

In addition to the contraindications presented in Table 12-11, iontophoresis should not be used when:
- The patient has a history of adverse reactions or hypersensitivity to electrical stimulation
- The patient has contraindications to the medication(s) being administered
- Pain or other symptoms of unknown origin are present

Precautions

- Controlled medications require a physician's prescription. Pay close attention to any notes or instructions provided by the pharmacist. State practice acts may further regulate the delivery of iontophoresis.
- The exact dosage of the medication delivered to the body is unknown.
- Erythema under the electrodes is common after the treatment.
- A treatment dose that is too intense (in amperage or duration) can result in burns beneath the delivery and/or return electrode.
- Do not reuse an electrode because medications remain in it, contaminating it for future use.

of the foot, are more difficult to penetrate than thinner skin. Deep structures such as the hip joint are located too deeply to be affected by iontophoresis.

In children, the anxiety caused by iontophoresis was not significantly less than that of an injection. Injections appear to be more tolerable over time. Also, cutaneous anesthesia derived from an injection is more tolerable than that obtained through iontophoresis.[178]

Many of the medications used during iontophoresis are controlled substances requiring a physician's prescription. The use of the iontophoresor may also be regulated by state practice acts.

Iontophoresis Mechanisms

Traditional iontophoresors deliver a low-voltage, high-amperage DC to the body. The generator's output ranges from 0 to 5 mA at skin impedances ranging from 500 ohms to 100 kilohms.

As we saw in the Phonophoresis section of Chapter 7, the stratum corneum is the primary barrier to the transfer of substances across the skin into the subcutaneous tissues. The electrical charge of the medication helps complete the circuit by carrying the current between the two electrodes. During iontophoresis, the primary path for current flow, and hence medication transfer, occurs through portals formed by hair follicles and skin pores.[1,61] Transfer occurs by an electromotive force, an electro-osmotic force, or a combination of both.[179]

For iontophoresis to occur, the applied current must be sufficient to overcome the skin/electrode resistance and still have enough energy to drive the medication through the skin's portals (typically an atomic weight less that 500 Da).[179,180,181] As the treatment progresses, the portals' resistance to electrical current flow and medication entry into the body decreases.[182] Once it is within the tissues, the medication is locally spread through passive diffusion that is not affected by the current source. The rate of this diffusion is such that the medication tends to remain more highly concentrated within those tissues directly subcutaneous to the introduction site and progressively less concentrated in the deeper tissues and in tissues peripheral to the treatment site.[183]

Iontophoresis uses a monopolar electrode arrangement in which the electrode containing the medication serves as the active electrode. The increased current density under the delivery electrode also decreases the resistance to the iontophoretic current; the higher the current density, the less resistance there is to electrical flow.[184] Although this trait seems to contradict Ohm's law, the decreased resistance is an artifact of an increase in the size of the skin pores or the creation of new ones.[185,186]

Local blood flow is increased for 1 hour after the treatment, and the stratum corneum is hydrated for 30 minutes after treatment. Although this assists in the subcutaneous diffusion of the medication, it may result in a wider-than-normal diffusion, spreading the medication systemically and lowering its concentration in the intended treatment area. The increased blood flow may also explain the **hyperemia** • after the treatment.[187]

Burns or severe skin irritation are problems inherent to the application of a DC on the human body. Either of these negative reactions is related to the hydrogen and hydroxide ions generated by the current. Experimental work using a low-frequency AC or a combination of ACs and DCs has been shown to be effective in delivering certain forms of medication to the body without the associated skin irritation.[188,189]

Medication Dosage

The medication dosage is measured in terms of milliamperes per minute (mA/min) and is based on the relationship between the amperage of the current and the treatment duration:

$$\text{Current amperage (mA)} \times \text{Treatment duration (min)} = \text{mA} \bullet \text{min}$$

Most iontophoresors use a dose-oriented treatment protocol where the user indicates the desired treatment dose and the generator calculates the duration and intensity of the treatment. A subsequent change in the output alters the treatment duration; increasing the amperage decreases duration and vice versa. If the treatment duration were shortened, the output intensity would be increased.

For example, if a medication were being used that was prescribed at a dose of 50 mA/min, the generator may default to an output of 5 mA and a treatment duration of 10 minutes (5 mA × 10 minutes = 50 mA/min). If this is the patient's first exposure to iontophoresis or if the patient has a history of sensitivity to this treatment, the intensity of the treatment would be decreased. Suppose the intensity was decreased to 3 mA. The generator would then recalculate the treatment duration to approximately 16 minutes and 40 seconds (3 mA × 16.67 minutes = 50 mA/min).

Immediately reduce the amperage when the patient reports any sensation other than tingling (e.g., reports of burning). The maximum treatment dosage depends on the polarity of the medication delivery electrode. Negative polarity can deliver up to an 80 mA/min dose; positive polarity can deliver up to a 40 mA/min dose.

The dose-oriented approach has led to the development of low-intensity, long-duration treatment in which the patient wears the patch for up to 24 hours (Fig. 13-7). Using a self-contained battery delivering 1 volt of charge, the patient wears the patch for 12 hours to deliver a dose equivalent to 40 mA/min and 24 hours to deliver a dose equivalent to 80 mA/min.

Hyperemia: A red discoloration of the skin caused by increased blood flow. The skin turns white when pressure is applied.

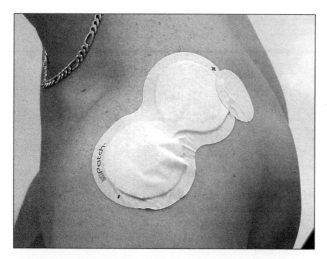

Figure 13-7. IontoPatch Extended Time-Release Iontophoresis System. This treatment is being applied for inflammation of the acromioclavicular joint. Note the "−" symbol on the lower left of the patch and the "+" symbol in the upper right. In this case, the medication was negatively charged, so it was loaded in the negative electrode. A buffering solution is loaded in the positive electrode to complete the circuit. The small round patch just next to the "+" symbol helps hold the electrode down should it begin to peel away. (IontoPatch courtesy of Birch Point Medical, Oakdale, MN.)

Medications

The type of medication used during iontophoresis depends on the nature of the pathology and the desired treatment outcome. Table 13-3 presents some common medications used during this treatment, indications for use, and typical treatment dosages. This information should not be viewed as recommended treatment protocols. Refer to the physician's

or pharmacist's recommended concentrations and treatment doses.

For the application of iontophoresis, water-soluble medications are dissolved in a carrier. The amount and rate of medication delivery are based on the total voltage applied, the duration of the treatment, the local pH, and the concentration of the medication in the delivery electrode. As the magnitude of each of these factors increases, the total dosage of the treatment increases. Increased concentrations (percentage) of the medication have the potential to clog the pores and decrease the delivery of the medications to the underlying tissues.[190] A vasoconstrictor such as epinephrine may be added to the medication to help maintain local concentration in the tissues.[179]

Certain reactions occur that complicate the delivery of medication into the tissues. The medication competes with other ions having the same polarity as the delivery electrodes. There is an equal chance that the medication ions will be driven into the tissues as other ions having the same molecular weight and size. Medications of larger ionic weight and mass require an increased output intensity to drive them through the tissues. Because of the amount of work (energy) required, smaller ions tend to be preferentially moved relative to larger ones.

Passive iontophoresis also alters the amount, rate, and quality of the phoresis. Recall that ions that have unlike charges attract each other. As a charged ion enters the tissues, it tends to "pull" ions having the opposite charge. Consider a negatively charged ion being pushed into the skin by the negative charge of the electrode. A nearby positively charged ion may be within the negative ion's field of attraction. The positively charged ion is pulled along with the negative ion as it enters the tissue.

TABLE 13-3   Sample Medications, Their Indications, and Treatment Dosages Used During Iontophoresis*†

MEDICATION(S)	PATHOLOGY	DELIVERY CONCENTRATION	DOSAGE	POLARITY
Acetic acid	Heterotopic ossification	2% mixed with distilled water	80 mA/min	Negative
Dexamethasone and lidocaine	Inflammation	4 mg Decadron (1 cm² suspension)	41 mA/min	Negative
	Pain control	4% Xylocaine (2 cm² suspension)	40 mA/min	Positive
Lidocaine and epinephrine	Pain control	4% Lidocaine 0.01 mL 1:50,000 epinephrine	30 mA/min	Positive
Lidocaine and epinephrine	Pain control	4% Lidocaine and 0.25 cc of 1:1000 epinephrine	20 mA/min	Positive
Dexamethasone	Inflammation	2 cc 4 mg/mL dexamethasone	41 mA/min	Negative

Refer to the physician's prescription for exact treatment parameters.
†Each size electrode has a maximum amperage that should not be exceeded. Consult the packaging information included with the electrodes.

Different types of medications may be mixed together so long as their ionic charges do cancel each other out or significantly weaken. To achieve equal doses of one medication of a relatively large molecular size and weight and another one of smaller mass, the concentration of the larger, less mobile medication must be increased.[183]

● BIOPHYSICAL EFFECTS OF IONTOPHORESIS

The exact biophysical effects obtained from the treatment depend on the type of medication used. Medications introduced into the body through iontophoresis can penetrate 6 to 20 mm below the skin and in most instances can reach the depth of tendinous structures and underlying cartilage. However, the exact dose of the medication reaching this depth is undetermined.[33,175,176,191]

When an anti-inflammatory or anesthetic mixture is used (e.g., dexamethasone [Decadron] and lidocaine [Xylocaine]), the onset of relief may take 24 to 48 hours, although immediate relief is sometimes reported. The latent effects may be attributed to a cumulative effect of the treatments.[33] Lidocaine, in concentrations of up to 50%, requires a minimum of 10 minutes of electrical current before the skin is anesthetized.[192] Superficial anesthesia can be achieved using iontophoresis, but the lack of depth of penetration prevents a total nerve block from being obtained.

The use of a direct current can potentially alter the pH of skin. However, changes in skin pH do not occur unless the treatment dosage exceeds 80 mA/min (beyond the range of normal dosage).[193]

Electrode Placement

The delivery of iontophoresis involves the use of a delivery electrode ("drug electrode") that serves as the active electrode and a return electrode that serves as the dispersive electrode (Fig. 13-8). Many application procedures use only one delivery electrode, but most units allow two to be used. The delivery electrode is placed over the target tissues. The return electrode is placed 4 to 6 inches away. When placing each electrode on the body, care should be taken to consider the underlying tissues. For example, if iontophoresis is being used to treat plantar fasciitis, the delivery electrode should be placed on the medial aspect of the arch, where the skin is relatively thin, rather than over the thick padding provided under the heel.

Instrumentation

Power: The POWER switch activates or deactivates the generator.

Reset: The RESET switch serves as an "emergency shutoff" in case of patient discomfort or a malfunction within the generator. At the conclusion of the treatment, pressing the

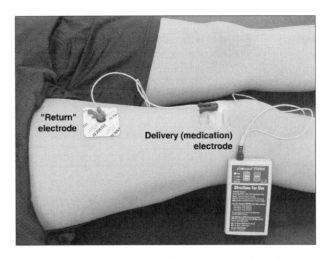

Figure 13-8. **Electrode Setup for Iontophoresis.** The appropriate medication is introduced to the delivery electrode, and the return electrode is saturated with an electrically neutral buffering solution. The polarity of the delivery electrode must have the same polarity as the medication being used.

RESET button decreases the dosage, output, and duration values to zero.

Dosage: This parameter sets the medication dosage in milliamperes per minute. Some units allow for the dosage to be keyed in directly (e.g., if a keypad is used, the numerical value is typed in) or set using INCREASE and DECREASE buttons.

Intensity (amperage): By setting the DOSAGE, the amperage increases to a preset level. Increasing the INTENSITY decreases the treatment DURATION; decreasing this value increases the DURATION while keeping the dosage at the level indicated.

Treatment duration: Decreasing the DURATION increases the treatment INTENSITY and vice versa.

Polarity: The polarity of the delivery electrode must be the same as that of the medication currently being applied (i.e., if a medication has a negative polarity, the delivery electrode must have a negative polarity). Units having a POLARITY switch change the polarity of the delivery electrode to either positive or negative. Other units require that the electrode leads be physically plugged into the positive and negative jacks.

Start-stop: Pressing this button the first time begins the current flow to the patient's body. For patient comfort, most generators are programmed so that the current is gradually ramped up from zero to the actual treatment duration. Pressing this button again either creates a pause in the treatment or terminates it, depending on the unit's design.

Setup and Application

Preheating the tissues may open skin pathways and ease the passage of the medication through the skin. The increased blood flow, however, may accelerate the removal of the medication from the area. Cold packs decrease blood flow and therefore theoretically maintain the medication concentration in the tissues. However, cold also may decrease the passage of medication into the tissue by tightening the skin portals. Do not apply hot packs or cold packs directly over the iontophoresis electrodes because uneven pressures can result in increased or decreased current densities or mask sensory feedback indicating thermal or chemical burning.

Refer to manufacturer's operating instructions for the procedures specific to the unit used.

Initiation of the Treatment

1. Clean the treatment site: Using alcohol, cleanse the area where the active and return electrodes are to be affixed to the body.
2. The areas where the electrodes are to be placed should be free of cuts, abrasions, and other open wounds and of excess body hair. Because shaving may cause nicks in the skin, clip excess body hair.
3. Prepare the ACTIVE electrode or electrodes: Fill the delivery electrode with the appropriate medication or medications in the manner applicable to the type of electrode being used. If indicated by the medication being used, add 1 mL of a buffering solution (0.9% saline and 0.5% potassium phosphate) to the active electrode. Buffering may only be required at higher treatment dosages (e.g., 80 mA/min).[193]
4. Wet the RETURN electrode with an appropriate buffering solution.
5. Position electrodes: Place the DELIVERY electrode over the treatment site and the RETURN electrode 4 to 6 inches away.
6. Set electrode polarity: Depending on the type of generator being used, either attach the electrode leads to the generator so that the polarity of the DELIVERY electrode matches the medication's charge or attach the electrode leads as indicated and adjust the POLARITY selector as needed.
7. Provide patient instructions: Inform the patient that tingling and itching may be experienced during the treatment, but the treatment should not be uncomfortable. Advise the patient to inform you of any pain, burning, or other unpleasant sensations.
8. Set treatment dose: Indicate the treatment dose recommended by the physician and pharmacist. Do not exceed the recommended dose or intensity for the electrode being used.
9. Adjust output parameters: Normally, the INTENSITY parameter is adjusted to suit the patient's comfort. If this is the patient's first treatment or if the patient has a history of sensitivity to this treatment or electrical stimulation in general, the output intensity should be decreased. The treatment intensity can be increased if indicated. Remember that decreasing the intensity increases the treatment duration and vice versa.
10. Supplemental treatment: Administer any appropriate follow-up treatments. Pulsed ultrasound (see Chapter 6) may be used after acetic acid iontophoresis for the reduction in the mass of traumatic myositis ossificans.[194]
11. Repeat treatment with the opposite polarity: If medications of different polarities are being used, repeat this procedure with the other medication using the appropriate polarity.
12. Apply a soothing ointment: A mild massage cream, aloe lotion, or skin-soothing ointment may be applied to the electrode sites to aid in reducing the amount of residual skin irritation associated with the treatment.
13. Discard electrodes: Iontophoresis electrodes may be used only for a single treatment.

■ Microcurrent Electrical Stimulation (Varied Currents)

Although there is no universally accepted definition of "microcurrent electrical therapy" (MET or MENS), some common denominators may be found. The current applied to the body uses a direct current or monophasic or biphasic pulse, an intensity that is usually below the depolarization threshold of sensory nerves, a current of less than 1000 mA.[31] These devices produce an electrical current that has approximately 1/1000 the amperage of TENS but a pulse duration that may be up to 2500 times longer. Microcurrent stimulation is used to restore the body's natural electrical potential to speed healing, reduce edema, and reduce pain. The efficacy of this technique has not been established.

Unlike the other electrical modalities described in this chapter, the distinguishing feature of microcurrent is that it does not attempt to excite peripheral nerves.[195] The subsensory current is thought to regulate cellular activity using a direct, alternating, or pulsed current (in a wide range of waveforms), with each possessing a broad band of pulse durations, frequencies, and treatment durations. Multiple channels may be used. This range of currents makes it difficult to analyze the theoretical and clinical effects of MET.

✱ Practical Evidence

The efficacy of MET has not been substantiated in professional literature. Few controlled studies report decreased pain, increased range of motion, and improved wound healing. However, more often than not, these effects were greater in experimental subjects than those seen in a control group, but less than other modalities, or they were conducted in an uncontrolled manner.[31,77,196,197,1987,199] Likewise, research exists that does not support microcurrent's efficacy as a therapeutic modality.[122,200-205]

At a Glance: **Microcurrent Electrical Stimulation**

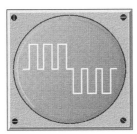

Parameters

CURRENT TYPE:	Monophasic, biphasic, direct, or alternating. Monophasic currents may regularly change the electrode polarity.
TOTAL CURRENT FLOW:	1–999 µA (peak current) 25 to 600 µA (RMS)
PULSE FREQUENCY:	0.1–1000 Hz
PULSE DURATION:	0.5–5000 µsec
PHASE DURATION:	0.5–5000 µsec

Wave form

Output Modulation

Intensity
Polarity/alternating polarity
Ramp
Threshold–Ohm meter

Treatment Duration

Most MET treatments range from 30 minutes to 2 hours and may be repeated up to four times per day.

Indications*

- Acute and chronic pain
- Acute and chronic inflammation
- Reduction of edema
- Sprains
- Strains
- Contusions
- Temporomandibular joint dysfunction
- Carpal tunnel syndrome
- Superficial wound healing
- Scar tissue
- Neuropathies

Contraindications

In addition to the contraindications presented in Table 12-11, the use of microcurrent electrical stimulation should not be used for:
- Pain or other symptoms of unknown origin
- **Osteomyelitis** •

Precautions

- The use of MET on dehydrated patients may result in nausea, dizziness, and/or headaches.
- Electrical "shocks" may be reported by the patient when MET is applied to scar tissue. This represents the decreased amount of current required to overcome the scar's electrical resistance.

The efficacy of these treatments has not been supported by published research.
RMS = root mean squared

Osteomyelitis: Inflammation of the bone marrow and adjacent bone.

● Biophysical Effects of Microcurrent Electrical Therapy

Tissue trauma affects the electrical potential of the involved cells, the previously described injury potential or current of injury.[82] Resistance to electrical current flow increases after trauma, so the body's intrinsic bioelectrical currents take the path of least resistance around, rather than through, the involved tissues. As a result of the diminished bioelectrical activity within the traumatized area, cellular capacitance is decreased, and the cell's homeostasis is further disrupted.[206,207,208] Theoretically, reestablishing the body's natural electrical balance allows the cell's adenosine triphosphate (ATP) supply to be replenished, thus providing the metabolic energy for healing to occur.

The theory supporting microcurrent's biophysical effects on the injury response process is based on the effect that a low-amperage current has on ATP levels. Currents below 500 mA increase the level of ATP, whereas higher amperages decrease the ATP level. Passing a low-amperage electrical current through mitochondria creates an imbalance in the number of proteins on either side of its cell membrane. As the protons move from the anode to the cathode, they cross the mitochondrial membrane, causing adenosine triphosphatase to produce ATP. The increased ATP production encourages amino acid transport and increased protein synthesis.[31,209]

Although it seems that a DC would best produce the effects described in this section, many MET protocols use an alternating or pulsed current.[209,210] It is unlikely that a DC is sufficient to overcome the skin's capacitive resistance because of the low amperage at which MET is applied. As you will recall, capacitive skin resistance decreases as the pulse frequency increases. Therefore, applying MET with an alternating or pulsed current lowers the current threshold required to overcome the skin's resistance. The distances used between the electrodes during treatment also serve to increase the amount of energy needed to complete the circuit.

Research has validated the effects of subthreshold electrical stimulation on cell membrane properties, neurological responses, and ionic responses.[195,211,212] These experimental designs most commonly use electrodes that are implanted within the tissues themselves. Other derivations have arisen from the benefits of sensory-level DC application. Unlike MET, the currents used in these studies did not have to overcome the resistance produced by the skin or have the electrical power needed to overcome the resistance posed by the tissues. Any interpolation between these effects and microcurrent may be inappropriate.

MET application has demonstrated increased collagen at the wound site, but this did not correlate to increased tensile strength or increased wound thickness.[198] Transient analgesia[199] and a decrease in post-exercise creatine kinase levels[213] have also been attributed to MET therapy.

Electrode Placement

The electrodes should be placed so that a line drawn through them transects the target tissues. This, in concept, is similar to the contiguous electrode placement technique described earlier in this chapter. However, proponents of MET view electrode placement in a three-dimensional rather than the traditional two-dimensional manner. This view holds that electrodes should also be placed on opposite sides of the torso or extremity and the current will flow through them. Perhaps if electricity flowed in a perfectly straight line between opposing electrodes, this would be true. However, remember that electricity follows the path of least resistance, which would most likely course the current around the body's circumference rather than straight through the core. Also remember that the greater the distance is between the electrodes, the greater the resistance, and the more current is required to overcome this resistance.

One technique for treating back pain places an electrode near the spinal cord at the same level as the painful tissues. The opposite electrode is then positioned on the contralateral side of the spinal cord on the anterior side of the body. When the axial skeleton is being treated, MET protocol suggests that treatment occur bilaterally.

The use of MET probes is described in the Setup and Application section.

Instrumentation

Power: When this switch is in its ON position, the current is allowed to flow to the internal components of the generator. Some units have a speaker that emits an audible sound when a certain electrical threshold is met. In this type of generator, the power switch often serves as a VOLUME control as well.

Timer: This control sets the duration of the treatment and subsequently displays the remaining time. On some units, the TIMER serves as the master power switch.

Start-stop: When this button is depressed to start the treatment, the circuit is closed, allowing the current to flow to the patient's tissues. When it is depressed again, the circuit is opened, interrupting the current flow. The START-STOP button may also set the treatment mode on some generators.

Amplitude: This control adjusts the current amperage from zero (OFF) to the maximal value of the unit. The output for each channel has its own AMPLITUDE control. The applied output is displayed on the OUTPUT meter.

Frequency (hertz): When a pulsed current is being applied, the FREQUENCY sets the number of pulses per second; when an AC is being administered, it sets the number of cycles per second. Each channel has its own output control.

Multiplier: A three-position switch that multiplies the output FREQUENCY by the value indicated. The output for each channel has its own multiplier control.

Polarity: This switch selects the output polarity in monophasic mode, or the rate at which the output polarity is alternated in biphasic mode.

Ramp: The ramp selects the rise time of the modulated output in biphasic mode.

Threshold: This button adjusts the level on the power meter at which audible output occurs.

Meter select: This control adjusts which channel is displayed on the power output meter.

Ohm meter: This device is used as a method of identifying stimulation points. When the probe is passed over an area of decreased electrical resistance (e.g., stimulation points, traumatized tissues), a tone, light, or numerical readout identifies the point on the skin at which stimulation should occur.

■ Setup and Application

Refer to manufacturer's operating instructions for the procedures specific to the unit used.

Initiation of the Treatment

1. Position the electrodes: Most MET stimulators require the use of silver electrodes. Unapproved carbon-rubber electrodes may present too much resistance to current flow and render the treatment ineffective.
2. Wet the electrodes: If felt-tipped electrodes or probes are being used, wet them with saline solution. Tap water should not be used because of its potentially high mineral content. Note that medicinal saline solution requires a physician's prescription. If this type of saline solution is not readily available, a saline-based contact lens cleaner may be used to wet the electrodes.
3. Select the output frequency: Most MET treatment protocols employ a 0.5-Hz frequency. If this frequency proves to be ineffective, a 1.5-Hz output may be attempted. Other protocols suggest using a frequency between 80 to 100 Hz for inflammatory conditions.
4. Increase the output intensity: Increase the intensity to the highest comfortable level, keeping in mind that most treatment applications occur at the subsensory level. Some protocols suggest a series of 5- to 10-minute treatments using a range of output intensities and varying pulse frequencies.
5. Reposition the electrodes: Each treatment bout with the electrode technique lasts from 5 to 10 minutes. At the end of each bout, the electrodes are removed, rewetted, and repositioned around the painful area.
6. Treat the contralateral side: Many MET protocols suggest that the same treatment that was delivered to the injured extremity or injured side of the body be repeated on the noninjured side.

Probe Technique

1. Set the timer: If the MET generator has a PROBE setting, select this. Otherwise, each treatment bout should last approximately 10 seconds.
2. Select output channel: Only one channel is used during the probe technique.
3. Identify target treatment area: Localize the center of pain as accurately as possible. Circle the area on the skin using a grease pencil or dry-erase marker.
4. Position probe: The area surrounding the target tissues is treated in an "X" manner. For example, the first treatment bout may have one probe positioned in the upper left-hand quadrant and the opposite probe in the lower right hand quadrant, relative to the mark identified in step 2. The next treatment bout would have the probes positioned in the upper right-hand and lower left-hand quadrant. The treatment progresses in this manner, with the probes being rotated around the target tissues in varying directions and distances, including anterior-posterior and medial-lateral placements.
5. Determine the number of bout sessions: Each bout in a single session persists for 10 seconds, and each session lasts approximately 2 minutes. Up to four sessions may be used during a single treatment.
6. Reevaluate the patient: The patient should be reevaluated after each bout session, and treatment parameters adjusted accordingly.

End of Section

Chapter Case Study

Diana's symptoms began with a sharp, stabbing pain that radiated into her right ear from her mid trapezius/levator scapulae insertion 3 weeks ago. She attributes symptoms to computer use at work, because data entry has dramatically increased in the past 2 months. Her skin temperature is normal, and there is moderate spasm of the levator scapulae with a highly sensitive trigger point at the scapula insertion.

1. What is the best therapeutic modality to consider in this situation?

2. What are the physiological effects on the injury response cycle from the application of this thermal agent?
3. What are the clinical symptoms that you hope to address with this intervention?

Case Study: **Continuation of Case Study From Section 1**

(The following discussion relates to Case Study 2 in Section 1.)

Based on this patient's condition, the availability of other modalities, and the lack of contraindications to the use of therapeutic modalities and therapeutic exercise, the most probable acute use of electrical stimulation would be that of pain control and trigger point therapy. However, the lack of access to electrotherapeutic modalities probably would not hinder this patient's progress. Other types of modalities could adequately address and resolve the patient's problems.

Pain Control
The problem of acute pain control has been addressed by the use of thermal agents, and the patient has received a prescription for muscle relaxants. If these approaches fail to reduce pain adequately, electrical stimulation could be incorporated into the program.

The acute nature of this injury, the lack of radicular symptoms, and the fact that the patient is taking medication for the pain would make sensory-level pain control an appropriate choice, especially if the patient's symptoms are alleviated during the application of heat and cold. In this case, the use of a portable TENS unit

should be considered and used as a part of the patient's home treatment program.

The electrodes would be positioned so that the current intersects over the primary area of pain. A short pulse duration, a high number of pulses per second, and a sensory-level intensity would be used. Because this unit would be used for long periods, its output must be modulated to help prevent accommodation. The patient would be instructed about how to connect and disconnect the unit, how to adjust the intensity, and, if indicated, how to modify the pulse characteristics.

Trigger Point Therapy
If the patient's trigger points do not subside after the other treatment approaches, electrical stimulation could be used to target them. High-voltage pulsed stimulation, delivered with a probe, a Neuroprobe, brief-intense TENS, or noxious-level stimulation can be used to attempt to break down the trigger point. Interrupting the local pain-spasm-pain cycle, decreasing the pain response, or causing the trigger point's fibers to fatigue can bring about long-term relief. The electrodes could safely be worn under the patient's cervical collar.

● ● ● **Section 4 Quiz**

1. Electrons travel from the _____, which has a _____ of electrons, to the _____, which has a _____ of electrons.
   A. Anode • high concentration • cathode • low concentration
   B. Anode • low concentration • cathode • high concentration
   C. Cathode • high concentration • anode • low concentration
   D. Cathode • low concentration • anode • high concentration

2. Monopolar stimulation involves the use of active and dispersive electrodes. The parameter that determines which electrode(s) will be active is:
   A. The POLARITY adjustment
   B. The average current
   C. The pulse duration
   D. The current density

3. What is the percent duty cycle for an electrical current that flows for 30 seconds and has no flow for 10 seconds?
   A. 33%
   B. 25%
   C. 75%
   D. 100%

4. All of the following are excitable tissues except:
   A. Muscle fiber
   B. Meniscal cartilage
   C. Sensory nerves
   D. Secretory cells

5. Which of the following electrical stimulation currents would cause physiochemical (i.e., galvanic) changes in the tissues?
   A. High-voltage pulsed stimulation
   B. Interferential stimulation
   C. Low-voltage alternating current
   D. Low-voltage direct current

6. Under normal circumstances, which of the following nerves would be the first to be depolarized by an electrical current?
   A. A superficial large-diameter nerve
   B. A deep large-diameter nerve
   C. A superficial small-diameter nerve
   D. A deep small-diameter nerve

7. Most tissues provide capacitive resistance to electrical current flow. Which of the following current types would meet the least amount of capacitive resistance?
   A. Direct current
   B. Monophasic current
   C. Biphasic current
   D. Alternating current

8. An electrical stimulation protocol that uses a high pulse frequency (e.g., 120 pps), short phase duration, and applied at the sensory level is thought to activate which pain control mechanism?
   A. Gate mechanism
   B. Endogenous opiate
   C. Central biasing
   D. Specificity

9. The electrodes from lead (A) have an area of 20 square inches; the electrodes originating from lead (B) have an area of 4 square inches. This type of application would be classified as:
   A. Monopolar
   B. Bipolar
   C. Quadripolar
   D. Polypolar

10. You are setting up an electrical stimulation unit to control pain through the endogenous opiate theory of pain modulation. The correct parameters for this are:
    A. High pulse rate, long phase duration, short treatment duration, motor level stimulation
    B. Low pulse rate, short phase duration, short treatment duration, sensory level stimulation
    C. High pulse rate, short phase duration, long treatment duration, sensory level stimulation
    D. High pulse rate, moderate phase duration, long treatment duration, noxious level stimulation

11. Iontophoresis is a technique that introduces medication into the tissues through the use of an electric current. For this method to work, the medication must:
    A. Have its outer valence shell filled
    B. Have a net ionic charge
    C. Be electrically neutral
    D. All are correct

12. Interferential stimulation is being applied with a carrier current of 4000 Hz and an interference current of 4130 Hz. The effective frequency of the current within the tissues would be:
    A. 8130 Hz
    B. 130 Hz
    C. 30 Hz
    D. None of these answers are correct

13. Which of the following conditions is a contraindication to the use of electrical stimulation?
    A. Post-traumatic pain
    B. Postsurgical pain
    C. Chronic pain
    D. Pain of unknown origin

14. A high-voltage pulsed stimulator uses what type of current?
    A. Monophasic
    B. Biphasic
    C. Polyphasic
    D. Direct

15. Which of the following duty cycles is most appropriate when attempting to reeducate the quadriceps muscle immediately postsurgery:
    A. 20%
    B. 40%
    C. 60%
    D. 80%

16. In general, a tonic contraction occurs when the number of pulses per second exceeds:
    A. 1
    B. 30
    C. 60
    D. 90

17. "The uninterrupted, bidirectional flow of electrons" best describes which of the following types of currents?
    A. Monophasic
    B. Biphasic
    C. Alternating
    D. Direct

18. In an electrical current, electrical flow consists of the movement of electrons; in the body's tissues, therapeutic current flow consists of the flow of:
    A. Protons
    B. Coulombs
    C. Electrons
    D. Ions

19. A POLARITY option would be found on which of the following modalities?
    A. High-voltage pulsed stimulator
    B. TENS unit
    C. Interferential stimulator
    D. Neuromuscular electrical nerve stimulator

20. Traumatized areas and stimulation points (e.g., motor points, trigger points) display a(n) _____ resistance to current flow.
    A. Increased
    B. Decreased

References

1. Kloth LC, Cummings JP: Electrotherapeutic Terminology in Physical Therapy. Section on Clinical Electrophysiology and the American Physical Therapy Association, Alexandria, VA, 1990.
2. Laufer Y, et al: Quadriceps femoris muscle torques and fatigue generated by neuromuscular electrical stimulation with three different wave forms. *Phys Ther.* 81:1307, 2001.
3. Lake DA: Neuromuscular electrical stimulation: An overview and its application in the treatment of sports injuries. *Sports Med.* 13:320, 1992.
4. Kantor G, et al: The effects of selected stimulus waveforms on pulse and phase characteristics at sensory and motor thresholds. *Phys Ther.* 74:951, 1994.
5. Petrofsky J, Prowse M, Bain M, et al: Estimation of the distribution of intramuscular current during electrical stimulation of the quadriceps muscle. *Eur J Appl Physiol.* 103:265, 2008.
6. Cook TM: Instrumentation. In Nelson RM, Currier DP (eds): Clinical Electrotherapy. Appleton & Lange, Norwalk, CT, 1987, pp 11–28.
7. Laufer Y, Elboim M: Effect of burst frequency and duration kilohertz-frequency alternating currents and of low-frequency pulsed currents on strength of contraction, muscle fatigue, and perceived discomfort. *Phys Ther.* 88:1167, 2008.
8. Baker LL: Neuromuscular electrical stimulation in the restoration of purposeful limb movements. In Wolf SL (ed): Electrotherapy. Churchill Livingstone, New York, 1981, pp 25–48.
9. Urbschait NL: Review of physiology. In Nelson RM, Currier DP (eds): Clinical Electrotherapy. Appleton & Lange, Norwalk, CT, 1987, pp 1–9.
10. Mödlin M, Forstner C, Hofer C, et al: Electrical stimulation of denervated muscles: First results of a clinical study. *Artif Organs.* 29:203, 2005.
11. DeVahl J: Neuromuscular electrical stimulation (NMES) in rehabilitation. In Gersh MR (ed): Electrotherapy in Rehabilitation. FA Davis, Philadelphia, 1992, pp 218–268.
12. Holcomb WR, Rubley MD, Miller MG, et al: The effect of rest intervals on knee-extension torque production with

neuromuscular electrical stimulation. *J Sport Rehabil.* 15:116, 2006.

13. Petrofsky J, Schawb E: A re-evaluation of modelling of the current flow between electrodes: Consideration of blood flow and wounds. *J Med Eng Technol.* 31;62, 2007.

14. Walsh DM: TENS: Clinical Application and Related Theory. Churchill Livingstone, New York, 1997.

15. Nolan MF: Conductive differences in electrodes used with transcutaneous electrical nerve stimulation devices. *Phys Ther.* 71:746, 1991.

16. Lieber RL, Kelly MJ: Factors influencing quadriceps femoris muscle torque using transcutaneous neuromuscular stimulation. *Phys Ther.* 71:715, 1991.

17. Alon G, et al: Effects of electrode size on basic excitatory responses on selected stimulus parameters. *J Orthop Sports Phys Ther.* 20:29, 1994.

18. Kuhn A, Keller T, Lawrence M, et al: The influence of electrode size on selectivity and comfort in transcutaneous electrical stimulation of the forearm. *IEEE Trans Neural Syst Rehabil Eng.* 18:255, 2010.

19. Miller MG, Cheatham CC, Holcomb WR, et al: Subcutaneous tissue thickness alters the effect of NMES. *J Sport Rehabil.* 17:68, 2008.

20. Ottoson D, Lundeberg T: Pain Treatment by Transcutaneous Electrical Nerve Stimulation: A Practical Manual. Springer-Verlag, New York, 1988.

21. Denegar CR, Huff CB: High and low frequency TENS in the treatment of induced musculoskeletal pain: A comparison study. *J Athl Train.* 23:235, 1988.

22. Berlant SR: Method of determining optimal stimulation sites for transcutaneous electrical nerve stimulation. *Phys Ther.* 64:924, 1984.

23. Cheing GLY, Hui-Chan CWY, Chan KM: Does four weeks of TENS and/or isometric exercise produce cumulative reduction of osteoarthritic knee pain? *Pain Rev.* 9:141, 2002.

24. Brown L, Holmes M, Jones A: The application of transcutaneous electrical nerve stimulation to acupuncture points (Acu-TENS) for pain relief: A discussion of efficacy an potential mechanisms. *Phys Ther Rev.* 14:93, 2009.

25. Yeh M, Chung Y, Chen K, et al: Acupoint electrical stimulation reduces acute postoperative pain in surgical patients with patient-controlled analgesia: A randomized controlled study. *Altern Ther Health Med.* 16:10, 2010.

26. Hall JE: Guyton and Hall Textbook of Medical Physiology. Saunders, New York, 2010.

27. Griffin JE, Karselis TC: Physical Agents for Physical Therapists, ed 2. Charles C Thomas, Springfield, IL, 1988.

28. Baker LL, et al: Effects of wave form on comfort during neuromuscular electrical. *Clin Orthop.* 223:75, 1988.

29. Scott WB, Causey JB, Marshall TL: Comparison of maximum tolerated muscle torques produced by 2 pulse durations. *Phys Ther.* 89:851, 2009.

30. Donadio V, Lenzi P, Montagna P, et al: Habituation of sympathetic sudomotor and vasomotor skin responses: Neural and non-neural components in healthy subjects. *Clin Neurophysiol.* 116:2542, 2005.

31. Johnson MI: Transcutaneous electrical nerve stimulation (TENS) and TENS-like devices: Do they provide pain relief? *Pain Rev.* 8:121, 2001.

32. Balogun JA, et al: High voltage electrical stimulation in the augmentation of muscle strength: Effects of pulse frequency. *Arch Phys Med Rehabil.* 74:910, 1993.

33. Harris PR: Iontophoresis: Clinical research in musculoskeletal inflammatory conditions. *J Orthop Sports Phys Ther.* 4:109, 1982.

34. De Domenico G: Interferential Stimulation (monograph). Chattanooga Group, Chattanooga, TN, 1988.

35. Han TR, Kim D, Lim SJ, et al: The control of parameters within the therapeutic range in neuromuscular electrical stimulation. *Intern J Neurosci.* 117:107, 2007.

36. Kim K, Croy T, Hertel J, et al: Effects of neuromuscular electrical stimulation after anterior cruciate ligament reconstruction of quadriceps strength, function, and patient-oriented outcomes: A systematic review. *J Orthop Sports Phys Ther.* 40:383, 2010.

37. Laufer Y, Tausher H, Esh R, et al: Sensory transcutaneous electrical stimulation fails to decrease discomfort associated with neuromuscular electrical stimulation in healthy individuals. *Am J Phys Med Rehabil.* 90:399, 2011.

38. Paillard T: Combined application of neuromuscular electrical stimulation and voluntary muscular contractions. *Sports Med.* 38:161, 2008.

39. Bircan C, Senocak O, Peker O, et al: Efficacy of two forms of electrical stimulation in increasing quadriceps strength: A randomized controlled trial. *Clin Rehabil.* 16:194, 2002.

40. Petrofsky J, Laymon M, Prowse M, et al: The transfer of current through skin and muscle during electrical stimulation with sine, square, Russian and interferential waveforms. *J Med Eng Technol.* 33:170, 2009.

41. Ferguson JP, et al: Effects of varying electrode site placements on the torque output of an electrically stimulated involuntary quadriceps femoris muscle contraction. *J Orthop Sports Phys Ther.* 11:24, 1989.

42. Delitto A, Rose SJ: Comparative comfort of three wave forms used in electrically eliciting quadriceps femoris muscle contractions. *Phys Ther.* 66:1704, 1986.

43. Holcomb WR, et al: A comparison of knee-extension torque production with biphasic versus Russian current. *J Sports Rehabil.* 9:229, 2000.

44. McLoda TA, Carmack JA: Optimal burst duration during a facilitated quadriceps femoris contraction. *J Athl Train.* 35:145, 2000.

45. Miller CR, Webers RL: The effects of ice massage on an individual's pain tolerance level to electrical stimulation. *J Orthop Sports Phys Ther.* 12:105, 1990.

46. Durst JW, et al: Effects of ice and recovery time on maximal involuntary isometric torque production using electrical stimulation. *J Orthop Sports Phys Ther.* 13:240, 1991.

47. Van Lunen BL, Carroll C, Gratias K, et al: The clinical effects of cold application on the production of electrically induced involuntary muscle contractions. *J Sport Rehabil.* 12:240, 2003.

48. Belanger AY, et al: Cutaneous versus muscular perception of electrically evoked tetanic pain. *J Orthop Sports Phys Ther.* 16:162, 1992.

49. Bowman BR, Baker LL: Effects of wave form parameters on comfort during transcutaneous neuromuscular electrical stimulation. *Ann Biomed Eng.* 13:59, 1985.

50. Gorgey AS, Dudley GA: The role of pulse duration and stimulation duration in maximizing the normalized torque during neuromuscular electrical stimulation. *J Orthop Sports Phys Ther.* 38:508, 2008.

51. Mandl T, Meyerspeer M, Reichel M, et al: Functional electrical stimulation of long-term denervated, degenerated human skeletal muscle: Estimating activation using T2-parameter magnetic resonance imaging methods. *Artif Organs.* 32:604, 2008.

52. Holcomb WR: A practical guide to electrotherapy. *J Sports Rehabil.* 6:272, 1997.

53. Parker MG, et al: Fatigue response in human quadriceps femoris muscle during high frequency electrical stimulation. *J Orthop Sports Phys Ther.* 7:145, 1986.

54. Holcomb WR, Kleiner DM: Versatile electrotherapy with the high-voltage pulsed stimulator. *Athl Ther Today.* 37, 1998.

55. Jensen JE: Stress fracture in the world class athlete: A case study. *Med Sci Sports Exercise.* 30:783, 1998.

56. Feil S, Newell J, Minoque C, et al: The effectiveness of supplementing a standard rehabilitation program with superimposed neuromuscular electrical stimulation after anterior cruciate ligament reconstruction: A prospective, randomized, single-blind study. *Am J Sports Med.* 39:1238, 2011.

57. Draper U, Ballard L: Electrical stimulation versus electromyographic biofeedback in the recovery of quadriceps femoris muscle function following anterior cruciate ligament surgery. *Phys Ther.* 71:455, 1991.

58. Gorgey AS, Mahoney E, Kendall T, et al: Effects of neuromuscular electrical stimulation parameters on specific tension. *Eur J Appl Physiol.* 97:737, 2006.

59. Delitto A, Snyder-Mackler, L: Two theories of muscle strength augmentation using percutaneous electrical stimulation. *Phys Ther.* 70:158, 1990.

60. Miller C, Thepaut-Mathieu C: Strength training by electrostimulation conditions for efficacy. *Int J Sports Med.* 14:20, 1993.

61. Sinacore DR, et al: Type II fiber activation with electrical stimulation: A preliminary report. *Phys Ther.* 70:416, 1990.

62. Petterson SC, Barrance P, Buchanan T, et al: Mechanisms underlying quadriceps weakness in knee osteoarthritis. *Med Sci Sports Exerc.* 40:422, 2008.

63. Walls RJ, McHugh G, O'Gorman DJ, et al: Effects of preoperative neuromuscular electrical stimulation on quadriceps strength and functional recovery in total knee arthroplasty. A pilot study. *BMC Musculoskelet Disord.* 11:119, 2010.

64. Schmitz RJ, et al: Effect of interferential current on perceived pain and serum cortisol associated with delayed onset muscle soreness. *J Sport Rehab.* 6:30, 1997.

65. Garrison DW, Foreman RD: Decreased activity of spontaneous and noxiously evoked dorsal horn cells during transcutaneous electrical nerve stimulation (TENS). *Pain.* 58:309, 1994.

66. Cox PD, et al: Effect of different TENS stimulus parameters on ulnar motor nerve conduction velocity. *Am J Phys Med Rehabil.* 72:294, 1993.

67. Oosterhof J, De Boo TM, Oostendorp RAB, et al: Outcome of transcutaneous electrical nerve stimulation in chronic pain: short-term results of a double-blind, randomised, placebo-controlled trial. *J Headache Pain.* 7:196, 2006.

68. Taylor K, et al: Effects of interferential current stimulation for treatment of subjects with recurrent jaw pain. *Phys Ther.* 67:346, 1987.

69. Longobardi AG, et al: Effects of auricular transcutaneous electrical nerve stimulation on distal extremity pain. *Phys Ther.* 69:10, 1989.

70. Jensen JE, et al: The use of transcutaneous neural stimulation and isokinetic testing in arthroscopic knee surgery. *Am J Sports Med.* 13:27, 1985.

71. Lewers D, et al: Transcutaneous electrical nerve stimulation in the relief of primary dysmenorrhea. *Phys Ther.* 69:3, 1989.

72. Gersh MR: Transcutaneous electrical nerve stimulation (TENS) for management of pain and sensory pathology. In Gersh MR (ed): Electrotherapy in Rehabilitation. FA Davis, Philadelphia, 1992, pp 149–196.

73. French S: Pain: Some psychological and sociological aspects. *Physiotherapy.* 75:255, 1989.

74. Sandberg ML, Sandberg MK, Dahl J: Blood flow changes in the trapezius muscle and overlying skin following transcutaneous electrical nerve stimulation. *Phys Ther.* 87:1047, 2007.

75. Miller BF, et al: Circulatory responses to voluntary and electrically induced muscle contractions in humans. *Phys Ther.* 80:53, 2000.

76. Chen C, Johnson MI, McDonough S, et al: The effect of transcutaneous electrical nerve stimulation on local and distal cutaneous blood flow following a prolonged heat stimulus in health subjects. *Clin Physiol Funct Imaging.* 27:154, 2007.

77. Carley PJ, Wainapel SF: Electrotherapy for acceleration of wound healing: Low intensity direct current. *Arch Phys Med Rehabil.* 66:443, 1985.

78. Feedar JA, et al: Chronic dermal ulcer healing enhanced with monophasic pulsed electrical stimulation. *Phys Ther.* 71:639, 1991.

79. Snyder-Mackler L: Electrical stimulation for tissue repair. In Snyder-Mackler L Robinson AJ (eds): Clinical Electrophysiology: Electrotherapy and Electrophysiologic Testing. Williams & Wilkins, Baltimore, 1989, pp 229–244.

80. Mehmandoust FG, Torkaman G, Firoozabadi M, et al: Anodal and cathodal pulsed electrical stimulation on skin would healing in guinea pigs. *J Rehabil Res Dev.* 44:611, 2007.

81. Newton R: High-voltage pulsed galvanic stimulation: Theoretical bases and clinical application. In Nelson RM, Currier DP (eds): Clinical Electrotherapy. Appleton & Lange, Norwalk, CT, 1987, pp 165–182.

82. Hart FX: Changes in the electric field at an injury site during healing under electrical stimulation. *J Bioelectricity.* 10:33, 1991.

83. Kloth LC: Physical modalities in wound management: UVC, therapeutic heating and electrical stimulation. *Ostomy Wound Manage.* 41:18, 1995.

84. Falanga V, et al: Electrical stimulation increases the expression of fibroblast receptors for transforming growth factor-beta (abstract). *J Invest Dermatol.* 88:488, 1987.

85. Gentzkow GD: Electrical stimulation to heal dermal wounds. *J Dermatol Surg Oncol.* 19:753, 1993.

86. Reich JD, et al: The effect of electrical stimulation on the number of mast cells in healing wounds. *J Am Acad Dermatol.* 25:40, 1991.

87. Szuminsky NJ, et al: Effect of narrow, pulsed high voltages on bacterial viability. *Phys Ther.* 74:660, 1994.

88. Litke DS, Dahners LE: Effects of different levels of direct current on early ligament healing in a rat model. *J Orthop Res.* 12:683, 1994.

89. Fujita M, et al: The effect of constant direct electrical current on intrinsic healing in the flexor tendon in vitro: An ultrastructural study of differing attitudes in epitendon cells and tenocytes. *J Hand Surg.* [Br]17:94, 1992.

90. Bettany JA, et al: Influence of high voltage pulsed direct current on edema formation following impact injury. *Phys Ther.* 70:219, 1990.

91. Mendel FC, Fish DR: New perspectives in edema control via electrical stimulation. *J Athl Train.* 28:1, 1993.

92. Reed BV: Effect of high voltage pulsed electrical stimulation on microvascular permeability to plasma proteins: A possible mechanism in minimizing edema. *Phys Ther.* 68:481, 1988.

93. Fish DR, et al: Effect of anodal high voltage pulsed current on edema formation in frog hind limbs. *Phys Ther.* 71:724, 1991.

94. Taylor K, et al: Effect of electrically induced muscle contractions on posttraumatic edema formation in frog hind limbs. *Phys Ther.* 72:127, 1992.

95. Mohr TM, et al: Effect of high voltage stimulation on edema reduction in the rat hind limb. *Phys Ther.* 67:1703, 1987.

96. Taylor K, et al: Effect of a single 30-minute treatment of high voltage pulsed current on edema formation in frog hind limbs. *Phys Ther.* 72:63, 1992.

97. Michlovitz S, et al: Ice and high voltage pulsed stimulation in treatment of lateral ankle sprains. *J Orthop Sports Phys Ther.* 9:301, 1988.

98. Griffin JW, et al: Reduction of chronic posttraumatic hand edema: A comparison of high voltage pulsed current, intermittent pneumatic compression, and placebo treatments. *Phys Ther.* 70:279, 1990.

99. Man IOW, Morrissey MC, Cywinski KJ: Effect of neuromuscular electrical stimulation on ankle swelling in the early period after ankle sprain. *Phys Ther.* 87:53, 2007.

100. Chakkalaka DA, et al: Electrophysiology of direct current stimulation of fracture healing in canine radius. *IEEE Trans Biomed Eng.* 37:1048, 1990.

101. Lilly-Masuda D, Towne, S: Bioelectricity and bone healing. *J Orthop Sports Phys Ther.* 7:54, 1985.

102. McLeod KJ, Rubin CT: The effect of low-frequency electrical fields on osteogenesis. *J Bone Joint Surg.* [Am]74:920, 1992.

103. Nash HL, Rogers CC: Does electricity speed the healing of non-union fractures? *Phys Sportsmedicine.* 16:156, 1988.

104. Stanish WD, et al: The use of electricity in ligament and tendon repair. *Phys Sports Med.* 13:110, 1985.

105. Driban JB. Bone stimulators and microcurrent: Clinical bioelectrics. *Athl Ther Today.* 9:22, 2004.

106. Pepper JR, et al: Effect of capacitive coupled electrical stimulation on regenerate bone. J *Orthop Res.* 14:296, 1996.

107. Needle AR, Kaminski TW: Effectiveness of low-intensity pulsed ultrasound, capacitively coupled fields, or extracorporeal shockwave therapy in accelerating stress fracture healing. *Athl Training Sports Health Care.* 1:133, 2009.

108. Nussbaum E, Rush P, Disenhaus L: The effects of interferential therapy on peripheral blood flow. *Physiother.* 76:803, 1990.

109. Currier DP, et al: Effect of graded electrical stimulation on blood flow to healthy muscle. *Phys Ther.* 66:937, 1986.

110. Houghton PE, Nussbaum EL, Hoens AM: Electrical stimulation. *Physiother Can.* 62:26, 2010.

111. Robinson AJ: Transcutaneous electrical nerve stimulation for the control of pain in musculoskeletal disorders. *J Orthop Sports Phys Ther.* 24:208, 1996.

112. Denegar CR, et al: Influence of transcutaneous electrical nerve stimulation on pain, range of motion, and serum cortisol concentration in females experiencing delayed onset muscle soreness. *J Orthop Sports Phys Ther.* 11:100, 1989.

113. Mohr T, et al: The effect of high volt galvanic stimulation on quadriceps femoris muscle torque. *J Orthop Sports Phys Ther.* 7:314, 1986.

114. Boutelle D, et al: A strength study utilizing the Electro-Stim 180. *J Orthop Sports Phys Ther.* 7:50, 1985.

115. Jette DU: Effect of different forms of transcutaneous electrical nerve stimulation on experimental pain. *Phys Ther.* 66:187, 1986.

116. Angulo DL, Colwell CW: Use of postoperative TENS and continuous passive motion following total knee replacement. *J Orthop Sports Phys Ther.* 11:599, 1990.

117. Cosgrove KA, et al: The electrical effect of two commonly used clinical stimulators on traumatic edema in rats. *Phys Ther.* 73:227, 1992.

118. Ralston DJ: High voltage galvanic stimulation: Can there be a "state of the art"? *J Athl Train.* 20:291, 1985.

119. Newton RA, Karselis TC: Skin pH following high voltage pulsed galvanic stimulation. *Phys Ther.* 63:1593, 1983.

120. Mohr T, et al: Comparison of isometric exercise and high volt galvanic stimulation on quadriceps femoris muscle strength. *J Orthop Sports Phys Ther.* 65:606, 1985.

121. Giles BE, Walker JS. Sex differences in pain and analgesia. *Pain Rev.* 7:181, 2000.

122. Wolcot C, et al: A comparison of the effects of high volt and microcurrent stimulation on delayed onset muscle soreness. *Phys Ther.* 71:S117, 1991.

123. Butterfield DL, et al: The effects of high-volt pulsed current electrical stimulation on delayed-onset muscle soreness. *J Athl Train.* 32:15, 1997.

124. Sandoval MC, Ramirez C, Camargo DM, et al: Effect of high-voltage pulsed current plus conventional treatment on acute ankle sprain. *Rev Bras Fisioter.* 14:193, 2010.

125. Snyder AR, Perotti AL, Lam KC, et al: The influence of high-voltage electrical stimulation on edema formation after acute injury: A systematic review. *J Sport Rehab.* 19:436, 2010.

126. Mendel FC, Dolan MG, Fish DR, et al: Effect of high-voltage pulsed current on recovery after grades I and II lateral ankle sprains. *J Sport Rehab.* 19:399, 2010.

127. Cook HA, et al: Effects of electrical stimulation on lymphatic flow and limb volume in the rat. *Phys Ther.* 74:1040, 1994.

128. Walker DC, et al: Effects of high voltage pulsed electrical stimulation on blood flow. *Phys Ther.* 68:481, 1988.

129. Heath ME, Gibbs SB: High-voltage pulsed stimulation: Effects of frequency of current on blood flow in the human calf. *Clin Sci (Colch).* 82:607, 1992.

130. Tracy JE, et al: Comparison of selected pulse frequencies from different electrical stimulators on blood flow in healthy subjects. *Phys Ther.* 68:1526, 1988.

131. Agren MS, et al: Collagenase during burn wound healing: Influence of a hydrogel dressing and pulsed electrical stimulation. *Plast Reconstr Surg.* 94:518, 1994.

132. Kincaid CB, Lavoie KH: Inhibition of bacterial growth in vitro following stimulation with high voltage, monophasic, pulsed current. *Phys Ther.* 69:651, 1989.

133. Fitzgerald GK, Newsome D: Treatment of a large infected thoracic spine wound using high voltage pulsed monophasic current. *Phys Ther.* 73:355, 1993.

134. Marchand S, et al: Effects of caffeine on analgesia from transcutaneous electrical nerve stimulation (letter to the editor). *N Engl J Med.* 333:325, 1995.

135. Palmer ST, Martin DJ, Steedman WM, et al: Alteration of interferential current and transcutaneous electrical nerve stimulation frequency: Effects on nerve excitation. *Arch Phys Med Rehabil.* 80:1065, 1999.

136. Roeser WM, et al: The use of transcutaneous nerve stimulation for pain control in athletic medicine. A preliminary report. *Am J Sports Med.* 4:210, 1976.

137. Walsh DM, et al: Transcutaneous electrical nerve stimulation: Relevance of stimulation parameters to neurophysiological and hypoalgesic effects. *Am J Phys Med Rehabil.* 74:199, 1995.

138. Barr JO, et al: Transcutaneous electrical nerve stimulation characteristics for altering pain perception. *Phys Ther.* 66:1515, 1986.

139. Indergand HJ, Morgan BJ: Effects of high-frequency transcutaneous electrical nerve stimulation on limb blood flow in healthy humans. *Phys Ther.* 74:361, 1994.

140. Walsh DM, et al: A double-blind investigation of the hypoalgesic effects of transcutaneous electrical nerve

stimulation upon experimentally induced ischaemic pain. *Pain*. 61:39, 1995.

141. Widerström EG, et al: Relations between experimentally induced tooth pain threshold changes, psychometrics and clinical pain relief following TENS. A retrospective study in patients with long-lasting pain. *Pain*. 51:281, 1992.

142. Dickie A, Tabasam G, Tashani O, et al: A preliminary investigation into the effect of coffee on hypolagesia associated with transcutaneous electrical nerve stimulation. *Clin Physiol Funct Imaging*. 29:293, 2009.

143. Gaid M, Cozens A: The role of transcutaneous electric nerve stimulation (TENS) for the management of chronic low back pain. *Int Musculoskelet Med*. 31:19, 2009.

144. Claydon LS, Chesterton LS: Does transcutaneous electrical nerve stimulation (TENS) produce "does-responses"? A review of systematic reviews on chronic pain. *Phys Ther Rev*. 13:450, 2008.

145. Altay F, Durmuş D, Cantürk F: Effects of TENS on pain, disability, quality of life, and depression in patients with knee osteoarthritis. *Turk J Rheumatol*. 25:116, 2010.

146. Pietrosimone BG, Saliba SA, Hart JM, et al: Effects of disinhibitory transcutaneous electrical nerve stimulation and therapeutic exercise on sagittal plane peak knee kinematics and kinetics in people with knee osteoarthritis during gait: A randomized controlled trial. *Clin Rehabil*. 24:1091, 2010.

147. Levin MF, Hui-Chan CWY: Conventional and acupuncture-like transcutaneous electrical nerve stimulation excite similar afferent nerves. *Arch Phys Med Rehabil*. 74:54, 1993.

148. Dean J, Bowsher D, Johnson MI: The effects of unilateral transcutaneous electrical nerve stimulation of the median nerve on bilateral somatosensory thresholds. *Clin Physiol Funct Imaging*. 26:314, 2006.

149. Buxton BP, et al: Self selection of transcutaneous electrical nerve stimulation (TENS) parameters for pain relief in injured athletes (abstract). *J Athl Train*. 29:178, 1994.

150. Tulgar M, et al: Comparative effectiveness of different stimulation modes in relieving pain. I. A pilot study. *Pain*. 47:151, 1991.

151. Tulgar M, et al: Comparative effectiveness of different stimulation modes in relieving pain. II. A double-blind controlled long-term study. *Pain*. 47:157, 1991.

152. Reib L, Pomeranz B: Alterations in electrical pain thresholds by use of acupuncture-like transcutaneous electrical nerve stimulation in pain-free subjects. *Phys Ther*. 72:658, 1992.

153. Aarskog R, Johnson MI, Demmink JH, et al: Is mechanical pain threshold after transcutaneous electrical nerve stimulation (TENS) increased locally and unilaterally? A randomized placebo-controlled trial in healthy subjects. *Physiother Res Int*. 12:251, 2007.

154. Chen CC, Johnson MI. An investigation the effects of frequency-modulated transcutaneous electrical nerve stimulation (TENS) on experimentally-induced pressure pain in healthy participants. *J Pain*. 10:1029, 2009.

155. Bechtel TB, Fan PT: When is TENS effective and practical for pain relief? *J Musculoskel Med*. 2:37, 1985.

156. Gersh MR, Wolf SL: Applications of transcutaneous electrical nerve stimulation in the management of patients with pain. *Phys Ther*. 65:314, 1985.

157. Somers DL, Somers MF: Treatment of neuropathic pain in a patient with diabetic neuropathy using transcutaneous electrical nerve stimulation applied to the skin of the lumbar region. *Phys Ther*. 79:767, 1999.

158. Sung P: The effect of Genesen® point stimulator: The median nerve conduction velocity (abstract). *Phys Ther*. 81:A5, 2001.

159. Paris DL, et al: Effects of the neuroprobe in the treatment of second-degree ankle sprains. *Phys Ther*. 63:35, 1983.

160. Selkowitz DM: Improvement in isometric strength of the quadriceps femoris muscle after training with electrical stimulation. *Phys Ther*. 65:186, 1988.

161. Laughman RK, et al: Strength changes in the normal quadriceps femoris muscle group as a result of electrical stimulation. *Phys Ther*. 63:494, 1983.

162. Snyder-Mackler L, et al: Strength of the quadriceps femoris muscle and functional recovery after reconstruction of the anterior cruciate ligament: A prospective, randomized clinical trial of electrical stimulation. *J Bone Joint Surg*. Am 77:1166, 1995.

163. Liu H, et al: Circulatory response of digital arteries associated with electrical stimulation of calf muscle in healthy subjects. *Phys Ther*. 67:340, 1987.

164. Ward AR, Robertson VJ: Sensory, motor, and pain thresholds for stimulation with medium frequency alternating current. *Arch Phys Med Rehabil*. 79:273, 1998.

165. Snyder-Mackler L: Electrical stimulation for pain modulation. In Snyder-Mackler L, Robinson AJ (eds): Clinical Electrophysiology: Electrotherapy and Electrophysiologic Testing. Williams & Wilkins, Baltimore, 1994, pp 205–227.

166. Kloth LC: Electrotherapeutic alternatives for the treatment of pain. In Gersh MR (ed): Electrotherapy in Rehabilitation. FA Davis, Philadelphia, 1992, pp 197–217.

167. Chen XH, et al: Electrical stimulation at traditional acupuncture sites in periphery produces brain opioid-receptor-mediated antinociception in rats. *J Pharmacol Exp Ther*. 227:654, 1996.

168. Ozcan J, Ward AR, Robertson VJ: A comparison of true and premodulated interferential currents. *Arch Phys Med Rehabil*. 85:409, 2004.

169. Kramer JF: Effect of electrical stimulation frequencies on isometric knee extension torque. *Phys Ther*. 67:31, 1987.

170. Hobler CK: Case study: Reduction of chronic posttraumatic knee edema using interferential stimulation. *J Athl Train*. 26:364, 1991.

171. Ward AR, Robertson VJ, Makowski RJ: Optimal frequencies for electric stimulation using medium-frequency alternating current. *Arch Phys Med Rehabil*. 83:1024, 2002.

172. Partridge CJ, Kitchen SS: Adverse effects of electrotherapy used by physiotherapists. *J Physio Ther*. 85:298, 1999.

173. Ford KS, Shrader MW, Smith J, et al: Full-thickness burn formation after the use of electrical stimulation therapy for rehabilitation of unicompartmental knee arthoplasty. *J Athroplasty*. 20:950, 2000.

174. Henley EJ: Transcutaneous drug delivery: Iontophoresis, phonophoresis. *Phys Rehabil Med*. 2:139, 1991.

175. Hasson SH, et al: Exercise training and dexamethasone iontophoresis in rheumatoid arthritis: A case study. *Physiother Canada*. 43:11, 1991.

176. Glass JM, et al: The quantity and distribution of radiolabeled dexamethasone delivered to tissue by iontophoresis. *Int J Dermatol*. 19:519, 1980.

177. Gundeman SD, et al: Treatment of plantar fasciitis by iontophoresis of 0.4% Dexamethasone: A randomized, double blind, placebo controlled study. *Am J Sports Med*. 25:312, 1997.

178. Zeltzer L, et al: Iontophoresis versus subcutaneous injection: A comparison of two methods of local anesthesia delivery in children. *Pain*. 44:73, 1991.

179. Brown MB, Martin GP, Jones SA, Akomeah FK: Dermal and transdermal drug delivery systems: Current and future prospects. *Drug Deliv*. 13:175, 2006.

180. Nimmo WS: Novel delivery systems: Electrotransport. *J Pain Symptom Manage.* 8:160, 1992.

181. Bertolucci LE: Introduction of antiinflammatory drugs by iontophoresis: A double blind study. *J Orthop Sport Phys Ther.* 4:103, 1982.

182. Scott ER, et al: Transport of ionic species in skin: Contribution of pores to the overall skin conductance. *Pharmacol Res.* 10:1699, 1993.

183. Bogner RB, Ajay, KM: Iontophoresis and phonophoresis. *US Pharmacist.* August 1994, H-10.

184. Kalia YN, Guy RH: The electrical characteristics of human skin in vivo. *Pharmacol Res.* 12:1605, 1995.

185. Pikal MJ, Shah S: Transport mechanisms in iontophoresis. II. Electroosmotic flow and the transference number measurements for hairless mouse skin. *Pharmacol Res.* 7:213, 1990.

186. Inada H, et al: Studies on the effects of applied voltage and duration on the human epidural membrane alteration/recovery and the resultant effects upon iontophoresis. *Pharmacol Res.* 11:687, 1994.

187. Grossmann M, et al: The effect of iontophoresis on the cutaneous vasculature: Evidence for current-induced hyperemia. *Microvasc Res.* 50:444, 1995.

188. Howard JP, et al: Effects of alternating current iontophoresis on drug delivery. *Arch Phys Med Rehabil.* 76:463, 1995.

189. Reinauer S, et al: Iontophoresis with alternating current and direct current offset (AC/DC iontophoresis): A new approach for the treatment of hyperhydrosis. *Br J Dermatol.* 129:166, 1993.

190. Evans TA, et al: The immediate effects of lidocaine iontophoresis on trigger-point pain. *J Sport Rehabil.* 10:287, 2001.

191. Nowicki KD, et al: Effects of iontophoretic versus injection administration of dexamethasone. *Med Sci Sports Exerc.* 34:1294, 2002.

192. Oshima T, et al: Cutaneous iontophoresis application of condensed lidocaine. *Can J Anaesth.* 41:667, 1994.

193. Guffey JS, et al: Skin pH changes associated with iontophoresis. *J Orthop Sports Phys Ther.* 29:656, 1999.

194. Wieder DL: Treatment of traumatic myositis ossificans with acetic acid iontophoresis. *Phys Ther.* 72:133, 1992.

195. Alon G: "Microcurrent": Subliminal electric stimulation. Does the research support its clinical use? *Sports Med Update.* 9:8, 1993.

196. Bertolucci LE, Grey T: Clinical comparative study of microcurrent electrical stimulation to mid-laser and placebo treatment in degenerative joint disease of the temporomandibular joint. *Craniology.* 13:116, 1995.

197. Lerner FN, Kirsch DL: A double-blind comparative study of microstimulation and placebo effect in short-term treatment of chronic back patients. *J Am Chiropr Assoc.* 15:S101, 1981.

198. Bach S, et al: The effect of electrical current on healing skin incision. An experimental study. *Eur J Surg.* 157:171, 1991.

199. Denegar CR, et al: The effects of low-volt microamperage on delayed onset muscle soreness. *J Sport Rehab.* 1:95, 1992.

200. Byl NN, et al: Pulsed microamperage stimulation: A controlled study of healing of surgically induced wounds in Yucatan pigs. *Phys Ther.* 74:201, 1994.

201. Leffmann DL, et al: The effect of subliminal transcutaneous electrical nerve stimulation of the rate of wound healing in rats. *Phys Ther.* 74:195, 1994.

202. Sinnreich MJ, et al: Microcurrent electrical nerve stimulation (MENS) and coracoacromial arch pain: The effects after one treatment. *Phys Ther.* 72:S68, 1992.

203. Ray R, et al: Microcurrent therapy versus a placebo for the control of symptoms in mild and moderate acute ankle sprains (unpublished manuscript). 1996.

204. Weber MD, et al: The effects of three modalities on delayed onset muscle soreness. *J Orthop Sports Phys Ther.* 20:236, 1994.

205. Allen JD, et al: Effect of microcurrent stimulation on delayed-onset muscle soreness: A double-blind comparison. *J Athl Train.* 34:334, 1999.

206. Becker RO: The Body Electric. William Morrow, New York, 1985.

207. Becker RO: Electrical control systems and regenerative growth. *J Bioelectricity* 1:239, 1982.

208. Windsor RE, et al: Electrical stimulation in clinical practice. *Phys Sportsmedicine.* 21:85, 1993.

209. Cheng N, et al: The effects of electric currents on ATP generation, protein synthesis, and membrane transport in rat skin. *Clin Orthop.* 171:264, 1982.

210. Stromberg BV: Effects of electrical currents on wound contraction. *Ann Plast Surg.* 21:121, 1988.

211. Swadlow HA: Monitoring the excitability of neocortical efferent neurons to direct activation by extracellular current pulses. *J Neurophysiol.* 68:605, 1992.

212. Pubols LM: Characteristics of dorsal horn neurons expressing subliminal responses to sural nerve stimulation. *Somatosens Mot Res.* 7:137, 1990.

213. Rapaski D, et al: Microcurrent electrical stimulation: A comparison of two protocols in reducing delayed onset muscle soreness. *Phys Ther.* 71S:116, 1991.

Mechanical and Light Modalities

This section presents the therapeutic agents that rely primarily on mechanical force and on chemical and/or bioelectrical properties to affect the injury response process.

Chapter 14

Intermittent Compression

Intermittent compression units assist in venous and lymphatic drainage by creating a pressure gradient that forces fluid out of the extremity through the venous system and spreads solid matter proximally along lymphatic ducts. The appliance may be filled with air (pneumatic compression) or chilled water (cryocompression) and may inflate as a single unit or sequentially. The ON/OFF cycle assists in milking or pumping edema out of the extremity.

● Intermittent compression units use mechanical pressure to encourage venous and lymphatic return from the extremities. Compression units consist of a nylon **appliance** designed to fit the body part (e.g., foot and/or ankle, half leg, full leg) that is connected to the unit through one or more hoses. The flow of air or cold water into the appliance creates the compression around the extremity.

The resulting compression is either circumferential or sequential. Circumferential compression applies an equal amount of pressure to all parts of the extremity simultaneously. The pressure is gradually increased to a level determined by the operator and held for a preset time during the ON cycle. The pressure then drops during the OFF cycle. The process then repeats.

Through this cycle, swelling is forced toward the torso through the venous and lymphatic return systems. Sequential compression increases the distal-to-proximal gradient through the sequential filling of pressure chambers within the appliance. The most distal compartment inflates, followed by the next compartment, and so on, until pressure is applied to the length of the appliance (Fig. 14-1).

✳ Practical Evidence

Constant compression is useful in preventing swelling and assisting in venous return. Intermittent compression is most effective in activating the lymphatic return mechanism.[1]

Compression devices work on two principles. Mechanical pressure waves force fluids within the venous system back toward the heart.[2] When the edema is confined to a local area, a limited number of lymphatic ducts are capable of reabsorbing the solid matter. Lymphatic uptake and return are assisted by spreading the edema over a larger area (usually proximally), allowing more lymphatic ducts to absorb the solid matter within the edema.

Intermittent cold compression units are used to treat acute injuries because of their ease of use and their ability to provide cold and compression while the limb is elevated (ice, compression, and elevation) (Fig. 14-2). Circumferential compression units may also be used

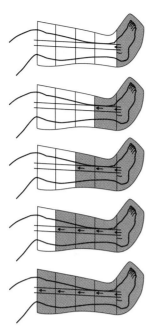

Figure 14-1. Sequential Compression. Compartments within the appliance fill distal to proximal, forcing the fluids toward the torso. Following the cycle, all the compartments deflate and the process repeats.

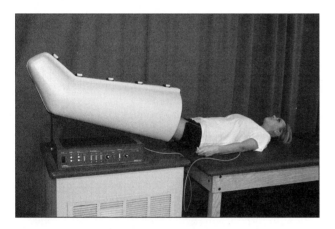

Figure 14-2. Sequential Cold Compression Unit. This device allows for simultaneous sequential cold compression and elevation. (The CRYO*Press*. Courtesy of Grimm Scientific Industries, Inc., Marietta, OH.)

immediately between ice bouts to prevent the formation of edema. However, compression units should not be used until the possibility of a fracture or compartment syndrome has been ruled out. In subacute or chronic conditions, intermittent or sequential compression is used to reduce edema and decrease ecchymosis from the area.

Cold compression therapy units, described in Chapter 6, deliver continuous compression and are useful in preventing edema. Intermittent compression units are used to remove edema that has already accumulated.

EFFECTS ON

The Injury Response Process

The movement of fluids out of the extremity is caused by the formation of a pressure gradient.[3,4] When external compression is applied, the gradient between the tissue hydrostatic pressure and the capillary filtration pressure is reduced, thus encouraging the reabsorption of interstitial fluids (Fig. 14-3). Because the tissues are being compressed, a second pressure gradient is formed between the distal portion of the extremity (high pressure) and the proximal portion (low pressure), forcing the fluids to move from the high-pressure area to a lower pressure area. If the extremity is elevated during this treatment, both of these pressures are enhanced by gravity, speeding venous drainage. Spreading the solid edematous matter over a larger area allows more lymphatic ducts to absorb the wastes and remove by-products from the extremity.[5]

During the compression sequence, blood flow to the treated area is decreased because of the external pressure on the extremity. The OFF time allows the venous and lymph vessels to reload, absorbing fluids and proteins from the tissues.

Although deep vein thrombosis (DVT) is a contraindication to intermittent compression, its use can prevent the onset of DVT. The increased venous flow helps prevent the accumulation of the substances that can lead to the formation of a thrombus.

Edema

Both circumferential and sequential compression units can significantly increase venous flow and reduce the swelling. During the treatment of lower leg edema, low pressure (35 to 55 mm Hg) increases the venous flow velocity 175%. When this pressure is increased to the range of 90 to 100 mm Hg, the venous flow accelerates to 336% of resting values (see Table 1-11).[5] Because extracellular debris is removed, the fresh blood flow to the area significantly increases following the treatment.[6]

Intermittent compression may be more effective in reducing fluid-rich post-traumatic edema than lymphedema. Reduced limb volume following intermittent compression may be the result of forcing fluids (water) through the venous system. Movement of protein molecules through the lymphatic system does not appear to be increased by intermittent compression. In this case, intermittent compression may limit the formation of edema by decreasing the blood capillary filtration pressure.[7] A study of post-acute ankle sprains that displayed **pitting edema** • found not only that simple elevation was more effective in reducing limb volume than intermittent compression and elastic wraps but also that the last two techniques actually increased the amount of edema.[8]

Pitting edema: An exudate-rich form of edema characterized by being easily indented ("pitted") by pressure.

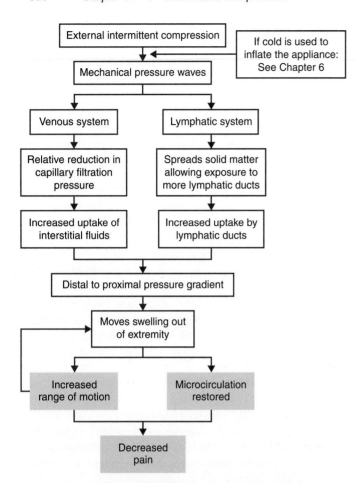

Figure 14-3. **Effects of Intermittent Compression.** Pressure waves replicate the venous and lymphatic milking associated with voluntary muscle contractions. Decreased swelling increases range of motion, restores microcirculation, and decreases pain.

✳ Practical Evidence

Venous blood flow from the leg is increased when sequential compression is applied to the foot and leg relative to intermittent compression of the calf alone.[9]

Intermittent compression is sometimes applied concurrently with an electrical stimulation muscle milking protocol. This approach combines the benefits of both edema reduction techniques into a single treatment session, but its efficacy has not been substantiated (Fig. 14-4).

The foot appears to rely on a mechanism other than muscle contractions or range of motion to initiate venous return. The venous foot pump is activated by pressure applied to the plantar aspect of the foot from the calcaneus to the metatarsal heads. This pressure, normally seen during weight bearing, decreases the long and transverse arches of the foot,

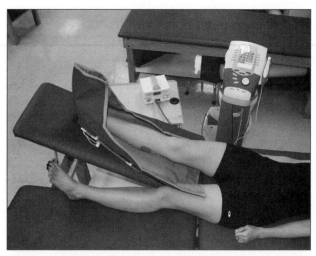

Figure 14-4. **Combination of Electrical Stimulation and Compression.** The electrodes (not visible) are positioned over the calf muscle.

stretching the veins and causing them to empty.[10] This implies that traditional compression techniques may not be successful for reducing foot edema. In this case, compression must be applied to the plantar aspect of the foot through weight bearing or simulated weight bearing by applying pressure to the plantar aspect of the foot.

To reduce the reaccumulation of edema, wrap the extremity or apply a compression garment and elevate the limb following treatment. To monitor the effectiveness of intermittent compression on edema reduction, pretreatment and posttreatment limb volume measurements should be taken. Once the edema is sufficiently reduced—and the patient's pathology permits—an active exercise regimen should be implemented.

Blood Flow

Blood flow is enhanced by decongesting the area. Intermittent compression increases the velocity of blood flow, which, in turn, enhances the production of nitric oxide, a strong vasodilator.[1]

Range of Motion

Synovial joints such as the knee, interphalangeal joints of the fingers and toes, and the elbow contain synovial fluid housed within a relatively dense joint capsule. This fluid must be able to move within the capsule for normal joint motion to occur, and moving from extension into flexion increases the amount of pressure within the joint.

When excess fluids form within a joint either as edema or **synovitis** ●, motion is limited because there is little if any room left within the joint capsule in which to displace the fluid. Excess fluids can trigger arthrogenic muscle inhibition (AMI), an inhibitory reflex that prevents active joint motion (see Chapter 1).[11,12] Reducing the joint volume assists in decreasing AMI and restoring

---

Synovitis: Inflammation of the synovial membrane.

normal active range of motion by reducing the hydraulic resistance to motion.[11,13]

Swelling of the distal joints decreases ROM. The decreased ROM further promotes distal swelling by limiting the muscle pump and reducing venous and lymphatic outflow.

Pain

Pain reduction is achieved by reducing the mechanical pressure caused by the edema and by restoring normal joint range of motion and function. Decreasing vascular clogging helps to restore normal arterial and vascular function. The subsequent increased arterial supply reduces ischemic pain by increasing the rate of delivery of oxygen and nutrients to the tissues.

■ Contraindications and Precautions

The primary contraindications to the use of intermittent compression are associated with the pressure applied to the extremity. The patient's arterial blood supply, including heart rate, blood pressure, and vessel continuity, must be sufficient to deliver oxygenated blood to the extremity during the treatment. Compression units are also contraindicated in compartment syndromes, such as anterior compartment syndrome, where the intracompartment pressure hinders normal blood perfusion. Other vascular insufficiencies such as gangrene, peripheral vascular disease, ischemic vascular disease, and arteriosclerosis are generally considered to be contraindications to treatment. On the physician's consent, patients with mild vascular insufficiency may be treated with reduced pressures and/or shortened ON times.

A bit of a paradox exists regarding DVT. Intermittent compression increases venous blood flow, thus helping to remove stagnant debris, thus decreasing the risk of a thrombus forming. However, because of the potential of dislodging a clot that has formed, do not apply intermittent compression on patients suffering from DVT or thrombophlebitis.

Congestive heart failure is a contraindication to the use of compression devices. The increased pressure on the vasculature may further damage the cardiovascular system or lead to decreased cardiac output. Patients suffering from congestive heart failure may experience increased sodium and water retention following compression therapy, both of which can increase bilateral peripheral edema. Pulmonary edema is aggravated by compression therapy because of the added load on the cardiorespiratory system similar to that described for congestive heart failure.

✳ Practical Evidence

Application of sequential pneumatic compression to the lower extremities resulted in slightly increased systemic blood pressure and reduced cardiac output and heart rate.[14] This creates the need for caution when applying compression devices to patients with cardiac and/or pulmonary impairments.

Insufficiency of valves within the venous network can result in gravity moving edema distally into the extremity.[3] Because these valves do not adequately close, the pressure from the compression appliance will force fluids both proximally and distally within the extremity (Fig 14-5). In the presence of known venous insufficiency, a full-extremity appliance should be used that maintains a distal to proximal pressure gradient.

The effects of intermittent compression on the reduction of lymphedema have not been conclusively substantiated. However, the treatment of lymphedema can result in edema proximal to the treatment site and the treatment of lower extremity lymphedema with intermittent compression can cause genital edema.[15]

Unhealed fractures, unresolved joint dislocations, or other musculoskeletal instabilities in the anteroposterior plane are contraindications to the use of compression devices over the involved joint. As the appliance inflates, it will attempt to move the joint into extension and place unwanted stresses on the structures in the area.

■ Overview of the Evidence

The efficacy of intermittent compression for increasing venous flow is widely accepted, but the effect of intermittent compression on lymphedema is not substantiated.[2] Conclusive evidence does not exist that intermittent compression is more effective than a compression wrap and elevation for reducing protein-rich pitting edema,[8] but evidence does support that compression units, elevation, and cold do reduce edema more than cryotherapy alone.[10]

No published research has conclusively determined the optimal treatment duration and duty cycles for reducing venous flow or lymphedema.

■ Clinical Application of Intermittent Compression

The instrumentation, setup, and application of circumferential and sequential intermittent compression units are similar. Before using an intermittent compression unit, refer to the manufacturer's documentation and protocol for the exact procedures for the model used.

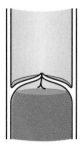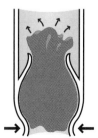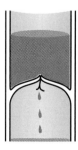

Figure 14-5. **Venous Insufficiency.** The one-way valves do not completely close, allowing venous blood to backfill and collect in the distal extremity, often resulting in swelling of the distal joints.

At a Glance: **Intermittent Compression**

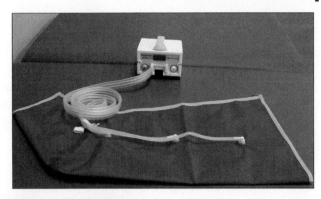

Description

An external pump forces air or water through an appliance fitted to the extremity. The changes in pressure force fluids through the venous system and solids through the lymphatic system to promote swelling reduction via increased venous return. Intermittent compression may increase lymphatic return. Protein-rich matter is less responsive to intermittent compression than fluids.[7]

Indications

- Post-traumatic edema
- Postsurgical edema
- Primary and secondary lymphedema
- Improving arterial circulation in the presence of arterial occlusive disease
- Vascular or lymphatic insufficiency including venous stasis ulcers
- *Prevention* of deep vein thrombosis. The presence of deep vein thrombosis is a contraindication to treatment.

Contraindications

- Acute conditions in which the possibility of a fracture has not been eliminated
- Conditions in which the pressure would further damage the structures (e.g., compartment syndromes)
- Peripheral vascular disease
- Arteriosclerosis
- Edema secondary to congestive heart failure
- Ischemic vascular disease
- Gangrene
- Dermatitis
- Deep vein thrombosis
- Thrombophlebitis
- Acute pulmonary edema

Treatment Duration

Intermittent compression can be applied once or twice a day for 20 minutes to several hours per session for post-traumatic edema. Treatment for lymphedema may be given for several hours. If the unit uses cold fluid, increase the temperature as the treatment duration increases.

Precautions

- Use care when treating the lower leg with a compression device. Even in the absence of a compartment syndrome, inflation devices can elevate intramuscular pressure to a level sufficient to cause ischemia.[16]
- Wrinkling of Stockinette may cause high-pressure areas and subsequent bruising as the pressure in the appliance increases.
- Application over superficial nerves may result in neuropathy and/or nerve palsy.[17]

Instrumentation

Refer to the operator's guide for the unit you are using.

Power: Turns the unit on or off.

Temperature: With cold compression units, regulates the temperature of the fluid flowing through a refrigeration device to the appliance. Some portable cold compression units use ice cubes for this purpose. The temperature of the fluid is displayed in the **TEMPERATURE GAUGE.**

Pressure: Adjusts the amount of compression in millimeters of mercury (mm Hg) applied to the extremity. This value should not exceed the patient's diastolic blood pressure. Many units have a digital or analog pressure display.

ON-OFF time: Controls the proportion of the time that the compression is on and off. This control may be a single switch with selectable duty cycles, or the **ON** (inflation time) and **OFF** (deflation time) times may be adjusted separately to set the duty cycle.

Pump: Turns on the pressure to the appliance.

Drain: Removes the pressure and deflates the appliance.

Setup and Application

Do not use intermittent compression devices in the presence of flammable gases such as anesthetics or oxygen.

Unit Preparation
1. Inspect the unit, garment, and hoses for obvious defects.
2. Plug the unit in or make sure that the batteries are fully charged.
3. Select the appropriate size of appliance for the extremity being treated (Fig. 14-6).
4. Check the appliance for tears or leaks. If a defect is found, repair the defect with an approved patch kit, return the appliance to the manufacturer for repair, or discard the appliance.

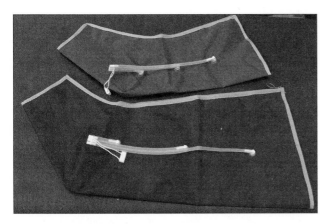

Figure 14-6. **Compression Appliances.** Top: Half-leg. Bottom: Full-leg. Other varieties and sizes are also available.

Patient Preparation
1. Establish the absence of contraindications.
2. Remove any jewelry on the patient's extremity being treated.
3. Determine the patient's diastolic blood pressure.
4. To evaluate the effectiveness of the treatment, mark one or more areas on the extremity, measure, and record the girth measurement of the body part being treated.[18]
5. For sanitary purposes, cover the area to be treated with Stockinette or similar material. Care must be taken to ensure that this inner layer is free of wrinkles.
6. Insert the injured limb into the appliance. When full-length appliances are used, avoid bunching the garment in the axilla or groin. To reduce the risk of neuropathy, do not overtighten the appliance and avoid placing straps and buckles over superficial nerves.[17]
7. For best results, elevate the limb during treatment. (With fluid-filled units it is easier to allow the appliance to initially fill and then to elevate the body part.)
8. Connect the appliance to the compression unit. Note that these units have input and exhaust tubes. The hoses must be properly connected to the appliance and the unit (Fig. 14-7). If a sequential compression unit is being used, the appliance and hoses must be connected so that the appliance fills from distal to proximal.

Initiation of the Treatment
1. If the intermittent compression unit uses a cold fluid, select the **TEMPERATURE** to be used, generally between 50°F and 55°F.
2. Select the maximal **PRESSURE** for the treatment. Normal pressure ranges are 30 to 60 mm Hg for the upper extremity and 60 to 100 mm Hg for the lower extremity (Table 14-1).[19] This pressure

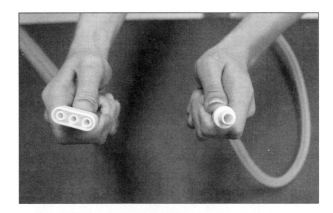

Figure 14-7. **Connectors for Intermittent and Sequential Compression Devices.** Sequential compression devices have two airways for each chamber in the appliance, one to inflate the chamber and the other to deflate it *(left connector).* Intermittent or constant compression devices usually only have one airway *(right).*

TABLE 14-1	**Intermittent Compression Treatment Parameters Used for Edema Reduction**

EXTREMITY	INFLATION PRESSURE	ON:OFF RATIO
Upper Extremity	40–60 mm Hg	3:1
Lower Extremity	60–100 mm Hg	3:1

should normally not exceed the diastolic blood pressure. If the treatment pressure must exceed the diastolic pressure, monitor the patient closely and use a lower duty cycle. Note that the actual pressure within the appliance is often significantly greater (up to 80% more) than the pressure displayed on the meter, especially in sequential units.[11,19] Because of the potential discrepancy between the metered pressure and actual pressure applied to the extremity, monitor the patient's distal neurovascular function.

3. Select the **ON-OFF** times. A 3:1 duty cycle (e.g., 45 seconds ON, 15 seconds OFF) is used, although the benefit of this protocol relative to others has not been substantiated. Individual manufacturers may recommend different protocols based on the characteristics of their machine.

4. Select the appropriate **TREATMENT TIME.** Treatment for post-traumatic edema may be given for 20 to 30 minutes. Treatment of lymphedema may be given for several hours.

5. Inform the individual about the sensations to be expected during the treatment. Instruct the patient to contact you if any unusual sensations, such as pain or a "tingling" feeling, are experienced during the treatment.

6. Encourage the patient to perform gentle range-of-motion exercises or wiggle the fingers (upper extremity treatments) or toes (lower extremity treatments) during the off cycle, if appropriate.

7. If long-term treatments (i.e., more than 60 consecutive minutes) are being administered, regularly interrupt the session and inspect the extremity being treated for proper capillary refill or the presence of unusual markings or unexpected pitting edema.

✳ Practical Evidence

There have been documented cases of peroneal neuropathy as the result of sequential compression application. To avoid this, assure that the appliance is of the appropriate length (evidence suggests that people of shorter stature are more predisposed to neuropathy).[17]

Termination of the Treatment
1. Reduce ON time or, if applicable, select the DRAIN mode to remove the air or fluid from the appliance.
2. Gently remove the body part from the appliance.
3. Remeasure the circumference of the extremity and determine the amount of edema reduction.
4. Apply a compression wrap or compression garment and any appropriate supportive devices. Instruct the patient to keep the limb elevated whenever possible between treatments.

Maintenance

Refer to the manufacturer's recommendations for maintenance intervals and procedures. Disconnect the compression unit from the electrical power source before cleaning.

Following Each Treatment
1. Clean the appliance using an approved cleanser.
2. If appliances are machine washable, turn them inside out and close them using the zipper.
3. Gas sterilization systems should be used when possible.
4. After cleaning, allow the appliance to dry, roll the hose(s), and store in a dry area.

Quarterly or as Indicated
1. Check air/water hoses for defects and replace if necessary.
2. Clean the external unit using an approved cleanser.
3. Check the electrical plug, electrical cord, and control cord (if present) for nicks, frays, or other visible damage.

Annually or as Required
1. A qualified service technician should perform an inspection and any subsequent maintenance, if necessary.

Chapter 15

Continuous Passive Motion

Continuous passive motion units are motorized devices that move one or more joints through a preset range of motion at a controlled speed. The joint movement is theorized to improve healing of soft tissue and certain articular pathologies and may prevent joint contractures and delay atrophy. Although these devices were originally designed for use on the knee, models have been developed for most joints.

● Continuous passive motion (CPM) is the antithesis of immobilization, a common postsurgical management technique. To deter the unwanted effects of immobilization, CPM devices deliver gentle stresses to the healing tissues. Still predominantly used for knee injuries, CPM units have been designed for the hand, wrist, hip, shoulder, elbow, and ankle (Fig. 15-1). Although passive motion can be applied through a dedicated CPM unit, it can be delivered manually by the clinician, but for a much shorter time.

Robert Salter,[20] a Canadian physician, originally proposed the use of CPM to assist in the healing of synovial joints. On the basis of his clinical observations, Salter hypothesized that the application of CPM would be beneficial in three ways:

- Enhancing the nutrition and metabolic activity of articular cartilage
- Stimulating tissue remodeling and regrowth of articular cartilage

- Accelerating the healing of articular cartilage, tendons, and ligaments

CPM devices are categorized into three types of design: free linkage, anatomical, and nonanatomical.[21,22] The free linkage design is similar to manually moving the patient's limb through the range of motion (ROM) by grasping it proximal and distal to the joint. Because the joint itself is not supported, free linkage units are not suitable for unstable joints.[22] CPM devices that incorporate an anatomical design attempt to mimic the natural motion of the involved joint and the proximal joints. Anatomical CPMs are the most suitable for the knee.

Nonanatomically designed CPM units make no attempt to replicate the natural joint motion, with compensatory movement occurring between the patient's extremity and the CPM's carriage. Table 15-1 summarizes the advantages and disadvantages of each of these styles of CPM units. Regardless of the type of CPM unit used, avoid placing unwanted stress on the joint's structures.

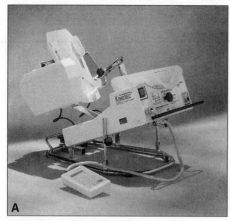
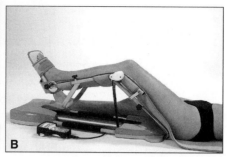
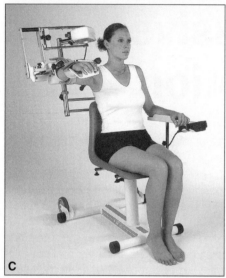
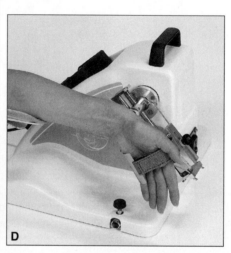

Figure 15-1. **Continuous Passive Motion Devices.** (A) Ankle. (B) Knee. (C) Shoulder. (D) Wrist and hand. (Kinetec courtesy of Sammons Preston Rolyan, an Ability One Company.)

TABLE 15-1 **Characteristics of Continuous Passive Motion Designs**

Continuous Passive Motion Linkage Design

PARAMETER	FREE LINKAGE	ANATOMICAL DESIGN	NONANATOMICAL DESIGN
Joint stability	Very poor	Good	Fair
Control of ROM	Very poor	Excellent	Fair
Total ROM	Poor	Excellent	Good
Multiaxis motion	Good	Poor	Fair
Adjustable to the patient	Excellent	Poor	Fair

ROM = range of motion.
Source: Adapted from Saringer.[22]

● EFFECTS ON

The Injury Response Process

The philosophy regarding the effects of CPM is "Motion that is never lost need never be regained. It is the regaining of movement that is painful."[23] Constant, gentle stresses applied to the injured structure encourage the remodeling of collagen along the lines of force and reduce the negative effects of joint immobilization.[24] When the injured joint is kept in motion, the unwanted effects of immobilization on muscle, tendons, ligaments, articular and hyaline cartilage, blood supply, and nerve supply are reduced (Fig. 15-2).

Under the stress of motion, collagen—normally deposited in a random order—aligns along the line of applied stress. This realignment reduces functional shortening, cross-linking of collagen, and capsular adhesions, thus maintaining the ROM,[21,25] enhancing the tensile strength of

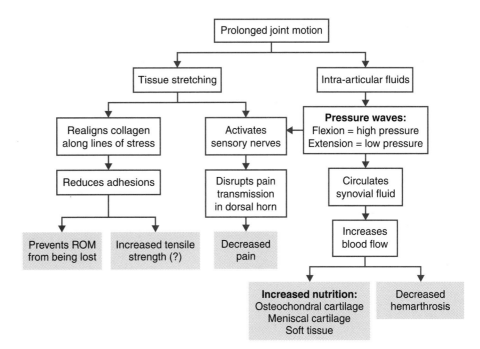

Figure 15-2. **Effects of Continuous Passive Motion.**

tendons, **allografts** •, and skin,[20] and stimulating repair of meniscal[26] articular cartilage.[26,27,28]

As the joint moves from extension to flexion and back, fluids within the capsule are exposed to low pressure where the joint volume is the greatest (normally extension) and high pressure where the joint volume is least. As the flexion angle increases, the pressures in the joint increase. As this cycle repeats, the change in pressure creates a pumping effect that circulates the synovial fluid. The circulating fluid may assist in the removal of joint **hemarthrosis** •, periarticular edema, and blood from the tissues surrounding the joint.[29] The circulation of synovial fluids activates anti-inflammatory mediators in meniscal cartilage.[26] The amount of ROM applied during the CPM sessions must be sufficient to increase intra-articular pressure but not be so great as to damage the surrounding soft tissue or graft.[30]

The effects and benefits associated with CPM are not universally substantiated or accepted. The decision to use CPM should be made on a patient-by-patient basis rather than for specific pathologies. The benefits derived from this treatment and the associated costs versus other treatment techniques should be considered when developing the treatment plan.[31,32] Active ROM exercises should be incorporated into the patient's treatment plan as soon as practical.[33]

Range of Motion

Introducing CPM early into the rehabilitation scheme may allow active motion and strength training routines to be incorporated earlier in the patient's program, an important consideration when dealing with an active population.[34,35,36]

When compared to patients receiving standard therapy, the benefits of CPM increasing the joint's ROM are seen early in the patient's rehabilitation program, but no long-term differences are realized.[28] When given free rein to control the ROM, patients, using comfort as their guide, increase their ROM by 6 to 7 degrees per day.[37]

CPM is more effective in increasing ROM caused by soft tissue restriction (for example, tightness of the Achilles' tendon during ankle dorsiflexion) than static stretching.[38] When applied immediately following surgery, CPM can be effective in increasing the amount of knee flexion, but this effect has not been substantiated following total knee **arthroplasty** •.[39,40] The need for manipulation of the knee joint following arthroplasty is significantly reduced or eliminated by the use of CPM.[29,41,42]

✱ Practical Evidence

Studies generally agree that CPM has limited utility following knee arthroplasty.[43,44,45,46] Only slight increases in knee flexion (2 degrees) and knee extension (3 degrees) are realized when CPM is applied immediately after surgery. The length of hospital stay is not affected, but the need for follow-up manipulation is reduced. The differing protocol, pathologies, and patient base used in these studies make reaching a firm conclusion regarding the efficacy of CPM on ROM impractical, although most studies demonstrate equivalency in the total ROM over the long term.

Allograft: A replacement or augmentation of a biological structure with a synthetic one.
Hemarthrosis: Blood in a joint.
Arthroplasty: Surgical reconstruction or replacement of an articular joint.

Increasing ROM may be contingent on the amount of time that the joint spends in the extremes of the ROM, or **total end-range time** (TERT). Increasing the TERT delivers a low-load, prolonged stress on the tissues, significantly increasing the ROM compared with a short-duration, high-load stress.[47]

The use of CPM alone does not fully restore ROM and has little effect on muscle strength. Manual or active therapy is required to fully restore strength and ROM. An undocumented benefit of the early application of CPM may be its assistance in helping the patient overcome the apprehension of moving the knee after surgery.

Lower extremity CPM has also been used to maintain the ROM in patients suffering from advanced cardiovascular pathology that restricts walking. CPM decreases the rate of atrophy and functional shortening of the quadriceps group with little increase in cardiovascular demands.[48]

Following rotator cuff repair, patients undergoing CPM demonstrated safe improvements in pain, ROM, and other functional measures.[28] However, these outcomes were no better than the results obtained from manual passive ROM exercises.[32]

Joint Nutrition

Both meniscal and articular cartilage are relatively avascular and derive most of their nutrients from synovial fluid. Meniscal and articular cartilage is sponge-like and is nourished by expansion and compression; through the natural movement of the joint, the synovial fluid is alternately absorbed by and squeezed out of the cartilage. During immobilization, synovial fluid is not distributed throughout the joint. The application of CPM is thought to stimulate the circulation of synovial fluids and causes the meniscal cartilage to increase its uptake of nutrients. The delivery and the subsequent absorption of nutrients assist both types of cartilage in the healing process.[49–51]

The use of early CPM for condylar cartilage defects assists in the healing process, maintains joint ROM, and has a better functional outcome than early active motion.[52–54] Active ROM can place unwanted compressive forces on the joint surfaces, as in the case of osteochondral defects or chondromalacia. By circulating synovial fluid, condylar cartilage healing is accelerated through the deposition of type II collagen,[50,53,54] but intra-operative inspection does not support these findings.[28] Healing of full-thickness defects may require up to 2 weeks of treatment.[50]

Edema Reduction

The effectiveness of CPM in the reduction of edema is not clearly understood and varies according to the body part and condition being treated.[55] The passive movements of the limb and the elevation of the body part should assist in venous and lymphatic return by milking the muscle.[56] Significant edema reduction after arthroplasty of the knee and ankle,[29,36,57] after anterior cruciate ligament (ACL) surgery, for knee inflammatory conditions,[58] and for hand edema[59,60] has been documented.

Pain Reduction

The movement of the joint activates afferent nerves located in the muscle, joint, and skin, and possibly provides pain control through the gate mechanism. Any associated reduction in edema or muscle spasm, as well as deterrence of functional shortening, would aid in limiting pain. However, CPM is not used as an acute pain-control technique.

✳ Practical Evidence

Studies show no significant difference in pain (as reported using a visual analog scale) and pain medication between patients receiving CPM and those not receiving CPM,[31,61] those receiving manual passive ROM treatments,[32] and those patients controlling their own medication dosage.[62]

Postoperatively, pain control medications may be administered to the patient during the CPM treatment. Narcotic injections or patient-controlled analgesia pumps, local anesthetic injection, or regional nerve blocks are employed to reduce the patient's post-operative pain and the discomfort associated with CPM.[30]

Ligament Healing

The early use of CPM promotes healing, often more so than surgical correction when a single ligament is involved and there is little rotational instability of the joint.[63] The physiological benefits of CPM application post–ACL surgery are not as promising as its use with other conditions. The ACL does not receive the same nutritional benefits from CPM as meniscal or articular cartilage.[64] The ACL is surrounded by its own synovial lining, which shields the ligament from gaining nutrition from the joint's synovial fluid. Instead, the ACL must rely on its intrinsic blood vessels.

✳ Practical Evidence

Although CPM is often used following ACL reconstruction and rotator cuff repair, a synthesis of published research does not support these practices versus active exercise alone, especially when costs are considered.[46,65–67]

Initial ROM immediately following surgery is increased in patients who receive CPM relative to those patients not receiving CPM. However, as long as proper follow-up therapy is received, there is no long-term difference in the joint's ROM.[68,69,70] CPM applied immediately following surgery has been demonstrated to be effective in increasing the biomechanical properties of allograft-augmented medial collateral ligament reconstruction.[71]

Many knee CPM units having a proximal posterior tibial bar cause an excessive amount of **translation** • of the tibia on the femur. In procedures such as ACL surgery, this movement could produce stress sufficient to damage the healing tissue and graft (Fig. 15-3).[72] After surgery, a properly fitted CPM can be used without increasing anterior ACL laxity.[73,74]

■ Contraindications

Unwanted joint motion and the associated stresses on bones and joint structures are the primary contraindications to CPM (see At a Glance: Continuous Passive Motion). CPM must not be applied in the presence of an unstable fracture. Because of the threat of causing it to spread, CPM should not be used in areas of uncontrolled infection. Likewise, CPM is contraindicated with spastic paralyses because the antagonistic motion may result in muscle damage.

CPM should be used with caution if the patient has a history of deep vein thrombosis. The pressure from the CPM cradle and increased venous return caused by limb motion and elevation may dislodge the clot. Intracompartmental pressures may be increased by the motion and/or supporting cradle straps.

Some CPM designs increase the amount of shear forces crossing the joint and unduly stress the soft tissues and graft. The type of CPM, arc of motion, and speed of motion should be adjusted based on the physician's recommendations for the pathology being treated.

■ Overview of the Evidence

Although the rationale for the use of CPM is sound, many published research articles question the efficacy for most clinical applications. Likewise, CPM has not been demonstrated to be more effective than traditional manual therapies (usually passive ROM).[31] The exception to this is the condition involving the articular cartilage in which compression of the joint surfaces must be avoided.[52,53]

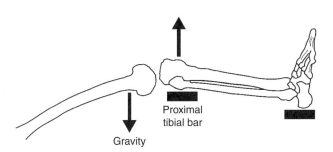

Figure 15-3. Tibial Translation During Continuous Passive Motion. A proximal bar supports the tibia while gravity allows the femur to move downward. This effect, coupled with the force of motion, can place unwanted stresses on the anterior cruciate ligament.

The effects of CPM on the healing of articular cartilage healing cannot be validated because of the lack of quality, controlled studies.[28]

CPM is often used following total knee arthroplasty and has subsequently been the focus of retrospective and prospective investigation. Some studies have concluded that CPM is beneficial in decreasing the length of hospital stay, decreased need for analgesic medication, earlier implementation of straight leg raises, and improved knee function/satisfaction scores at the time of discharge.[75] Evidence also suggests that the need for knee manipulations following arthroplasty is reduced.[41,42]

Following total knee arthroplasty, ROM in higher degrees of knee flexion (70 to 110 degrees) required less pain medication than patients receiving CPM within 0 to 50 degrees of flexion or no CPM, but these differences were not statistically significant.[61] Other studies have demonstrated that effects on length of hospital stay [40–42] and Knee Society Score (a measure of knee function and patient satisfaction) followed similar patterns.[40,61]

Nearly all studies conclude that there is no significant long-term difference in pain or ROM between patients who received postoperative CPM and those who did not.[29,32,40–42,61,75–79] The decision to include CPM in the early treatment protocol must be made by considering the immediate and long-term benefits relative to the associated costs and potential hazards.[31,39]

■ Clinical Application of Continuous Passive Motion

Instrumentation

Refer to the operator's guide for the unit you are using.

Power: This switch activates the internal circuits of the CPM unit.

Reset: This button clears all previous settings from the CPM unit's memory.

Timer: This control sets the duration of the treatment. A CONTINUOUS setting is provided for long-term treatments.

ROM: This control adjusts the ROM from slight hyperextension (approximately +5 degrees) to full flexion (approximately 130 degrees). Some units have separate controls to adjust the amount of flexion and extension.

Speed: This knob adjusts the rate of motion between 10 and 120 degrees per second. Slow speeds are used immediately postsurgery or postinjury. Increased speed (cycles per second) has been theorized to produce better tensile properties of healing tendons than lower speeds.[80]

Deceleration/Acceleration: Adjusts the number of degrees per second the joint accelerates at the beginning of the motion and decelerates during the terminal phase of motion.

Translation: Sliding or gliding of opposing articular surfaces.

At a Glance: **Continuous Passive Motion**

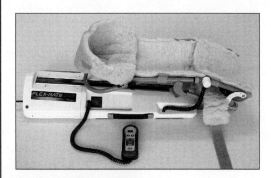

Description

A motorized device that moves one or more joints at a controlled speed through a preset range of motion. Continuous passive motion is used to restore early range of motion, delaying atrophy and improving joint nutrition.

Indications

- After surgical repair of stable intra-articular or extra-articular joint fractures
- After joint surgery, including surgery on the ACL[74]
- Following open reduction–internal fixation fracture management
- After joint arthroplasty
- After surgery or chronic pathology to the knee extensor mechanisms
- Joint contractures
- Following meniscectomy
- After knee manipulations
- After joint débridement for **arthrofibrosis** ●
- Tendon lacerations
- After osteochondral repair
- For enhancing the reabsorption of a hemarthrosis
- Thrombophlebitis
- Following surgical correction of chondromalacia patellae

Primary Effects

- Improved nutrition of articular structures
- Increased metabolic activity of articular structures
- Increased remodeling of collagen along the lines of stress
- Increased tensile strength of healing tendons, ligaments, and other soft tissue
- Improved early range of motion
- Potential edema reduction
- Pain reduction via secondary mechanisms (e.g., increased ROM)

Contraindications

- Cases in which the device causes an unwanted translation of opposing bones, overstressing the healing tissues
- Unstable fractures
- Spastic paralyses
- Uncontrolled infection

Treatment Duration

Continuous passive motion may be applied in long-term bouts where the patient is continuously attached to the unit, or the device may be applied in 1-hour treatment bouts three times a day. After surgery, use is for 6 to 8 hours a day, although the duration preferred by patients is 4 to 8 hours.[37] Patients may also be instructed in the use of CPM for in-home treatments, or a home-care visit may be required.

Precautions

- The use of continuous passive motion in conjunction with anticoagulation therapy may produce an intracompartmental hematoma[81] or deep vein thrombosis.[30]
- Skin irritation from the straps or carriage cover may develop. Overtightening of the straps and/or dressing can lead to necrosis of the incision sites or other local tissue.[10]

Arthrofibrosis: The repair and replacement of inflamed joint tissue by connective tissues.

TERT: Total end range time. The amount of time the joint is held in the end of flexion and extension ROM.

Pause (Extension/Flexion Delay): This button stops the motion at the extreme ROM (flexion and/or extension) to allow a passive stretching of the fibers to occur.

Interrupt Switch: This control allows the patient to discontinue the CPM.

Trigger jack: Some units allow synchronization of CPM and electrical stimulation. The TRIGGER JACK allows the neuromuscular electrical stimulation unit to be activated during the PAUSE function.

Program: Microprocessor-controlled CPM devices may have preprogrammed protocols that are selected from a menu. User-defined protocol may also be stored and recalled for later use. Refer to the operator's manual for step-by-step instructions.

Setup and Application

Often, the CPM unit is applied in the recovery room after surgery by a CPM technician. The following protocol is provided as an example for a post–ACL reconstructive surgery. Refer to the operator's manual for other knee protocols and/or the operation of CPM units designed for other body parts. Advanced units, especially those for the shoulder, may require specialized training to assure proper setup and protocol selection. CPM devices should not be used in the presence of flammable gases such as anesthetics or oxygen.

Preparation for the Treatment

1. Confirm that the patient is free of contraindications to the use of CPM (see At a Glance: Continuous Passive Motion).
2. Ensure that the unit is clean and fit the CPM unit with a clean carriage cover.
3. Most CPM devices can be adjusted to fit the involved extremity even when the patient is wearing a brace or surgical bandages.
4. The physician may elect to remove circumferential wraps (e.g., cotton batting, elastic wraps) and cover the limb with a single cotton or elastic sleeve.[30]
5. Measure the length of the patient's thigh from the ischial tuberosity to the joint line of the knee. Adjust the proximal carriage so that the proximal end meets the bottom of the buttocks and, if applicable to the unit, aligns with the coxofemoral joint.
6. Determine the length of the lower leg by measuring from the joint line of the knee to approximately 1/4 inch beyond the heel. Adjust the distal portion of the carriage accordingly.
7. Place the lower extremity in the unit with the joint line of the knee aligning to the articular hinge of the CPM unit (Fig. 15-4).
8. Adjust the foot in the footplate so that the tibia is placed in the neutral position. Internally or

externally rotating the tibia can result in increased stress on the ACL.

Initiation of the Treatment

1. Give the patient the handheld control and provide instruction on how and when to use it, including adjusting the speed and ROM and terminating the treatment.
2. Set the ROM as prescribed by the physician. Generally this protocol is started with a limited ROM (0 to 60 degrees) and progresses to the full ROM as healing occurs and pain decreases. The programmed ROM and the actual ROM imposed on the joint may be up to 20 degrees different.[22,82] Confirm the actual joint motion using a goniometer.
3. Set the SPEED of the treatment (e.g., cycle time of 4 minutes; 15 cycles per hour). Units may have preprogrammed protocols that are chosen from a menu.
4. The patient may be instructed to increase the ROM at regular intervals as tolerated. Some units do not allow the protocol to be changed once the treatment has been initiated.
5. Instruct the patient and those tending the patient (including family members) to recognize pressure-related problems caused by the CPM carriage. Adjust the carriage accordingly.
6. If this is a home-based treatment, the patient should be provided with written instructions and an emergency contact number.
7. Regularly check the patient for signs of intracompartmental hemorrhage or deep vein thrombosis.

Termination of the Treatment

1. Position the carriage to best suit removing the limb from the unit, usually just short of full extension.

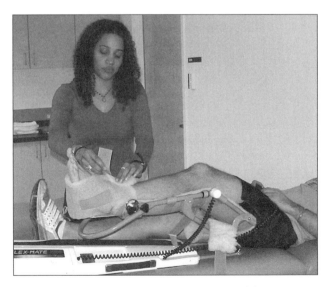

Figure 15-4. **Setup for Continuous Passive Motion.** The joint axis must be aligned with the hinges on the CPM cradle.

2. Loosen the restraining straps, footplate, or other supports.
3. Carefully lift the extremity and have an assistant remove the CPM unit.
4. Cut or remove the sleeve from the extremity.
5. Inspect the extremity for pressure sores, distal redness, or swelling that is indicative of increased compartmental pressure or deep vein thrombosis, and the surgical sites for proper healing. Notify a physician if any abnormal findings are noted.
6. Clean the extremity according to the physician's protocol.
7. If indicated, redress the surgical wounds and reapply a sterile dressing or compression wrap.

Maintenance

Refer to the manufacturer's recommendations for maintenance intervals and procedures. Disconnect the CPM unit from the electrical power source prior to cleaning.

Following Each Treatment
1. Clean the surfaces with a disinfectant soap. If the unit becomes soiled with blood or other bodily fluids use a 10% solution of household chlorine bleach to clean the surfaces.
2. Clean or replace the carriage cover. Some covers can be sterilized by using an **autoclave** ● at 225°F (125°C). Check the manufacturer's recommendations for additional hygiene concerns. Covers may be reused for the same patient, but patient-to-patient reuse is not recommended.

Quarterly or as Indicated
Some units have an automatic alert that maintenance is needed.
1. Lubricate all moving parts (e.g., joints, ball bearings, threaded rods).
2. Check the electrical plug, electrical cord, and control cord (if present) for nicks, frays, or other visible damage.

Autoclave: A device used to sterilize medical instruments using steam heat at 250°F (121°C).

16

Cervical and Lumbar Traction

Cervical and lumbar traction are applications of a force that separates the vertebrae and opens the intervertebral space in the treated area. The increased space reduces pressure on the intervertebral disks and spinal nerve roots, opens the facet joints, and elongates the soft tissue.

● Traction is a technique that applies a longitudinal force to the spine and associated structures, distracting the vertebrae. The distractive force can be administered by gravity (weights or body weight), a machine, the clinician, or by the position of the patient's body. Mechanical force is applied with either continuous or intermittent tension using several different methods. The force of the traction can occur in one plane or multiple planes (polyaxial traction).

Traction is indicated in conditions in which the patient's pain is caused by mechanical pressure on the vertebrae, facet joints, or spinal nerve roots, or other conditions in which removing the mechanical stress results in pain reduction. Unless specifically prescribed by a physician, traction should not be used for acute injuries, hypermobile vertebrae, or other instances when the stability of the vertebral column is in question.

Traction, immobilization, and bed rest were once the common treatments of choice for spinal and back pain. Contemporary practice frequently emphasizes active exercise with traction being used to provide short-term,

mechanical relief of pressure placed on nerve roots, articular facets, and other structures.

■ Principles of Traction

The effect and effectiveness of traction is related to the position of the body part, the position of the patient, the force and duration of the traction, and the angle of pull.[83] To distract the vertebrae, the force applied must be sufficient to overcome the sum of resistance of the weight of the body part being treated, the tension of the surrounding soft tissues, the force of friction between the patient and the table, and the force of gravity. Friction is negligible during cervical traction and lumbar/pelvic traction when a split table is used. Gravity works against cervical spine traction when the patient is seated; when the patient is supine, gravity is not a factor.

Traction is an appropriate treatment modality for hypomobile vertebrae. Traction should not be used in the presence of hypermobility of vertebral segments. The tension may lead to subluxation or dislocation of the vertebra or further increase the hypermobility of the segment.

Types of Traction

Traction maintains the cervical or lumbar spine in an elongated position and can be delivered continuously or intermittently (Table 16-1). **Sustained traction** is applied with relatively small force for 45 minutes or less; the tension in **continuous traction** does not change over the course of hours or days. These methods of application stimulate the supporting and stabilizing functions of the spinal structures, allowing the muscles to relax.

Sustained traction is applied through a weight-and-pulley system, pneumatic system, motorized device, or patient positioning. **Manual traction** is administered by the clinician. During **auto-traction** the patient controls the amount of traction applied.

Intermittent traction alternates periods of traction force with intervals of relaxation in the tension by way of an ON/OFF duty cycle. During the ON cycle, the vertebral segments are distracted and the soft tissues are elongated. The OFF or relaxation phase allows a relative decrease in the amount of neuromuscular activity. Intermittent traction is most commonly applied through the use of a motorized system or manually by the clinician (Fig. 16-1).

The patient may also self-administer **positional traction** techniques (Fig. 16-2). Body position is used to elongate—stretch—the involved tissues or reduce pressure on the vertebral structures.

Angle of Pull

The angle of the applied traction is described relative to the long axis of the vertebral column and must be appropriate for the pathology being treated. Traction angles are described as neutral (transverse plane), flexion or extension (frontal plane), or unilateral (sagittal plane). Multiaxial (sometimes referred to as polyaxial) traction applies a distractive force in both the frontal and sagittal plane.

TABLE 16-1 Types of Traction

Type	Description
Continuous	Constant tension applied for more an extended time (i.e., days) delivered using mechanical means such as weights and pulleys. Traction is delivered at a low load and is used to slightly lengthen soft tissues or for immobilization.
Sustained	Constant tension applied for less than 45 minutes delivered using mechanical means (e.g., motorized unit, weights and pulleys). Tension is administered with a higher load than continuous traction, allowing for separation of bony structures.
Intermittent	Alternates bouts of tension with no tension. Tension is delivered for 15 to 120 seconds and is followed by an interval of decreased or no tension. Delivered using a motorized unit or manual techniques, intermittent traction delivers a relatively high traction load that stretches soft tissues and separates the vertebra.
Manual traction	Sustained or intermittent traction applied by the clinician.
Positional traction	Traction placed on the spine based on the patient's posture and/or gravity. Positional traction stretches soft tissue and affects the pressure on bony surfaces.
Auto-traction	Mechanical traction where the patient controls the amount of tension

Note: Some of the above traction types can be applied in combination.

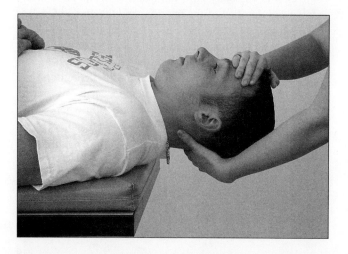

Figure 16-1. **Manual Cervical Traction.** The clinician grasps the patient's occiput to apply traction along the length of the entire cervical spine.

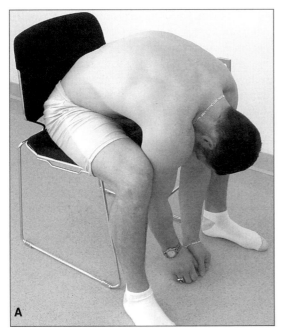
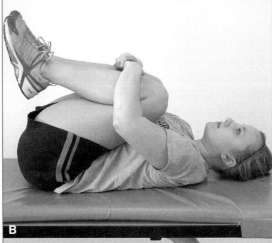

Figure 16-2. **Positional Traction Techniques.** (A) For the thoracic and cervical spine. (B) For the lumbar spine.

Sagittal Angle

In healthy tissue, the application of an equal amount of tension on the right and left side of the body should result in an approximately equal amount of separation on both sides of the vertebrae. Hypomobile conditions such as unilateral muscle spasm or adhesions can cause increased opening on the non-involved side when traction is applied; unilateral soft-tissue laxity can result in increased opening on the involved side (Fig. 16-3). The patient's physical examination should identify the bilateral balance of traction to be used during the treatment.

Unilateral tension can be placed on the vertebrae by the use of a polyaxial harness or patient positioning. This method increases the amount of tension applied to the structures on the right or left side of the vertebrae and is useful with unilateral facet joint pathology, nerve root impingement, or muscle spasm.

Unilateral traction can often be achieved simply through patient positioning. This method of traction is used when lateral bending of the spine reduces the patient's symptoms.

Frontal Angle

The effect of the angle of pull in the frontal plane produces different results on the facet joints in the cervical and lumbar spine. In the cervical inferior facet joints are angled anteriorly; in the lumbar spine, they are angled posteriorly. Placing the cervical spine in flexion opens the facet joints and increases

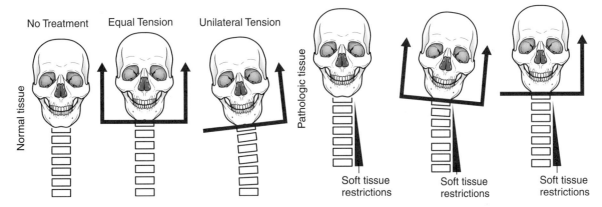

Figure 16-3. **Tension in the Sagittal Plane.** In the absence of hyper- or hypomobile tissues, equal tension during traction should cause an equal amount of separation between the vertebra. Unbalanced tension should result in an increased opening on the side with the greater tension. In the presence of pathologic tissue, in this example hypomobility on the patient's left side, equal tension will result in an increased separation on the nonaffected side. If the tension is greater on the hypomobile side, an equal amount of separation should occur. In the case of hypermobile tissue, the opposite would occur.

the intervertebral space, but too much flexion will result in a decrease in the anterior space. Because the lumbar facets are angled posteriorly, placing the lumbar spine in extension will open the facet joints. When the traction is applied in the neutral position, the intervertebral disk is allowed to elongate.

Tension

The amount of tension applied to the body is expressed in terms of pounds (or kilograms) or as a percentage of the patient's body weight. Once the traction force overcomes the effects of gravity, friction, and body weight, the force is then absorbed and dissipated by the patient's muscle tone and soft-tissue tension. Less force is needed to distract the cervical spine than the lumbar spine. The vertebrae closest to the source of the traction, C1–C2 during cervical traction or L5–S1 during lumbar traction for example, require less force to separate than those farther from the harness.

There is no clear formula used to determine the amount of tension to apply during the treatment. The general guideline is to use the least amount of tension needed to relieve the symptoms or produce the desired effects. The intensity of the traction should be inversely related to the duration of the treatment. Patients can tolerate more tension if the duration of the traction is reduced.

As we all know, more is not always better. This is certainly the case with traction, especially in the presence of unstable joints. Too much force can produce muscle guarding or can further injure the soft tissue. As discussed in the following section, too much force or too great a treatment duration can cause an overhydration of the intervertebral disks and increase their chance of rupture.[84]

■ General Uses for Cervical and Lumbar Traction

The fundamental effects of cervical traction and lumbar traction arise from the distraction of the vertebral segments. Before significant bony separation can occur, the force of the traction must first overcome the resistance exerted by the soft tissues. The benefits of traction tend to be short-lived but may be sufficient to break the pain-spasm-pain cycle (Fig. 16-4).

This section presents the common therapeutic benefits of treatment (Table 16-2). Specific effects or influences are described in the appropriate section.

Disk Protrusions

Disk protrusions can place pressure on a spinal nerve root, usually the one immediately below the involved disk, or

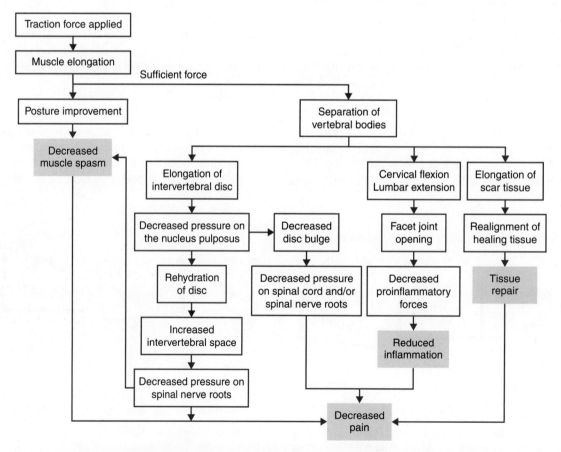

Figure 16-4. **General Effects of Traction.** The primary benefits of traction occur from decreasing the compressive forces between adjacent vertebrae. After overcoming muscle tension, the resulting effects decrease pressure on the intervertebral disks, open facet joints, and elongate ligaments and other intrinsic soft tissue. Note that placing the cervical spine in flexion opens the facet joints; applying a traction force with the lumbar spine in extension will open the facet joints.

compress the spinal cord. Because of their anatomical structure and high water content, disks have the ability to deform (Box 16-1). In the presence of a disk protrusion, body weight and muscle tone compress the disk and force the **nucleus pulposus** ● outward (Fig. 16-5).

Traction affects the disks by decreasing the pressure between contiguous vertebrae. Given sufficient tension, the vertebrae separate and elongate the disks. Negative pressure within the disk removes the forces on the nucleus pulposus, thereby decreasing pressure on the spinal cord

TABLE 16-2   **Guidelines for the Treatment of Various Pathologies With Traction**

PATHOLOGY	ANGLE	TYPE
Facet joint	Cervical: Flexion	Intermittent
	Lumbar: Extension	
	Unilateral (if pathology is unilateral)	
Intervertebral space (e.g., degenerative disk disease)	Cervical: Flexion (too much will result in decreased anterior space)	Sustained
	Lumbar: Neutral	
Nerve root impingement	Bilateral: Neutral	Sustained
	Unilateral: Neutral with spine laterally flexed to the opposite side	
Disk protrusion	Extension, neutral, or flexion (based on pain relief obtained)	Intermittent
Muscle spasm	Position the traction to elongate the affected tissues	Sustained
	Bilateral—Equal	
	Unilateral—Unilateral	

BOX 16-1. INTERVERTEBRAL DISKS AND DISK LESIONS

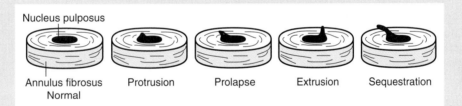

Vertebral disks consist of two distinct portions. The outer portion of the disk, the annulus fibrosus, is a relatively inflexible, dense, collagen-rich substance. The middle section, the nucleus pulposus, is a shock-absorbing material having a gelatinous consistency. Each disk is composed of 60 to 70% water, allowing it to be deformable, yet not easily compressed.[85]

During the day, the weight of the body slowly compresses the disks, causing them to dehydrate. At night—or when the body is reclined for long periods—the load is taken off the disks, and they expand and reabsorb fluids. For this reason, you are slightly taller in the morning than at night.[86] Over time the disks also lose proteoglycan, a molecule that attracts and retains water. The disks become more and more dehydrated between the ages of 40 and 60, resulting in decreased range of motion and a narrowing of the intervertebral **foramen** ●.[85,87]

Dehydration also weakens the annulus fibrosus, which allows the nucleus pulposus to protrude through and place pressure on the spinal nerve root. Protrusions, as used in this chapter, describe anything from a bulge in the disk to a complete rupture of the disk where the nucleus pulposus exits the disk. A definitive **diagnosis** ● of these conditions is made using an MRI, CT scan, or other imaging technique.

Traction helps reduce disk protrusions by separating the vertebrae, creating negative pressure within the disk, causing the nucleus pulposus to retreat away from the spinal nerve root and spinal cord.

Nucleus pulposus: The gelatinous middle of an intervertebral disk.

Foramen: An opening (e.g., in a bone) to allow the passage of blood vessels or nerves.

Diagnosis: A physician's determination of the nature and scope of an injury or illness.

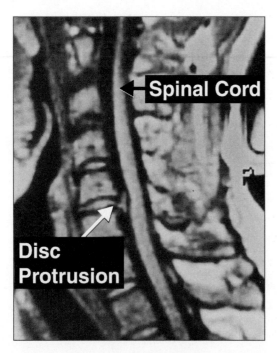

Figure 16-5. **Cervical Disk Herniation.** Note the posterior protrusion of the nucleus pulposus that places pressure on the spinal cord. Cervical traction can decrease the amount of pressure caused by a disk herniation.

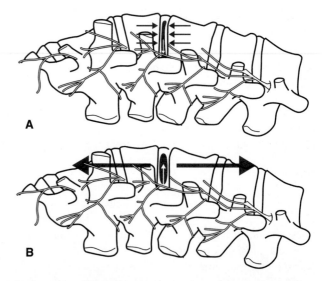

Figure 16-6. **Nerve Root Compression Caused by a Disk Protrusion.** (A) When the vertebrae are load bearing, the intervertebral disk compresses, forcing the nucleus pulposus posteriorly and laterally outward (similar to squeezing a tube of toothpaste), often placing pressure on a spinal nerve root. (B) Removing the weight-bearing forces causes the pulposus to return into the disk and relieve pressure on the nerve root.

and nerve root (Fig. 16-6).[88,89] Pressure from the tightening posterior longitudinal ligament may also force the pulposus inward.[90] Acute disk injuries respond better to traction than chronic lesions.[91] A displaced disk fragment may also be allowed to realign itself on the disk—and subsequently heal—by reducing the pressure and increasing the disk's hydration. Treatment of disk conditions typically require a long "ON" cycle (e.g., 60 seconds) and a short "OFF" cycle (e.g., 20 seconds).

Disk compression is often reproduced by patient positioning. In Figure 16-6A, if the patient flexes the spine, the nucleus pulposus is forced posteriorly, placing pressure on the nerve root. If the symptoms move outwardly (peripheralization), avoid that position during treatment. Educate the patient to always change positions or avoid activities that cause the peripheralization of symptoms.

Traction applied for too long can cause the disk to absorb too much fluid (imbibe). Similarly to an overfilled water balloon, an overly hydrated disk may be predisposed to rupture.[84] Sustained traction can also increase the amount of pressure at the end of the treatment, especially if the tension is not gradually reduced.

Degenerative Disk Disease and Nerve Root Compression

Degenerative disk disease is the gradual, progressive wasting of the intervertebral disks. As the disks lose their mass, the space between the disks decreases (Box 16-2). With time,

the vertebrae begin to form spurs and other **osteophytes** •, causing the vertebral column to straighten, creating a "bamboo pole" appearance (Fig. 16-7).

Increasing the intervertebral space opens the intervertebral foramen and reduces the amount of pressure on the nerve root. Removing the mechanical pressure on the nerve root allows the opportunity for inflammation of the nerve root to decrease.[88,89] Further nerve root compression can be prevented by reducing adhesions within the dural sleeve by elongating the surrounding structure.[91] In the lumbar nerve roots, traction can also reduce radicular symptoms by restoring the normal slack in the neuromeningeal structures.[92]

Facet Joint Pathology

The inferior facet of the superior vertebrae articulates with the superior facet of the vertebrae below (see Box 16-2). The facet joints significantly contribute to the spine's motion and decrease the stress placed on the vertebral bodies and disks. In healthy vertebrae, approximately 20% of the spine's weight-bearing load is transmitted through the facet joints. When the lumbar spine facet joints are inflamed they bear up to 47% of the load.[93]

When the angle of pull places the lumbar spine in extension or the cervical spine in flexion, the resulting tension opens the facet joints. Hypomobility of the facet joints is reduced by placing the spine in its neutral position. The resulting traction produces glide between the superior and inferior facets.

Osteophyte: A branching bony outgrowth.

Box 16-2. STENOSIS OF THE INTERVERTEBRAL FORAMEN

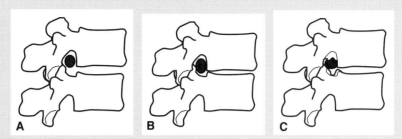

Thirty-one pairs of spinal nerve roots branch off the spinal cord, 8 in the cervical region, 12 in the thoracic region, 5 in the lumbar spine, and 6 in the sacrum. In the mobile spine, these roots exit the vertebral column via the intervertebral foramen, an opening formed by pairs of notches on the inferior surface of one vertebra with a corresponding notch on the superior surface of the vertebrae below. The intervertebral foramen normally allows plenty of room for the nerve root to exit between the vertebrae (Fig. A).

A narrowing of the intervertebral space, the area between the vertebral bodies, such as in the case of disk degeneration (see Box 16-1), can cause a decrease in the diameter of the intervertebral foramen (Fig. B). In some instances, this narrowing is sufficient to produce **radicular** ● symptoms along the involved nerve root's distribution.

Changes in the weight-bearing load on the vertebral bodies and the facet joints and biomechanical changes can result in the formation of osteophytes (Fig. C). The presence of this bony outgrowth not only decreases the size of the intervertebral foramen, it can cause inflammation of the nerve's sheath. Inflamed nerves occupy more space than healthy nerves, thus increasing the chance of impingement.

Although stenosis of the intervertebral foramen can occur at any level, this condition is most prevalent in the cervical and lumbar regions.

In the lumbar spine, approximately twice the tension required to elongate the lumbar spine is required to distract the facet joints.[94] Although less tension would be required in the cervical spine, the proportions of force required to obtain facet distraction would be expected to be reduced. The resulting reduced load can decrease inflammation and other compressive problems.

Muscle Spasm

Traction may be useful in the relief of muscle spasm caused by nerve root impingement or arising from postural disorders. Long, slow stretching can reduce tonic muscle contractions by elongating the involved fibers.[91] Stimulating the muscle's mechanoreceptors can decrease pain and spasm by activating the spinal gate.[92] Intermittent traction promotes relaxation during the OFF phase. Decreased pressure on the spinal nerve roots achieved by increasing the diameter of the intervertebral foramen also results in decreased muscle spasm (see Degenerative Disk Disease and Nerve Root Compression).

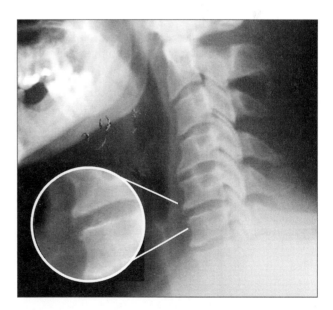

Figure 16-7. **Radiographic View of Degenerative Disk Disease.** Note the absence of the normal spinal curvature and the "beaking" appearance of the anterior and posterior aspects of the vertebral bodies *(inset).*

Radicular: Distally radiating pain caused by spinal nerve root involvement.

Other Effects

Although largely unsubstantiated, traction may also provide other benefits to the paraspinal structures. Improved circulation, increased metabolism, and enhanced nutrition of the structures have all been attributed to the application of cervical or lumbar traction.[90,91,95]

■ Cervical Traction

The human head accounts for approximately 8.1% of the total body weight (approximately 14 pounds for the average adult), but more force is needed to produce widening of the vertebral structures because of the cervical musculature and other soft tissues. For most pathologies, separation of the cervical spine begins to occur with an applied force equal to about 20% of the body weight with the patient reclined.[96] When the patient is in the seated, gravity-dependent position, a greater proportion of the total body weight is required before separation occurs. The effect of friction during cervical traction is, for the most part, negligible.

Motorized units can be used to administer intermittent or sustained traction. Intermittent traction may be delivered manually (see Fig. 16-1). Sustained traction can also be administered through a weight-and-pulley system or by a pneumatic device (Fig. 16-8).

Mechanical traction is applied to the cervical spine via a harness affixed to the skull. There are two basic types of harnesses: the mandibular-occipital harness and the occipital harness (Fig. 16-9). The mandibular-occipital harness can place too much pressure on the temporomandibular joint (TMJ) and may cause discomfort, especially if there is a pre-existing TMJ pathology. Occipital halters place all of the force on the skull's occipital bone and can place the cervical

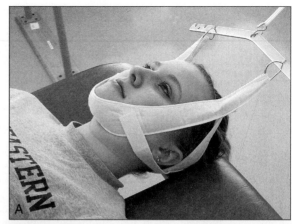
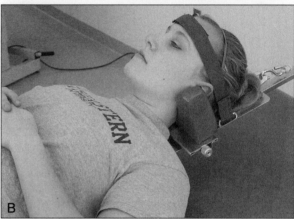

Figure 16-9. **Harnesses Used During the Application of Mechanical Cervical Traction.** (A) Mandibular-occipital harness. (B) Occipital harness.

spine in various degrees of flexion, extension, or lateral bending. Other specific styles of halters are designed to allow for specificity of spinal separation at a lower percentage of the body weight.[97] In general, patients experience less mouth and jaw discomfort when they wear a mouthguard during treatment. This technique is particularly useful in patients with periodontal health issues (e.g., tooth decay).[98]

Treatment Parameters

This section describes the variables of patient positioning and the type and amount of traction used during cervical traction. These variables must be consistent with the treatment goals needed to resolve the patient's disability. Refer to Table 16-2 for general treatment guidelines for common pathologies. Except for where noted, this section refers to mechanical traction techniques.

Patient Position

Cervical traction may be applied with the patient in one of several positions, but the two most common are the seated and supine positions. When the patient is seated, the traction must first overcome the force of gravity before therapeutic forces are placed on the cervical structures. Because of this, more tension is required to separate the

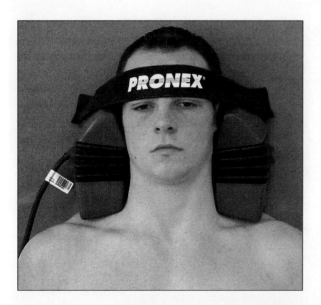

Figure 16-8. **Sustained Traction Using Pneumatic Pressure.** This method has the advantage over door-mounted units because the patient is placed in the horizontal, gravity-eliminated position. (Pronex courtesy of Glacier Cross, Inc., Kalispell, MT.)

vertebrae when the patient is seated than when the patient is horizontal.

The supine position has several advantages. With the patient supine, the cervical muscles are allowed to relax because they are not supporting the weight of the head. Therefore, a lower amount of tension is required to separate the vertebra and obtain therapeutic effects.[99]

Angle of Pull

To open the intervertebral space, place the cervical spine in approximately 25 to 30 degrees of flexion. This position straightens the normal cervical **lordotic** ● curvature, opening the posterior articulations, widening the intervertebral foramen, and stretching the posterior soft tissues. The anterior portions of the intervertebral disks are compressed, and the posterior portion elongates when the neck is placed in flexion. When the cervical spine is placed in extension, the opposite effect occurs.

To separate the facet joint surfaces, the traction must be administered in at least 15 degrees of flexion (Table 16-3).[100] When the patient is being treated in the seated position, vertebral separation is significantly increased when the patient is seated in the anterior lean position, increasing the angle of pull.[101]

Tension

Although cervical traction treatment bouts can last for hours, the mechanical benefits appear to occur in the first few minutes of treatment. When the patient is placed supine, vertebral separation begins when tension equal to 7% of the patient's body weight is applied.[102,103] Because of the weight of the structures and associated soft tissue, the upper vertebrae, C1–C2, require less force to separate than the lower cervical spine. The least amount of force necessary to produce the desired effects (e.g., decrease in symptoms) should be used. There is a significant increase in the opening of the intervertebral foramen between 5 kg and 10 kg of traction force; however, there is no additive benefit when the force is increased to 15 kg.[104]

Excess force applied to the cervical spine during traction may be transmitted to the lumbar area via the dural covering of the spinal cord. This can lead to residual lumbar nerve root impingement and subsequent pain, especially when the patient has a history of lumbar osteoarthritis or other lumbar degenerative changes.[83] During the treatment, question the patient about sensations in the cervical, thoracic, and lumbar spine and the extremities.

● EFFECTS ON

The Injury Response Process

The basic effects of cervical traction are similar to those presented in the biophysical effects section of this chapter.

TABLE 16-3 **Amount of Cervical Intervertebral Separation Based on the Angle of Traction**

		Traction Angle		
STRUCTURE	SPINAL SEGMENT	NEUTRAL	30° FLEXION	15° EXTENSION
Anterior intervertebral	C2–C3	6%	21%	2%
separation	C3–C4	8%	10%	-1%
	C4–C5	12%	16%	-1%
	C5–C6	5%	15%	-2%
	C6–C7	0%	9%	-2%
Posterior intervertebral	C2–C3	15%	5%	4%
separation	C3–C4	22%	4%	-14%
	C4–C5	19%	17%	-26%
	C5–C6	19%	19%	-37%
	C6–C7	37%	20%	-50%
Facet joint separation	C2–C3	2%	–12%	7%
	C3–C4	2%	–14%	3%
	C4–C5	5%	–19%	15%
	C5–C6	3%	–10%	17%
	C6–C7	10%	–5%	6%

Negative percentages indicate a decrease in the intervertebral space.
Source: Adapted from Wong, AM, et al: Clinical trial of a cervical traction modality with electromyographic biofeedback. Am J Phys Med Rehabil 76:19, 1997.

Lordosis: The forward curvature of the cervical and lumbar spine.

This section presents the research regarding the specific effects of cervical traction.

Application of cervical traction reduces the pressure on the cervical nerve roots caused by mechanical pressure from bony protuberances or intervertebral disk protrusions. Elongating the cervical spine separates the vertebrae and decompresses these structures.

Intermittent cervical traction is incorporated into the treatment plan to reduce the pain and paresthesia associated with cervical nerve root impingement, muscle spasm, or articular dysfunction. The most significant improvements are seen in patients who had symptoms for less than 12 weeks.[90] This passive treatment can be combined with active exercise to enhance the benefits of the treatment.

✳ Practical Evidence

A clinical prediction rule has been developed to identify patients who are most likely to benefit from cervical traction and exercise. Based on the following clinical findings:

- Age 55 or older
- Peripheralization of symptoms with mobilization of the C4–C7 vertebrae
- Positive shoulder abduction test
- Positive upper extremity nerve tension test
- Positive cervical distraction test

Patients who demonstrate three of these findings increase positive outcomes to 79%. When four of these findings are present the outcomes increase to 95%.[105] However, in most cases of cervical radiculopathy the addition of cervical traction does not improve patient outcomes.[106]

Muscle Spasm

Traction may be used to alleviate cervical muscle spasm by reducing the pressure on the cervical nerve roots or stretching the muscle in an effort to interrupt the pain-spasm-pain cycle. An analysis of **electromyograms** ● following treatment bouts of intermittent cervical traction showed no decrease in the amount of spasm in the treated tissues when compared with pretreatment activity.[96,107,108] However, another study did show reduced excitability of the alpha-motoneuron pool.[109]

The reduction of cervical muscle spasm is contingent on finding the optimal amount of traction force. Too little force will not sufficiently elongate the musculature or open the intervertebral foramen, and little or no benefit will be gained. If too much force is applied, an unwanted muscle contraction will ensue as the body attempts to protect itself, resulting in the opposite effect of that desired.

Pain

In addition to breaking the pain-spasm-pain cycle, as described in the previous section, several other factors have been associated with the reduction of pain. Traction can reduce pain by decreasing the amount of mechanical pressure placed on the cervical nerve roots. Intermittent traction is thought to improve blood flow and to decrease myofascial adhesions. This same rhythm may also stimulate joint and muscular sensory nerves and inhibit the transmission of pain through the gate mechanism.[110] In clinical practice, however, the addition of intermittent cervical traction in the treatment of chronic neck pain does not appear to improve patient outcomes.[111]

Cervical traction decreases the radicular symptoms associated with cervical nerve root impingement.[91] If the pain results from a disk lesion, the bulging nucleus pulposus is encouraged to centralize or return to its normal position. Although a disk lesion is not normally responsive to intermittent traction, sustained traction can provide the time necessary for reabsorption of the nucleus pulposus.

✳ Practical Evidence

Individuals diagnosed with cervical radiculopathy respond favorably to a treatment regime of manual therapy, cervical traction, and neck flexor muscle strengthening when the following predictors are present: younger than age 54, nondominant arm is affected, and looking down does increase the symptoms.[112]

Contraindications to the Use of Cervical Traction

Clinical cervical traction is absolutely contraindicated in the presence of vertebral fracture or dislocation. The exception to this is the use of traction immobilization such as a halo splint applied by a physician. All acute cervical spine trauma should be evaluated by a physician to rule out fractures, dislocations, or other spinal instability before clinical treatment (see At a Glance: Cervical Traction). Unless specifically ordered by a physician, cervical traction should not be used on patients with diseases, infection, or tumors that affect the cervical vertebrae. Care must also be taken to avoid cervical motions that are contraindicated.

Electromyogram: A recording of the electrical charges associated with the contraction of a muscle.

Traction applied to hypermobile joints can elongate the stabilizing tissues and lead to increased instability.[92] Do not use traction in the presence of severe disk herniations because of the possibility of increasing the rate of degeneration. Rheumatoid arthritis and osteoarthritis are contraindications because necrosis can cause ligamentous weakness. The force of the applied traction could result in vertebral subluxation or dislocation and further weaken the soft tissue structures.

Vertebral artery dysfunction is a contraindication to cervical traction, by using unilateral or polyaxial techniques. Cervical traction should not be used on patients who experience dizziness during treatment or when the head is extended or rotated, or who demonstrate a positive vertebral artery test.

Initial treatments should be administered with relatively low tension to determine the patient's response. Discontinue the use of traction if the patient's symptoms increase or if new symptoms develop.

Overview of the Evidence

Although the effects of patient position and angle of pull on the vertebrae have been substantiated, the other treatment parameters are less clear. The exact amount of tension and the duration of the treatment are relatively undefined. Parameters used for individual patients are often derived by trial and error. For this reason, patient interviews to determine the effects of the treatment take on an added level of importance in determining the protocol.

Studies investigating the effects of lumbar and cervical traction indicate that this treatment approach is no better or worse than other modalities in reducing the symptoms of disk compression, but patients receiving treatment showed improvements versus those not receiving treatment.[95] The actual amount of reabsorption of the cervical nucleus pulposus has not been established.

The additional benefit of including cervical traction to an intervention program that includes multiple exercises and therapeutic modalities has been questioned. In a randomized clinical trial the group receiving cervical traction in addition to other courses of care demonstrated no additional relief in pain, loss of function, or disability.

■ Clinical Application of Intermittent Cervical Traction

The following protocol describes the setup and application of motorized intermittent cervical traction with the patient in a reclined position. Manual traction may be used before mechanized traction to determine the potential benefits of the treatment.

Instrumentation

Refer to the operator's manual for the particular unit being used.

Mode: This setting allows the traction to be applied intermittently or continuously.

Type: For multipurpose units that treat both the lumbar and cervical spine. If "Cervical" is selected, the TYPE function presets a maximum amount of tension that can be produced.

Cable release: Eliminates the tension on the traction cable. On some units the CABLE RELEASE is disabled if the cable is under a load. In this case, to reduce the traction force on the cervical spine, have the patient slide toward the unit.

Hold time: This control adjusts the duration of the traction phase (in seconds).

Rest time: This control adjusts the duration of the relaxation phase (in seconds). It is applicable only to intermittent traction.

Tension: Controls the amount of tension, in pounds, applied to the halter.

Low tension: Sets the minimum amount of tension to be applied during the OFF cycle.

Tension increase/decrease: Adjusts the rate of traction force increase and decrease (in seconds).

Tension steps: Provides for the incremental increase and/or decrease in the amount of tension. The tension at each step is held for a predetermined time until tension is increased or decreased.

Duration: Selects the total treatment time.

Harness (halter): The "standard" halter applies force to the mandible and **occiput** •. Modified halters have been designed that place the force on the occiput and may allow specificity regarding the cervical level where the separation occurs, and decrease the forces placed on the TMJ (see Fig. 16-9).

Spreader bar: This device connects the older style halter to the traction device through a pulley cable and prevent the cables from rubbing against the patient's face and ears.

Safety switch: This switch allows the patient to interrupt the treatment and decrease tension.

EMG electrodes: Some units allow for the concurrent use of EMG. Refer to Chapter 18 for more information on the clinical use of EMG biofeedback.

Alarm: Sounds when the patient triggers the safety switch. Will also sound if the amount of tension selected is too great for the cervical spine or a malfunction is detected by the unit.

Occiput: The posterior base of the skull.

At a Glance: **Cervical Traction**

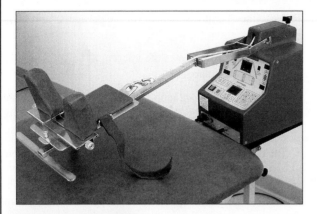

Description

Cervical traction distracts the cervical vertebrae and can be applied continuously or intermittently. This traction can be delivered by way of a motorized unit, weights, gravity, or manually by the clinician.

Indications

- Degenerative disk diseases
- Herniated or protruding intervertebral disk
- Nerve root compression/radicular pain and associated muscle spasm
- Osteoarthritis or facet joint inflammation
- Facet joint pathology limiting range of motion including hypomobile facet joints
- Capsulitis of the vertebral joints
- Pathology of the anterior or posterior longitudinal ligaments
- Cervical muscle spasm

Primary Effects

- Elongation of the cervical vertebrae, relieving pressure on the intervertebral disks and assisting in the reabsorption of the nucleus pulposus that places pressure on cervical nerve roots
- Relieves pressure on the spinal nerve roots caused by narrowing of the intervertebral foramen
- Reduces pressure on the facet joints
- Elongates cervical musculature

Contraindications

- Acute injury
- Unstable spine
- Diseases affecting the vertebrae or spinal cord, including cancer and **meningitis** •
- Vertebral fractures
- Extruded disk fragmentation
- Spinal cord compression
- Positive vertebral artery test
- Conditions in which vertebral flexion and/or extension is contraindicated
- Osteoporosis
- Rheumatoid arthritis
- Conditions that worsen after traction treatments or motion

Treatment Duration

- Facet joint pathology: 25 min
- Degenerative disk disease: 10 min
- Disk protrusion: 8–10 min
- Muscle spasm: 20 min
- (Approximate treatment durations)

Precautions

- Cervical traction should never be attempted in traumatic conditions that have not been evaluated to rule out a fracture or dislocation.
- The patient must be closely monitored throughout the treatment, and the treatment should be immediately discontinued if symptoms increase or if pain or paresthesia is experienced.
- Improper extension traction can result in a rupture of the cervical esophagus.[113]
- Excessive duration and/or traction weight can cause thrombosis of the internal jugular vein.[114]
- Low tension should be used when hypermobility is present (check with a physician prior to treatment).
- Only sustained or continuous traction should be used when motion is contraindicated.
- Mandibular-occipital harnesses should not be used if the patient is suffering from temporomandibular joint pathology.

Meningitis: Inflammation of the membranes of the brain or spinal cord.

Setup and Application

Digital units can display force in pounds (lb) or kilograms (kg). Familiarize yourself with the units of measure used by the facility.

Motorized traction devices should not be used in the presence of flammable gas such as oxygen, nitrous oxide, and many anesthetic gases. The unit may interfere with sensitive electrical equipment.

Patient Preparation

1. Determine the presence of any contraindications. In some cases the **vertebral artery test** should be performed to rule out the presence of conditions that occlude the blood supply to the brain.
2. Determine the patient's body weight.
3. The cervical musculature may be pretreated with moist heat to decrease muscle spasm.
4. Instruct the patient to remove any earrings, glasses, or other clothing that may interfere with the placement of the halter.
5. Lay the patient on the treatment table in the supine position.
6. Place a pillow or other support under the patient's knees.
7. Ensure that the motor unit is firmly attached to its base.
8. Certain individuals, including those with periodontal disease, may experience less discomfort if they wear a mouthguard during treatment.[98]
9. For bilateral traction, position the unit so that the line of pull is aligned with the midline of the body (i.e., so that the head is not laterally flexed). For unilateral traction, adjust the halter or position the patient accordingly.
10. Secure the halter to the cervical region according to the manufacturer's instructions. Normally the pressure points are on the occipital processes. Older style halters also place pressure on the chin. To avoid pressure on the mandible or TMJ, use an occipital harness (see Fig. 16-9).
11. Connect the halter to the spreader bar.
12. Align the unit so that the angle of pull corresponds to the pathology being treated (see Table 16-2).
13. Give the patient the SAFETY switch and explain its purpose and use. **The SAFETY switch must be in the patient's possession throughout the duration of treatment.**
14. Explain to the patient the sensations to be expected during the treatment and to report pain, discomfort, or worsening of symptoms.

Initiation of the Treatment

1. Reset all controls to zero and turn unit ON.
2. If applicable, set the TYPE switch to "Cervical."
3. Remove any slack in the pulley cable.
4. Adjust the RATIO to the appropriate on-off sequence, normally a 3:1 or 4:1 ratio.
5. Adjust the TENSION to approximately 10 pounds or 7% of the patient's body weight. If this is the patient's first exposure to intermittent cervical traction, or if the person is displaying apprehension about the treatment, use a lower than normal TENSION.
6. If the control is adjustable, set the LOW tension (this value is often set to zero or 10% of the maximum tension).
7. Instruct the patient as to what to expect during the treatment and to inform you if any discomfort is experienced. Explain that the force of the pull is felt at the occiput and not at the chin.
8. Set the appropriate treatment DURATION, and initiate the treatment (refer to Table 16-2).
9. Allow the unit to cycle through its first tension cycle. The TENSION may be gradually increased during subsequent cycles. If pain is experienced at any time during the treatment, decrease the amount of force or discontinue the treatment.
10. Instruct the patient to remain relaxed during both the on and off cycles.
11. If the pressure placed on the mandible causes discomfort in the teeth or TMJ, gauze or a mouthpiece may be placed between the teeth to dissipate the force.
12. At regular intervals, question the patient about abnormal sensations in the cervical, thoracic, and lumbar spine and the extremities.

Termination of the Treatment

1. If the traction unit does not automatically do so, gradually reduce the TENSION over a period of three or four cycles.
2. Gain some slack in the cable and turn the unit off.
3. Remove the SPREADER BAR and HALTER.
4. Question the patient regarding any perceived benefit or complications derived from the treatment.
5. Have the patient remain sitting or lying supine for 5 minutes after the conclusion of the treatment. Record the pertinent information (tension, duration, duty cycle) in the patient's medical file.

Maintenance

Discontinue the treatment and turn off the unit if unusual noises or abnormal function is noticed during the treatment. Contact an authorized technician for service.

After Each Use

1. Clean the unit according to the manufacturer's recommendation.
2. Avoid allowing liquids (including cleaning solutions) from entering the unit.

At Regular Intervals

1. Check the electrical power cord for kinks, frays, or cuts.

2. Check the traction cable for knots, twisting, and if applicable, damage to its protective (usually nylon) coating.
3. Recalibrate the unit. Follow the manufacturer's recommended procedures and timetable for recalibrating the traction device.
4. Clean the harness according to the manufacturer's instructions.

Annual

The traction device must be inspected and serviced by an authorized technician.

■ Lumbar Traction

To be effective, lumbar traction must overcome the weight of the lower extremities (approximately half of the total body weight), pelvis, and the soft tissue tension produced by the paraspinal muscles and ligaments. As with cervical traction, the benefits of lumbar traction are obtained by separating the lumbar vertebrae. Unlike cervical traction, friction is a strong counterforce against the force of the traction and increases the total amount of tension that must be applied during the treatment. A split table (also referred to as a lumbar traction table) in which the lower extremity portion of the table is free to glide on a track reduces the influence of friction between the body and the table (Fig. 16-10).

Lumbar traction is commonly applied using a motorized unit. Manual traction can be applied using a belt that allows the clinician's body weight to help deliver the force. An optional force meter will assist in delivering more precise tension. Each of these methods requires that the patient wear a pelvic traction harness and a thoracic stabilization harness that fixates the patient to the table (Fig. 16-11). The effectiveness of the treatment is diminished if there is not good contact between the harness and the patient's skin.

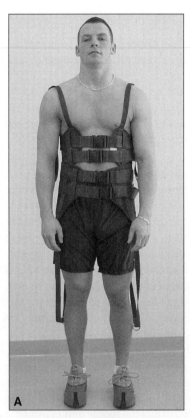

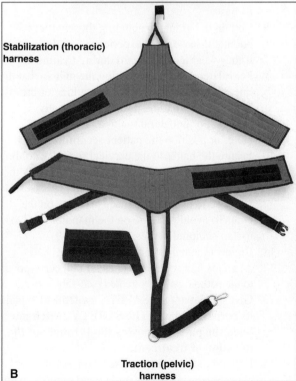

Stabilization (thoracic) harness

Traction (pelvic) harness

Figure 16-11. **Pelvic and Thoracic Harness Used During Lumbar Traction.** (A) Older style harness using bilateral pulls (note the straps hanging next to each leg). (B) A contemporary harness system that uses a single axis of pull. (B, Courtesy of the Chattanooga Group, Hixson, TN.)

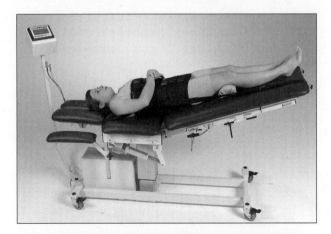

Figure 16-10. **Multiaxial Split Table for Lumbar Traction.** In addition to the lower half of the table gliding on rollers, to eliminate friction and permit vertebral separation to occur at a lower applied force, this unit also flexes, extends, and rotates the lower extremity, allowing for unilateral traction. (Used with permission of the Saunders Group, Inc.)

The patient's body weight can be used to deliver traction to the lumbar spine. Inversion traction—in which the patient is suspended upside down by the ankles or legs—was a popular method of elongating the lumbar spine. However, this method is hazardous for patients who have hypertension, and other cardiovascular disorders and glaucoma.[90]

Gravitational traction can be administered with the patient upright, although some patients cannot tolerate the discomfort caused by the torso harness.[90] This method does not carry with it the cardiovascular problems associated with inversion traction, only slightly increasing systolic blood pressure and having no effect on diastolic blood pressure. Gravitational traction is capable of increasing the posterior disk space between L1 and S1 (the length of the lumbar spine) by 31 mm.[90]

The patient can also self-administer gravitational traction, called autotraction. Hanging from a bar or supporting the weight of the body on the arms of a chair or between parallel bars while relaxing the spinal muscles can distract the vertebrae (Fig 16-12). This method is limited by the patient's upper body strength.

Treatment Parameters

The fundamental parameters for lumbar traction are presented in Table 16-2. The primary difference between cervical and lumbar traction is the increased amount of tension required to separate the lumbar vertebrae. Except where noted, this section refers to mechanical traction techniques.

Tension

Friction, muscle and soft tissue tension, and the weight of the lower extremity require significantly more tension to separate the lumbar vertebrae than that required for the cervical spine. When lumbar traction is applied using a standard plinth, approximately one half of the force applied is required to overcome the weight of the body part. For example, if a patient's lower extremity and pelvis weighs 100 lb, vertebral separation does not begin until at least 50 lb of tension is applied. Split traction tables remove the effect of friction (see Fig. 16-10).

The range of tension used during lumbar traction is quite variable, and the efficacy of various weights has not been established. Published ranges for the amount of tension used are from 10% to 300% of the patient's body weight.[92,115]

Over 90% of the increase in intervertebral separation occurs during the first 15 minutes of static traction.[90,115] After 25 minutes of static traction, mean torso length increased by an average of 8.9 mm.[115]

Patient Position and Angle of Pull

Patient position has more influence on the angle of pull during lumbar traction than cervical traction. Lumbar traction can be applied with the patient prone or supine (Fig. 16-13). Each of these positions equally decreases the amount of myoelectric

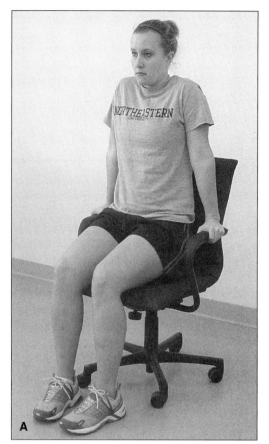

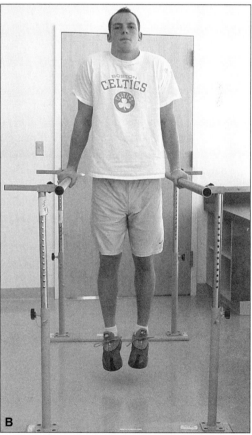

Figure 16-12. **Methods of Self-Administered Autotraction.** (A) Sitting in a chair for the sacroiliac joint. (B) Using parallel bars for the sacroiliac joint and lumbar spine.

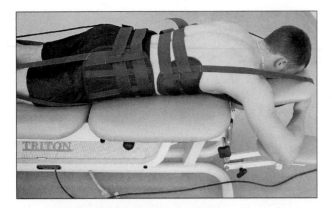

Figure 16-13. Lumbar Traction Applied in the Prone Position. This position permits other modalities to be applied concurrently with the traction.

activity of the paraspinal muscles.[116] Patient comfort, the pathology being treated, and the spinal segments and structures being treated also help determine the patient position.

Positioning the patient supine increases lumbar flexion of the lumbar spine. Flexing the hip and knees further increases flexion of the lumbar spine and pelvis, flattening the lumbar spine. Flexing the hips from 45 to 60 degrees of flexion increases the laxity in the L5–S1 segment, 60 to 75 degrees in the L4–L5 segment, and 75 to 90 degrees in the L3–L4 segment.[117] Flexing the hips to 90 degrees also increases the posterior intervertebral space.[117] In the lumbar spine, extension opens the facet joint and increases distraction in the upper lumbar and, possibly, the lower thoracic segments.

The prone position is used when excessive flexion of the lumbar spine and pelvis or lying supine causes pain or increases peripheral symptoms. An increased amount of distraction occurs in the lower lumbar segments when the patient is prone, a beneficial effect with lower disk protrusions. This position has the advantage of allowing other modalities to be applied concurrently with the traction.[95]

The patient's position and angle of pull should maximize the separation and elongation of the target tissues. An anterior angle of pull increases the amount of lumbar lordosis. A posterior angle of pull increases lumbar kyphosis, but too much flexion can impinge on the posterior spinal ligaments.

Determining the optimal position and angle of pull is often derived by trial and error and depends on the patient and the pathology (see Table 16-2). For example, a posterior disk protrusion may respond best with the patient prone and the spine placed in extension or neutral. However, if no pain relief is obtained in either of these positions, positioning the patient supine with the lumbar spine placed in flexion may produce beneficial results.

Relief of symptoms caused by nerve root impingement should be obtained with the patient supine and the spine flexed. If the impingement is unilateral, additional pain relief may be obtained by rotating the involved side slightly upward by placing a folded towel or bolster under the involved side.

Unilateral traction is used for the treatment of **functional scoliosis** ● of the lumbar and thoracic spine (Fig. 16-14). The tension is applied to the convex side of the curvature, straightening the vertebral column and elongating the muscles on the opposite, concave side of the column.[118] Traction is not considered to be effective for the treatment of **structural scoliosis** ● .

● Effects on

The Injury Response Process

Lumbar traction is useful in treating many of the same conditions as cervical traction, resulting in a decrease

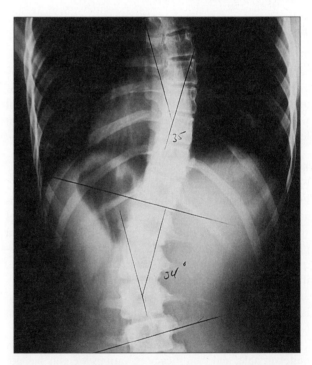

Figure 16-14. Spinal Scoliosis (posterior view). Scoliosis is the lateral curvature of the spinal column in the frontal plane. Focusing on the lumbar segment, this radiograph shows a convex curvature on the left side, elongating the soft tissue on that side. The right lumbar curvature is concave. The muscles on this side are shortened. Note that this radiograph depicts structural scoliosis caused by misshaped vertebrae. Traction is only effective on functional scoliosis.

Functional scoliosis: Lateral curvature of the spinal column in the frontal plane caused as the spinal column attempts to compensate for postural deficits such as leg length discrepancy. Functional scoliosis is also known as protective scoliosis.

Structural scoliosis: Lateral curvature of the spinal column caused by malformed vertebrae and/or intervertebral disks.

in lumbar lordosis, distraction of the vertebral bodies, increase in disk height, stretching of lumbar muscles, and widening of the intervertebral foramina.[90] The effects of lumbar traction are similar to those described in the General Uses for Cervical and Lumbar Traction section of this chapter.

✱ Practical Evidence

A clinical prediction rule has been developed to identify patients who are most likely to benefit from lumbar traction. Based on the following clinical findings:

 – Age older than 30 years
 – No neurological deficit involvement
 – Patient is not involved in manual labor
 – Fear-avoidance belief questionnaire work score of less than 21

Patients who are positive on all four variables have a probability of 69% for successful traction, the presence of three variables decreases the probability to 42%, two variables 30%, and one variable 20%.[119]

Muscle Spasm

Lumbar traction can be effective in reducing muscle spasm caused by nerve root impingement from narrowing of the intervertebral foramen, stenosis, or disk protrusions. To a lesser degree, traumatic muscle spasm can be reduced secondary to stretching of the muscles, although the amount of elongation is less than that obtained by standard stretching routines. EMG analysis demonstrates that the angle of pull does not affect muscle activity in healthy adults. Increased mobility following treatment may be associated with disk rehydration.[120]

Pain Associated With Disk Degeneration

Increasing the amount of separation between the vertebrae can reduce impingement of the lumbar nerve roots. Nerve entrapment as a result of a disk protrusion can be reduced by allowing the disk to return to its original shape, decompressing the nucleus pulposus to below 100 mm Hg (Fig. 16-15).[88,121] Radicular pain caused by lumbar disk herniation is reduced with forces of 30 and 60% of the body weight.[88,89,92] Prone traction applied for 30 minutes over 8 weeks (five 30-min sessions a week for 4 weeks followed by one 30-min treatment a week for 4 weeks) demonstrated significant improvement in pain and disability scores in patients with lumbar disk degeneration.[122]

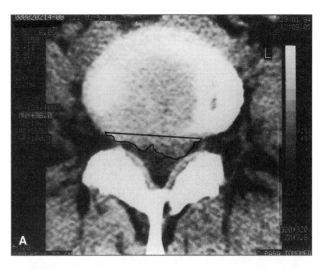

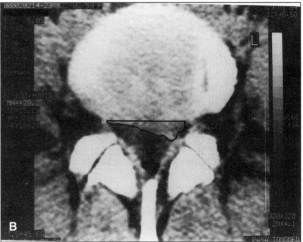

Figure 16-15. **CT Scan Demonstrating Uptake of the Nucleus Pulposus of the L4–L5 Disk During Lumbar Traction.** (A) The nuclear material can be seen intruding into the spinal canal and left neural foramia (shaded area). (B) When 45 kg of traction force is applied to the lumbar spine, the nuclear material regresses into the disk, decreasing pressure on the spinal canal and left neural foramia.

Contraindications to the Use of Lumbar Traction

The contraindications to the use of lumbar traction are similar to those described for cervical traction. Vertebral body fractures or unstable spinal segments are an absolute contraindication to lumbar traction unless the treatment is specifically approved by the patient's physician.

Lumbar traction has been used for **spondylolisthesis** ● and **spondylolysis** ●, but this should be done with caution and diligence (Fig. 16-16). Spondylolisthesis can lead to hypermobility of the vertebral segment, a contraindication to sustained and intermittent traction. Too much tension can speed the degeneration associated with spondylolysis.

Spondylolisthesis: Forward slippage of the lower lumbar vertebra on the vertebra below.
Spondylolysis: The breaking down of a vertebral structure.

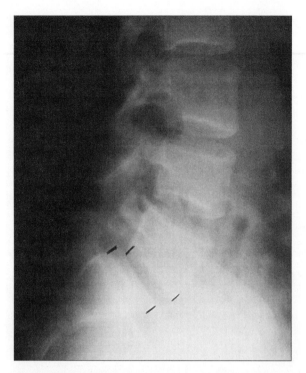

Figure 16-16. **Spondylolisthesis of the L5–S1 Vertebrae.** Spondylolisthesis is the forward slippage of a vertebra on the one below it. This condition results in pain in the lumbar spine and buttocks that increases when the lumbar spine is placed in extension. Lumbar traction should not be used when the vertebral segment is hypermobile.

* Practical Evidence

Lumbar traction is not an effective treatment approach for patients with nonspecific low back pain.[123]

Do not use lumbar traction for patients with pain of unknown origin or pain caused by diseases, infections, or tumors (see At a Glance: Lumbar Traction). Traction applied to severely herniated disks may increase the rate of degeneration. Discontinue use if the treatment increases the severity of the patient's symptoms.

Rheumatoid arthritis and osteoarthritis are contraindicated because necrosis can cause ligamentous weakness. The force of the applied traction could result in vertebral subluxation or dislocation and further weaken the soft tissue structures.

Controversies in Treatment

The efficacy of lumbar traction has been supported for several types of pathology. Lumbar traction is not considered to be effective in decreasing nonspecific low back pain.[123,124]

Computed tomographic imaging indicates that lumbar traction increases the reabsorption of the nucleus pulposus.

However, the location of the protrusion does affect the efficacy of the treatment. Protrusions closer to the body's midline are more likely to have positive treatment outcomes than lateral protrusions. Factors such as the calcification of the disk also decrease the effectiveness of the treatment.[125] A comparison of lumbar traction and isometric exercise indicated that neither of the interventions was more effective in decreasing pain caused by disk herniations than placebo.[126]

Clinical Application of Intermittent Lumbar Traction

The following section describes the use of motorized lumbar traction. The patient position and angle of pull must be appropriate for the condition being treated. Manual traction may be used before mechanized traction to determine the potential benefits of the treatment.

Instrumentation
Refer to the operator's manual for the particular unit being used.

Traction harness: Sometimes referred to as the pelvic "corset." Fits around the patient's pelvis and attaches to the traction unit's pulley cable.

Stabilization harness: Fits around the patient's torso and attaches to the treatment table.

Split table: The lower half of the table glides on rollers, thus eliminating friction and allowing vertebral separation to occur at a lower applied force.

Mode: This setting allows the traction to be applied intermittently or continuously.

Type: For multipurpose units that treat both the lumbar and cervical spine.

Hold time: This control adjusts the duration of the traction phase (in seconds).

Rest time: This control adjusts the duration of the relaxation phase (in seconds). Applicable only to intermittent traction.

Tension: Controls the amount of tension, in pounds, applied to the halter.

Cable release: Eliminates the tension on the traction cable.

Low tension: Sets the minimum amount of tension to be applied during the OFF cycle.

Tension increase/decrease: Adjusts the rate of traction force increase and decrease (in seconds).

Tension steps: Provides for the incremental increase and/or decrease in the amount of tension. The tension at each step is held for a predetermined time until tension is increased or decreased.

At a Glance: **Lumbar Traction**

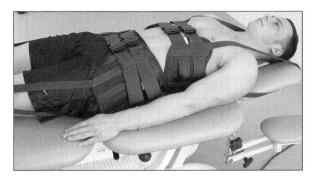

Description

Lumbar traction distracts the lumbar and possibly the lower thoracic vertebrae. Using a motorized unit (shown above), lumbar traction can be applied continuously or intermittently. Lumbar traction can also be applied manually by the clinician, by weights, or by gravity (autotraction).

Indications

■ Nerve root compression
■ Radicular pain
■ Herniated or protruding intervertebral disk
■ Degenerative disk disease
■ Lumbar muscle spasm
■ Osteoarthritis or facet joint inflammation
■ Facet joint pathology including hypomobile facet joints

Primary Effects

■ Elongation of the lumbar vertebrae, relieving pressure on the intervertebral disks. Aids in the reabsorption of the nucleus pulposus.
■ Relieves pressure on the spinal nerve roots caused by narrowing of the intervertebral foramen
■ Reduces pressure on the facet joints

Contraindications

■ Acute injury
■ Unstable spinal segments
■ Cancer, meningitis, or other diseases affecting the spinal cord or vertebrae
■ Extruded disk fragmentation
■ Advanced disk degeneration or advanced herniation
■ Spinal cord compression
■ Rheumatoid arthritis
■ Conditions that worsen after treatment

Treatment Duration

■ Facet joint pathology: 25 min
■ Degenerative disk disease: 10 min
■ Disk protrusion: 8 to 10 min
■ Muscle spasm: 20 min

Precautions

■ Monitor the patient closely during the treatment. Discontinue use if symptoms increase.
■ Low-tension traction should be used if ligamentous damage is suspected.
■ Use only sustained or continuous traction if lumbar motion is contraindicated.

Duration: Selects the total treatment time.

Safety switch: Allows the patient to interrupt the treatment and immediately decrease the tension if pain or other discomfort is experienced.

Alarm: Sounds when the patient triggers the safety switch or a malfunction in the unit is detected.

Setup and Application

The following protocol describes the setup and application of motorized intermittent lumbar traction with the patient supine and the knees and hip flexed (e.g., for treatment of nerve root impingement) on a split traction table (therefore negating the effect of friction between the patient and the tabletop).

Digital units can display force in pounds (lb) or kilograms (kg). Familiarize yourself with the unit of measure that is used by the facility.

Motorized traction devices should not be used in the presence of flammable gases such as oxygen, nitrous oxide, and many anesthetic gases. The unit may interfere with sensitive electrical equipment.

Patient Preparation
1. Determine the presence of any contraindications.
2. Calculate the patient's body weight.

3. If a split table is being used, unlock the lower section to allow it to slide.

4. The patient's clothing must not interfere with the fit of the halter and not allow the traction or stabilization halter to slide during the treatment.

5. Fit the traction halter on the patient's pelvis. Depending on the type of harness being used, a towel or other type of padding may need to be placed between the harness and the patient's skin.

6. Fit the stabilization harness to the patient's torso, normally fitting over the 8th through 10th ribs. There may be slight overlap between the stabilization and traction harness.

7. If necessary, drape the patient for modesty.

8. If a split table is being used, align the target spinal segment over the opening between the fixed and mobile portion of the table.

9. Position the patient, the patient's hip and knee position, and the angle of pull appropriate for the treatment being treated (refer to Table 16-2). If the patient is supine and lumbar/pelvic flexion is indicated, elevate the lower legs.

10. Align the angle of pull according to the patient's pathology (refer to Table 16-2).

11. Give the patient the SAFETY switch and explain its purpose and use. **The SAFETY switch must be in the patient's possession throughout the duration of treatment.**

12. Explain to the patient the sensations to be expected during the treatment and to report pain, discomfort, or worsening of symptoms.

Initiation of the Treatment

1. Reset all controls to zero and turn the unit ON.

2. If applicable, set the TYPE switch to "Lumbar."

3. Remove any slack in the pulley cable.

4. Adjust the RATIO to the appropriate ON-OFF sequence (refer to Table 16-2).

5. Adjust the tension to approximately 25% of the patient's body weight. Radicular pain caused by lumbar disk herniation is often reduced with forces of 30 and 60% of the body weight.[92,102]

6. If the setting is adjustable, set the LOW tension (this value is often set to zero or 10% of the maximum tension).

7. Instruct the patient as to what to expect during the treatment and to inform you if any discomfort is experienced.

8. Set the appropriate treatment DURATION, and initiate the treatment (refer to Table 16-2).

9. Allow the unit to go through its first tension cycle. The TENSION may be gradually increased during subsequent cycles. Increase the amount of tension as indicated. If pain is experienced at any time during the treatment, decrease the amount of force or discontinue the treatment.

10. Instruct the patient to remain relaxed during both the on and off cycles.

11. At regular intervals question the patient about abnormal sensations in the cervical, thoracic, and lumbar spine and the extremities.

Termination of the Treatment

1. If the traction unit does not automatically do so, gradually reduce the TENSION over a period of three or four cycles.

2. Gain some slack in the cable, and turn the unit off.

3. Remove the traction and stabilization halter.

4. Question the patient regarding any perceived benefit or complications derived from the treatment.

5. Have the patient remain lying for 5 minutes after the conclusion of the treatment.

6. Record the pertinent information (tension, duration, duty cycle) in the patient's medical file.

Maintenance

After Each Use

1. Clean the unit according to the manufacturer's recommendation.

2. Avoid allowing liquids (including cleaning solutions) from entering the unit.

At Regular Intervals

1. Check the electrical power cord for kinks, frays, or cuts.

2. Check the traction cable for knots, twisting, and if applicable, damage to its protective (usually nylon) coating.

3. Recalibrate the unit. Follow the manufacturer's recommended procedures and timetable for recalibrating the traction device.

4. Clean the harness according to the manufacturer's instructions.

Annual

The traction device must be inspected and serviced by an authorized technician.

Chapter 17

Therapeutic Massage

Kerry Gordon, MS, ATC, CMT, CSCS

Massage is one of the oldest forms of healing techniques. Using therapeutic touch, the body's tissues are manipulated to reduce muscle spasm, promote relaxation, improve blood flow, and increase venous drainage. The scope of massage theories, techniques, and effects is broad. This chapter addresses massage techniques that are most frequently used in the treatment of musculoskeletal conditions.

● Massage, the systematic manipulation of the body's tissues, has been present in most cultures and can be traced back as far as the ancient Olympics. Regional variations have contributed to the different forms of massage used today. This diverse background leads to differences in application protocol and theory (Table 17-1).

Massage and myofascial release are forms of soft tissue mobilization in which the tissues are manipulated to produce the desired effects. Joint mobilization, another form of manual therapy, is not discussed in this text.

Massage is an effective treatment method for promoting local and systemic relaxation or invigoration, increasing local blood flow, breaking down adhesions, and encouraging venous and lymphatic return. Because it is a time-consuming task that requires the full attention of the clinician, massage is infrequently used in multi-function health-care facilities. Still, massage has increased in popularity and massage therapy is a continually growing profession.

Massage is a skill- and knowledge-based technique, and because of the possibility for misuse, many states require licensure for massage therapists. Most other healing professions, including athletic training and physical therapy, incorporate massage techniques into their professional preparation. Massage therapists often work cooperatively with other health-care providers or may be dual credentialed.

■ Massage Strokes

There are several different types of massage strokes, and each may be varied by adding more or less pressure, using different parts of the hand, or changing the direction and frequency of the strokes (Table 17-2). These elements are then sequenced to produce different effects. The following sections describe the basic elements of several techniques and discuss how they can be varied.

TABLE 17-1 Selected Methods of Manual Therapy Techniques

Technique	Description
Acupressure	Pressure is applied along acupuncture meridians, altering the body's energy pattern.
Craniosacral therapy	Alters the flow of cerebrospinal fluid by lightly massaging points along the spinal column.
Deep tissue massage	Targets individual deep muscle fibers and attempts to release adhesions and increase blood flow to restricted areas.
Lymphatic massage	Targets the lymphatic system and attempts to remove edema, waste products, and toxins from the body using light, rhythmic strokes.[127] This is one of few techniques that can be used for acute musculoskeletal injuries. Activation of the lymphatic system may limit acute inflammation.[128]
Myofascial release	Breaks adhesions and other restrictions in the body's fascial network to restore normal function.
Neuromuscular therapy	Focuses on reducing pain and muscle spasm by identifying trigger points and treating with ischemic compression.
Instrumented Assisted Soft-Tissue Mobilization	Use of a tool to address myofascial dysfunction and soft-tissue adhesions.
Shiatsu	Use of various forms of compression strokes and stretches based on physiology or traditional Chinese medicine.
Swedish massage	Traditional massage techniques used for increasing muscle relaxation.

TABLE 17-2 Summary of Basic Massage Strokes and Their Physiological Effect

Stroke	Technique	Effect
Effleurage	Stroking of the skin	**Deep stroking:** stimulates deep tissues, forces fluids in the direction of the stroke. **Superficial stroking:** slow strokes: promotes relaxation. **Fast strokes:** stimulates tissues and encourages blood flow.
Pétrissage	Lifting and kneading	Stretches and separates muscle fiber and fascia, from the skin and scar tissue.
Friction	Deep pressure cross fiber stroking	Stimulates the body's natural healing process, separates tissues, and breaks up scar tissue.
Active Assisted	Combination of compression with broadening and muscle stripping	Stretches and lengthens the affected muscles to increase range of motion and decrease restriction.
Neuromuscular	Ischemic compression	Decrease hypersensitivity and hypertonicity in taut muscle bands.
Tapotement	Tapping or pounding	Promotes relaxation and the desensitization of the skin's nerve endings.
Vibration	Rapid shaking	Increases blood flow and provides systemic invigoration of tissues.

Effleurage

Effleurage, the stroking of the skin, is performed with the palm of the hand or knuckles to stimulate deep tissues, or with the fingerpads to stimulate sensory nerves. This stroke is categorized as being either superficial or deep. Superficial stroking may either follow the contour of the body itself, or follow the direction of the underlying muscles, but does not attempt to move the underlying muscle. Deep stroking requires more pressure to target and elongate the muscle fiber and stretch the fascia.

A slow, light stroke promotes relaxation, introduces the patient to the treatment, and is used to spread the massage lubricant over the area to be treated. Rapid strokes encourage blood flow and stimulate the tissues. Deep strokes can be used to elongate muscles and should follow the course of veins and lymph vessels from distal to proximal to force fluids back toward the heart.

Light effleurage is generally performed at both the beginning and end of the massage and may be used between pétrissage strokes. During the initial stages of the treatment, effleurage relaxes the patient and indicates the areas that will be massaged. At the conclusion of the treatment, effleurage can "calm down" nerves that become irritated during the massage.

CLINICAL TECHNIQUES: EFFLEURAGE

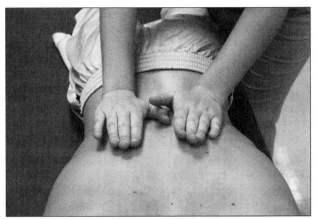

Basic technique

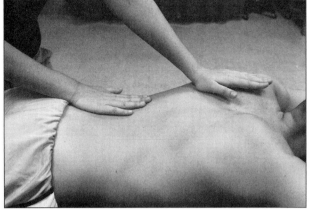

Shingling technique

Indications
- Muscle strains
- Shingling technique is recommended for large muscles

- Improve circulation
- Prior to or following competition in conjunction with sports massage techniques

Technique
- All effleurage strokes are performed in a rhythmic manner.
- Strokes should be directed toward the heart.
- The thumbs can be used to fit into anatomical contours (e.g., between the metatarsals, the posterior portion of the malleoli).

- Ideally, at least one hand should be in contact with the skin at any given point.

Basic effleurage:
1. Place the hands (palms, fingers, or knuckles) parallel to the body part being treated and symmetrical to its long axis.
2. Apply the appropriate amount of pressure for the desired effects.
3. Using a mirrored motion, stroke the body part along its long axis—the strokes may also follow the course of veins and lymph vessels or large muscle masses (e.g., the latissimus dorsi).

4. While still mirroring each other, lightly glide the hands back to the starting point using a light stroke of the fingerpads.
5. Repeat procedures 1 through 4 until the target tissues have been covered and/or the desired effects have been obtained.

"Shingling" technique:
1. Place one palm over the target tissue.
2. Using the palm, make short (e.g., 8-inch) to moderate (e.g., 12-inch) strokes following the path of the underlying muscle or vein, using the amount of pressure appropriate for the desired effects.
3. Just prior to the hand leaving the body, repeat the stroke using the opposite hand, starting approximately one-half the distance between the starting and ending point of the prior stroke, thus overlapping the strokes similar to shingles on a roof and provide the patient with the sensation of unbroken contact.

4. Continue along the length of the treatment area. Keeping the strokes in the original position, progress back toward the starting point.
5. Repeat procedures 1 through 4 until the target tissues have been covered and/or the desired effects have been obtained.

Pétrissage

Pétrissage is the lifting, kneading, and rolling of the skin, subcutaneous tissue, and muscle with the fingers or hand. This stroke has some similarity to myofascial skin rolling technique, but pétrissage targets the underlying muscle and is particularly useful in superficial, mobile muscles such as the upper trapezius or the muscles of the forearm. Pétrissage frees adhesions by stretching and separating muscle fiber, fascia, and scar tissue. This technique milks the muscle of waste products, assists in venous return, and can lead to muscular relaxation.

CLINICAL TECHNIQUES: PÉTRISSAGE

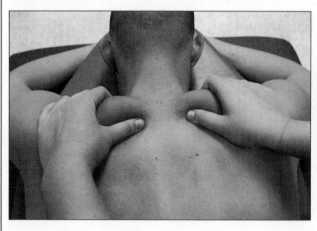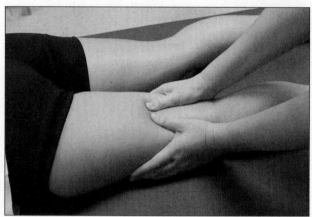

Indications
- Injuries in the late stages of healing/chronic conditions
- Areas having multiple muscles
- Superficial muscles

Technique
1. If pétrissage is the only technique being performed, it may be performed without the use of a lubricant.
2. Pétrissage is often administered following effleurage and/or moist heat pack application.
3. Using one or two hands, gently grip and lift the underlying muscle and move the tissue back and forth.
4. Repeat step three for a few repetitions before progressing to a new location.

Friction Massage

Friction massage mobilizes muscle fibers and separates adhesions in muscle, tendon fibers, or scar tissue that restrict motion and cause pain, and is used to facilitate local blood perfusion.[129] Transverse friction massage is also used for the treatment of trigger points, tendinitis, postsurgical scars or other forms of joint adhesions to promote functional realignment of the fibers.[130]

There are two basic types of friction massage: circular and cross-fiber massage. Both are used with the intention of addressing the underlying muscle structure as compared to the overlying epidermis (as in effleurage). **Circular friction massage** is applied with the thumbs working in circular motion and is often effective in the treatment of trigger points (see Chapter 1). Deep and precise work such as trigger point release should be avoided pre-event. In **transverse friction massage,** the thumbs or fingertips stroke the tissue from opposite directions targeting the underlying tissue structure. Friction massage can be painful to receive but may produce a temporary analgesic effect post treatment. When treating a large muscle mass the elbow or a commercial deep-kneading device can be used in place of the thumbs.[131]

The deep pressure applied during friction massage is used to evoke mechanical changes in the tissue, leading to the development of functional scar tissue and minimizing adhesions. A temporary analgesic effect occurs as the result of the stimulation of sensory nerves and increasing local blood circulation. The treatment should be followed by stretching of the treated muscle group.[131]

■ Neuromuscular Techniques

A trigger point is an area of tissue hyperirritability that, when compressed, is locally tender. If the point is sufficiently hypersensitive it will give rise to referred pain and tenderness (also known as "referred autonomic phenomena" and "distortion of proprioception").[132] The different types

CLINICAL TECHNIQUES: FRICTION MASSAGE

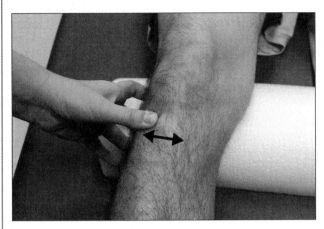 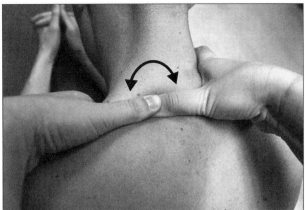

Indications
- Musculotendinous adhesions
- Realignment of scar tissue
- Trigger point therapy

Technique
1. The area may be preheated using a moist heat pack or ultrasound.
2. Position the patient so that the muscle is in a relaxed position.
3. Use the thumb to "pin" the tissue and locate the adhesions

4. Begin lightly and gradually progress to firmer, deeper circular strokes or strokes that run perpendicular or parallel to the underlying target tissue.
5. The force must be applied so that the pressure will reach and separate the deep tissues.
6. Friction massage can be followed by a stretching routine to further facilitate range of motion.

Comments
This method of massage is to be avoided in conditions in which the underlying tissues would be further injured by the pressure, such as acute injuries where an unwanted acceleration of the inflammatory response may occur.

Friction massage can be performed by the patient as a part of a home-treatment program.
To reduce soreness, this treatment may be followed by ice or ice massage.

---

of trigger points include myofascial, cutaneous, fascial, ligamentous, and periosteal.

Ischemic Compression

Once a trigger point within a palpable taut band is located, it may be treated using **ischemic compression.** This technique consists of applying direct pressure to a trigger point with the thumb, fingertips, or elbow. This technique can be painful. The amount of pressure applied is determined by the patient's pain tolerance and should not exceed a 7 or 8 (out of 10) on the pain scale.[133] The compression is maintained for 30 to 90 seconds or until there is a decrease in pain or hypertonicity. Both short duration (30 seconds), high-intensity and long duration (90 seconds), moderate intensity ischemic compression techniques reduce the pain and sensitivity of trigger points.[134] Do not use this technique on acute injuries.

✳ Practical Evidence

In patients diagnosed with carpal tunnel syndrome, treatment of trigger points in the arm using ischemic compression reduced patient self-reported symptoms for 6 months.[135]

Sports Massage

"Sports massage" is a broad term used to describe a combination of efflurage, pétrisssage, and friction massage. This technique is used for balancing muscle groups, shortening recovery time, and increasing functional range of motion in preparation for activity or following activity. Vigorous strokes are applied through clothing to help stimulate the nervous system to prepare for activity. The pressure should progressively increase from light to deep and the duration should be shorter than 30 minutes.

Muscle stripping is a sport-specific massage technique that exerts sustained pressure along the muscle fibers, usually applied from the insertion (distal) to the origin (proximal) and parallel to the muscle fibers being worked. Muscle stripping is effective in large muscle groups such as the hamstrings or quadriceps.

Active assisted techniques use compression and broadening (stretching perpendicular to the muscle fibers) techniques applied while the muscle is concentrically contracting. Muscle stripping is performed against an antagonist contraction to further release restrictions within the muscle and surrounding fascia. With the patient prone and the knee flexed to 90 degrees, apply compression and broadening strokes perpendicular to the muscle fiber (Fig. 17-1). Repeat several times until the length of the muscle has been treated. The patient then actively extends the knee as longitudinal stripping with the thumbs is applied from the insertion to the origin. Repeat until the length of the muscle as been treated. This technique is most efficiently used when applied to the extremities. An active stretch or warm-up after this massage technique will have a positive neuromuscular effect on the elasticity of the muscle.

■ Myofascial Release

Myofascial release involves the combination of traditional effleurage, pétrissage, and friction massage strokes with simultaneous stretching of the muscles and fascia to obtain relaxation of tense or adhered tissues and restore tissue mobility. Fascia forms an interconnected network that connects and surrounds muscle, tendons, and nerves, and separates the skin and adipose tissue from the underlying muscle. Fascial adhesions or restrictions in one area can affect function elsewhere. Abnormalities of the myofascial system are thought to be linked to fibromyalgia, chronic fatigue syndrome, myofascial pain syndrome, postural deviations, and decreased muscular function.[136–139]

Myofascial release attempts to restore normal function by breaking adhesions and restoring normal fascial length. Imagine fascia as your clothing. Wet clothes tend to stick to your skin and do not allow free movement underneath. This mimics fascial restrictions. Myofascial release is analogous to separating the wet clothing from your skin. It allows for efficiency of movement in the underlying structures that are restricted. Fascia does not deform when it is exposed to a quick, high-intensity force. Fascia will, however, elongate when a slow, moderate-intensity force is applied to it, an effect referred to as **creep.** The pressures used for most myofascial techniques take advantage of this phenomenon to stretch the underlying fascia. These myofascial techniques should be followed by traditional muscle stretching techniques.

The actual application of myofascial release techniques tends not to follow a structured pattern. Rather, the clinician receives cues and feedback from the patient's tissues that indicate what strokes and stretches are appropriate. The basic myofascial release techniques involve pulling the tissues in opposite directions, stabilizing the proximal or superior position with one hand while applying a stretch with the opposite hand, or using the patient's body weight to stabilize the extremity while a longitudinal stress is applied.

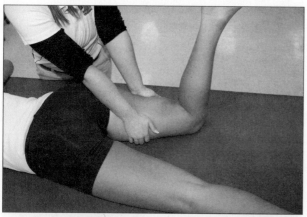
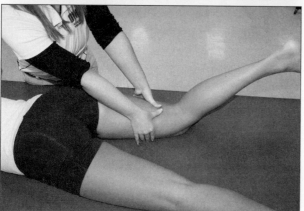

Figure 17-1. **Active Assisted Muscle Stripping.**

✱ Practical Evidence

High-quality research supports the premise of myofascial release; fascia has contractile properties that allows it to constrict or elongate, it is capable of being stretched through the skin, and it contains nerve endings and capillaries. However, the lack of high-quality studies cannot support or refute the clinical benefits of myofascial release.[140]

Areas of myofascial adhesions or shortening are found by gently gliding the skin in multiple directions, seeking to identify areas of restricted motion, or observing the patient's posture and noting areas of possible fascial shortening. Once the restriction is identified, myofascial release can be used to restore mobility. For example, a seated patient may feel a stretch or pull in the thoracic and lumbar spine when asked to flex the head and thorax. This identifies a fascial restriction that, once treated, can be immediately re-evaluated to determine the results of the treatment.

Specialized training in myofascial release techniques is needed to become proficient in these procedures.

The **J-stroke** is one of the most fundamental forms of myofascial release and is used to mobilize superficial fascial restrictions. **Skin rolling** also reduces superficial myofascial adhesions. Depending on the amount and depth of the pressure applied, **focused stretching** can release both superficial and deep fascial restrictions. The **arm pull, leg pull,** and **diagonal release** attempt to stretch large areas of fascia in the extremities and torso.

CLINICAL TECHNIQUES: MYOFASCIAL TECHNIQUES: J-STROKES

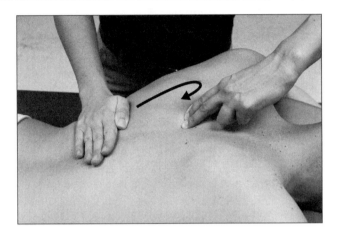

Description
Breaks adhesions and other restrictions in the body's fascial network to restore normal function

Indications
Treatment of chronic soft tissue malalignment including chronic neck/back pain and scar tissue adhesions.

Effects
Release localized superficial fascial restrictions.

Technique
After locating the adhesion:
1. One hand moves the skin to place the adhesion on stretch.
2. Using the second and third fingers of the other hand, stroke in the opposite direction of the force, terminating in a curl, forming a J. Hold for 90 to 120 seconds or until restriction releases. You may feel a heat or pulsating sensation underneath your fingers.
3. Repeat until all adhesions have been reduced.

CLINICAL TECHNIQUES: MYOFASCIAL TECHNIQUES: FOCUSED STRETCHING

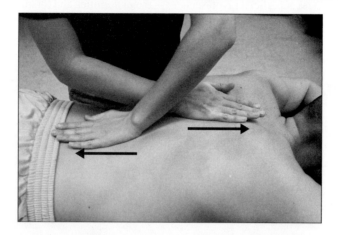

Description

Focused stretching is used to reduce superficial or deep adhesions by moving the skin and fascia in opposite directions. In the case pictured, the force is parallel to the line of the muscles, but this technique can also be performed perpendicular to the muscle fibers.

Indications

Large muscle groups such as the back.

Technique

After identifying the area of restriction:
1. Place the heel of one hand in the area of the restriction.
2. The opposite arm is crossed in front and the hand is placed below the first hand.
3. Stretch the tissues to take up the slack.
4. Using slow, deep pressure, stretch the tissues.
5. Repeat the above steps in opposite directions until no restrictions are felt.

CLINICAL TECHNIQUES: MYOFASCIAL TECHNIQUES: SKIN ROLLING

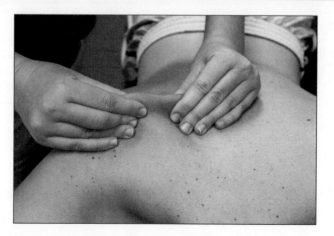

Description

Outwardly, skin rolling in myofascial therapy is similar to pétrisssage except that it specifically addresses the fascia instead of the underlying muscle (see Clinical Techniques: Pétrisssage).

The skin is lifted and rolled between the fingers, identifying and focusing on areas of superficial myofascial adhesions.

Indications
Release of superficial myofascial adhesions.

Technique
1. Begin by progressing from the inferior and lateral segment of the body area being treated and progress medially and superiorly.[133]
2. Using the fingers and thumb, lift and separate the skin from the underlying tissues.
3. Roll the skin between the fingers, noting any adhesions, tightness, or other limitations.
4. When an area of adhesion is identified:
   • Lift the skin and move it in the direction of the restriction.
   • Move the skin in the direction of the restriction.
   • If the adhesion is still present, move the skin diagonal to the restriction.
   • Repeat until the restriction has been resolved.
5. Repeat the above steps, this time progressing from the superior and lateral portion of the body segment to the inferior and medial portion.

CLINICAL TECHNIQUES: MYOFASCIAL TECHNIQUES: ARM PULL/LEG PULL

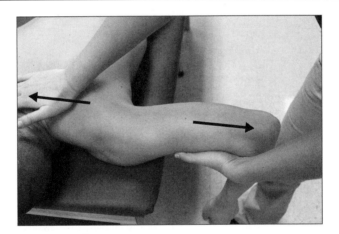

Description
Extremity pulls stretch the fascia first as a single unit and then focus on local areas of adhesion. The theory and technique for the leg pull is similar to the arm pull.

Indications
Stretch large areas of fascia in the extremities.

Technique
1. Position the patient supine with the arm relaxed at the side.
2. Grasp the extremity either at the thenar and hypothenar eminence or just proximal to the wrist.
3. Apply a gentle traction force (5 to 10 lb, depending on the size of the patient) that is in line with the anterior deltoid.
4. Hold the stretch until relaxation is felt in the arm.
5. Abduct the shoulder approximately 10 to 15 degrees and repeat the procedure. Continue until full abduction is reached or pain or glenohumeral pathology limits motion.
6. During this process, identify any areas of regional restriction and use the appropriate myofascial techniques to reduce the adhesion.

CLINICAL TECHNIQUES: MYOFASCIAL TECHNIQUES: DIAGONAL RELEASE

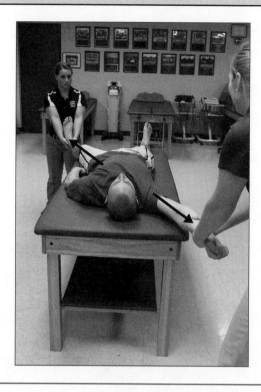

Description

The diagonal release is similar to the arm or leg pull, but affects a larger area of tissue.

Indications

Stretch large areas of fascia from contralateral extremities.

Technique

1. Position the patient prone or supine. If the prone position is used, the face should be padded.
2. One clinician grasps the leg just proximal to the talocrural joint.
3. The other clinician grasps the opposite arm proximal to the wrist.
4. Keeping the arm and leg horizontal to each other, one clinician stabilizes the extremity while the other moves the limb until adhesions are felt. A gentle traction force is then applied.
5. Step 4 is repeated until all adhesions have been identified and released (or reduced).
6. Repeat this process with the opposite limb and/or the opposite clinician providing the stabilizing force.

Self-myofascial release is an effective way to address fascial restrictions when there is limited time for manual soft tissue mobilization techniques. Autogenic inhibition can help improve soft tissue extensibility by relaxing the muscle, thus allowing for activation of the antagonist muscle. There is a variety of equipment available, ranging from foam rollers to golf balls that can be used to effectively release myofascial adhesions. The smaller and denser the equipment is, the more intense the pressure will be.[141]

The patient should start with a low-density foam roller until an appropriate tolerance can be built up to progressively increase the intensity. The patient should roll perpendicular to the muscle fiber direction and locate an area of hypersensitivity and hold for a minimum of 30 seconds and up to 90 seconds before moving to another position. As this can cause some muscle soreness, similar to the feeling of a bruise, this technique should not repeated until the soreness resolves. Typically this can be 1 to 2 days.

Active release techniques can also be very effective in the treatment of soft tissue adhesions especially where a muscle strain or injury has healed. Active release can help a healed muscle strain by encouraging a more functional realignment of the scar tissue. There are three stages to this technique:

1. Locate the structure and passively shorten the muscle.
2. Apply tension directly on the adhesion with the thumb.
3. Have the patient actively contract the antagonist muscle while the tissue glides underneath your thumb.

Active release can be very painful and should be limited to three glides per treatment area and there should be a minimum of 48 hours between treatments. Active release can also be effective in treating nerve entrapments. An extensive knowledge of anatomy will help increase the efficacy of this treatment as it is very specific to the structure being mobilized. Advanced certification is required to become proficient in the active release technique.

◼ Instrument-Assisted Soft-Tissue Mobilization

Instrument-assisted soft-tissue mobilization (IASTM) is used to identify and treat myofascial dysfunctions such as chronic tendinopathies, scars that have healed improperly, restrictions such as soft-tissue fibrosis, and other chronic inflammatory disorders. IASTM can encourage realignment of end-phase scarring and myofascial restrictions that cause improper tensile forces on musculotendinous attachments.

The general concept of IASTM is based on Gua Sha, an ancient Eastern medicine healing technique, and Cyriax's theory of manual deep soft-tissue mobilization.[142] There are several types of commercial instruments constructed from stainless steel, ceramic, or plastic. Examples include Sound Assisted Soft Tissue Mobilization (SASTM®), Augmented Soft Tissue Mobilization (ASTYM®), and Graston®. These instruments assist the clinician in identifying areas of fascial adhesions by amplifying the underlying unhealthy tissue texture and enhancing the sensation to the clinician's hands, thus increasing the efficacy of treatment (Fig. 17-2). This helps to isolate treatment to the affected tissue and to protect the clinician from repetitive manual therapy techniques that can be physically taxing.

The mechanical load caused by the instruments appears to be the primary mechanism that initiates the healing response.[143] The instruments are thought to cause local inflammatory response including capillary hemorrhage and a fibroblastic response that reactivates the healing process.[144] The intention is to create a permanent change in the elasticity of the tissue treated. The red petechiae markings are not to be confused with bruising. If treatment is done improperly, it can cause damage to healthy tissue or exacerbate unhealthy tissue. Therefore, this treatment is contraindicated for use on acute injuries. To maximize the benefits of this intervention, the involved soft tissues should be stretched immediately following treatment. The external tensile load of stretching helps the collagen realignment via increased collagen synthesis and proteoglycan, the "filler" substance

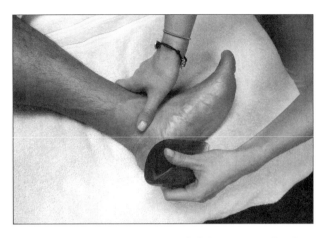

Figure 17-2. **Instrument-Assisted Soft-Tissue Mobilization.**

in most soft tissue.[143,145] IASTM is also used before rehabilitation exercises and/or training. Subsequent exercise assists in stressing the tissue positively in its newly aligned state. Positive outcomes have been found in degenerated tissue following IASTM.[146] Patients in clinical studies suffering from carpal tunnel syndrome or plantar fasciitis reported decreased pain and increased range of motion and function following conclusion of the treatment battery. Some patients may report increased soreness immediately following IASTM and bruising some time following treatment. However, these effects are short-lived.[146]

● EFFECTS ON

The Injury Response Process

Massage is promoted to elicit a number of responses within the body. These responses are related to the direct mechanical effects on the tissue (e.g., breaking adhesions), reflexive responses that occur secondary to stimulation of the nerves (e.g., pain reduction), or by psychological means (e.g., systemic relaxation).

In general, massage strokes can produce various responses, depending on the body part, amount of pressure applied, and the speed of the stroke. Light, slow stroking of the skin results in systemic relaxation. Fast, deep strokes cause an increase in blood flow to the area, invigorating the person in preparation for competition.

Cardiovascular Effects

Deep friction or vigorous massage is thought to produce vascular changes similar to those of inflammation, with the treated area being marked by increased blood flow, histamine release, and an increased temperature. Light massage may activate the sympathetic nervous system that causes temporary capillary vasodilation. Deeper, more vigorous massage is used to produce longer lasting vasodilation of the capillaries and arterioles, thus increasing blood flow to the area. Massage may evoke an initial spike in blood pressure, presenting a precaution for its application to individuals having uncontrolled high blood pressure.

Massage applied for the purpose of inducing systemic relaxation does produce physiological changes in the cardiovascular system. Decreased heart rate, respiratory rate, and blood pressure have been observed in patients after 30 minutes of massage.[147] Massaging acupressure points is reported to decrease systolic and diastolic blood pressure, decrease heart rate, and reduce cutaneous blood flow.[148] Trigger point massage can also reduce systolic and diastolic blood pressure and heart rate and promote systemic relaxation.[149]

Neuromuscular Effects

Pétrissage has been shown to decrease neuromuscular excitability, but only during the massage, and the effects are confined to the muscles being massaged.[150,151,152] A massage routine, consisting of deep effleurage, circular friction, and transverse friction applied to the hamstrings, can increase hamstring flexibility.[153] This effect is a result of the combined decrease in neuromuscular excitability (relaxation) and stretching of muscle and scar tissue. Massage or myofascial techniques designed to increase muscular, fascial, or capsular extensibility should be followed by manual stretching of the limb.

Massage is less effective in decreasing muscular recovery time after exercise but may be effective in reducing the amount of delayed-onset muscle soreness (when applied 2 hours after explosive exercise or endurance training) by reducing the **emigration** ● of neutrophils and by increasing serum cortisol levels.[154,155]

Edema Reduction

When properly performed, massage increases venous and lymphatic flow that assists in the removal of venous and lymphatic edema and increases lymphatic uptake by spreading the extravasated substances, exposing them to more lymphatic absorption points.[156] Laboratory studies suggest that activation of the lymphatic system may limit acute inflammation.[128] Manual or mechanical massage (see Chapter 14) forces fluids within the vessels to move toward the heart. Because of the associated pressures, edema reduction massage should not be used directly on acutely injured tissues.

✱ Practical Evidence

Manual edema reduction massage is often added to the conventional intervention of elevation, compression, and functional training. Although there were no long-term differences in the results, the group receiving massage had a faster resolution of edema.[157]

The key to reducing edema is first to mobilize the proximal area of edema before attempting to move the distal areas. This procedure, known as "uncorking the bottle," can be

visualized as removing a traffic jam. Cars at the back of the pack cannot move forward until the car at the front of the line moves. Clinically, this is performed by first applying the technique proximal to the injured area, then working distally toward it. To maintain the level of edema reduction and prevent rebound swelling, apply a compression wrap following treatment and keep the limb elevated whenever possible.[158,159]

Treatment Strategies
Edema Reduction Massage

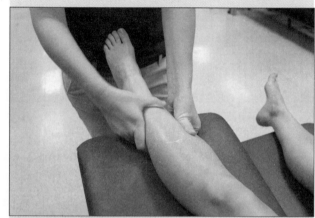

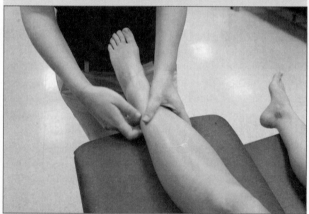

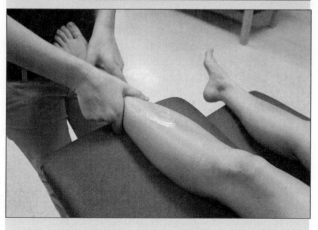

Emigration: Passage of white blood corpuscles through the walls of capillaries and veins during inflammation.

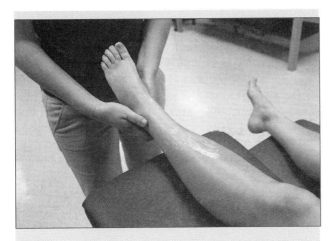

Edema reduction massage is begun proximal to the swollen area, progressing distally to the edema, and then works proximally again, repeating as many times as needed. This effect, "uncorking the bottle," increases lymphatic uptake and venous flow by first mobilizing the proximal fluids, thus allowing the distal edema to flow proximally.

1. Elevate the body part to be treated using an incline board, pillow, or other device.
2. Cover the entire surface to be treated with a lubricating massage lotion.
3. Position yourself distal to the limb. For example, if the ankle is being massaged, stand so that you see the bottom of the foot.
4. Begin by making long, slow strokes toward the heart, starting proximal to the injured area. Every fourth or fifth stroke, move the starting point of the massage slightly distal.
5. Continue stroking longitudinally, with the starting point gradually being moved distally.
6. When the distal portion of the edematous area is reached, begin working back to the original starting point.

Pain Control

Pain reduction obtained from massage is the result of several different mechanisms, but the primary effect is derived through the stimulation of cutaneous sensory receptors, activating the spinal gate and the release of endogenous opiates, interrupting the pain-spasm-pain cycle. The benefits of massage-mediated pain reduction can last up to 24 hours after the treatment.[160]

Mechanical pain is reduced through interrupting muscle spasm and reducing edema. Chemical pain is thought to be diminished by increasing blood flow and by encouraging the removal of cellular wastes, but these responses are unsubstantiated. However, simply touching the skin can also reduce the pain by activating cutaneous receptors. Gentle massage activates sensory nerves and, therefore, inhibits pain through the gate mechanism.[161,162] Massage has also been shown to activate the autonomic nervous system and

pacinian receptors, both of which assist in hindering nociceptive impulses[156] and decrease H-reflex amplitude of spinal cord–injured patients, but only during the actual massage administration.[163,164] Massage has not been shown to significantly affect serum levels of endogenous opiates, such as β-endorphin, in a treatment group compared with a control group.[165] Further pain reduction may occur secondary to mediation of neural reflexes.[166]

Psychological Benefits

Despite the lack of empirical evidence for many of the physiological benefits that are claimed to be associated with massage, support for the psychological benefits does exist. Much of this benefit extends from the one-on-one interaction required between the clinician and the patient.[161,167] This interaction reduces patient anxiety, depression, and mental stress.[147,168] Although pain reduction can be attributed to stimulation of sensory nerves and decreased spasticity within the treated area, administering massage to uninvolved areas also brings about pain relief.[169] Patient compliance in reporting for treatment sessions is greatly enhanced when massage is included as a part of the treatment regimen.[170]

■ Contraindications to Therapeutic Massage

Therapeutic massage requiring deep pressure is contraindicated in acute injury or inflammation, including sprains, fractures, joint dislocations, and other conditions in which the pressure or motion would worsen the condition. Massage should not be applied directly to open skin wounds or skin conditions (e.g., cellulitis, dermatitis) that should not be touched otherwise or infected areas. Vascular conditions such as varicose veins or hematoma where direct pressure on the vessels should be avoided or the pressure could loosen a clot are also contraindications to therapeutic massage. Massage is not indicated for the reduction of all forms of edema. Acute edema could cause more inflammation and more swelling. Swelling caused by cardiovascular insufficiency including uncontrolled high blood pressure, kidney or liver disease, or pleural effusion is contraindicated.

■ Controversies in Treatment

Massage is often therapeutic because of its "healing touch" effect, spiritual aspects, and other emotional or cognitive effects. As such, the holistic benefits of this treatment approach should not be discounted. However, empirical evidence does call into question many of the effects attributed to therapeutic massage.

The effects of massage on blood flow are unclear. Massaging the forearm and quadriceps muscle groups with effleurage, pétrissage, and tapotement failed to increase the arterial blood flow supplying these groups.[171] Massage before submaximal treadmill testing revealed no significant differences in cardiac output, blood pressure, and lactic acid concentration in a treatment group compared with a group receiving no massage before testing.[172]

Although massage is often used before athletic competition to improve performance, a study examining the effects of massage before competition concluded that this technique does not significantly increase the stride frequency of sprinters.[173] Massaging muscles between exercise bouts, be it a sprinter's legs between races or a pitcher's shoulder between innings, does little to reduce muscular fatigue.[153,174] However, psychological benefits may still be gained from these techniques.

Athletic activity may result in muscle damage, delayed-onset muscle soreness, and decreased strength, conditions for which massage is often used to treat. However, it appears that "sports massage" techniques fail to address any of these detrimental effects[175] and do not significantly reduce blood lactate concentration.[176]

Recovery from exercise does not appear to be enhanced following massage treatment. Massage has little physiological effect on blood lactate concentrations or other metabolic byproducts.[171,172,176] The effect of massage on delayed-onset muscle soreness is mixed.[154,155,177] Low-intensity active exercises such as stationary bike riding or walking should be used to accelerate the removal of the metabolic byproducts of exercise.[176]

Although anecdotal evidence indicates otherwise, transverse friction massage has not been found to be effective in the treatment of iliotibial band friction syndrome[130] or lateral epicondylitis during controlled studies.[178]

■ Clinical Application of Massage

Massage is as much an art as it is a science. There are multiple ways to perform therapeutic massage, but most sessions begin with warming, superficial strokes and conclude with slow, superficial strokes. The proportion of strokes and techniques used in the remainder of the session is based on the patient's pathology and the desired treatment outcomes.

Preparation

To be performed properly, the patient must be comfortably positioned and, if applicable, a massage lubricant must be used. Before administering the massage, the patient must be appropriately draped for modesty and the area to be treated must be exposed.

Massage Media

Most massages incorporate some type of lubricant to decrease the friction between the patient's skin and the hand; however, massage can be given without any lubricant being used. Lubricants, including massage lotion, peanut oil, coconut oil, powder, and even counterirritants allow the hands to glide smoothly over the skin and focus the effects on the underlying muscle. If the massage is being given over hairy areas, lubricants are needed to keep from pulling body hair.

The least amount of massage lubricant required to perform the massage should be applied to the patient. Using too much lubricant makes it difficult to adequately manipulate the tissues. Too little lubricant can cause skin irritation or pull the patient's body hair. Patients who have dry skin require that lubricant be added throughout the course of the treatment. Lubricant should not be applied to the face.

Various massage and myofascial release techniques are enhanced when performed without the use of a lubricant. In addition, friction assists in mobilizing the skin over the underlying tissues, making the use of lubricants contraindicated with this style of massage.

Tables and Chairs

Specialized massage tables that have a cutout to comfortably fit the patient's face and upper extremities can be used for treatment. Standard treatment plinths can also be used, but a face bolster or rolled towel should be used when the patient is placed prone while bolsters are placed under the abdomen and let to decrease tension on the low back. Massage chairs can be used for thoracic, cervical spine, and upper extremity massage sessions (Fig. 17-3).

General Considerations

1. Establish the absence of contraindications.
2. Explain the type of massage that will be applied and the expected sensations.
3. If an adjustable-height table is being used, the height should allow the clinician to keep the spine straight during the massages. Any bending or motion should occur at the knees, not at the waist.
4. Cover the table with a sheet.
5. The position of the patient relative to the clinician is important to both parties. When treating small areas the clinician should stand in a place that requires little or no repositioning. Likewise, long strokes, such as those applied to the back or hamstrings, should be performed by taking small steps rather than by bending the back.
6. Position the patient so that the muscles being massaged are relaxed. If an extremity is being massaged to reduce edema, it should be elevated.
7. If a massage lubricant is being used, warm it slightly between the hands so that it is not uncomfortable when applied (i.e., not too hot or too cold). Then spread the lubricant on the skin. Do not pour the lubricant directly on the body.
8. When a painful area is being treated, the massage begins in a nonpainful area, works through the area of pain, and concludes on another pain-free area.
9. Drape the patient to ensure modesty and expose the area to be treated.

At a Glance: Therapeutic Massage

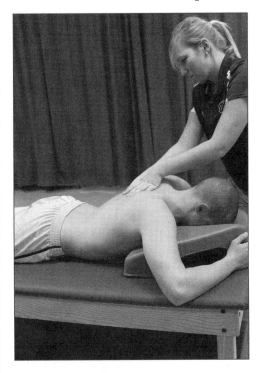

Description

Massage uses touch to produce muscular, nervous, and cardiovascular changes. Targeted techniques are used to break up adhesions and muscle spasm.

Indications

- To relieve fibrosis and other myofascial adhesions
- To increase venous return
- Edema reduction
- Reduction of lymphatic or venous edema
- To break the pain-spasm-pain cycle
- To evoke systemic relaxation
- Trigger points
- To improve or stimulate local blood flow
- To increase range of motion

Primary Effects

- Increased blood flow
- Increased venous and lymphatic drainage
- Sedation
- Pain reduction
- Elongation of muscle fibers and other soft tissue
- Hypotonicity

Contraindications

- Areas of active inflammation
- Sites where fractures have failed to heal
- Skin conditions in area to be treated
- Open wounds in the area to be treated
- Infection causing **lymphangitis** •
- Phlebitis, thrombophlebitis, or hematoma
- Varicose veins
- Arteriosclerosis
- Cellulitis
- Abscess or other forms of infection

Treatment Duration

- The duration of the massage ranges from a few minutes up to an hour. The duration is dependent on the type of massage being applied and the clinical setting in which it is given.
- Massage for edema reduction is given once a day for an average duration of 5 to 10 minutes.
- Friction massage is performed once a day for 5 minutes or as needed.

Precautions

- Areas of sensory deficit
- Acute sprains or strains—avoid the application of deep pressure.
- Massage may increase the inflammatory response when used early in the acute or subacute stage of the injury response cycle.
- Use decreased pressure when applying massage over areas having decreased sensation.
- Do not use massage for swelling caused by cardiovascular insufficiency, kidney or liver disease, or pleural effusion.

Lymphangitis: Inflammation of the lymphatic vessels draining an extremity. This condition is most often associated with inflammation or infection.

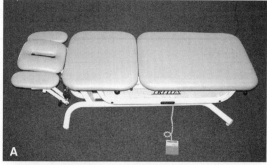

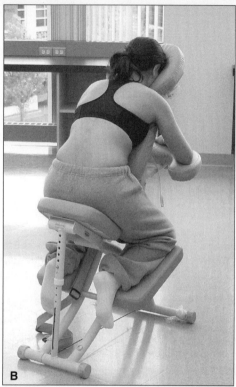

Figure 17-3. **Massage Table (A) and Chair (B).**

Traditional Massage

1. The area may be preheated with moist heat to promote relaxation of the musculature.
2. A bolster may be placed under the ankles and a small pad, such as a folded towel or small pillow, placed under the abdomen to assist in the relaxation of the lumbar musculature.
3. If applicable, apply the massage lubricant on the body parts to be treated.
4. Follow the application of the lubricant with a light, slow effleurage.
5. Gradually build up to deeper effleurage.
6. Begin pétrissage strokes.
7. Using a towel, wipe the lubricant off the patient's skin before applying deep friction massage where (and if) applicable.
8. Apply tapotement to the back and extremities (if treated).
9. Reapply pétrissage and deep effleurage.
10. End the treatment with light effleurage.

Termination of the Treatment

1. If a lubricant was used, remove it with a towel.
2. If appropriate for the stage of injury, encourage active range-of-motion exercises.
3. Following edema reduction massage, apply a compression wrap and keep the extremity elevated whenever possible.
4. To assist in flushing metabolic waste from the body, the patient should be encouraged to drink water after the treatment.
5. Remove the sheet from the table and launder properly.

Chapter 18

Electromyographic Biofeedback

Unlike other therapeutic modalities presented in this text, electromyographic biofeedback does not deliver energy to the body. Instead, biofeedback measures the amount of a specific type of physiological activity that is occurring. In the case of muscle contractions, the amount of motor nerve activity is being observed. The biofeedback unit then converts this activity into a visual or audible form that can be interpreted by the patient and clinician.

● Biofeedback is the process of detecting physiological activity in the body and converting that activity into visual and/or auditory cues that the patient can use. With electromyographic (EMG) biofeedback, the unit amplifies the body's neuromuscular electrical activity and converts it to auditory and/or visual signals. The patient then uses this feedback to modify further activity such as increasing muscle contraction.

Consider, for example, a patient who is recovering from anterior cruciate ligament (ACL) surgery who is unable to voluntarily contract the vastus medialis oblique (VMO) muscle. Because of swelling, lack of use (disuse atrophy), and pain, the patient does not contract this muscle. With time, the normal neurological loop used to innervate the VMO is lost; the patient "forgets" how to contract the muscle. When biofeedback is used over the VMO, the feedback indicates when motor nerve impulses are being directed to the muscle (Fig. 18-1).

Biofeedback measures at least one of five biophysical properties (Table 18-1). The resulting feedback can be used to reeducate muscle, facilitate muscular relaxation, control blood pressure and heart rate, and decrease the physical signs of emotional stress.

Biofeedback does not monitor the actual response itself (e.g., the strength of the contraction), but rather it measures the conditions associated with response (e.g., neurological activity). The normal proprioceptive input is amplified through the use of sound, light, or meters. The strength of the feedback increases as the number of motor units recruited into the contraction increases. This information can be used to increase the strength of healthy muscle and restore normal function.[180]

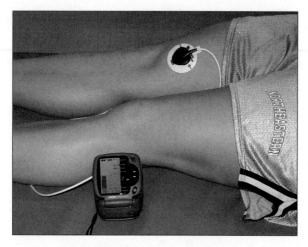

Figure 18-1. **Electromyographic Biofeedback.** Electrode placement for the vastus medialis oblique muscle.

TABLE 18-1	Types of Biofeedback
TYPE	PRINCIPLE
Electromyographic (EMG)	Measures the electrical activity in skeletal muscle.
Mechanomyographic	Measures the transverse displacement of the skin over the target muscle based on the sound produced and/or skin tension. Quantifies oscillations in skin caused by changes in muscle fibers.[179]
Peripheral temperature	Measures temperature changes in the distal extremities (e.g., fingers). Increased temperature indicates a relaxed state (increased superficial blood flow). Decreased temperature indicates stress, fear, or anxiety (decreased superficial blood flow).
Photoplethysmography	Measures the amount of light reflected by subcutaneous tissues based on the amount of blood flow.
Galvanic skin response	Measures the amount of perspiration on the skin by passing a small current through the fingers and/or palm. Sweaty skin contains salt and is a better conductor than dry skin.

Because most clinical applications of EMG biofeedback use superficial electrodes, that technique will be the focus of this chapter. Conceptually, biofeedback functions by[181]:

- Monitoring the physiological process.
- Objectively measuring the process.
- Converting what is being monitored into feedback that optimizes the desired effects.

With orthopedic patients, biofeedback is most often used as an adjunct to muscle reeducation and training or to encourage the relaxation of a muscle group. Biofeedback is also used for patients suffering central nervous system trauma such as spinal cord injury or stroke. Functional patterns such as gait and grasping and strength training may also be reestablished using biofeedback.

■ Measurements

The electronic and physiological mechanisms associated with EMG biofeedback are covered in the next section. At this point, a clarification must be made between "monitoring" and "measuring" the electrical activity. **Monitoring** involves determining whether neuromuscular activity is present and, if so, whether it is increasing or decreasing. **Measuring** the activity involves placing an objective scale on the monitored readout.

Consider the two meters depicted in Figure 18-2. The meter in Figure 18-2A shows that activity is taking place, and we can tell if it is increasing, decreasing, or holding steady by observing the relative position of the needle. When a scale is placed on the meter, the amount of activity,

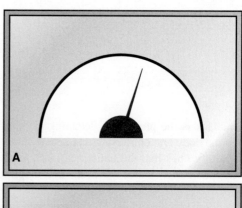

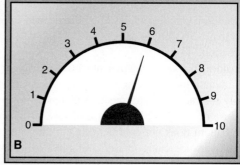

Figure 18-2. **Measuring Versus Monitoring of Biofeedback.** Meter (A) indicates if activity is occurring and the change over time. Meter (B) provides objective measures through the use of a numeric scale.

and therefore the degree of change, can be objectively measured (Fig. 18-2B). The scale on a biofeedback unit may use the number of microvolts, a simple 0-to-10 scale, or a bar graph or other visual representation as the measure. Because of the lack of a standard biofeedback scale, measurements made on a unit used by one brand cannot be compared with measurements on a unit used by another brand.[181,182] Also, placement of skin electrodes from treatment to treatment affects the measurement's reliability.[183]

The meter is only one form of meaningful information that biofeedback units can provide. Most units can convert the signals into sound waves, an advantage because they allow the patient to focus on the muscle rather than looking at the biofeedback unit. The pitch of the sound increases and decreases based on the amount of neuromuscular activity. Computer interfaces are also used to create larger renditions of the feedback and may provide increased motivation by creating a game-like, competitive atmosphere.

■ Biophysical Processes and Electrical Integration

Application of EMG biofeedback involves the use of three electrodes positioned over the target muscle or muscle group. Basic EMG biofeedback units have one channel composed of three surface electrodes combined on a single self-adhesive electrode. Two of these electrodes are "active electrodes" that measure the amount of electrical activity within the muscle. The third electrode, the "reference electrode" is used to filter out nonmeaningful electrical activity. The most sensitive EMG surface monitors have electrodes made with silver (Fig. 18-3). Surface electrodes are more sensitive to electrical activity in superficial muscles than in deeper muscles. Needle electrodes implanted directly in the muscle are used with EMG units for diagnostic and research purposes.

The electrodes monitor the electrical activity within a local area of a muscle, usually the muscle belly (Fig. 18-4).

Some EMG units have two or more channels that allow multiple muscles to be monitored or a single muscle to be monitored in different areas. The amount of electrical activity within the muscle increases as more motor units are recruited into the contraction. These signals are then picked up by the electrodes, amplified, and converted into visual or auditory signals. Although this process seems straightforward, it is complicated by the presence of other electromagnetic energy in our environment. We are always being bombarded by electromagnetic energy. A small portion of this energy is absorbed by the body and subsequently detected by the biofeedback unit. This unwanted energy, "noise," must be filtered out before the meaningful activity can be determined (Box 18-1).

Although EMG biofeedback requires three electrodes, they are often found on a single self-adhesive patch with the active electrodes spaced approximately 3 cm apart, although some units require that each electrode be applied individually (see Fig. 18-3). Locating the active electrodes close to each other targets the specific muscle, but the raw signal is relatively weak. Increasing the distance between the active electrodes increases the strength of the raw signal and monitors a greater proportion of the muscle. However, as the distance is increased, the reliability of the signal decreases because electrical activity in the surrounding muscles and external electrical interference will be detected by the biofeedback unit.[182]

● EFFECTS ON

The Injury Response Process

EMG biofeedback itself does not affect the injury response process. Unlike other modalities presented in this text, biofeedback units assist voluntary functions to produce the desired results. Other types of biofeedback units monitor autonomic nervous system function such has heart rate.

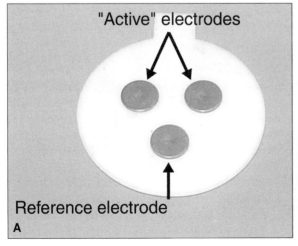

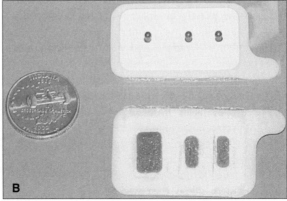

Figure 18-3. **EMG Biofeedback Surface Electrodes.** (A) Standard self-adhesive modeling showing the active and reference electrodes. (B) Silver electrodes. A U.S. quarter is used for size reference.

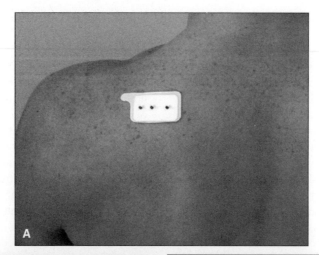

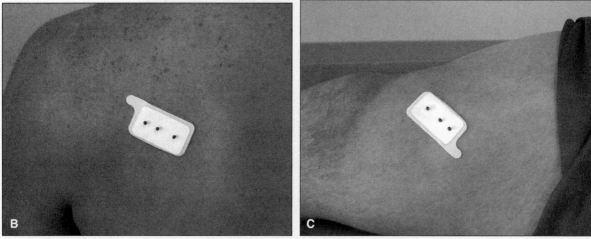

Figure 18-4. **Placement of Biofeedback Electrodes.** (A) Supraspinatus. (B) Infraspinatus. (C) Vastus medialis oblique.

Because of this, the effectiveness of biofeedback is judged on a case-by-case basis.[182] Biofeedback facilitates muscle reeducation and promotes relaxation. Increased muscle strength can then increase range of motion. In turn, these effects can lead to a reduction in pain and an increase in function (Figure 18-5).[183]

Because EMG biofeedback detects the electrical activity associated with muscle contractions, there must be an intact nerve supply to and from the muscle. Adjunct strategies can be used to help facilitate a muscle contraction (Table 18-2). The injured tissues must be able to withstand the tension and stresses associated with the motion, and there must be some level of nerve supply to the target muscle or muscle groups.

Biofeedback can be used with electrical stimulation to further restore neuromuscular function. The electrical stimulation unit is programmed to produce a muscle contraction once the patient has reached the threshold established with the biofeedback unit.

The benefits of biofeedback are enhanced by educating the patient on the concept of biofeedback, incorporating learning strategies, and setting patient goals.[184,185]

Verbal feedback can reinforce the neuromuscular reeducation and provide positive cognitive reinforcement to the patient. However, this type of feedback while the patient is concentrating on producing a muscle contraction can distract the patient from the task at hand, so refrain from talking to the patient until the exercise has been completed.[186]

Neuromuscular Effects

Biofeedback is most often incorporated into an orthopedic treatment and rehabilitation program after surgery or long-term immobilization. Edema, pain, and decreased input from joint receptors inhibit voluntary muscle contractions. The use of biofeedback shapes the response that enables the central nervous system to reestablish sensory-motor loops "forgotten" by the patient.[187,188] On reaching the brain, the sound or visual cues stimulate cerebral areas that normally receive proprioceptive information. These artificial signals, combined with the visual cue of actually watching the muscle contract, assist in reopening a neural loop that sends efferent signals to the appropriate muscles.

Box 18-1. EMG BIOFEEDBACK SIGNAL PROCESSING

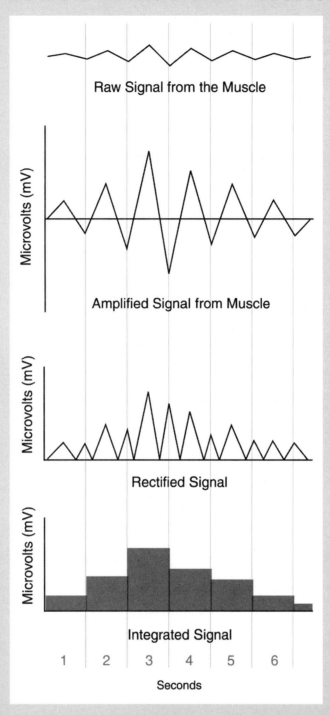

Raw Signal from the Muscle

Amplified Signal from Muscle

Rectified Signal

Integrated Signal

Five steps are required to process and provide feedback of the body's neuromuscular electrical activity:

Identify ⇒   **Amplify** ⇒   **Rectify** ⇒   **Integrate** ⇒   **Output**
Signal   **Signal**   **Signal**   **Signal**   **Signal**

The EMG unit filters out electrical noise and identifies the raw signal, positive and negative electrical activity associated with the depolarization and repolarization of the involved cells. Referring to Figure 18-3, you will notice that two electrodes are labeled "active" and one as "reference." The reference electrode serves as a measurement point for a very small current passed between the two active electrodes. This results in two sources supplying input to a differential amplifier within the unit. Here, the meaningful

Continued

Box 18-1. EMG BIOFEEDBACK SIGNAL PROCESSING—cont'd

information is separated from the meaningless noise. Because the extraneous noise is produced by electromagnetic sources, it occurs at a constant frequency and is detectable anywhere in the body. The differential amplifier compares the input from two sources and eliminates any activity that is common to both. In theory, the remaining activity represents the **raw signal** of the neuromuscular activity. However, the integrity of the final signal depends on the quality of the unit and the number of filters used (more filters lead to a more precise signal). The amplitude of the raw signal is small and must be **amplified** by the unit. **Rectification** involves taking the absolute value of the negative electrical activity and making it a mathematically positive number, causing the plot to move to the positive side of the baseline. The final EMG signal is formed by calculating the root-mean-square average of the electrical activity per unit of time, **integration.** The integrated signal is then converted into an **output signal** that is normally a visual display or auditory tone.

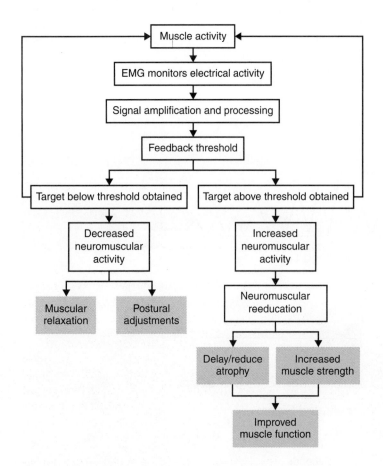

Figure 18-5. **Effects of Electromyographic biofeedback.** The EMG unit detects and amplifies the electrical activity associated with motor nerves and muscle contractions. The feedback threshold indicates the amount of EMG activity that increases or decreases the feedback. Activity above the threshold represents increased muscular activity (muscle recruitment); below the threshold indicates decreased muscular activity (relaxation).

TABLE 18-2   Methods to Facilitate a Muscle Contraction

- Have the patient contract the muscle on the opposite limb, then attempt to contract the involved muscle.
- Apply the biofeedback unit to the opposite limb so that the person will "learn" the biofeedback technique.
- Watch and/or touch the contracting muscle.
- Contract surrounding or opposing muscles.
- Contract the proximal portion of the muscle to facilitate neuromuscular activity in the distal motor units.
- Use electrical stimulation to evoke a muscle contraction (note: disconnect the biofeedback device prior to using this technique).

Facilitative biofeedback can modify contraction timing patterns.[189]

✳ Practical Evidence

During neuromuscular rehabilitation, EMG biofeedback is most beneficial when it is incorporated early in the patient's program, especially when active motions are involved.[190,191]

Improvements in the quality and quantity of a muscle contraction can be seen following a single treatment session. To help the patient retain the newly learned neurological pathways, the patient should perform active muscle contractions without the biofeedback unit immediately following each session. Home exercise programs that target the involved muscles will facilitate the retention of muscle memory.

The cognitive process of neuromuscular relaxation is similar to that of evoking muscle contractions. However, rather than attempting to reestablish neural loops, the goal is to quiet these pathways. The goal of relaxation therapy is to decrease the number of motor impulses being relayed to the muscle in spasm. Orthopedically, this technique is best used with cases of subconscious muscle guarding. Biofeedback can be used during the activities of daily living to reinforce proper posture and biomechanics[179] and has been successfully used to control prehypertension.[192]

The use of relaxation biofeedback does not significantly increase flexibility in healthy individuals when compared with standard flexibility exercises. However, athletes combining flexibility with biofeedback displayed a greater retention of improvement than those training without the aid of biofeedback.[193]

Pain Reduction

Long-term pain reduction stems from restoring normal function of the body part. Reeducating muscle and reducing atrophy helps to restore normal biomechanics. Decreasing muscle spasm reduces the amount of mechanical pressure placed on nociceptors.

Inhibitory biofeedback has also been successfully used in the reduction of myofascial pain, the pain associated with migraine and tension headaches, as well as in general stress reduction.[194] Most inhibitory pain-control approaches also involve cognitive and behavioral aspects that build on the biofeedback sessions.[195,196]

■ Contraindications

The primary contraindications to the use of biofeedback are those conditions where muscle tension or joint motion would cause further injury. A general guideline is not to use biofeedback if the patient is prohibited from moving the joint or if isometric contractions are contraindicated.

Unhealed tendon grafts, avulsed tendons, and second- or third-degree strains may be damaged by the tension associated with even moderate muscle contractions. Injuries to the joint structures or unstable fractures are also contraindications to biofeedback.

■ Overview of the Evidence

The efficacy of EMG biofeedback is clinically well-accepted neuromuscular reeducaton. The primary concern relates to the unit's accuracy in detecting the muscle's raw signal. Surface electrodes are most sensitive to superficial muscles. Electrode placement, electromagnetic noise, and tissue variability (e.g., the amount of hydration) cause significant variability in the signals produced even by the same subject.[182]

Despite the physiological basis for the use of EMG biofeedback in muscular reeducation, the clinical benefits of this technique have not been substantiated in the literature. The primary reason is the lack of published research and methodological differences in those studies.[197]

■ Clinical Application of Biofeedback

Instrumentation

Biofeedback units range from the very simple to the complex. Portable "take-home" units have fewer features and are easier to use than clinical models. The following description is of the typical midrange unit. Consult the user's manual of your particular unit for a more detailed description of its operation.

Alarm: Identifies a target range for EMG activity. Feedback is triggered when the EMG activity is within a specified range of the target value or is significantly above or below preset levels (see **Sensitivity range**).

Output: Determines the type of feedback available. Visual feedback appears by way of a meter or bar graph. The audio output is normally adjustable between various frequencies. Many models allow for a computer interface that presents the feedback in a graphical method on the computer's monitor. Computers can store results of the session.

Sensitivity range: This control provides coarse adjustments on the neuroelectrical level needed to obtain feedback. The feedback may be **threshold,** a constant alarm or visual cue that is elicited once the threshold has been reached, or **progressive,** where the level of feedback increases with the intensity once the threshold has been reached.

Statistics: Some biofeedback units calculate the statistics of the patient's muscular activity. These data can be used to assess the rehabilitation program. Measures such as the mean, maximum, and standard deviation of the amount of EMG activity provide quantitative information for evaluating the patient's progress.

At a Glance: **Electromyographic Biofeedback**

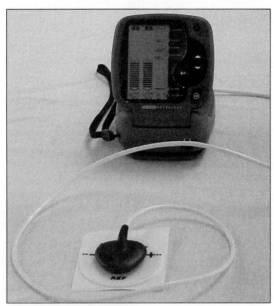

Description

Electromyographic biofeedback detects the amount of electrical activity associated with a muscle contraction and converts it to visual and/or auditory feedback that promotes the strength of the muscular contraction or facilitates relaxation.

Indications

- To facilitate muscular contractions
- To regain neuromuscular control
- To decrease muscle spasm
- To promote systemic relaxation

Treatment

Biofeedback can be performed daily as needed either in the clinical setting or at home. Be aware of any muscle soreness that may occur after exercise and adjust the treatment protocol accordingly.

Contraindications

- Conditions in which muscular contractions would insult the tissues
- Conditions where the contraction will cause joint movement and motion

Precautions

- Do not exceed the prescribed range of motion.
- Avoid undue muscle tension that may affect grafts or other tissue restrictions.

Tuner: Allows fine adjustments on the threshold required to obtain feedback.

Volume: Adjusts the audible output of the feedback. Audible feedback may come from a built-in speaker or through an earpiece or headphones.

Setup and Application

Patient Preparation

1. Question the patient to rule out the presence of contraindications.
2. Remove any dirt, oil, or makeup in the area where the electrodes are to be applied by wiping the skin with alcohol. These substances impede the conduction of the bioelectric signals, as may excess body hair where the electrodes are to be placed. Shave the area if applicable.
3. Very sensitive biofeedback units may require that the electrode site be mildly abraded with an emery cloth.
4. Apply a suitable conductive gel to the electrodes.
5. Secure the electrodes over a motor point near the belly of the muscle targeted in this therapy (see Appendix C). If a motor point chart is not available, locate the electrodes over the muscle belly. Note that the active electrodes must be applied

over the target muscle. The reference electrode may be placed anywhere on the body, but by convention, it is normally placed between the two active electrodes (see Figure 18-3).

6. Plug the common electrode leads into the INPUT jacks on the unit.
7. Turn the unit ON.
8. Adjust the OUTPUT to the desired mode of feedback (visual, audio, or both).
9. Provide instructions to the individual regarding the proper use of biofeedback, including goal setting.
10. The patient should be free of visual and auditory distractions during the course of the session.

Facilitation of Isometric Muscle Contraction

1. Instruct the patient to relax the body part as much as possible.
2. Place the body part in the desired position.
3. Instruct the patient to maximally contract the muscle.
4. Adjust the **Sensitivity range** to the lowest value that does not provide feedback and note the value.
5. Have the patient relax as best as possible.
6. Set the **Sensitivity range** to approximately two-thirds of the value.
7. Instruct the patient to contract the muscle until maximum feedback is obtained and then hold the contraction for 6 seconds.
8. Have the patient completely relax so that the meter resets to the baseline before the next contraction.

9. If the patient will use an earphone during the treatment, complete two or three contractions using the speaker while the patient is under supervision to familiarize the patient with the treatment prior to its use.
10. Repeat the contractions as indicated. If the muscle group is severely atrophied, the number of contractions is normally limited to 10 to 15 contractions because of fatigue.
11. By decreasing the sensitivity, the patient will have to elicit a stronger contraction to receive feedback.
12. If the individual is unable to evoke a contraction, refer to the strategies presented in Table 18-2.

Termination of the Procedure

1. Remove the electrodes, and wipe away any excess gel.
2. If disposable electrodes are being used, discard after use.
3. To avoid dependency on biofeedback, have the patient perform additional sets of contractions without the aid of the unit to "remember" how to perform the contractions.

Maintenance

Following Each Use

Clean the biofeedback case, lead wire, and earphones following each treatment using a mild cleanser.

At Regular Intervals

Regularly inspect the electrode lead wires and jacks for kinks, frays, and defects.

Chapter 19

Low-Level Laser Therapy

The light spectrum encompasses ultraviolet, visible, and infrared energy. Although some thermal effects may be obtained from these modalities, the primary benefits are derived from photochemical effects.

● Electromagnetic energy is the most abundant form of energy in the universe. The energy found in the electromagnetic spectrum, including radio waves, and x-rays, is categorized by the frequency and length of its wave (Appendix B). Light, a form of electromagnetic energy, has three general classifications: ultraviolet, visible, and infrared (Fig. 19-1). Energy having a wavelength greater than 780 **nanometers** ● (nm) (the upper end of visible light) is infrared energy. The ultraviolet (UV) spectrum is located in the area below the range of visible light (380 nm).

Many therapeutic modalities presented in this text use energy within the light range of the electromagnetic spectrum, although the light energy may not be visible to humans. UV light is used for the treatment of certain skin conditions. Medical lasers produce beams of energy that can cause either tissue destruction or therapeutic effects within the tissues.

■ Therapeutic Lasers

Lasers produce highly refined, **monochromatic** ● light in the ultraviolet, visible, or infrared range. Lasers, an acronym for *L*ight *A*mplification by *S*timulated *E*mission of *R*adiation, consist of highly organized light **(photons)** ● that elicits physiological events in the tissues. **Low-level laser therapy (LLLT)** does not normally cause tissue destruction.[198] The U.S. Food and Drug Administration (FDA) has approved LLLT for the treatment of **carpal tunnel syndrome** ● and musculoskeletal shoulder and neck pain; however, clinically it is used for a wide range of conditions.

The energy produced by therapeutic lasers can have a wavelength between 650 and 1200 nanometers (nm).[199] This range includes UV, visible, and infrared light on the electromagnetic spectrum. The frequency (wavelength) determines the color of the laser light. Frequency and wavelength, often

---

Nanometer: One-billionth (10^{-9}) of a meter.

Monochromatic: Light that consists of only one color.

Carpal tunnel syndrome: Compression of the median nerve that produces pain, numbness, and weakness in the palm and ring and index fingers.

Photon: A unit of light energy that has zero mass, no electrical charge, and an indefinite life span.

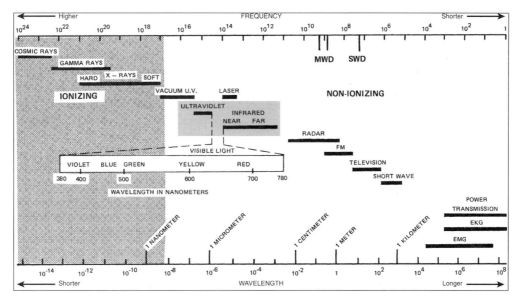

Figure 19-1. **The Electromagnetic Spectrum.** The visible portion of the light spectrum consists of energy having a wavelength of approximately 380 to 780 nm. Infrared light has a wavelength between 780 and 12,500 nm; energy with a wavelength between 180 and 400 nm is in the ultraviolet range. There is a slight amount of overlap between the visible light range and that of ultraviolet and infrared light.

used interchangeably, are inversely related to each other: as frequency increases, wavelength decreases (and vice versa). The photons emitted during LLLT activate certain skin receptors that stimulate or inhibit physiological events. These effects are caused by activation of **chromophores,** parts of a molecule (generally **melanin** • and hemoglobin) that absorb light having a specific color (wavelength). Because of the specificity of chromophores in absorbing light energy, wavelength is thought to determine which skin receptors are affected.[200]

Class 4 lasers ("hot lasers") produce thermal changes in the tissues, causing the tissues to be destroyed, evaporated, or dehydrated or causing protein coagulation (see Table 19-1).[201] Hot lasers are used for surgery, capsular shrinkage, ocular surgery, and wrinkle and tattoo removal. Because of their destructive potential, high-power lasers are not found in the rehabilitation setting.

Other forms of light therapy include ultraviolet lamps, superluminous diodes (SLDs), and light-emitting diodes (LEDs). These types of light modalities are reported to evoke some of the effects of phototherapy, but their biophysical effects are different. A laser applicator may include LEDs and SLDs to produce visible light to assist in targeting the laser, especially when the laser output is not in the visible light range. Some manufacturers may include LEDs and SLDs to promote an additive effect to the laser treatment.

■ Laser Characteristics

Lasers produce a refined, homogeneous beam of light characterized by three features: the light is (1) monochromatic, (2) coherent, and (3) collimated. **Monochromatic** means all

of the light energy has the same wavelength, thereby producing the same color. Sunlight passing through a prism creates a rainbow of colors because it has light of different wavelengths. A laser light passed through a prism simply bends and the color leaving the prism the same as that entering it.

Light photons travel in waves having different lengths. This wavelength determines the color of the light. When all of the light waves are in phase, they are said to be **coherent** (Fig 19-2). Light from a light bulb spreads—diverges—as it travels. Laser light is **collimated** because the beam does not tend to diverge as it travels through space.

Lasers are classified by the FDA's Center for Devices and Radiological Health (CDRH) based on the **Accessible Emission Limit** (AEL). The AEL is the maximum permissible power level for each class, ranging from 1 (minimum risk of causing harm) to 4 (extreme risk) (Table 19-1).

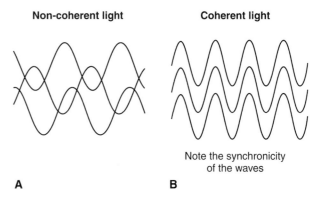

Figure 19-2. **Light Waves In and Out of Phase.** Light having the same wavelength, but the photons are out of phase. With coherent light the photons are in phase.

Melanin: Pigmentation of the hair, skin, and eye produced by melanocytes.

TABLE 19-1 U.S. Food and Drug Administration's Center for Devices and Radiological Health Laser Classification System

CLASSIFICATION	DESCRIPTION
1	These lasers are exempt from most control measures.
	The laser output is either safe to the human eye or contained within the device in a manner that keeps the laser from escaping.
	No special labeling is required.
2	Low-power lasers—visible light may be emitted.
	Output does not exceed 1 mW.
	The normal eye blink reflex (approximately 0.25 s) will protect the eye from direct contact with the laser output.
	Must be labeled with **"CAUTION—Laser Radiation: Do not stare into beam."**
2a	Visible laser is produced (e.g., a bar code scanner).
	Eye damage can occur if the laser enters the eye for more than 1000 seconds.
	The labeling is the same as for type 2 lasers.
3a	Produces an output up to 5 mW.
	Direct contact with the eye for short periods is not hazardous. Viewing the laser through magnifying optics such as eyeglasses can present a hazard.
	Must be labeled with **"CAUTION—Laser Radiation: Do not stare into beam or view directly with optical instruments."**
	Class 3a lasers do not require that the patient and clinician wear goggles during treatment.
3b	Medium power lasers producing an output of 5 mW to 500 mW.
	Direct contact of the laser output with the eyes can result in damage.
	Must be labeled with **"DANGER—Visible and/or invisible laser radiation—avoid direct exposure to beam."**
	The patient and the clinician (and anyone in the immediate area) must don goggles during treatment.
4	High power lasers having an output of greater than 500 mW.
	Direct or indirect contact with the skin and eyes can be hazardous.
	Toxic airborne contaminants may be produced.
	The output creates a fire hazard.
	Must be labeled with **"DANGER—Visible and/or invisible laser radiation—avoid eye or skin exposure to direct or scattered beam."**

Laser Output Parameters

In the United States therapeutic lasers have a wavelength of 650 nm to 1200 nm. The low and medium power output associated with LLLT does not cause significant thermal changes in the tissues, so therapeutic benefits are thought to be related to photochemical events.[199,202] The magnitude of the tissue's reaction to laser light is based on the physical characteristics of the output frequency/wavelength (absorption, reflection, and transmission), power density (irradiance), the duration of the treatment, and the vascularity of the target tissues.[199,203] The depth of penetration is also affected by the skin's melanin and blood hemoglobin content, both of which absorb photons.[200]

Effects that occur from the absorption of photons are termed the **direct effect.** An **indirect effect** is produced by chemical events caused by the interaction of the photons emitted from the laser and the tissues. The indirect effect may produce changes that occur deeper in the tissues than those caused by the direct effect.

In some cases therapeutic lasers require a base unit that houses the laser generator (Box 19-1). The output is delivered to the body through a fiber optic cable and a hand-held applicator. The laser medium (e.g., gallium aluminum arsenide, argon, helium-neon) determines the wavelength—and therefore the effects of—the laser output.

Wavelength and Frequency

Wavelength and frequency are inversely related. Long wavelengths have a lower frequency than shorter wavelengths (see Appendix B). LLLT has a frequency of up to 5000 Hz, a duration of 1 to 500 milliseconds, and an interpulse interval of 1 to 500 milliseconds, although there is variability depending on the make and model of the unit.[204]

The laser's depth of penetration, the point where photons are absorbed by the tissues, depends on the wavelength of the light. Longer wavelengths (800 to 1000 nm) penetrate deeper into the tissues than lasers

Box 19-1. PRODUCTION OF LASER

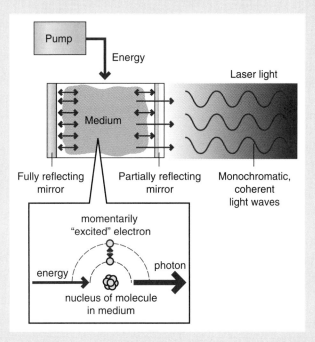

Laser production requires four essential components: (1) an active (amplifying) medium, (2) a mechanism for exciting the medium (a pump), (3) a reflective mirror, and (4) a partially reflective mirror that allows for some transmission of light and reflects the rest.

Lasers are referred to by the type of active medium (the atoms that are stimulated to produce the light) they use, HeNe (helium-neon) or GaAs (gallium-arsenic), for example. The active medium is a solid, liquid, or gas that contains atoms, molecules, or ions that are capable of storing energy that, when stimulated, release their energy as light. Any subsequent increase in light energy through the lasing mechanism is known as **gain.**

Through a process known as **pumping,** energy is introduced into the active medium. For a solid medium, the pumping is obtained by irradiating the medium with a bright light; gaseous mediums are energized by passing an electrical current through the medium.

When a photon of light is absorbed by an atom, molecule, or ion, an outer electron moves from its normal orbit, its **ground state,** to a higher orbit termed the **excited state.** By being moved to a higher orbit, the electron, and therefore the atom, reaches a higher energy state. After a brief stay (less than a millionth of a second) in the higher orbit, the electron spontaneously returns to its ground state and in the process releases another photon. The released photon will have the same wavelength (and therefore frequency) as the photon that was absorbed.

Stimulated response occurs when a photon strikes an atom that is already in the excited state and causes the electron that is in the higher orbit to move to a lower one. In this case, instead of a single photon being released, two photons are released. Each of these photons has the same wavelength and is in phase. When more atoms are in an excited state than in the ground state, a **population inversion,** more photons are emitted than absorbed, forming the basis for the emission of laser.

A laser generator consists of an **oscillator,** the active medium located between two mirrors. One mirror reflects 100% of the photons that strike it and the other mirror is only partially reflective. Photons that reflect off the mirrors are reflected back into the medium for further amplification. Those photons that transmit through the partially reflective mirror form the laser output.

having shorter wavelengths (600 to 700 nm). There is an "optical window" where the penetration of light energy through the tissues is maximized. This window is contingent on the type and consistency of the tissues.[199] The amount of power—discussed in the next section—also affects the depth of penetration.

✱ Practical Evidence

Helium-neon (HeNe) lasers have been demonstrated to be the most effective for stimulating tissue healing; gallium aluminum arsenide (GaAlAs) lasers appear to be more effective in reducing pain.[205,206]

The laser's wavelength depends on the medium used (Table 19-2). New evaluation methods have indicated that some low-power lasers can affect tissues up to 2 cm deep secondary to indirect responses, especially when applied over bony prominences such as the cervical spine and skull.[207]

Helium-neon (HeNe) lasers stimulate a mixture of helium and neon gases, producing light with a wavelength of 632.8 nm, within the visible red light range. The maximum output of HeNe lasers is usually 1 mW or less (although some models may produce output between 0.5 to 35 mW), and the energy can penetrate up to 0.8 to 15 mm deep.[208] The indirect effect may produce tissue changes deeper than 15 mm. HeNe lasers typically have an output in the range of 14 to 29 mJ (millijoule, 10^{-3} joule). The clinical availability of HeNe laser is limited because of their relative expense.

Gallium arsenide (GaAs) laser is produced by a semiconductor diode chip and delivers a light wave between 904 to 910 nm. This wavelength places the GaAs laser within the infrared spectrum (invisible to the human eye). The energy can penetrate the tissues up to 2 cm. GaAs lasers may produce up to 2 mW output that is often pulsed, delivering a significantly lower average power than HeNe lasers (see Power and Treatment Dosage). GaAs lasers have a visible light pointing system that illuminates when the laser output is being emitted to target the treatment effects.

Gallium aluminum arsenide (GaAlAs) laser multiple diodes with each diode producing up to 30 mW of power at a wavelength of 830 nm. The outputs of the diodes combine to produce a total treatment output of 90 mW, theoretically producing a deeper depth of penetration.[209] Although multidiode systems produce an increased output, their dosage specifications are unclear.[202]

Power

Dosage, the amount of energy applied to the tissues, is similar to that used for therapeutic ultrasound. The power density of the treatment is expressed in milliwatts per square centimeter (mW/cm^2) and is based on the laser output (expressed in mW) and the surface area (circumference) of the emitted energy. This calculation is based on the formula:

$$\text{Power density (mW/cm}^2) = \text{Watts (mW)/Target area (cm}^2)$$

Laser output is described in joules, and is the most meaningful output measure when pulsed laser output is used. This calculation factors in the actual amount of time that the energy produced and is expressed in terms of joules per square centimeter (J/cm^2):

$$\text{Energy density (J/cm}^2) = \text{Watts (W)} \times \text{Time (Sec)/Target area (cm}^2)$$

Treatment Dosage

Most LLLT treatments are based on dose-oriented treatments per unit of area. The treatment duration is based on the energy density (joules per square centimeter [J/cm^2]), the average power of the output, and the area of the output beam. Most generators perform the following calculation to determine the treatment duration:

$$\text{Treatment duration} = (\text{J/cm}^2\text{/Average power}) \times \text{Target area (cm}^2)$$

✳ Practical Evidence

Similar to therapeutic ultrasound, many LLLT treatments are delivered at a dosage that is well below that expected to evoke biological responses.[210] Proper dosing is required to produce the desired physiological effects.

For example, assume a treatment dosage of 5.0 J/cm^2 with an average output of 1 mW over an area of 1 square centimeter. The total treatment time would be:

Treatment duration = (5 J/cm^2/0.001 W) × 0.01 cm^2
Treatment duration = 5000 × 0.01 cm^2
Treatment duration = 50 seconds

Common clinical dosage of LLLT ranges from 0.5 to 10.0 J/cm^2. As with most therapeutic modalities, the Arndth-Schultz principle dictates appropriate dosing (see Appendix A).[211] Insufficient dosages will not stimulate the desired response; doses that are too intense will cause tissue damage or hinder the healing process.

Acute conditions are treated with an output of less than 0.5 J/cm^2. The dosage for chronic conditions is normally less than 3.0 J/cm^2 (Table 19-3). Individual

TABLE 19-2   Types of Therapeutic Lasers

NAME	ABBREVIATION	WAVELENGTH (NM)	LIGHT BAND
Argon	Ar	488	Blue
Gallium-arsenide	GaAs	904	Infrared
Gallium aluminum arsenide*	GaAlAs	830	Infrared
Helium-neon	HeNe	632.8	Red
Indium gallium aluminum phosphate	InGaAlPO$_4$	670	Red

* Gallium aluminum arsenide can be manipulated to create different wavelengths.

TABLE 19-3	Treatment Dosing Based on the Pathology	
	Inflammatory State	
CONDITION	ACUTE	CHRONIC
Tendinopathy	24 to 30 J	35 to 40 J
Sprains	25 to 30 J	35 to 45 J
Strains	25 to 35 J	35 to 45 J

The applied treatment dosage should be based on the density of the energy (J/cm².

This table is provided as a sample. Refer to the manufacturer's recommendation and the current literature for the recommended dosage.

Adapted from McLeod IA. Low-level laser therapy in athletic training. Athl Ther Today. 9:17, 2004.

laser manufacturers publish recommended treatment intensity and durations, although the evidence base for making this decision is currently lacking. On units that combine laser and LED and/or SLD emitters, the dosage and application should be determined only by the number of laser diodes.

● EFFECTS ON

The Injury Response Process

Laser energy can stimulate tissues at depths up to 2 cm below the surface of the skin.[212,213] Although several studies have demonstrated positive effects of LLLT, the exact mechanism of action has yet to be identified. Current evidence suggests that the biophysical benefits are related to photomechanical or photochemical, rather than photothermal effects.[204] This response is based on the **first law of photobiology,** which states that for light to affect tissue, it must be absorbed by specific receptors (Fig. 19-3).[199]

In human tissues the primary photoreceptors (chromophores) include hemoglobin, COX, **myoglobin** ● , and **flavoproteins** ● . The energy from the absorbed photons affects the mitochondria, which stimulates the production of adenosine triphosphate (ATP).[205] The energy produced by ATP alters molecular-level activity, including short-term stimulation of the electron transport chain, stimulation of

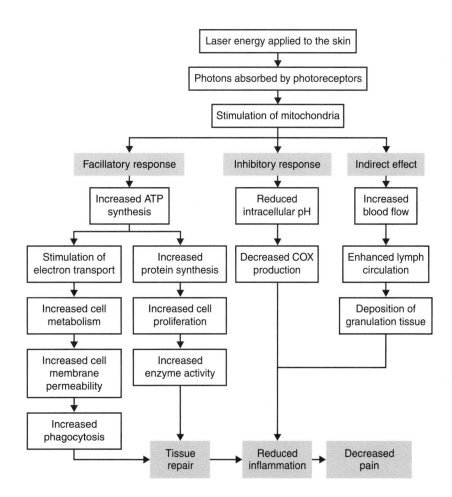

Figure 19-3. **Proposed Mechanism of Low-Level Laser Therapy.**

Myoglobin: A blood-based protein that stores oxygen in the tissues.
Flavoprotein: A protein involved in oxidation within a cell.

the mitochondrial respiratory chain, increased synthesis of adenosine triphosphate (ATP), and a reduction in intracellular pH and COX production.[199,202]

These actions are theorized to affect pain-producing tissue, such as areas of muscle spasm, by restoring the normal properties of muscle tissue via the increased formation of ATP and increased enzyme activity.[213,214] The effects of laser energy are most pronounced when the cells are traumatized, possibly explaining the lack of physiological changes noted in subjects using healthy subjects.[204,209,215]

Inflammation and Tissue Repair

Although the exact mechanism of action is yet to be substantiated, LLLT can produce anti-inflammatory or proinflammatory responses that affects healing. The biophysical effects depend on the type of laser applied and the power applied (Fig. 19-4).[216] There are overlapping areas where multiple effects occur. In the range of approximately 2.5 to 5 J, an anti-inflammatory effect and fibroblast stimulation occurs. Between the range of approximately 7 to 14 J anti-inflammatory effects continue, but fibroblast production is inhibited.[210,216] Anti-inflammatory effects appear to be more pronounced in laser in the high red or infrared bands (e.g., HeNe, GaAs, and GaAlAs).[210]

GaAs lasers promote muscle healing in the active inflammatory phase.[217] HeNe laser applied 2 days post injury and applied at 48-hour intervals is more effective in promoting healing than placebo for the first 21 days.[205]

✳ Practical Evidence

When applied at a sufficient and appropriate dosage, LLLT yields pain relief and produces anti-inflammatory markers that are significantly better than markers observed using a placebo.[210]

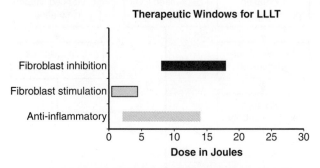

Therapeutic Windows for LLLT

Figure 19-4. **Dosage in Joules Required to Affect Tissue Repair.** Adapted from Lopes-Martin RAB, Penna SC, Joensen J, Iversen VV, et al: Low level laser therapy [LLLT] in inflammatory and rheumatic diseases: A review of therapeutic mechanisms. *Curr Rheumatol Rev.* 3:147, 2007.

Wound Healing

Lasers are used to assist in the healing of superficial wounds including skin ulcerations, surgical incisions, and burns. Because of their relatively low power output, HeNe lasers are less effective in destroying bacteria than indium gallium aluminum phosphate (InGaAlPO$_4$) lasers.[218]

The healing process is enhanced by the accelerated phagocytic activity and the selective destruction of bacteria.[218,219] The absorption of photons is believed to cause increased ATP synthesis that accelerates cell metabolism and encourages the release of free radicals.[218,220] Cell membrane permeability is altered and there is an increase in fibroblast, lymphocyte, and macrophage activity.[221] Blood and lymph circulation is improved in the area surrounding the treatment area, promoting the growth of granulation tissue[222] and the growth of new capillaries.[210] Increased fibroblast proliferation has been associated with LLLT; the response appears to be tissue and wavelength-specific.[204] Laser therapy is also thought to increase collagen content and increase tensile strength of healing wounds.[223]

The bactericidal effects of low-power lasers are enhanced by the preapplication of photosensitizers. These substances, not to be confused with photosensitizing medications such as tetracycline, absorb light having a specific frequency, increasing the intensity of the laser output. The increased laser uptake increases cell membrane permeability and enhances the production of free radicals and **singlet oxygen** • , and selective cell death occurs.[218]

Pain Reduction

LLLT has been used to decrease acute and chronic pain. Proposed mechanisms of pain reduction include altering nerve conduction velocity or decreasing muscle spasm.[224] These pain control approaches have been augmented with the use of sympathetic blocks and antidepressant medication.[225] Low-intensity laser can reduce the rate and velocity of sensory nerve impulses in inflamed nerves, but changes are seldom observed in healthy nerves.[210] Decreased prostaglandin synthesis may also account for decreased pain.[215,216]

Theories on how laser disrupts sensory nerve condition include effects similar to that seen during cold application but without the thermal changes.[208] Low-intensity GaAlAs laser having a wavelength of 830 nm and applied at 9.6 J/cm^2 [227] and HeNe having a wavelength of 632.8 nm applied at 19 mJ/cm^2 [208] reduced the rate of nerve conduction at the site of the treatment and distally. These effects had a significant latency period following the treatment.

Decreased skin resistance indicates the presence of local hypersensitive areas such as trigger points and acupuncture points. HeNe laser applied to cervical trigger points[228] and acupuncture points corresponding to pain caused by

---

Singlet oxygen: An uncharged form of oxygen that can selectively destroy cells.

fibromyalgia[229] resulted in increased skin resistance and decreased pain. GaAlAs laser applied at 50 mW (total dose = 2 J) for 1 minute (total dose = 2 J) at each tender joint demonstrated significant decrease in pain and improved clinical function following 10 days of treatment (5 days per week for 2 weeks).[215]

Laser therapy has demonstrated the ability to reduce the pain associated with post-herpetic neuralgia[225] and to resolve neurapraxia.[222] Another possible explanation for pain reduction following laser treatment is the release of endogenous opiates.[210,230]

✴ Practical Evidence

Laser having a wavelength of 904 nm (GaAs) has demonstrated effectiveness in the short-term relief of pain associated with lateral epicondalygia.[231]

Fracture Healing

Many of the same biophysical effects that assist soft tissue healing are theorized to enhance fracture healing and bone remodeling via an indirect effect. These effects, including increased capillary formation, calcium deposition, increased callus formation, and reduction of hematoma, may be associated with the direct or indirect effect. Photons striking the tissues may create micropressure waves that affect the healing bone in a manner similar to ultrasonic bone growth stimulators.[221,232]

Using an animal model, both GaAs and GaAlAs lasers applied daily at 4.0 J/cm² increased the density of the healing callus relative to a control group. However, the longer wavelength GaAs laser group had significantly denser callus than the GaAlAs group, but there was no improvement in the bones' tensile strength.[232,233] Laboratory studies have also demonstrated that GaAlAs improves bony fixation to titanium implants.[234] A higher-power carbon dioxide (CO_2) laser increased the rate of hematoma absorption and the removal of necrotic tissue, leading to enhanced fracture healing in laboratory animals.[221]

The preponderance of studies comparing the effects of laser-induced fracture healing relative to other bone growth stimulation techniques involves animal studies. At this point these studies are limited and inconclusive. One study suggests that there is no difference in healing between laser and pulsed ultrasound (US),[235] while other studies suggest improved healing relative to pulsed US.[236,237] These limited results prevent them from being applied to human bone growth stimulation.

■ Contraindications and Precautions

Laser produces nonionizing radiation, greatly reducing the possibility of causing permanent damage to cellular structures or damaging DNA. The retina is sensitive to low-power laser exposure; even brief (1 second) contact can result in permanent damage to the retina. Infrared energy is invisible, negating the eye's protective blink reflex. Depending on the type of laser being used, appropriate safety goggles should be worn by both the patient and the clinician (refer to the manufacturer's instructions regarding eye protection). Because of the risk of increasing the rate of cancerous cell growth, low-power laser therapy must not be applied to tumors or cancerous lesions.

Some medications such as tetracycline, antihistamines, oral contraceptives, and antidepressants increase the skin's sensitivity to sunlight. In these cases begin the patient with a below normal LLLT dosage and note any adverse reaction. If a question exists about the potential contraindication to laser therapy, contact the patient's physician or a pharmacist.

Some tattoo inks function as a photosensitizer, potentially predisposing the patient to adverse treatment effects. When possible, avoid the application of laser directly over tattoos. If direct application over tattoos is unavoidable, decrease the intensity of the initial treatment and monitor the patient for signs of "burning" (similar to a sunburn) or increased inflammation. These signs may take up to 48 hours to be seen.

■ Overview of the Evidence

LLLT is an evolving treatment approach that must be considered in the context of unclear treatment protocol, different forms of laser energy applied, conflicting results, and unknown biophysical effects. Although the evidence is building to support the use of LLLT, it is difficult to make an informed decision because of methodological issues associated with several studies. The application of laser energy to the tissues with a power well below that needed to evoke physiological changes is perhaps the single largest confounder in substantiating the efficacy of laser therapy.[210] Another confounding factor is that healthy tissue appears not to react to laser energy, negating the findings of studies performed on healthy subjects.[204,210,215]

Although therapeutic laser has been used to control pain and otherwise alter nerve conduction velocity, research studies using various types of lasers and a range of output parameters have not significantly substantiated this effect.[202,209,212,239] The anti-inflammatory benefits of GaAs laser was substantiated by a well-designed, controlled study.[226] However, several prior studies have concluded that laser treatment was not effective in treating musculoskeletal pain[210] including myofascial pain,[240] lateral epicondylagia,[239] traumatic orthopedic pain,[241] rheumatoid arthritis,[230] and tooth extraction.[242] Two early meta-analyses of the effect of laser therapy in treating orthopedic and skin conditions strongly suggest that this is not an effective modality in the treatment of these conditions.[243,244]

A study investigating the effects of HeNe laser, GaAs laser, and standard treatment protocol on pain and range of motion associated with **tendinopathies** ● demonstrated that all three treatment groups improved over a 2-week period, but the laser treatment groups had no significant benefits relative to the control group.[245] Other studies, however, do demonstrate improved function and reduced pain following LLLT.[215,231,246]

Several studies investigating the effect of laser on wound healing have questioned the efficacy of this technique.[204] Using human subjects, no significant difference in the healing rates of chronic venous leg ulcers was found between a group receiving standard treatment protocol augmented by HeNe laser (applied at 6 mW) and a group receiving standard treatment and sham laser.[247] A laboratory study investigating the healing characteristics of straight-line incisions in rat skin concluded that HeNe laser application demonstrated slight increases in tensile strength and other healing measures early, but these differences were only statistically significant, not clinically significant. There was no long-term difference in healing characteristics between irradiated and nonirradiated groups.[248]

Although cellular level effects and increased callus formation in fractures treated with GaAs and GaA1As,[232] and CO_2 [221] lasers have been identified, these effects were not replicated using the more common HeNe lasers applied at 2 or 4 J.[211] The evidence that laser improves fracture healing is lacking.[232]

The lack of a substantiated biological mechanism of action in response to LLLT, identification of the specific wavelength for use with certain conditions, and evidence of adequate treatment dosages must be addressed for LLLT to be accepted by mainstream medicine.[210]

■ Clinical Application of Therapeutic Lasers

Setup and Application

The setup, application, and dosage are device-specific. Refer to the user's manual for the exact application procedures. The following is provided as a general overview and should not replace formal training on the device being used. Most units have preprogrammed protocol based on the clinical problem being treated (e.g., pain, muscle spasm, wound healing).

Laser therapy should be administered in a space that prevents unintended exposure to laser output by others in the facility. Class II and III lasers should be administered only by those who have been trained to use these devices.[238]

Instrumentation

Although there are a limited number of laser units marketed in the United States, the available functions and types of laser output produced (e.g., HeNe, GaAs) create diversity in the instrumentation. When units produced outside of the United States are considered, the difference in instrumentation becomes even greater.

Timer: Selects the duration of the treatment. On some units, the timer function may be overridden by selecting the **MANUAL** switch.

Frequency: For pulsed output, adjusts the frequency or duration, or both, of the laser pulses. Do not confuse this parameter with the output frequency of the laser. Wavelength is the best description of the energy being administered.

Source: Selects the type of laser, typically GaAlAs, GaAs, or HeNe.

Power: Adjusts the output in watts. The total amount of energy is equal to the output wattage and the treatment duration (joules = power × duration). The total output per unit of area is measured as joules per square centimeter (J/cm^2).

Preparation of the Generator
1. If applicable, clean the laser lens(es) with an approved cleaner and/or polish.
2. Determine the treatment dosage and technique to be administered during the treatment.
3. Select the appropriate size laser applicator head.
4. If laser is being applied to open wounds, cover the applicator face with a clear plastic wrap to prevent transmission of contaminants. This technique results in the loss of approximately 8% of the total laser energy.[249]
5. Select the desired power output display. Joules per square centimeter (J/cm^2) is the recommended output measure.

Preparation of the Patient
1. Assure that the patient is free on any contraindications to the application of LLLT.
2. If applicable to the type of laser being used, the patient and clinician should wear goggles.
3. Clean the area to be treated with soap and water or alcohol swabs. Allow the area to dry thoroughly before initiating the treatment.
4. Cryotherapy may be administered prior to LLLT. The decreased blood flow and decreased tissue profusion are believed to increase the depth of laser penetration and decrease the inflammatory effects of the treatment. Heating the area prior to the application increases blood flow, thereby decreasing the depth of penetration and increasing the inflammatory effects.[200]
5. Determine the application technique to be used:

   Point technique: Laser is applied to predetermined points for a duration sufficient to deliver the appropriate amount of energy

---

Tendinopathy: Any disease or trauma involving a muscle's tendon, tissues surrounding the tendon, or the tendon's insertion into the bone.

At a Glance: Therapeutic "Cold" Lasers

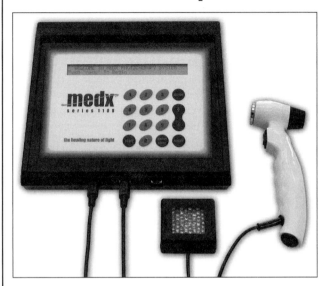

Description

Laser is a highly organized form of ultraviolet, visible, or infrared light. Photons that are absorbed by the cells produce direct changes in their function. Indirect effects occur secondary to photochemical events.

Primary Effects

- Altered nerve conduction velocity
- Vasodilation of microvessels
- Increased ATP production
- Increased collagen production
- Increased macrophage activity

Treatment Duration

The treatment duration depends on the type of laser being used (e.g., helium-neon), the pathology being treated, and the power of the output.

Indications

- Wound healing
- Fracture healing
- Musculoskeletal pain
- Myofascial pain/fibromyalgia[215]
- Trigger points
- Inflammatory conditions
- Osteoarthritis
- Rheumatoid arthritis
- Arthritis
- Carpal tunnel syndrome

Contraindications

- Application to the eyes
- Application over the thyroid gland
- High-intensity application over areas of hemorrhage
- Over areas of active deep vein thrombosis or thrombophlebitis
- Over cancerous areas
- Do not apply to the low back or abdomen during pregnancy
- Do not apply to the testicles

Precautions

- LLLT should not be applied within 6 months of radiation therapy.
- Because of unknown effects, lasers should not be applied over unfused epiphyseal plates, or be administered to small children.
- The patient may experience dizziness during the treatment. If this occurs, discontinue the treatment. If the episode recurs, laser therapy should not be applied to the patient.
- Caution should be used with patients who are taking medications that increase sensitivity to light including certain antihistamines, oral contraceptives, NSAIDs, tetracyclines, and antidepressants.
- Some tattoo inks may increase the absorption of laser energy.

Grid technique: Used for larger areas, an imaginary grid with points spaced 1 cm apart is placed over the treatment area. The laser is then applied to each point.[200]

Scanning technique: This method of laser application resembles traditional US application. The laser probe is slowly moved over the target tissues until the desired treatment dosage is reached. This method of application can decrease energy transmission.

6. When treating a joint, position it in the open-packed position (usually flexion) within patient comfort.

Initiation of the Treatment

1. Determine the treatment **DOSAGE** in J/cm^2.
2. Select the treatment **DURATION** (seconds). If the generator uses a dose-oriented treatment, the output (J/cm^2) will change in response to changes in the treatment duration.
3. Select the output mode. If the pulsed mode is selected, use the **FREQUENCY** control to select the number of pulses. Low pulse frequencies (1 to 20 pps) are used to promote tissue healing; pain is treated with a frequency greater than 20 pps.
4. View the dosage based on the treatment duration, frequency, and duty cycle used. If the dosage is out of range of the desired treatment parameters make adjustments as needed.
5. Hold the applicator so that the laser energy strikes the skin at a 90-degree angle.
6. Press the **START** button. If the laser head requires charging a countdown timer will indicate the time until the treatment actually begins.
7. Unless otherwise indicated, the applicator should remain in contact with the patient's skin throughout the treatment.

Maintenance
Following Each Treatment

1. Clean the head using a manufacturer-approved cleanser.

At Regular Intervals
1. Check all cords and cables for kinks, frays, and cuts.
2. Check lens for dirt, grime, and/or oil buildup.

Annually
1. Have the unit inspected and calibrated by an authorized technician. LED lasers may need to be recalibrated every 6 months.[238]

End of Section

Case Study: Bertha

Bertha is a 62-year-old female who sustained a right wrist fracture 6 weeks ago, which was medically managed with immobilization of a fiberglass cast. The cast was removed 3 days ago by the physician, and today you are the treating therapist for this patient. Her primary limitations are pain 4/10 rest, 10/10 activity; greater than 50% limited active and passive wrist range of motion; and poor strength due to pain and edema. Her edema measures 3 cm greater midpalm right versus left. She is medically healthy, except for a history of ovarian cancer 20 years ago that was treated successfully.

1. What are some edema management options to consider in this situation?

2. What are the physiological effects on the injury response cycle from the application of this thermal agent?
3. What are the clinical symptoms that you hope to address with this intervention?
4. What other interventions may be appropriate over the following 2 weeks for this diagnosis? Why?

Case Study: Sam

Sam is a 40-year-old man who is diagnosed with a herniated lumbar disk with left leg radiculopathy. He has mild osteoarthritis. His evaluation shows limited trunk active range of motion, moderate spasm in his lumbosacral paraspinals, and pain that radiates into the left buttock. The physician would like him to receive a course of treatment of lumbar traction.

1. What are the indications for traction?
2. What are the physiological effects on the injury response cycle from the application of this agent?

3. What are the clinical symptoms that you hope to address with this intervention?
4. What other thermal modalities may be appropriate over the following 2 weeks for this diagnosis? Why?

Case Study: Mr. Smith

Mr. Smith is a 77-year-old man with 10 years of progressive degenerative joint disease at the knee. He is currently 2 days out of surgery for a total knee arthroplasty. A continuous passive machine is requested by the physician.

1. What are three contraindications to the use of a continuous passive machine?

2. What are the physiological effects on the injury response cycle from the application of this thermal agent?
3. What are the clinical symptoms that you hope to address with this intervention?

Case Study: Continuation of Case Study From Section 1

(The following discussion relates to Case Study 2 in Section 1.)

Two of the modalities presented in this section, cervical traction and massage, would be appropriate for our patient's cervical trauma.

Massage

Soft tissue massage using effleurage and pétrissage strokes can promote relaxation of the involved muscles. Depending on the clinician's preference, the patient could be placed in the supine, prone, or seated position, with the head resting on a table to promote relaxation. The massage strokes should run parallel to the muscle fibers to help lengthen them. The patient would further benefit from massage by increased local blood flow and decreased neuromuscular excitability. Deep, localized friction massage can be used to help break up trigger points.

Cervical Traction

Cervical traction would be used only in the later stages of this patient's treatment protocol. Recall that the patient has been diagnosed as having a cervical strain and sprain. If traction were used too soon after the injury, the force may cause further damage to the cervical ligaments. Likewise, the patient does not show signs of radiating pain, decreasing the likelihood of cervical nerve root impingement.

Intermittent cervical traction, applied in two 5-minute intervals with a maximum of 25 pounds of tension, will assist in decreasing muscle spasm and pain, especially if the treatment is preceded by the application of moist heat packs. Placing the patient in the supine position lowers the amount of tension needed to elongate the muscles by decreasing motor activity in the cervical musculature.

● ● ● Section 5 Quiz

1. All of the following effects have been attributed to continuous passive motion (CPM) except:
   A. Increased nutrition to the meniscus
   B. Increased nutrition to the articular cartilage
   C. Increased tensile strength of tendons and allografts
   D. Increased nutrition to the anterior cruciate ligament

2. Intermittent cervical traction can be useful in relieving the pain associated with intervertebral disk herniations. This reduction of pain occurs by reducing the bulge of the _____ through the _____.
   A. Fibrous pulposus • nucleus pulposus
   B. Annulus fibrosus • nucleus pulposus
   C. Nucleus pulposus • annulus fibrosus
   D. Nucleus pulposus • fibrous pulposus

3. When applying intermittent compression to an extremity, the pressure in the appliance should not exceed:
   A. The diastolic blood pressure
   B. The systolic blood pressure
   C. The difference between the diastolic and systolic blood pressure
   D. The resting heart rate

4. Electromyographic biofeedback measures:
   A. The amount of tension produced by a muscle group
   B. The amount of electrical activity within a muscle
   C. The amount of myelin activity within a muscle
   D. All of the above

5. Which of the following techniques produces the greatest amount of femoral blood flow?
   A. Pneumatic sleeve
   B. Manual calf compression
   C. Straight-leg raises
   D. Anatomic CPM

6. All of the following are indications for the use of intermittent compression except:
   A. Postsurgical edema
   B. Gangrene
   C. Lymphedema
   D. Venous stasis ulcers

7. Which of the following types of continuous passive motion designs provides for the most joint stability?
   A. Free linkage
   B. Anatomical
   C. Nonanatomical

8. Light having a wavelength of 780 to 12,500 nm would be classified as:
   A. Ultraviolet
   B. Blue
   C. Red
   D. Infrared

9. Therapeutic laser is being applied at a total of 5 watts for 10 seconds over an area of 10 square centimeters. What is the energy density (J/cm²)?
   A. 5 J/cm²
   B. 25 J/cm²
   C. 0.5 J/cm²
   D. 50 J/cm²

10. The depth that laser energy penetrates into the body is related to:
    A. Total watts
    B. Duty cycle
    C. Wavelength
    D. Total joules

11. The body's fascia can be elongated using a _____ force.
    A. Quick, high-intensity
    B. Slow, high-intensity
    C. Quick, moderate-intensity
    D. Slow, moderate-intensity

12. In addition to the amount of force applied, what other parameters influence the effect of cervical traction?
    A.
    B.
    C.
    D.

13. List two reasons why separation of the vertebral column occurs at a lower percentage of the patient's body weight in the reclining position than in the sitting position.
    A.
    B.

14. Match the following massage strokes to method of delivery:
    A. Pétrissage   _____ Pounding of the skin
    B. Tapotement   _____ Kneading of the skin
    C. Effleurage   _____ Stroking of the skin

References

1. Capps SG: Cryotherapy and intermittent pneumatic compression for soft tissue trauma. *Athl Ther Today.* 14:2, 2009.
2. Partsch H: Intermittent pneumatic compression in immobile patients. *Int Wound J.* 5:389, 2008.
3. Pierce C, McLeod KJ: Feasibility of treatment of lower limb edema with calf muscle pump stimulation in chronic heart failure. *Eur J Cardiovasc Nurs.* 8:345, 2009.
4. Goddard AA, Pierce CS, McLeod KJ: Reversal of lower limb edema by calf muscle pump stimulation. *J Cardiopulm Rehabil Prev.* 28:174, 2008.
5. Muhe E: Intermittent sequential high-pressure compression of the leg: A new method of preventing deep vein thrombosis. *Am J Surg.* 147:781, 1984.
6. Olavi A, et al: Edema and lower leg perfusion in patients with posttraumatic dysfunction. *Acupunct Electrother Res.* 16:7, 1991.
7. Miranda F, et al: Effect of sequential intermittent pneumatic compression on both leg lymphedema volume and on lymph transport as semi-quantitatively evaluated by lymphoscintigraphy. *Lymphology.* 34:135, 2001.
8. Rucinski TJ, et al: The effects of intermittent compression on edema in postacute ankle sprains. *J Orthop Sports Phys Ther.* 14:65, 1991.
9. Iwama H, Obara S, Ohmizo H: Changes in femoral blood flow velocity by intermittent pneumatic compression: calf compression device versus plantar-calf sequential compression device. *J Anesth.* 18:232, 2004.
10. Stöckle U, et al: Fastest reduction of posttraumatic edema: Continuous cryotherapy or intermittent impulse compression? *Foot Ankle Int.* 18:432, 1997.
11. Hopkins JT, et al: Cryotherapy and transcutaneous electric neuromuscular stimulation decrease arthrogenic muscle inhibition of the vastus medialis after knee joint effusion. *J Athl Train.* 37:25, 2001.
12. Hopkins JT, Ingersoll CD: Arthrogenic muscle inhibition: A limiting factor in joint rehabilitation. *J Sports Rehabil.* 9:135, 2000.
13. Hopkins JT, et al: The effects of cryotherapy and TENS on arthrogenic muscle inhibition of the quadriceps. *J Athl Train.* 36:S49, 2001.
14. Fanelli G, Zasa M, Baciarello M, et al: Systemic hemodynamic effects of sequential pneumatic compression of the lower limbs: A prospective study in healthy volunteers. *J Clin Anesth.* 20:388, 2008.
15. Boris M, et al: The risk of genital edema after external pump compression for lower limb lymphedema. *Lymphology.* 31:15, 1998.
16. Gilbart MK, et al: Anterior tibial compartment pressures during intermittent sequential pneumatic compression therapy. *Am J Sports Med.* 23:769, 1995.
17. Wright RC, Yacoubian SV: Sequential compression device may cause peroneal nerve palsy. *Orthopedics.* 9:444, 2010.
18. Mayrovitz HN, Macdonald J, Davey S, et al: Measurement decisions for clinical assessment of limb volume changes in patients with bilateral and unilateral limb edema. *Phys Ther.* 87:1362, 2007.
19. Segers P, Belgrado JP, Leduc A, et al: Excessive pressure in multichambered cuffs used for sequential compression therapy. *Phys Ther.* 82:1000, 2002.
20. Salter RB: The biologic concept of continuous passive motion of synovial joints: The first 18 years of basic research. *Clin Orthop.* 12, May, 1989.
21. McCarthy MR, et al: The clinical use of continuous passive motion in physical therapy. *J Orthop Sports Phys Ther.* 15:132, 1992.
22. Saringer J: Engineering aspects of the design and construction of continuous passive motion devices for humans. In Salter RB (ed): Continuous Passive Motion (CPM): A Biological Concept for the Healing and Regeneration of Articular Cartilage, Ligaments, and Tendons—From Origination to Research to Clinical Applications. Williams & Wilkins, Baltimore, 1993, pp 403–410.
23. Diehm SL: The power of CPM: Healing through motion. *Patient Care* 8:34, 1989.
24. O'Donoghue PC, et al: Clinical use of continuous passive motion in athletic training. *J Athl Train.* 26:200, 1991.
25. Jordan LR, et al: Early flexion routine: An alternative method of continuous passive motion. Clin Orthop. 231, June, 1995.

26. Ferretti M, Srinivasan A, Deschner J, et al: Anti-inflammatory effects of continuous passive motion on meniscal fibrocartilage. *J Orthop Res.* 23:1165, 2005.

27. Williams JM, et al: Continuous passive motion stimulates repair of rabbit knee cartilage after matrix proteoglycan loss. *Clin Orthop.* 252, July, 1994.

28. Plessis MD, Eksteen E, Jenneker A, et al: The effectiveness of continuous passive motion on range of motion, pain and muscle strength following rotator cuff repair: A systematic review. *Clin Rehabil.* 25:291, 2011.

29. McInnes J, et al: A controlled evaluation of continuous passive motion in patients undergoing total knee arthroplasty. *JAMA.* 268:1423, 1992.

30. O'Driscoll SW, Nicholas JG: Continuous passive motion (CPM): Theory and principles of clinical application. *J Rehabil Res Dev.* 37:178, 2000.

31. Ring D, et al: Continuous passive motion following metacarpophalangeal joint arthroplasty. *J Hand Surg AJ.* 23:505, 1998.

32. LaStayo PC, et al: Continuous passive motion after repair of the rotator cuff. A prospective outcome study. *J Bone Joint Surg Am.* 80:1002, 1998.

33. Trumble T, Vedder NB, Seiler JG, et al: Zone-IT flexor tendon repair: A randomized prospective trial of active place-and-hold-therapy compared with passive motion therapy. *J Bone Joint Surg.* 92A:1381, 2010.

34. Gates HS, et al: Anterior capsulotomy and continuous passive motion in the treatment of posttraumatic flexion contracture of the elbow: A prospective study. *J Bone Joint Surg Am.* 74:1229, 1992.

35. Nadler SF, et al: Continuous passive motion in the rehabilitation setting: A retrospective study. *J Phys Med Rehabil.* 72:162, 1993.

36. Montgomery F, Eliasson M: Continuous passive motion compared to active physical therapy after knee arthroplasty: Similar hospitalization times in a randomized study of 68 patients. *Acta Orthop Scand.* 67:7, 1996.

37. Chiarello CM, et al: The effect of continuous passive motion duration and increment on range of motion in total knee arthroplasty patients. *J Orthop Sports Phys Ther.* 25:119, 1997.

38. McNair PJ, et al: Stretching at the ankle joint: Viscoelastic responses to holds and continuous passive motion. *Med Sci Sports Exerc.* 33:354, 2001.

39. London N, et al: Continuous passive motion: Evaluation of a new portable low cost machine. *Physiother.* 85:610, 1999.

40. Chin B, et al: Continuous passive motion after total knee arthroplasty. *Am J Phys Med Rehabil.* 79:421, 2000.

41. Ververeli PA, et al: Continuous passive motion after total knee arthroplasty: Analysis of costs and benefits. *Clin Orthop.* 208, December, 1995.

42. Lachiewicz PF: The role of continuous passive motion after total knee arthroplasty. *Clin Orthop.* 380:144, 2000.

43. Harvey LA, Brosseau L, Herbert RD: Continuous passive motion following total knee arthoplasty in people with arthritis. *Cochrane Database Sys Rev.* 2:CD004260, 2003.

44. Leach W, Reid J, Murphy F: Continuous passive motion following total knee replacement: A prospective randomized trial with follow-up to 1 year. *Knee Surg Sports Traumatol Arthrosc.* 14:922, 2006.

45. Lenssen TAF, van Steyn MJA, Crijins YHF, et al: Effectiveness of prolonged use of continuous passive motion (CPM), as an adjunct to physiotherapy, after total knee arthroplasty. *BMC Musculoskelet Disord.* 9:60, 2008.

46. Bruun-Olsen V, Heiberg KE, Mengshoel AM: Continuous passive motion as an adjunct to active exercises in early rehabilitation following total knee arthroplasty—a randomized controlled trial. 31:277, 2009.

47. Flowers KR, LaStayo, P: Effect of total end range time on improving passive range of motion. *J Hand Ther.* 7:150, 1994.

48. Wright A, et al: An investigation of the effect of continuous passive motion and lower limb passive movement on heart rate in normal volunteers. *Physiother Theory Pract.* 9:13, 1993.

49. Gershuni DH, et al: Regional nutrition and cellularity of the meniscus. Implications for tear and repair. *Sports Med.* 5:322, 1988.

50. Kim HKL, et al: The potential for regeneration of articular cartilage in defects created by chondral shaving and subchondral abrasion: An experimental investigation in rabbits. *J Bone Joint Surg Am.* 73:1301, 1991.

51. Kim HKW, et al: Effects of continuous passive motion and immobilization on synovitis and cartilage degeneration in antigen induced arthritis. *J Rheumatol.* 22:1714, 1995.

52. Alfredson H, Lorentzon R: Superior results with continuous passive motion compared to active motion after periosteal transplantation. A retrospective study of human patella cartilage defect treatment. *Knee Surg Sports Traumatol.* 7:232, 1999.

53. Mussa R, et al: Condylar cartilage response to continuous passive motion in adult guinea pigs: A pilot study. *Am J Orthod Dentofacial Orthop.* 115:360, 1999.

54. Moran ME, Salter RB: Biological resurfacing of full-thickness defects in patellar articular cartilage of the rabbit. Investigation of autogenous periosteal grafts subjected to continuous passive motion. *J Bone Joint Surg Br.* 74:659, 1992.

55. Namba RS, et al: Continuous passive motion versus immobilization: The effect on posttraumatic joint stiffness. *Clin Orthop.* 218, June, 1991.

56. Von Schroeder HP, et al: The changes in intramuscular pressure and femoral vein flow with continuous passive motion, pneumatic compression stockings, and leg manipulations. *Clin Orthop.* 218, May, 1991.

57. Grumbine NA, et al: Continuous passive motion following partial ankle joint arthroplasty. *J Foot Surg.* 29:557, 1990.

58. Mullaji AB, Shahane MN: Continuous passive motion for prevention and rehabilitation of knee stiffness: A clinical evaluation. *J Postgrad Med.* 35:204, 1989.

59. Giudice ML: Effects of continuous passive motion and elevation on hand edema. *Am J Occup Ther.* 44:914, 1990.

60. Dirette D, Hinojosa J: Effects of continuous passive motion to the edematous hands of two persons with flaccid hemiplegia. *Am J Occup Ther.* 48:403, 1994.

61. Macdonald SJ, et al: Prospective randomized clinical trial of continuous passive motion after total knee arthroplasty. *Clin Orthop.* 380:30, 2000.

62. Barthelet Y, et al: Effects of perioperative analgesic technique on the surgical outcome and duration of rehabilitation after major knee surgery. *Anesthesiology.* 91:8, 1999.

63. Kannus P: Immobilization or early mobilization after an acute soft-tissue injury? *Phys Sports Med.* 28:55, 2000.

64. Skyhar MJ, et al: Nutrition of the anterior cruciate ligament: Effects of continuous passive motion. *Am J Sports Med.* 13:415, 1985.

65. Smith TO, Davies L: The efficacy of continuous passive motion after anterior cruciate ligament construction: A systematic review. *Phys Ther Sport.* 8:141, 2007.

66. Wright RW, et al: A systematic review of anterior cruciate ligament reconstruction rehabilitation. Part I: Continuous passive motion, early weight bearing, postoperative

bracing, and home-based rehabilitation. *J Knee Surg.* 21:217, 2008.

67. Wright RW, Preston E, Flemming BC, et al: A systematic review of anterior cruciate ligament reconstruction rehabilitation. Part I: Continuous passive motion, early weight bearing, postoperative bracing, and home-based rehabilitation. *J Knee Surg.* 21:217, 2008.

68. Engstrom B, et al: Continuous passive motion in rehabilitation after anterior cruciate ligament reconstruction. *Knee Surg Sports Traumatol Arthrosc.* 3:18, 1995.

69. McCarthy MR, et al: The effect of immediate continuous passive motion on pain during the inflammatory phase of soft tissue healing following anterior cruciate ligament reconstruction. *J Orthop Sports Phys Ther.* 17:96, 1993.

70. Witherow GE, et al: The use of continuous passive motion after arthroscopically assisted anterior cruciate ligament reconstruction: Help or hindrance? *Knee Surg Sports Traumatol Arthrosc.* 1:68, 1993.

71. Zarnett R, et al: The effect of continuous passive motion on knee ligament reconstruction with carbon fiber. *J Bone Joint Surg Br.* 73:47, 1991.

72. Drez D, et al: In vivo measurement of anterior tibial translation using continuous passive motion devices. *Am J Sports Med.* 19:381, 1991.

73. Rosen MA, et al: The efficacy of continuous passive motion in the rehabilitation of anterior cruciate ligament reconstructions. *Am J Sports Med.* 20:122, 1992.

74. McCarthy MR, et al: Effects of continuous passive motion on anterior laxity following ACL reconstruction with autogenous patellar tendon grafts. *J Sports Rehabil.* 2:171, 1993.

75. Wasilewski SA, et al: Value of continuous passive motion in total knee arthroplasty. *Orthopedics.* 13:291, 1990.

76. Yashar AA, et al: Continuous passive motion with accelerated flexion after total knee arthroplasty. *Clin Orthop.* 345:38, 1998.

77. Chen B, et al: Continuous passive motion after total knee arthroplasty: A prospective study. *Am J Phys Med Rehabil.* 79:421, 2000.

78. Sperber A, Wredmark T: Continuous passive motion in rehabilitation after anterior cruciate ligament reconstruction. *Knee Surg Sports Traumatol.* 3:18, 1995.

79. Richmond JC, et al: Continuous passive motion after arthroscopically assisted anterior cruciate ligament reconstruction: Comparison of short- versus long-term use. *Arthroscopy.* 7:39, 1991.

80. Takai S, et al: The effects of frequency and duration of controlled passive mobilization on tendon healing. *J Orthop Res.* 9:705, 1991.

81. Graham G, Loomer RL: Anterior compartment syndrome in a patient with fracture of the tibial plateau treated by continuous passive motion and anticoagulants: Report of a case. *Clin Orthop.* 197, May, 1985.

82. Bible JE, Simpson AK, Biswas D, et al: Actual knee motion during continuous passive motion protocols is less than expected. *Clin Orthop Relat Res.* 467:2656, 2009.

83. LaBan MM, et al: Intermittent cervical traction: A progenitor of lumbar radicular pain. *Arch Phys Med Rehabil.* 73:295, 1992.

84. Saunders H: The use of spinal traction in the treatment of neck and back conditions. *Clin Orthop Rel Res.* 179:31, 1983.

85. Roberts S, Evans H, Trivedi J, et al: Histology and pathology of the human intervertebral disc. *J Bone Joint Surg Am.* 88:S10, 2006.

86. Lundon K, Bolton K: Structure and function of the lumbar intervertebral disk in health, aging, and pathologic conditions. *J Orthop Sports Phys Ther.* 31:291, 2001.

87. Murakami H, Yoon TS, Attallah-Wasif ES, et al: Quantitative differences in intervertebral disc-matrix composition with age-related degeneration. *Med Biol Eng Comput.* 48:469, 2010.

88. Sari H, Akarirmak U, Karacan I, et al: Computed tomographic evaluation of lumbar spinal structures during traction. *Physiother Theory Pract.* 21:3, 2005.

89. Ozturk B, Gunduz OH, Ozoran K, et al: Effect of continuous lumbar traction on the size of herniated disc material in lumbar disc herniation. *Rheumatol Int.* 26:622, 2006.

90. Tekeoglu I, et al: Distraction of lumbar vertebrae in gravitational traction. *Spine.* 23:1061, 1998.

91. Moeti P, Marchetti G: Clinical outcome from mechanical intermittent cervical traction for the treatment of cervical radiculopathy: A case series. *Phys Ther.* 31:207, 2001.

92. Meszaros TF, et al: Effect of 10%, 30%, and 60% body weight traction on the straight leg raise test of symptomatic patients with low back pain. *J Orthop Sports Phys Ther.* 30:595, 2000.

93. Yang KH, King AI: Mechanism of facet load transmission as a hypothesis for low-back pain. *Spine.* 9:557, 1984.

94. Judovich B, Nobel GR: Traction therapy: A study of resistance forces. *Am J Surg.* 93:108, 1957.

95. Werners R, et al: Randomized trial comparing interferential therapy with motorized lumbar traction and massage in the management of low back pain in a primary care setting. *Spine.* 24:1579, 1999.

96. Wong AM, et al: Clinical trial of a cervical traction modality with electromyographic biofeedback. *Am J Phys Med Rehabil.* 76:19, 1997.

97. Walker GL: Goodley polyaxial cervical traction: A new approach to a traditional treatment. *Phys Ther.* 66:1255, 1986.

98. Demir T, Canakci V, Eltas A, et al: Effectiveness of mouthguards on tooth pain and mobility in cervical traction treatment. *J Back Musculoskelet Rehabil.* 21:91, 2008.

99. Fater DCW, Kernozek TW: Comparison of cervical vertebral separation in the supine and seated positions using home traction units. *Physiother Theory Pract.* 24:430, 2008.

100. Wong AM, et al: The traction angle and cervical intervertebral separation. *Spine.* 17:136, 1992.

101. Chung CT, Tsai SW, Chen CJ, et al: Comparison of the intervertebral disc spaces between axial and anterior lean cervical traction. *Eur Spine J.* 18:1669, 2009.

102. Deets D, et al: Cervical traction: A comparison of sitting and supine positions. *Phys Ther.* 57:225, 1977.

103. Fater DC, Kernozek TW: Comparison of cervical vertebral separation in the supine and seated position using home traction units. *Physiother Theory Pract.* 24:430, 2008.

104. Liu J, Ebraheim NA, Sanford CG, et al: Quantitative changes in the cervical neural foramen resulting from axial traction: In vivo imaging study. *Spine J.* 8:619, 2008.

105. Raney NH, Peterson EJ, Smith TA, et al: Development of a clinical prediction rule to identify patients with neck pain likely to benefit from cervical traction and exercise. *Eur Spine J.* 18:382, 2009.

106. Young IA, Michener LA, Cleland JA, et al: Manual therapy, exercise, and traction for patients with cervical radiculopathy: A randomized clinical trial. *Phys Ther.* 89:632, 2009.

107. Jette DU, et al: Effect of intermittent, supine cervical traction on the myoelectric activity of the upper trapezius muscle in subjects with neck pain. *Phys Ther.* 65:1173, 1985.

108. Murphy, MJ: Effects of cervical traction on muscle activity. *J Orthop Sports Phys Ther.* 13:220, 1991.

109. Bradnam L, et al: Manual cervical traction reduces alpha-motoneuron excitability in normal subjects. *Electromyogr Clin Neurophysiol*. 40:259, 2000.

110. DeLacerda FG: Effect of angle of traction pull on upper trapezius muscle activity. *J Orthop Sports Phys Ther*. 1:205, 1980.

111. Borman P, Keskin D, Ekici B, et al: The efficacy of intermittent cervical traction in patients with chronic neck pain. *Clin Rheumatol*. 27:1249, 2008.

112. Cleland JA, Fritz JM, Whitman JM, et al: Predictors of short-term outcome in people with a clinical diagnosis of cervical radiculopathy. *Phys Ther*. 87:1619, 2007.

113. Latimer EA, et al: Tear of the cervical esophagus following hyperextension from manual traction: Case report. *J Trauma*. 31:1448, 1991.

114. Simmers TA, et al: Internal jugular vein thrombosis after cervical traction. *J Int Med Res*. 241:333, 1997.

115. Bridger RS, et al: Effect of lumbar traction on stature. *Spine*. 15:522, 1990.

116. Letchuman R, Deusinger RH: Comparison of sacrospinalis myoelectric activity and pain levels in patients undergoing static and intermittent lumbar traction. *Spine*. 18:1361, 1993.

117. Harrison DE, Cailliet R, Harrison DD, et al: A review of biomechanics of the central nervous system—Part III: Spinal cord stresses from postural loads and their neurologic effects. *J Manipulative Physiol Ther*. 22:399, 1999.

118. Saunders HD: Unilateral lumbar traction. *Phys Ther*. 61:221, 1981.

119. Cai C, Pua YH, Lim KC: A clinical prediction rule for classifying patients with low back pain who demonstrate short-term improvement with mechanical lumbar traction. *Eur Spine J*. 18:554, 2009.

120. Cholewicki J, Lee AS, Reeves NP, et al: Trunk muscle response to various protocols of lumbar traction. *Man Ther*. 14:562, 2009.

121. Ramos G, Martin W: Effects of vertebral axial decompression on intradiscal pressure. *J Neurosurg*. 81:350, 1994.

122. Beattie PF, Nelson RM, Michener LA, et al: Outcomes after a prone lumbar traction protocol for patients with activity-limiting low back pain: A prospective case series study. *Arch Phys Med Rehabil*. 89:269, 2008.

123. Beurskens AJ, et al: Efficacy of traction for nonspecific low back pain. 12-week and 6-month results of a randomized clinical trial. *Spine*. 22:2756, 1997.

124. Beurskens AJ, et al: Efficacy of traction for non-specific low back pain. A randomized clinical trial. *Lancet*. 346:1596, 1995.

125. Onel D, et al: Computer tomographic investigation of the effect of traction on lumbar disc herniations. *Spine*. 14:82, 1989.

126. Ljunggren AE, et al: Manual traction versus isometric exercises in patients with herniated intervertebral lumbar discs. *Physiother Theory Pract*. 8:207, 1992.

127. Schillinger A, et al: Effect of manual lymph drainage on the course of serum levels of muscle enzymes after treadmill exercise. *Am J Phys Med Rehabil*. 85:516, 2006.

128. Huggenberger R, Siddiqui SS, Brander D, et al: An important role in lymphatic vessel activation in limiting acute inflammation. *Blood*. 117:4667, 2011.

129. Cyriax, JH: Clinical applications of massage. In Rogoff JB (ed): Manipulation, Traction, and Massage, ed 2. Williams & Wilkins, Baltimore, 1980.

130. Brasseau, L, et al: Deep transverse friction massage for treating tendinitis. *Cochrane Database Syst Rev*. 1:CD003528, 2002.

131. Sefton J: Myofascial release for athletic trainers, part 3: Specific techniques. *Athl Ther Today*. 9(3):40, 2004.

132. Simons D, Travell J, Simons L: Upper Half of the Body. Travell & Simons' Myofascial Pain and Dysfunction: The Trigger Point Manual, ed. 2 vol. 1. Williams & Wilkins, 1999.

133. Sefton J: Myofascial release for athletic trainers, part 2: Guidelines and techniques. *Athl Ther Today*. 9(2):52, 2004.

134. Hou C, Tsai L, Cheng K, et al: Immediate effects of various physical therapeutic modalities on cervical myofascial pain and trigger-point sensitivity. *Arch Phys Med Rehabil*. 83:1406, 2002.

135. Hains G, Descarreaux M, Lamy A, et al: A randomized controlled (intervention) trial of ischemic compression therapy for chronic carpal tunnel syndrome. *J Can Chiropr Assoc*. 54: 155, 2010.

136. Goldenberg DL: Fibromyalgia, chronic fatigue syndrome, and myofascial pain syndrome. *Curr Opin Rheumatol*. 3:247, 1991.

137. Wolfe F, et al: The fibromyalgia and myofascial pain syndromes: A preliminary study of tender points and trigger points in persons with fibromyalgia, myofascial pain syndrome and no disease. *J Rheumatol*. 19:944, 1992.

138. King JC, Goddard MJ: Pain rehabilitation: II. Chronic pain syndrome and myofascial pain. *Arch Phys Med Rehabil*. 75:S9, 1994.

139. Sefton J: Myofascial release for athletic trainers, part 1: Theory and session guidelines. *Athl Ther Today*. 9(1):48, 2004.

140. Remvig L, Ellis RM, Patijn J: Myofascial release: An evidence-based treatment approach? *Int Musculoskelet Med*. 30:29, 2008.

141. Curran PF, Fiore RD, Crisco JJ: A comparison of the pressure exerted on soft tissue by 2 myofascial rollers. *J Sport Rehabil*. 17:432, 2008.

142. Stasinopoulos D, Johnson MI: Cyriax physiotherapy for tennis elbow/lateral epicondylitis. *Br J Sports Med*. 38:675, 2004.

143. Hammer WI, Pfefer MT: Treatment of a case of subacute lumbar compartment syndrome using the Graston technique. *J Manipulative Physiol Ther*. 28:199, 2005.

144. Gehlsen GM, Ganion LR, Helfst RH: Fibroblast responses to variation in soft tissue mobilization pressure. *Med Sci Sports Exerc*. 31:531, 1999.

145. Hammer WI: The effect of mechanical load on degenerated soft tissue. *Journal of Bodywork and Movement Therapies*. 12:246, 2008.

146. Burke J, Buchberger DJ, Carey-Logmani T, et al: A pilot study comparing two manual therapy interventions for carpal tunnel syndrome. *J Manipulative Physiol Ther*. 30:50, 2007.

147. Ferrell-Torry AT, Glick OJ: The use of therapeutic massage as a nursing intervention to modify anxiety and the perception of cancer pain. *Cancer Nurs*. 16:93, 1993.

148. Felhendler D, Lisander B: Effects of non-invasive stimulation of acupoints on the cardiovascular system. *Complement Ther Med*. 7:231, 1999.

149. Delaney JP, et al: The short-term effects of myofascial trigger point massage therapy on cardiac autonomic tone in healthy subjects. *J Adv Nurs*. 37:364, 2002.

150. Morelli M, et al: Changes in H-reflex amplitude during massage of triceps surae in healthy subjects. *J Orthop Sports Phys Ther*. 12:55, 1990.

151. Sullivan SJ, et al: Effects of massage on alpha motoneuron excitability. *Phys Ther*. 71:555, 1991.

152. Morelli M, et al: H-reflex modulation during manual muscle massage of human triceps surae. *Arch Phys Med Rehabil*. 72:915, 1991.

153. Crosman LJ, et al: The effects of massage to the hamstring muscle group on range of motion. *J Orthop Sports Phys Ther.* 6:168, 1984.

154. Smith LL, et al: The effects of athletic massage on delayed onset muscle soreness, creatine kinase, and neutrophil count: A preliminary report. *J Orthop Sports Phys Ther.* 19:93, 1994.

155. Tiidus PM, Shoemaker JK: Effleurage massage, muscle blood flow and long-term post exercise strength recovery. *Int J Sports Med.* 16:478, 1995.

156. Nalilbolff BD, Tachiki KH: Autonomic and skeletal muscle response to nonelectrical cutaneous stimulation. *Percept Motor Skills.* 72:575, 1991.

157. Knygsand-Roenhoej K, Maribo T: A randomized clinical controlled study comparing the effect of modified manual edema mobilization treatment with traditional edema technique in patients with a fracture of the distal radius. *J Hand Ther.* 24:184, 2011.

158. Kriederman B, et al: Limb volume reduction after physical treatment by compression and/or massage in a rodent model of peripheral lymphedema. *Lymphology.* 35:23, 2002.

159. Howard SB, Krishnagiri S: The use of manual edema mobilization for the reduction of persistent edema in the upper limb. *J Hand Ther.* 14:291, 2000.

160. Nixon M, et al: Expanding the nursing repertoire: The effect of massage on post-operative pain. *Australian J Adv Nurs.* 14:21, 1997.

161. Malkin K: Use of massage in clinical practice. *Br J Nurs.* 3:292, 1994.

162. Furlan AD, et al: Massage for low back pain. *Cochrane Database Syst Rev.* 2:CD001929, 2002.

163. Goldberg J, et al: The effect of two intensities of massage on H-reflex amplitude. *Phys Ther.* 72:449, 1992.

164. Goldberg J, et al: The effect of therapeutic massage on H-reflex amplitude in persons with a spinal cord injury. *Phys Ther.* 74:728, 1994.

165. Day JA, et al: Effect of massage on serum level of a-endorphin and a-lipotropin in healthy adults. *Phys Ther.* 67:926, 1987.

166. Goats GC, Keir KA: Connective tissue massage. *Br J Sports Med.* 25:131, 1991.

167. Ching M: The use of touch in nursing practice. *Australian J Adv Nurs.* 10:4, 1993.

168. Field T, et al: Massage therapy reduces anxiety and enhances EEG pattern of alertness and math computations. *Int J Neurosci.* 86:197, 1996.

169. Weinrich SP, Weinrich MC: The effect of massage on pain in cancer patients. *Appl Nurs Res.* 3:140, 1990.

170. Ferrell BA, et al: A randomized trial of walking versus physical methods for chronic pain management. *Aging* (Milano). 9:99, 1997.

171. Shoemaker JK, et al: Failure of manual massage to alter limb blood flow: Measures by Doppler ultrasound. *Med Sci Sports Exer.* 29:610, 1997.

172. Boone T, et al: A physiologic evaluation of the sports massage. *J Athl Train.* 26:51, 1991.

173. Harmer PA: The effect of pre-performance massage on stride frequency in sprinters. *J Athl Train.* 26:55, 1991.

174. Cafarelli E, et al: Vibratory massage and short-term recovery from muscular fatigue. *Int J Sports Med.* 11:474, 1990.

175. Tiidus PM: Manual massage and recovery of muscle function following exercise. A literature review. *J Orthop Sports Phys Ther.* 25:107, 1997.

176. Martin NA, Zoeller RF, Robertson RJ, et al: The comparative effects of sports massage, active recovery, and rest in promoting blood lactate clearance after supramaximal leg exercise. *J Athl Train.* 33:30, 1998.

177. Striggle JM, et al: Effects of vibrational massage on delayed onset muscle soreness and H-reflex amplitude. *J Athl Train.* 37(S):S105, 2002.

178. Lehmann JF, et al: Effect of therapeutic temperatures on tendon extensibility. *Arch Phys Med Rehabil.* 51:481, 1970.

179. Madeleine P, Vedsted P, Blangsted K, et al: Effects of electromyographic and mechanomyograpic biofeedback on upper trapezius muscle activity during standardized computer work. *Ergonomics.* 49:921, 2006.

180. Croce RV: The effects of EMG biofeedback on strength acquisition. *Biofeedback Self Regul.* 11:299, 1986.

181. Peek CJ: A primer of biofeedback instrumentation. In Schwartz MS (ed): Biofeedback: A Practitioner's Guide. Guilford Press, New York, 1987.

182. Araujo RC, et al: On the inter- and intra-subject variability of the electromyographic signal in isometric contractions. *Electromyogr Clin Neurophysiol.* 40:225, 2000.

183. Intiso D, et al: Rehabilitation of walking with electromyographic biofeedback in drop-foot after stroke. *Stroke.* 25:1189, 1994.

184. Utz SW: The effect of instructions on cognitive strategies and performance in biofeedback. *J Behav Med.* 17:291, 1994.

185. Segreto J: The role of EMG awareness in EMG biofeedback learning. *Biofeedback Self Regul.* 20:155, 1995.

186. Vander Linden DW, et al: The effect of frequency of kinetic feedback on learning an isometric force production task in nondisabled subjects. *Phys Ther.* 73:79, 1993.

187. Draper V: Electromyographic biofeedback and recovery of quadriceps femoris muscle function following anterior cruciate ligament reconstruction. *Phys Ther.* 70:25, 1990.

188. Wolf SL: Neurophysiological factors in electromyographic feedback for neuromotor disturbances. In Basmajian JV (ed): Biofeedback: Principles and Practice for Clinicians. Williams & Wilkins, Baltimore, 1983.

189. Ingersoll CD, Knight KL: Patellar location changes following EMG biofeedback or progressive resistive exercises. *Med Sci Sports Exerc.* 23:1122, 1991.

190. Coleborne GR, et al: Feedback of ankle joint angle and soleus electromyography in the rehabilitation of hemiplegic gait. *Arch Phys Med Rehabil.* 74:1100, 1993.

191. Yip SLM, Ng GYF: Biofeedback supplementation to physiotherapy exercise programme for rehabilitation of patellofemoral pain syndrome: A randomized controlled pilot study. *Clin Rehabil.* 20:1050, 2006.

192. Wang S, Li S, Xu X, et al: Effect of slow abdominal breathing combined with biofeedback on blood pressure and heart rate variability in prehypertension. *J Altern Complement Med.* 16:1039, 2010.

193. Cummings MS, et al: Flexibility development in sprinters using EMG biofeedback and relaxation training. *Biofeedback Self Regul.* 9:395, 1984.

194. Flor H, Birbaumer N: Comparison of the efficacy of electromyographic biofeedback, cognitive-behavioral therapy, and conservative medical interventions in the treatment of chronic musculoskeletal pain. *J Consult Clin Psychol.* 61:653, 1993.

195. Newton-John TR, et al: Cognitive-behavioural therapy versus EMG biofeedback in the treatment of chronic low back pain. *Behav Res Ther.* 33:691, 1995.

196. Valeyen J, et al: Behavioural rehabilitation of chronic low back pain: Comparison of an operant treatment, an operant-cognitive treatment and an operant-respondent treatment. *Br J Clin Psychol.* 34:95, 1995.

197. Silkman C, McKeon J: The effectiveness of electromyographic biofeedback supplementation duration knee rehabilitation after injury. *J Sport Rehabil.* 19:343, 2010.
198. Bischko JJ: Use of the laser beam in acupuncture. *Acupunct Electrother Res.* 5:29, 1980.
199. Huang YY, Chen AC, Carroll JD, et al: Biphasic dose response in low level light therapy. *Dose Response.* 7:358, 2009.
200. McLeod IA. Low-level laser therapy in athletic training. *Athl Ther Today.* 9:17, 2004.
201. Perkins SA, Massie JE: Patient satisfaction after thermal shrinkage of the glenohumeral-joint capsule. *J Sports Rehabil.* 10:157, 2001.
202. Bartlett WP, et al: Effect of Gallium-aluminum-arsenide triple-diode laser irradiation on evoked motor and sensory action potentials of the median nerve. *J Sports Rehabil.* 11:12, 2002.
203. Lehmann JF, De Lateur BJ: Laser as a physical treatment modality. In Lehmann JF (ed): Therapeutic Heat and Cold, ed 4. Williams & Wilkins, Baltimore, 1990, p. 582.
204. Posten W, Wrone DA, Dover JS, et al: Low-level laser therapy for wound healing: Mechanism and efficacy. *Dermatol Surg.* 31:3, 2005.
205. McBrier N, Olczak JA: Low level laser therapy for stimulating muscle regeneration following injury. *Athl Ther Today.* 14:20, 2009.
206. Enewemeka C, Parker J, Dowdy D, et al: The efficacy of low-power lasers in tissue repair and pain control: A meta-analysis study. *Photomed Laser Surg.* 22:323, 2004.
207. Ohshiro T, et al: Penetration depths of 830 nm diode laser irradiation of the head and neck assessed using a radiographic phantom model and wavelength-specific imaging film. *Laser Ther.* 8:197, 1996.
208. Snyder-Mackler L, Bork CE: Effect of helium-neon laser irradiation on peripheral sensory nerve latency. *Phys Ther.* 68:223, 1988.
209. Bartlett WP, et al: Effect of gallium aluminum arsenide triple-diode laser on median nerve latency in human subjects. *J Sports Rehabil.* 8:99, 1999.
210. Bjordal JM, Johnson MI, Iversen V, et al: Low-level laser therapy in acute pain: A systematic review of possible mechanisms of action and clinical effects in randomized placebo-controlled trials. *Photomed Laser Surg.* 24:158, 2006.
211. David R, et al: Effect of low-power He-Ne laser on fracture healing in rats. *Lasers Surg Med.* 19:458, 1996.
212. Greathouse DG, et al: Effects of clinical infrared laser on superficial radial nerve conduction. *Phys Ther.* 65:1184, 1985.
213. King CE, et al: Effect of helium-neon laser auriculotherapy on experimental pain threshold. *Phys Ther.* 70:24, 1990.
214. Pires Oliveria DAA, De Oliveria RF, Magini M, et al: Assessment of cytoskeletan and endoplasmic reticulum of fibroblast cells subjected to low-level laser therapy and low-intensity pulsed ultrasound. *Photomed Laser Surg.* 27:461, 2009.
215. Armagan O, Tascioglu F, Ekim A, et al: Long-term efficacy of low level laser therapy in women with fibromyalgia: A placebo-controlled study. *J Back Musculoskelet Rehabil.* 19:135, 2006.
216. Lopes-Martin RAB, Penna SC, Joensen J, et al: Low level laser therapy [LLLT] in inflammatory and rheumatic diseases: A review of therapeutic mechanisms. *Curr Rheumatol Rev.* 3:147, 2007.
217. Rizzi CF, et al: Effects of low-level laser therapy (LLLT) on the nuclear factor (NF)-kB signaling pathway in traumatized muscle. *Lasers Surg Med.* 38:704, 2006.
218. DeSimone NA, et al: Bactericidal effect of 0.95-mW helium-neon and 5-mW indium-gallium-aluminum-phosphate laser irradiation at exposure times of 30, 60, and 120 seconds on photosensitized *Staphylococcus aureus* and *Pseudomonas aeruginosa* in vitro. *Phys Ther.* 79:839, 1999.
219. Hawkins D, Houreld N, Abrahamse H: Low level laser therapy (LLLT) as an effective modality for delayed would healing. *Ann NY Acad Sci.*1056:486, 2005.
220. Ricevuti G, et al: In vivo and in vitro HeNe laser effects on phagocyte functions. *Inflammation.* 13:507, 1989.
221. Tang XM, Chai BP: Effect of CO_2 laser irradiation on experimental fracture healing: A transmission electron microscope study. *Lasers Surg Med.* 6:346, 1986.
222. Hamilton GF, et al: The effects of helium-neon laser upon regeneration of the crushed peroneal nerve. *J Orthop Sports Phys Ther.* 15:209, 1992.
223. Wood VT, Pinfildi CE, Neves MAI, et al: Collagen changes and realignment induced by low-level laser therapy and low-intensity ultrasound in the calcaneal tendon. *Lasers Surg Med.* 42:559, 2010.
224. Ilbuldu E, Cakmak A, Disci R, et al: Comparison of laser, dry needling, and placebo laser treatments in myofascial pain syndrome. *Photomed Laser Surg.* 22:306, 2004.
225. Numazawa R, et al: The role of laser therapy in intensive pain management of postherpetic neuralgia. *Laser Ther.* 8:143, 1996.
226. Bjordal JM, Lopes-Martins RAB, Iversen VV: A randomised, placebo controlled trial of low level laser therapy for activated Achilles tendinitis with microdialysis measurement of peritendinous prostaglandin E_2 concentrations. *Br J Sports Med.* 40:76, 2006.
227. Baxter GD, et al: Effects of low intensity infrared laser irradiation upon conduction in the human median nerve in vivo. *Exp Physiol.* 79:227, 1994.
228. Snyder-Mackler L, et al: Effects of helium-neon laser irradiation on skin resistance and pain in patients with trigger points in the neck or back. *Phys Ther.* 69:336, 1989.
229. Sprott H, Mueller W: Efficiency of acupuncture in patients with fibromyalgia. *Reumatologia* (Warsaw). 32:414, 1994.
230. Heussler JK, et al: A double blind randomized trial of low power laser treatment in rheumatoid arthritis. *Ann Rheum Dis.* 52:703, 1993.
231. Bjordal J, Lopes-Martins RAB, Joensen J, et al: A systematic review with procedural assessments and meta-analysis of low level laser therapy in lateral elbow tendinopathy (tennis elbow). *BMC Musculoskelet Disord.* 9:75, 2008.
232. Glinkowski W, Rowinski, J: Effect of low incident levels of infrared laser energy on the healing of experimental bone fractures. *Laser Ther.* 7:67, 1995.
233. Shakouri SK, Soleimanpour J, Salekzamani Y, et al: Effect of low-level laser therapy on the fracture healing process. *Lasers Med Sci.* 25:73, 2010.
234. Khadra M, Lyngstadaas SP, Haanaes HR, et al: Effect of laser therapy on attachment, proliferation and differentation of human osteoblast-like cells cultured on titanium implant material. *Biomaterials.* 26:3503, 2005.
235. Oliveria P, Sperandio E, Fernandes KR, et al: Comparison of the effects of low-level laser therapy and low-intensity pulsed ultrasound on the process of bone repair in the rat tibia. *Rev Bas Fisioter.* 15:200, 2011.
236. Fávaro-Pipi E, Feitosa SM, Riberio DA, et al: Comparative study of the effects of low-intensity pulsed ultrasound and low-level laser therapy on bone defects in tibias of rats. *Lasers Med Sci.* 25:727, 2010.

237. Lirani-Galvão AP, Jorgetti V, da Silva OL: Comparative study of how low-level laser therapy and low-intensity pulsed ultrasound affect bone repair in rats. *Photomed Laser Surg.* 24:735, 2006.

238. Houghton PE, Nussbaum EL, Hoens AM: Low-level laser therapy (LLLT)/non-coherent light. *Physiother Can.* 62:39, 2010.

239. Lundeberg T, et al: Effect of laser versus placebo in tennis elbow. *Scand J Rehabil Med.* 19:135, 1987.

240. Thorsen H, et al: Low level laser therapy for myofascial pain in the neck and shoulder girdle. A double-blind cross-over study. *Scand J Rheumatol.* 21:139, 1992.

241. Mulcahy D, et al: Low level laser therapy: a prospective double blind trial of its use in an orthopaedic population. *Injury.* 26:315, 1995.

242. Fernando S, et al: A randomized double blind comparative study of low level laser therapy following surgical extraction of lower third molar teeth. *Br J Oral Maxillofac Surg.* 31:170, 1993.

243. Gam AN, et al: The effect of low-level laser therapy on musculoskeletal pain: A meta-analysis. *Pain.* 52:63, 1993.

244. Beckerman H, et al: The efficacy of laser therapy for musculoskeletal and skin disorders: A criteria-based meta-analysis of randomized clinical trials. *Phys Ther.* 72:483, 1992.

245. Siebert W, et al: What is the efficacy of soft and mid lasers in therapy of tendinopathies? A double-blind study. *Arch Orthop Trauma Surg.* 106:358, 1987.

246. Ay S, Dogan SK, Evcik D: Is low-level laser therapy effective in acute or chronic low back pain? *Clin Rheumatol.* 29:905, 2010.

247. Lundeberg T, Malm M: Low-power HeNe laser treatment of venous leg ulcers. *Ann Plastic Surg.* 27:537, 1991.

248. Surinchak JS, et al: Effects of low level energy lasers on the healing of full thickness skin defects. *Lasers Surg Med.* 2:267, 1983.

249. Chen C, Diven DG, Lockart S, et al: Laser transmission through transparent membranes used in cutaneous laser treatment. *J Am Acad Dermatol.* 45:919, 2001.

Appendix A

Physical Properties Governing Therapeutic Modalities

The laws of physics govern the energies used by therapeutic modalities. This appendix presents an overview of these physical properties. Modality-specific physical properties are discussed in the relevant chapters of this text.

■ The Electromagnetic Spectrum

Various forms of energy are constantly bombarding us: the light from the sun, the heat from a fire, and the waves emitted from radio transmitters. This energy, known as **electromagnetic radiation,** is produced by virtually every element in the universe and is characterized by the following traits:

- Transports energy through space
- Requires no transmission medium
- Travels through a vacuum at a constant rate of 300 million meters per second
- Does not have mass and is composed of pure energy

Each form of energy is ordered on the electromagnetic spectrum on the basis of its wavelength or frequency (Fig. A-1).

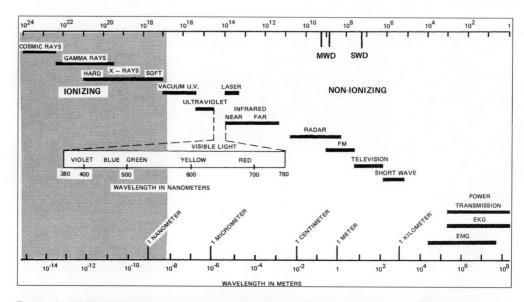

Figure A-1. **A Graphical Representation of the Electromagnetic Spectrum.** (Adapted from Illuminating Engineering Society of North America Lighting Handbook, New York, ed 8, 1993.)

■ Regions of the Electromagnetic Spectrum

The energy's wavelength uniquely defines each portion of the electromagnetic spectrum. The reference measure for wavelength is the meter (Table A-1).

■ Ionizing Range

Energy within the ionizing range of the electromagnetic spectrum is characterized by the relative ease with which atoms can release free electrons, protons, or neutrons. Ionizing radiation can easily penetrate the tissues and deposit its energy within the cells. If this energy is sufficiently high, the cell loses its ability to divide, eventually killing the cell.

Ionizing radiation is used diagnostically in obtaining radiographs (below the threshold required for cell death) and therapeutically in radiation treatment for some forms of cancer (above the threshold). Because ionizing radiation is hazardous, the total dose of exposure must be tightly monitored and controlled. Energy found in this portion of the electromagnetic spectrum is used only under closely controlled circumstances.

■ The Light Spectrum

This portion of the spectrum encompasses ultraviolet, visible, and infrared light energy. Electromagnetic radiation possessing a wavelength between 380 and 780 nm forms the spectrum of **visible "white" light.** White light is the combination of seven colors, each representing a different wavelength on the spectrum. These seven colors, ranked from the shortest to the longest wavelength, are violet, indigo, blue, green, yellow, orange, and red.

Light energy having a wavelength greater than 780 nm is termed **infrared light** or infrared energy. Because this wavelength is greater than the upper limits of what the human eye is capable of detecting, infrared energy is invisible. Any object possessing a temperature greater than absolute zero emits infrared energy proportional to its temperature. Hotter sources transmit more infrared energy because they possess a shorter wavelength than cooler objects.

The infrared spectrum is divided into two distinct sections. The near infrared is the portion of the spectrum that is closest to visible light, with wavelengths ranging between 780 and 1500 nm. The far-infrared portion is located between 1500 and 12,500 nm. Energy in the near infrared range is capable of producing thermal effects 5 to 10 mm deep in tissue, whereas far infrared energy results in more superficial heating of the skin (less than 2 mm deep).

Light with a wavelength shorter than visible light is **ultraviolet light.** Like infrared energy, ultraviolet light is undetectable by the human eye. Energy in the near ultraviolet range has wavelengths ranging between 290 and 400 nm, whereas the far ultraviolet range encompasses wavelengths between 180 and 290 nm. Both of these forms of ultraviolet light produce superficial chemical changes in the skin. Sunburn is an example of the effect of an overdose of ultraviolet radiation.

Many therapeutic modalities use energy within the light range of the electromagnetic spectrum. Ultraviolet light is used for the treatment of certain skin conditions. Depending on the relative temperatures involved, transfer of infrared energy is used to heat or cool the body's tissues. Medical lasers produce beams of energy in the ultraviolet, visible, and infrared light regions that can result in either tissue destruction or therapeutic effects within the tissues.

TABLE A-1 Units of Measure for Wavelengths Relative to the Meter (39.37 in.)		
NAME	SYMBOL	WAVELENGTH
Angstrom	Å	10210 m
Nanometer	nm	1029 m
Micrometer	mm	1026 m
Millimeter	mm	1023 m
Centimeter	cm	1022 m
Meter	m	—
Kilometer	km	103 m

Diathermy and Electrical Currents

Electromagnetic radiation of longer wavelengths has an intensity sufficient to cause an increase in tissue temperature. Collectively known as "diathermy," these types of electromagnetic energies create a magnetic field that is changed into heat through the process of conversion. The two most common types of therapeutic diathermy are microwave and shortwave diathermy.

In the range above shortwave diathermy and extending on to infinity are electrical stimulating currents. These devices use the direct flow of electrons and ions to elicit physiological changes within the tissues. It should be noted that the physical manipulations done to the electrical current do not allow for its precise location on the electromagnetic spectrum. The exception to this is un-interrupted direct current, possessing the theoretical wavelength of infinity.

Physical Laws Governing the Application of Therapeutic Modalities

The efficacy of a particular treatment depends on the proper choice and application of a modality. The modality must be capable of producing the desired physiological changes at the intended tissue depth. A superficial heating agent has little positive effect on a deep-seated injury. The proper modality will not produce optimal results if it is applied incorrectly.

For physiological changes to occur, the energy applied to the body must be absorbed by the tissues. Across the electromagnetic spectrum, there is little correlation between wavelength and the ability to penetrate the body's tissues.[1] Both x-rays and radio waves penetrate the tissues despite their polar positions on the spectrum.

Heat Transfer

Conductive heat transfer to or from the body is governed by the laws of thermodynamics. The amount of energy exchanged during a cold or superficial heat treatment can be calculated using the following equation:

$$H = k \, A \, t \, (\Delta T/\Delta L)$$

where:

$$H = \text{Total heat transfer}$$
$$k = \text{Thermal conductivity of the tissues}$$
$$A = \text{Area through which the energy is being transmitted}$$
$$t = \text{Total time that the modality is applied}$$
$$\Delta T = \text{Temperature gradient between the modality and the tissues}$$
$$\Delta L = \text{Distance separating the thermal gradient}$$

When applying modalities such as moist heat or ice packs, the area (A) represents the surface area where the modality contacts the skin. Increasing the surface area increases the amount of energy exchanged. The thermal conductivity (k) differs from tissue layer to tissue layer, with adipose tissue representing the lowest exchange rate. The distance separating the thermal gradient (ΔL) is the distance from the modality to the target tissues.

Adding an insulating layer between the modality and the skin reduces the energy exchange two ways. Insulators have a low thermal capacity that decreases the amount of energy exchanged. The insulating material also increases the distance between the modality and the skin, increasing the value of ΔL, thus reducing the total energy exchange.

Cosine Law

Electromagnetic energy is most efficiently transmitted to the tissues when it strikes the body at a right angle (90 degrees). Because this angle (the angle of incidence) deviates away from 90 degrees, the efficiency of the energy affecting the tissues is decreased by the cosine of the angle. The cosine law defines this relationship as:

$$\text{Effective energy} = \text{Energy} \times \text{Cosine of the angle of incidence}$$

With radiant energy, a difference of ±10 degrees from the right angle is considered within accept-able limits during treatment.[2]

Inverse Square Law

The intensity of radiant energy depends on the distance between the source and the tissues and is described by the inverse square law. The intensity of the energy striking the tissues is proportional to the square of the distance between the source of the energy and the tissues:

$$E = Es/D^2$$

where:

E = the amount of energy received by the tissue
Es = the amount of energy produced by the source
D^2 = the square of the distance between the target and the source

Doubling the distance between the tissue and the energy decreases the intensity at the tissue by a factor of four (Fig. A-2).

Arndt-Schultz Principle

To enable energy to affect the body, it must be absorbed by the tissues at a level sufficient to stimulate a physiological response. As described by the general adaptation syndrome (see Chapter 1), if the amount of energy absorbed is too little, no reaction takes place, and if the amount of energy is too great, damage results. This concept applied to the application of therapeutic modalities is known as the Arndt-Schultz principle and is translated into clinical practice through the application of the proper modality at the proper intensity for the appropriate duration.

Law of Grotthus-Draper

The law of Grotthus-Draper describes an inverse relationship between the penetration and absorption of energy by which any energy that penetrates the body and is not absorbed by one tissue layer is passed along to the next layer. The more energy that is absorbed by the superficial tissues, the less remains to be transmitted to underlying tissues.

Consider, for example, the application of moist heat to the quadriceps muscle group. Some of the energy is absorbed by the skin, decreasing the amount of energy delivered to the adipose tissue. Some of the remaining energy is absorbed by the adipose tissue, leaving only a fraction of the initial energy left to heat the muscle. This example also illustrates the fact that adipose tissue can act as an insulator, inhibiting the thermal heating of muscle. This concept applies to most therapeutic modalities, with the difference being the layer or layers in which the majority of energy loss occurs.

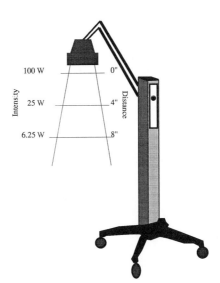

Figure A-2. **An Example of the Inverse Square Law.** Each time the distance between the source of infrared energy and the tissue is doubled, the intensity of the energy delivered to the tissue is reduced by a factor of four.

■ Measures

Distance Conversion

The basis of measurement in the metric system is the meter (m), a distance of 39.37 inches. The exact distance of 1 m is the wavelength associated with a specific frequency in the electromagnetic spectrum. The inch, according to history, was derived from the length of the middle phalanx of a king's index finger.

Comparison Between English and SI Measures of Length

	MILLIMETERS	CENTIMETERS	METERS	INCHES	FEET	YARDS
1 mm =	1.0	0.1	0.001	0.03937	0.00328	0.0011
1 cm =	10.0	1.0	0.01	0.3937	0.03281	0.0109
1 in. =	25.4	2.54	0.0254	1.0	0.0833	0.0278
1 ft =	304.8	30.48	0.3048	12.0	1.0	0.333
1 yd =	914.4	91.44	0.9144	36.0	3.0	1.0
1 m =	1000.0	100.0	1.0	39.37	3.2808	1.0936

Source: Adapted from Venes D, Thomas CL (eds): Taber's Cyclopedic Medical Dictionary, ed 21. FA Davis, Philadelphia, 2009, p 2585.

To convert English measures to meters, multiply the unit by the following conversion constants. To convert meters to the English system, divide by the constant.

ENGLISH MEASURE	CONSTANT
Inches	0.0254
Feet	0.3048

Weight and Mass Conversion

ENGLISH MEASURE	CONSTANT
Ounces	0.0283495
Pounds	0.4535924

Temperature Conversion

To convert Fahrenheit to centigrade:

$$C° = (F° − 32) × 5/9$$

To convert centigrade to Fahrenheit:

$$F° = (C° × 9/5) + 32$$

References

1. Kloth LC, Ziskin MC: Diathermy and pulsed electromagnetic fields. In Michlovitz SL (ed): Thermal Agents in Rehabilitation, ed 2. FA Davis, Philadelphia, 1990, pp 170–199.
2. Griffin JE, Karselis TC: Physical Agents for Physical Therapists, ed 3. Charles C Thomas, Springfield, IL, 1988, pp 229–263.

Appendix B

Trigger Points and Pain Patterns

"Trigger points" are small areas of localized sensitivity and pain found in muscles and connective tissue.[1] They may be produced by acute trauma, chronic inflammation, or ischema, or they may be developed as a result of stress from daily activities or postural habits. Although the pain and sensitivity are localized, reports in the literature suggest that the discomfort may be referred to other parts of the body ("referred pain") through the autonomic nervous system.

These areas may be located by palpation, with the aid of the eraser end of a pencil, or by means of electrical currents. It has been suggested that the combination of electrical stimulation and ultrasound is beneficial in both locating and treating the involved areas. A tetanizing current within the comfortable intensity range of the patient is normally used for both location and treatment, offering "massage-like" contraction to the muscles to which it is applied.[2]

Illustrations are from Mettler Electronics Corporation, Anaheim, California, with permission.

References
1. Alvarez DJ, Rockwell PG: Trigger points: Diagnosis and management. *Am Fam Physician* 65:653, 2002.
2. Travel J, Rinzier SH: The myofascial genesis of pain. *Postgrad Med.* II(5): May 1952.

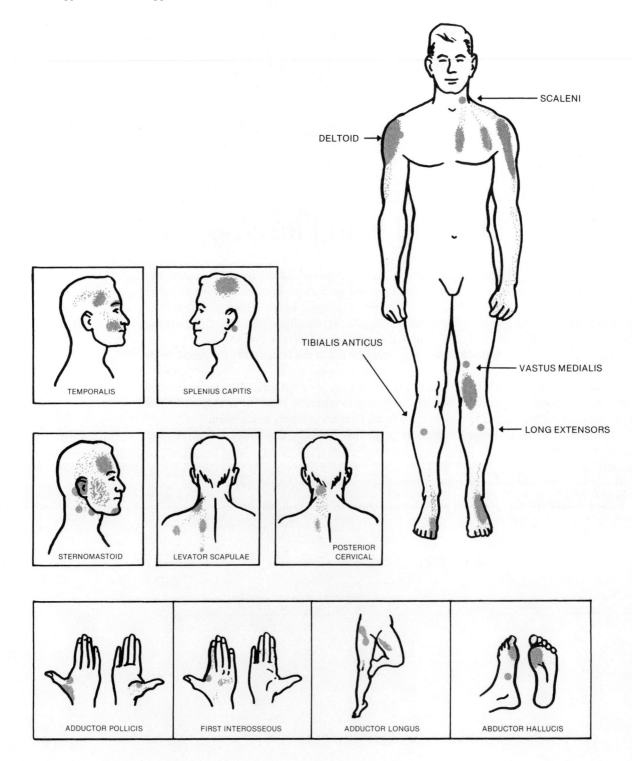

SCALENI

DELTOID

TEMPORALIS

SPLENIUS CAPITIS

STERNOMASTOID

LEVATOR SCAPULAE

POSTERIOR CERVICAL

TIBIALIS ANTICUS

VASTUS MEDIALIS

LONG EXTENSORS

ADDUCTOR POLLICIS

FIRST INTEROSSEOUS

ADDUCTOR LONGUS

ABDUCTOR HALLUCIS

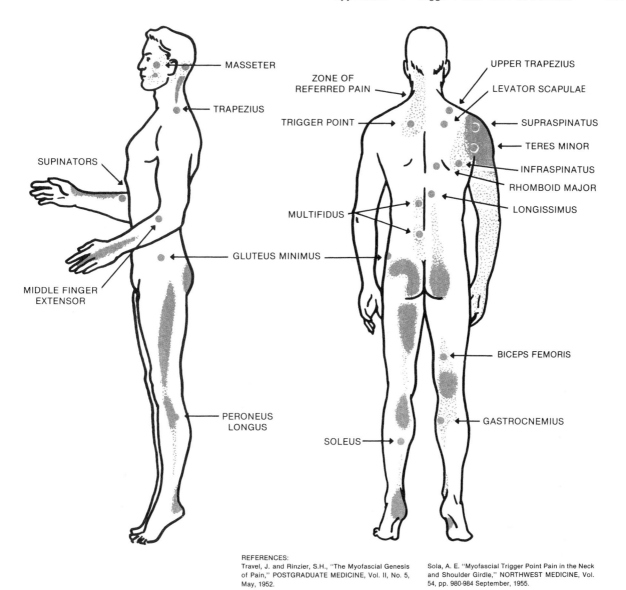

MASSETER

TRAPEZIUS

SUPINATORS

MIDDLE FINGER
EXTENSOR

GLUTEUS MINIMUS

PERONEUS
LONGUS

ZONE OF
REFERRED PAIN

TRIGGER POINT

MULTIFIDUS

SOLEUS

UPPER TRAPEZIUS

LEVATOR SCAPULAE

SUPRASPINATUS

TERES MINOR

INFRASPINATUS

RHOMBOID MAJOR

LONGISSIMUS

BICEPS FEMORIS

GASTROCNEMIUS

REFERENCES:
Travel, J. and Rinzier, S.H., "The Myofascial Genesis of Pain," POSTGRADUATE MEDICINE, Vol. II, No. 5, May, 1952.

Sola, A. E. "Myofascial Trigger Point Pain in the Neck and Shoulder Girdle," NORTHWEST MEDICINE, Vol. 54, pp. 980-984 September, 1955.

STERNALIS

SERRATUS ANTERIOR

PECTORALS

GLUTEUS MEDIUS   ILIOCOATALIS

Appendix C

Medical Shorthand

The following represent examples of medical shorthand for note taking and medical records. Because of both the similarities and differences between different abbreviations, facilities should develop an approved institutional list of abbreviations and have them readily available for staff and administrators.

◼ Therapeutic Modalities or Treatments

CWP	Cold whirlpool	MT	Manual therapy
EMS	Electrical muscle stimulation	MWD	Microwave diathermy
ES	Electrical stimulation	RICE	Rest, ice, compression, elevation
HP	Hot pack	SWD	Shortwave diathermy
HT	Hubbard tank	TENS	Transcutaneous electrical nerve stimulation
HVPS	High-voltage pulsed stimulation		
HWP	Hot whirlpool	TFM	Transverse friction massage
ICE	Ice, compression, elevation	TX	Traction
IFS	Interferential stimulation	US	Ultrasound
IM	Ice massage	UV	Ultraviolet
MENS	Microcurrent electrical neuromuscular stimulation	WP	Whirlpool

◼ Dosage/Administration

AC	Before meals	PER OS, PO	By mouth
AD LIB	At discretion/as desired	PRN	Whenever necessary
ASA	Aspirin	Q	Every
ASAP	As soon as possible	QD	Every day
BID	Twice daily	QH	Every hour
BIW	Biweekly	QID	Four times a day
MAX	Maximum	QOD	Every other day
MED	Minimal erythemal dose (ultraviolet light)	QN	Every night
		$Q\Rightarrow$	Every X hours (e.g., Q3HR = every 3 hours)
	Medium		
MIN	Minimal	SED	Suberythemal dose (ultraviolet light)
MOD	Moderate	SIG	Directions for use
NOC	Night, nocturnal	SOS	When necessary, if necessary
NPO	Nothing by mouth	ST	Start
OD	Once daily	TID	Three times a day
PC	After meals	TIW	Three times a week
PCA	Patient-controlled anesthesia	W/cm^2	Watts per square centimeter
PER	By or through		

◼ Range of Motion, Exercise, and Activity

//	Parallel bars		NWB	Non-weight-bearing
AAROM	Active assistive (assisted) range of motion		OOB	Out of bed
			OOW	Out of work
ABD	Abduction		PWB	Partial weight-bearing
ADD	Adduction		PNF	Proprioceptive neuromuscular facilitation
ADL	Activities of daily living		PREs	Progressive resistance exercises
amb	ambulation		PROM	Passive range of motion
AP	Ankle pumps		PRON	Pronation
AROM	Active range of motion		QS	Quadriceps muscle sets
BR	Bed rest		REHAB	Rehabilitation
CWI	Crutch walking instruction/exercise		REPs	Repetitions
EV	Eversion		ROM	Range of motion
EXT	Extension		ROT	Rotate, rotational
FARM	Full active range of motion		RROM	Resistive range of motion
FLX	Flexion		RTW	Return to work
FWB	Full weight-bearing		SB	Side bending
GT	Gait training		SLR	Straight-leg raise
HEP	Home exercise program		SUP	Supination
INV	Inversion		TTW	Toe touch weight-bearing
MMT	Manual muscle test		WBAT	Weight-bearing as tolerated
MVT	Movement			

◼ Surgical and Medical Procedures

ACLR	Anterior cruciate ligament reconstruction		OREF	Open reduction, external fixation
BX	Biopsy		ORIF	Open reduction, internal fixation
CBC	Complete blood count		THA	Total hip arthroplasty
CT/CAT	Computer-assisted tomography		THR	Total hip replacement
CTR	Carpal tunnel release		TKA	Total knee arthroplasty
MRI	Magnetic resonance imaging		TKR	Total knee replacement

◼ Assistive Devices and Braces

AFO	Ankle-foot orthosis		LAC	Long arm cast
CR	Crutches		LLC	Long leg cast
CW	Crutch walking		SAC	Short arm cast
HAC	Half arm cast		WC	Walking cast
HLC	Half leg cast		w/c	Wheelchair
KAFO	Knee-ankle-foot orthosis			

◼ Measurements and Time

+, pos	Positive		doa	Date of admission
–, neg	Negative		doi	Date of injury
<	Less than		dos	Date of surgery
=	Equals		DTD	Dated
>	Greater than		ft	Foot/feet
a.m.	Morning (just after midnight to just before noon)		GA	Gestational age
			g	Gram
BLA	Baseline assessment		h, hr	Hour
C	Centigrade, Celsius		hs	At bedtime
cm	Centimeter		ht.	Height
cont.	Continue		H&P	History and physical
DA	Developmental age		in.	Inch

kg	Kilogram	sec	Seconds
L, l	Liter	stat	Immediately
lb	Pounds	TBSP	Tablespoon
m	Meter	TSP	Teaspoon
min	Minutes	UNK	Unknown
mg	Milligram	wk	Week
mL	Milliliter	wt	Weight
mm	Millimeter	WNL	Within normal limits
mo	Month	X	Number of times performed (e.g., 2×)
oz	Ounce	yr	Year
PTA	Prior to admission	y/o	Years old
p.m.	Afternoon (just past noon to just prior to midnight)		

■ Grades

1	First degree	N	Normal
2	Second degree	P	Poor
3	Third degree	T	Trace
ABN	Abnormal	N/A	Not applicable
F	Fair	WNL	Within normal limits
G	Good		

■ Body Area

L	Left	FT	Foot/feet
R	Right	GH	Glenohumeral joint
ACJ	Acromioclavicular joint	INF	Inferior
ACL	Anterior cruciate ligament	JT	Joint
AE	Above elbow	L	Lumbar spine
AIIS	Anterior inferior iliac spine	L#	Lumbar spine level (e.g., L1, L2)
AK	Above knee	LB	Low back (lumbar)
ANT	Anterior	LCL	Lateral collateral ligament
AP	Anteroposterior	LE	Lower extremity
ASIS	Anterosuperior iliac spine	MCL	Medial collateral ligament
ATF	Anterior talofibular ligament	P	Proximal
B	Bilateral/both	P/#	Proximal range (e.g., p/3 = proximal third)
BE	Below elbow		
Bilat.	Bilaterally	PA	Posteroanterior
BK	Below knee	PCL	Posterior cruciate ligament
BLE	Bilateral lower extremities	PIP	Proximal interphalangeal joint
C	Cervical spine	PSIS	Posterior superior iliac spine
C#	Cervical spine level (e.g., C1, C2)	PTF	Posterior talofibular ligament
CF	Calcaneofibular ligament	SCJ	Sternoclavicular joint
CV	Cardiovascular	T	Thoracic spine
D	Distal	T#	Thoracic spine level (e.g., T1, T2)
D/#	Distal range (e.g., d/1 = distal third)	UE	Upper extremity
DIP	Distal interphalangeal joint		

■ General Note Taking

$\bar{p}$	After	,,	Female
~	Approximately	,	Male
$\bar{a}$, a	Before	1°	Primary
Δ	Change	2°	Secondary
↓	Down, decreasing	3°	Tertiary

↑	Up, increasing	P:	Plan
c̄	With	PATH	Pathology
s̄	Without	PALP	Palpation
A:	Assessment	PE	Physical examination/evaluation
ADM	Admission	PH	Past history
AMA	Against medical advice	PMH	Prior medical history
c/o	Complains of	POMR	Problem-oriented medical record
CC	Chief complaint	POSS	Possible
cc	Cubic centimeter	POST	Following, after
D/C	Discontinue	POSTOP	After surgery
DNK	Did not keep appointment	PREOP	Before surgery
Dx	Diagnosis	PROG	Progress/progressing
EVAL	Evaluation	re:	Regarding, relating to, pertaining to
FH	Family history	RE-ADM	Re-admission
Hx, hx	History	RO, r/o	Rule out
IC	Informed consent	Rx	Treatment, prescription
imp.	Impression	S/P	Status post (condition following)
IN SITU	In its natural place	S:	Subjective
indep	Independent	SCP	Standard care plan
LTG	Long-term goals	SOP	Standard operating procedure
M&R	Measure and record	SOAP	Subjective, objective, assessment plan; format of note taking
MA	Medical assistance		
Meds	Medication	SSN	Social security number
MRN	Medical record number	STG	Short-term goals
N/A	Not applicable	Sx	Symptoms
NKA	No known allergies	t.o.	Telephone order
NKI	No known injuries/illnesses	TPR	Temperature, pulse, and respiration
O.P., OP	Outpatient	v.s.	Vital signs
O.R., OR	Operating room	vo	Verbal orders
O:	Objective		

■ Injuries and Diseases

AIDS	Acquired immunodeficiency syndrome	LAC	Laceration
AODM	Adult onset diabetes mellitus	LBP	Low back pain
ARF	Acute renal failure	LOC	Loss of consciousness
CA	Cancer	MCA	Motorcycle accident
CAD	Coronary artery disease	MI	Myocardial infarction
COLD	Chronic obstructive lung disease	MS	Multiple sclerosis
COPD	Chronic obstructive pulmonary disease	MTBI	Mild traumatic brain injury
CP	Cerebral palsy	NIDD	Non–insulin-dependent diabetes
CVA	Cerebrovascular accident	OA	Osteoarthritis
DDD	Degenerative disc disease	PARA	Paraplegic
DJD	Degenerative joint disease	PID	Pelvic inflammatory disease
DM	Diabetes mellitus	PFJS	Patellofemoral joint syndrome
DVT	Deep vein thrombosis	PNI	Peripheral nerve injury
FUO	Fever, unknown origin	PVD	Peripheral vascular disease
FX	Fracture	QUAD	Quadriplegic
HA, H/A	Headache	RA	Rheumatoid arthritis
HBP	High blood pressure	SCI	Spinal cord injury
HCVD	Hypertensive cardiovascular disease	SIW	Self-inflicted wound
HI	Head injury	SOB	Shortness of breath
HIV	Human immunodeficiency virus	SPR	Sprain
HNP	Herniated nucleus pulposus	STR	Strain
HTN	Hypertension	TBI	Traumatic brain injury

■ Personnel

AT, ATC, LAT	Athletic trainer	OT	Occupational therapist/occupational therapy
COTA	Certified occupational therapy assistant		
CVT	Cardiovascular technologist	OTC	Orthopedic technologist, certified
DC	Doctor of chiropractic	PA, P.A.	Physician assistant
DO	Doctor of osteopathy	PT	Physical therapist/physical therapy
EENT	Eye, ears, nose, and throat	PTA	Physical therapy assistant
ENT	Ears, nose, and throat	Pt, pt	Patient
GYN	Gynecology	RD	Registered dietitian
MD	Medical doctor	RN	Registered nurse
MT	Massage therapist	RT	Respiratory therapist
NP	Nurse practitioner	RTR	Registered technologist, Radiology
OB	Obstetrics		

Appendix D

Motor Points

A motor point is the place in a muscle where the muscle is most easily excited with a minimum amount of electrical stimulation; the motor point is usually located near the center of the muscle mass, where the motor nerve enters the muscle. For each muscle, the motor point may vary from patient to patient, or even at different times for the same patient, depending on the pathology. The accompanying charts are guides to the motor points.

Illustrations are from Mettler Corporation, Anaheim, California, with permission.

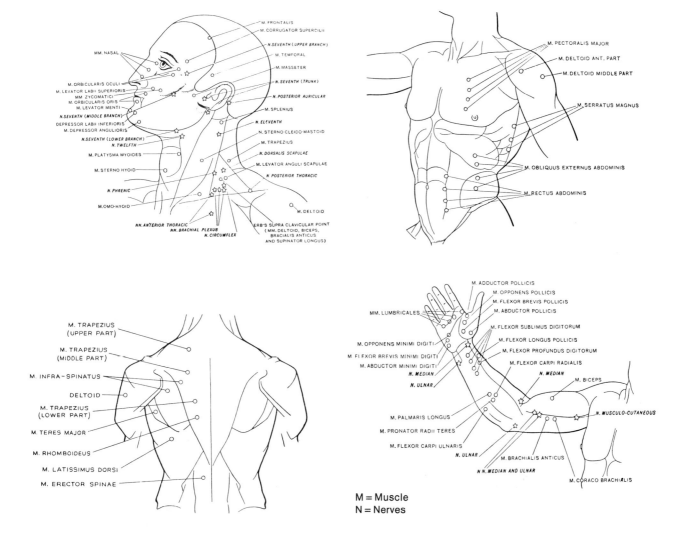

M = Muscle
N = Nerves

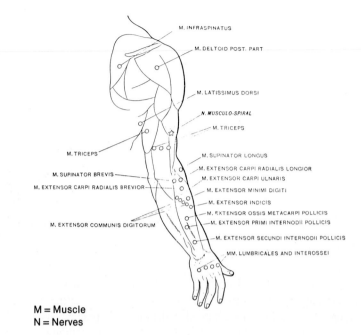

M = Muscle
N = Nerves

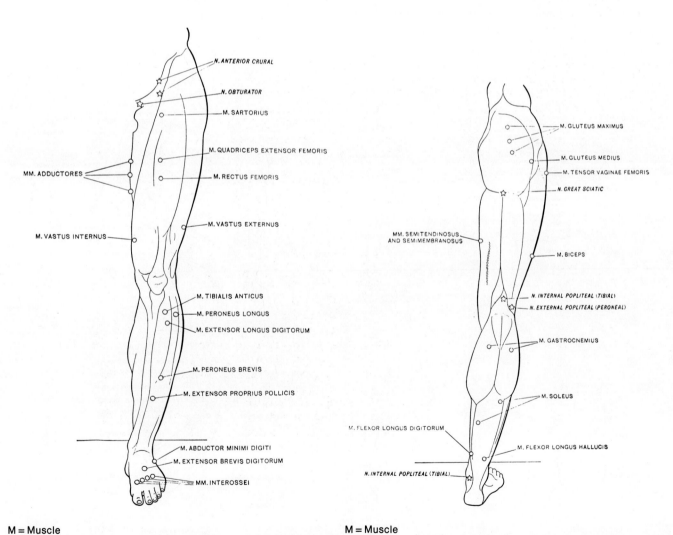

M = Muscle
N = Nerve

M = Muscle
N = Nerve

Appendix E

Ohm's Law

■ Calculation of Ohm's Law in Series and Parallel Circuits

In a Series Circuit:

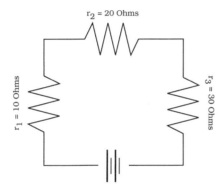

If we know that a potential of 120 V is applied to a circuit with 60 ohms of resistance, the amperage can be calculated by using Ohm's law. Using the values in the figure above, the equation for calculating the current flow through the series of resistors is:

$$I = V/R_t$$
$$I = 120 \text{ V}/60 \text{ ohms}$$
$$I = 2A$$

If each of three resistors has a different resistance (say, 10 ohms, 20 ohms, and 30 ohms), the voltage will fluctuate between resistors. By applying a derivation of Ohm's law, $V = IR$, the voltage across each resistor may be calculated as:

$V_1 = Ir_1$ $V_2 = Ir_2$ $V_3 = Ir_3$
$V_1 = 2A \times 10$ ohms $V_2 = 2A \times 20$ ohms $V_3 = 2A \times 30$ ohms
$V_1 = 20$ V $V_2 = 40$ V $V_3 = 60$ V

By adding $V_1 + V_2 + V_3$, you can see that the sum of the potential across the individual resistors equals the total power applied to the circuit. The current (amperage) remains the same throughout a series circuit. The voltage and the resistance vary.

In a Parallel Circuit:

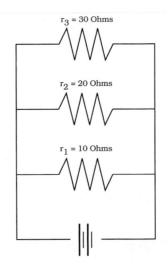

To calculate the total resistance for a parallel circuit, we must keep in mind that the flow in each pathway is inversely proportional to its resistance. Because voltage is constant, this value may be canceled out and the mathematical reciprocal (1/n) of the resistance may be used:

$$I = V/R_t$$
$$I = 120 \text{ V}/5.56 \text{ ohms}$$
$$I = 21.6 \text{ A}$$

The amount of current flowing across each resistor (and path) is calculated by:

$i_1 = v/r_1$	$i_2 = v/r_2$	$i_3 = v/r_3$
$i_1 = 120 \text{ V}/10 \text{ ohms}$	$i_2 = 120 \text{ V}/20 \text{ ohms}$	$i_3 = 120 \text{ V}/30 \text{ ohms}$
$i_1 = 12 \text{ A}$	$i_2 = 6 \text{ A}$	$i_3 = 4 \text{ A}$

where:

$$i_n = \text{Amperage across resistor n}$$
$$v = \text{Voltage applied to the circuit}$$
$$r_n = \text{Resistance in ohms}$$

Unlike series circuits, the parallel circuits have the same voltage across each path. The amperage and resistance differ from path to path. Therefore, if the voltage across one path can be calculated, the voltage for the entire circuit is known.

Appendix F

Section Quiz Answers

Section 1

1. B	7. A	13. A	19. C
2. C	8. C	14. B	20. D
3. C	9. C	15. B, D	21. B
4. B	10. A	16. D	22. C
5. C	11. D	17. B	23. A
6. A	12. C	18. A	24. D

Section 2

1. B	6. B	11. B	16. C
2. D	7. C	12. C	17. D
3. B	8. B	13. B	
4. D	9. B	14. D	
5. D	10. D	15. C	

Section 3

1. C	10. B
2. A	11. B
3. D	12. B
4. D	13. C
5. A	14. C
6. A	15. A
7. C	16. A
8. D	17. B
9. A	18. A

20.

19. Any of the following are acceptable answers:

Hydration
Age
Composition
Vascularity
Thickness

	ULTRASOUND	SHORTWAVE DIATHERMY
Type of energy	Acoustical	Electromagnetic
Tissue heated	Collagen-rich	C: Adipose tissue, skin I: Muscle, blood vessels
Volume of tissue heated	Small (~20 cm^2)	Large (~200 cm^2)
Temperature increase	1 MHz: > 6.3°F (3.5°C)	C: > 7.0°F (3.9°C) (adipose tissue)
	3 MHz: > 14.9°F (8.3°C)	I: > 18.0°F (10°C) (intramuscular tissue)
Heat retention	Short (approximately 3 minutes)	Long (approximately 9 minutes)

■ Section 4

1. C	6. A	11. B	16. B
2. D	7. D	12. B	17. B
3. C	8. A	13. D	18. D
4. B	9. A	14. A	19. A
5. D	10. A	15. A	20. B

■ Section 5

1. D
2. C
3. A
4. B
5. C
6. B
7. B
8. D
9. A
10. C
11. D

12. Position of the cervical spine

   Patient position
   Angle of pull
   Treatment duration

13. The force of gravity is eliminated
   The cervical muscles are placed in
   a more relaxed position

14. B
   A
   C

Appendix G

Case Study Discussion

Section Two

Cold therapy application is the intervention of choice. The ideal combination of ice, compression, and elevation to limit post-injury fluid collection is best obtained with ice bags or conventional gel ice packs. The physiological changes reduce the release of inflammatory mediators, decrease prostaglandin synthesis, and decrease capillary permeability.

The clinical symptoms in this case are from a prevention standpoint, because the injury just occurred. The ice application is aimed at limiting swelling accumulation, minimizing pain, limiting muscle spasm, and limiting range of motion loss.

Ice application may be implemented after acute reinjury episodes ("rolling" ankle incident, or exercise or activity in excess), to reduce pain on a "bad" day, to reduce muscle spasm, or to assist in restoration of range of motion. Other thermal agents can include ice immersion, whirlpool (cold-warm temperature), and ice massage. The ice immersion allows range of motion to be performed simultaneously to increase patient's active role in recovery; the whirlpool will allow range-of-motion exercise, and the temperature can be increased as the injury moves into the subacute phase of recovery to enhance metabolism to promote healing. Ice massage works best for small, uneven local regions of injury (such as the lateral ligaments or foot intrinsics) where the trauma primarily occurred. Thermal agents may be an option if acute inflammation has resolved, but low intensity is recommended owing to high ratio of bone to soft tissue in the injured region.

Section Three

Shortwave diathermy induction coil drum is the best option owing to large surface area of involved tissues, marked muscle spasm, and the open wound in the lumbar region. The clinician should be certain that there is no metal within the field of the shortwave diathermy. If the patient has scoliosis with a rod implanted in his spine, for example, the treatment may need application of a sterile dressing to minimize the risk of infection and sterile towels used as a hot pack cover.

During heating, the following physiological responses are stimulated: local cellular metabolism, blood flow, fibroblastic activity, collagen deposition, and new capillary growth.

Heating agents may place the patient at higher risk for infection with contact from nonsterile towels or hot pack covers. Ultrasound can only be applied to a portion of the problem area, due to the wound.

Clinically, treatment is addressing marked muscle spasm, range-of-motion loss, pain, and wound healing.

Section Four

In a clinical setting, the best option for this patient varies tremendously according to the clinician's previous success rate, patient preference, and concurrent treatment approaches implemented. Much success comes from removing the source, the computer workstation ergonomics. Until the workstation is adjusted for proper body mechanics, the problems are unlikely to resolve. Intervention options could include thermal ultrasound, massage, cryostretch (e.g., spray and stretch), and neuromuscular or interferential electrical stimulation. Physiologically, the main effect would be to reduce the muscle spasm by inhibiting muscle contraction.

The clinical symptoms that should be addressed are range of motion, pain, spasm, tenderness, and muscle strength and endurance.

■ Section Five

Commentary—Bertha

Edema management can be addressed with massage, electrical stimulation, and warm and cold thermal agents. The physiological effects are to assist venous and lymphatic return, reduce viscosity of fluid, remove cellular debris, and increase delivery of nutrients for the healing of the soft tissues. Clinical goals would be based on her deficits, and treatment is rendered to reduce edema, improve range of motion, decrease pain, and improve function. Owing to her history of cancer, ultrasound should be avoided. Interferential electrical stimulation and heat packs would be appropriate.

Commentary—Sam

Indications include muscle spasm, degenerative disc disease, nerve root compression, capsulitis of the vertebral joint, and herniated intervertebral disks. Traction can be used to try to interrupt the pain-spasm-pain cycle. The pressure on the nerve roots should be reduced by the distraction force of the traction unit. Clinically, the centralization of symptoms is a sign of progress, by one man's opinion. The clinical symptoms that should be reduced are pain, range of motion, and radicular pain. Other interventions to ease the muscle spasm, without compromising the disc pressure, could include heat therapy, electrical stimulation, ice packs, and ultrasound, if symptoms are localized to a small area.

Commentary—Mr. Smith

Contraindications include peripheral vascular disease, deep vein thrombosis, dermatitis, gangrene, and compartment syndromes. Constant, gentle range of motion will increase remodeling of collagen in an orderly fashion and promote nutrient exchange. Clinical gains are expected in range of motion, edema reduction, pain management, and diminished soft-tissue spasm.

Book Glossary

Absolute refractory period: The period after a nerve's depolarization during which a subsequent depolarization cannot occur, used for recharging the electrical potential.

Absolute zero: Theoretically, the lowest possible temperature, equal to $-273°C$ or $-460°F$. At this point, all atomic and molecular motion ceases.

Absorption: The process of a medium collecting thermal energy and changing it to kinetic energy.

Accommodation: The decrease in a nerve's action potential frequency over time when exposed to an unchanging depolarization stimulus.

Acetylcholine: Neurotransmitter responsible for transmitting motor nerve impulses.

Acoustical interface: A surface where two materials of different densities meet.

Acoustical spectrum: Energy transmitted through mechanical waves.

Acoustical streaming: The unidirectional flow of fluids within the tissues caused by the application of therapeutic ultrasound.

Actin: A contractile muscle protein.

Actinomycosis: A disease state of actin caused by a fungus.

Action potential: The change in the electrical potential of a nerve or muscle fiber when stimulated.

Activities of daily living: Fundamental skills required for a certain lifestyle, including mobility, self-care, and grooming.

Acupuncture points: Points on the skin theorized to control systemic functions. These points lie along 12 main channels, eight secondary channels, and a network of subchannels.

Acute: Of recent onset. The period after an injury when the local inflammatory response is still active.

ADA: See Americans With Disabilities Act.

A-delta fibers: A type of nerve that transmits painful information that is often interpreted by the brain as burning or stinging pain.

Adenosine triphosphate (ATP): An important source of energy for intracellular metabolism.

Adriamycin: An antibiotic medication.

Aerobic: Requiring the presence of oxygen.

Afferent: Carrying impulses toward a central structure, for example, the brain.

Alarm stage: The first stage in the general adaptation syndrome in which the body readies its defensive systems.

Albinism: A condition in which the individual lacks pigmentation of the skin, hair, and eyes. The skin is prone to sunburns and the eyes are particularly sensitive to light (photophobia).

Allograft: A replacement or augmentation of a biological structure with a synthetic one.

Alpha-motoneurons: Efferent motor neurons that innervate muscle fibers.

ALS: See Anterior lateral system.

Alternating current: The uninterrupted flow of electrons marked by a change in the direction and magnitude of the movement.

Americans With Disabilities Act: Legislation passed in 1990 (Public Law 101-336) that protects the rights of disabled individuals by creating standards to ensure access and prohibit discrimination in transportation, accommodation, public services, and so on.

Amino acids: Building blocks of protein.

Amperage: The rate of flow of an electrical current. One ampere is equal to the rate of flow of 1 coulomb per second.

Amplitude: The maximum departure of a wave from the baseline.

Amplitude ramp: The gradual rise or fall in a pulse train's amplitude.

Anabolic: The synthesis of molecules from its component elements, constructive metabolism.

Anaerobic: Able to survive in the absence of oxygen. Anaerobic systems derive their energy through the breakdown of adenosine triphosphate (ATP) into adenosine diphosphate (ADP).

Analgesia: Absence of the sense of pain.

Analgesic: A pain-reducing substance.

Analog: A readout on a continuously variable scale. A clock with hands is a type of analog display.

Anesthesia: A loss of, or decrease in, sensation.

Angiogenesis: Formation of new blood vessels.

Angstrom (Å): A distance equal to 10^{-10} m or one-billionth of a meter.

Annulus fibrosus: The dense, inflexible outer layers of an intervertebral disk.

Anode: The positive pole of an electrical circuit. It has a low concentration of electrons and is the opposite of the cathode.

Antabuse: A medication (generic name: disulfiram) used in treating alcoholism. Consumption of alcoholic drinks while taking antabuse results in severe nausea and vomiting.

Antalgic gait: A gait resulting from pain on weight bearing. The stance phase of gait is shortened on the affected side.

Anterior lateral fasciculus: The large bundle of fibers in the anterolateral spinal cord and brain stem that carry second-order pain fibers to the brain stem and thalamus.

Anterior lateral system: The ascending fiber system that conveys pain and temperature sensation from spinal cord to the thalamus.

Antibiotic: A substance that inhibits the growth of, or kills, microorganisms.

Arndt-Schultz principle: A principle stating that for energy to affect the body, it must be absorbed by the tissues at a level sufficient to stimulate a physiological response.

Arteriole: A small artery leading to a capillary at its distal end.

Arthrofibrosis: The repair and replacement of inflamed joint tissue by connective tissues.

Arthrogenic muscle inhibition: Denervation of a muscle or muscle group caused by joint swelling.

Arthroplasty: Surgical reconstruction or replacement of an articular joint.

Asymmetrical: Lacking symmetry (e.g., two halves of unequal size or shape).

Atmospheres absolute (ATA): Water (or air) pressure exerted on the body. One ATA is the standard pressure placed on the body at sea level. Each 33-ft immersion from sea level equals an increase of 1 ATA. For example, immersion to a depth of 33 feet exerts 2 ATA, 66 feet exerts 3 ATA, 99 feet exerts 4 ATA, and so on.

ATP: See Adenosine triphosphate.

Attenuation: The decrease in a wave's intensity resulting from the absorption, reflection, and refraction of energy.

Autoclave: A device used to sterilize medical instruments using steam heat at 250°F (121°C).

Average current: The average amplitude of a current. When the current can be represented by a sine wave, the average current is calculated by multiplying the amplitude by 0.637.

Axon: The stem of a nerve.

Axonotmesis: Damage to nerve tissue without physical severing of the nerve.

Bacterium (plural bacteria): A microscopic organism.

Basement membrane: Extracellular material that separates the base of epithelial cells from connective tissue.

Basic fibroblast growth factor (bFGF): Increases the size of the callus and mechanical strength of the repair during fracture healing.

Battery (criminal): The unwanted touching of one person by another.

Beam nonuniformity ratio (BNR): The ratio between the highest intensity in an ultrasonic beam and the output reported on the meter.

Beat pattern: The frequency formed when two electrical circuits of two different frequencies are mixed.

β-Endorphin: A neurohormone similar to morphine.

Bilateral: On both sides of the body.

Biphasic current: A pulsed current possessing two phases, each of which occurs on opposite sides of the electrical baseline. The bidirectional flow of electrons that is marked by discrete periods of noncurrent flow.

Bipolar stimulation: Electrical stimulation using electrodes of approximately equal surface area from each lead. The resulting current density under the electrodes from each lead is approximately equal.

Breach of duty: A departure from the implied duty based on the reasonable and prudent doctrine.

Calorie: The amount of energy needed to raise the temperature of 1 g of water by 1°C. One calorie equals 4.1860 joules of energy.

Capacitance: The frequency-dependent ability to store a charge. The symbol for capacitance is C and is expressed in farads (F).

Capillary filtration pressure: The pressure that moves the contents of a capillary outward to the tissues.

Capitated: The provision of health care services for a fixed cost or flat fee.

Cardinal signs of inflammation: Heat, redness, swelling, pain, and loss of function in the area; used as a gauge in determining the extent and stage of the injury response process.

Carotid sinus: An enlargement of the carotid artery near the branch of the internal carotid artery, located distal to the inferior arch of the mandible. Baroreceptors at this site monitor and assist in the regulation of blood pressure.

Carpal tunnel syndrome: Compression of the median nerve that produces pain, numbness, and weakness in the palm and ring and index fingers.

Catabolic: A metabolic process that breaks a molecule into its component elements, thereby releasing energy.

Catalyst: A substance that accelerates a chemical reaction.

Cathode: The negative pole of an electrical circuit. It has a high concentration of electrons and carries the opposite charge to the anode.

Cavitation: The formation of microscopic bubbles during the application of therapeutic ultrasound.

C fiber: A type of nerve that transmits painful information that is often interpreted by the brain as throbbing or aching.

Change of state: Transformation from one physical state to another (e.g., ice to water).

Channel (electrical): An electrical circuit consisting of two poles that operate independently of other circuits.

Chassis: The framework to which electrical components are attached.

Chemosensitive pain receptors: Nerves that are excited by the presence of certain chemical substances.

Chemotaxis: Movement of living protoplasm toward or away from a chemical stimulus.

Chronic: Continuing for a long period; with injury, extending past the primary hemorrhage and inflammation cycle.

Cingulate gyrus: A large region of the cerebral cortex that lies superior to the corpus callosum. It is important in affective responses to pain.

Circuit, closed: A complete pathway that allows electrons to flow to and from the electrical source.

Circuit, open: An incomplete pathway that does not allow electrons to flow to or from the electrical source.

Circumferential compression: Compression applied in a manner that provides even pressure around the circumference of the body part.

Coagulation: The process of blood clotting.

Cold-induced vasodilation: An unsubstantiated theory suggesting that cold application results in a net increase in the cross-sectional diameter of blood vessels.

Collagen: A protein-based connective tissue.

Collagenase: A substance that causes collagen to break down.

Collateral compression: A form of compression that provides pressure on only two sides of the body part.

Collimated: Possessing a beam of parallel rays or waves that form a column of energy.

Commission: Response to a situation in a manner that is not reasonable and prudent.

Compartment syndrome: Increased pressure within a muscular compartment, causing decreased blood flow to and from the distal extremity, decreased distal nerve function, and decreased local muscular blood perfusion and pain.

Compression (mechanical): An external force applied to the body (e.g., an elastic wrap) that serves to decrease the pressure gradient between the blood vessels and tissue.

Compression (ultrasonic): A decrease in the size of a cell during high-pressure peaks.

Conduction: The transfer of heat from a high temperature to a low temperature between two objects that are touching each other.

Conductive properties: The ability of a tissue to transfer heat (from a high temperature to a low temperature) or electrical energy.

Conductor (electrical): A material having the ability to transmit electricity. Conductors have many free electrons and provide relatively little resistance to electrical flow. Within the body, tissues having a high water content are considered conductors.

Connective tissue: Tissue that supports and connects other tissue types.

Consensual touching: A situation in which the person being touched has agreed to be touched. Consensual agreements negate the charge of battery.

Constructive interference: Two waves that, perfectly synchronized, combine to produce a single wave of greater amplitude.

Continuous interference: Two waves that are slightly out of phase interacting to produce a single wave whose amplitude and/or frequency varies.

Contracture: A condition resulting from the loss of a tissue's ability to lengthen.

Contraindications (Contraindicate): To make inadvisable.

Contralateral: Pertaining to the opposite side of the body. The left side is contralateral to the right.

Convection: The cooling of one object and the subsequent heating of another by the circulation of a fluid, usually water, or air.

Convergent: Two or more input routes reduced to a single route.

Conversion: Transformation of high-frequency electrical energy into heat.

Cortisol: A cortisone-like substance produced in the body.

Cosine law: A law stating that, as an angle deviates away from 90 degrees, the effective energy is reduced by the multiple of the cosine of the angle: Effective energy = Energy × Cosine of the angle. A deviation of ±10 degrees is considered within acceptable limits for therapeutic treatments.

Coulomb: The amount of charge produced by 6.25×10^{18} electrons (negative charge) or protons (positive charge).

Coulomb's law: A law stating that opposite charges attract and like charges repel each other.

Counterirritant: A substance causing irritation of superficial sensory nerves to reduce the transmission of pain from underlying nerves.

CPT Codes: See Current procedural terminology codes.

Crepitus: A grinding or crunching sound or sensation.

Cryoglobulinemia: A condition in which abnormal blood proteins, cryoglobulins, group together when exposed to cold. This condition can lead to skin color changes, hives, subcutaneous hemorrhage, and other disorders.

Cryokinetics: A treatment technique that involves moving the injured body part while it is being treated with cold, thus decreasing pain while increasing range of motion.

Cryotherapy: The application of therapeutic cold to living tissues.

Current procedural terminology codes: Codes used to describe the care provided for the patient and used for billing purposes.

Cyanosis (cyanotic): A blue-gray discoloration of the skin caused by a lack of oxygen.

Cyclooxygenase-2 (COX-2): Inflammatory agent that encourages bone healing.

Cytokine: A protein produced by white blood cells.

DC/ML: See Dorsal columns/Medial lemniscus.

Defamation of character: Mistruths said about a person that cause harm.

Degassed water: Water that has boiled for 30 to 45 minutes and then allowed to sit undisturbed for 4 to 24 hours, allowing gaseous bubbles to escape.

Degeneration (muscular): The decrease in size and strength of a muscle that occurs secondary to atrophy.

Delayed-onset muscle soreness: Residual muscle soreness, caused secondary to damage of the muscle cells, that appears within 24 hours after heavy muscular activity, particularly with eccentric muscle actions.

Dementia: The progressive loss of cognitive and intellectual functions without impairment of perception or consciousness. Symptoms include disorientation, memory impairment, impaired judgment, and impaired intellectual ability.

Dendrite: Synaptic connections of a nerve arising from a body.

Denervated: Lack of the proper nerve supply or nerve function to, for example, an area or muscle group.

Deoxyribonucleic acid: Carries genetic information for all organisms except RNA.

Dependent position: An arrangement in which the body part is placed lower than the heart, increasing the intravascular pressure.

Dermal ulcer: A slowly healing or nonhealing break in the skin.

Dermatome: A segmental skin area supplied by a single nerve root.

Destructive interference: Two waves that are exactly out of phase, interacting to cancel each other out.

Diagnosis: The determination of the nature and scope of an injury or illness.

Dialysis: An external device that is used to assist or replace the kidney's function of filtering blood.

Diapedesis: Part of the inflammatory response characterized by movement of white blood cells and other substances through gaps formed in vascular walls to enter the tissues.

Diastolic blood pressure: The lowest level of pressure in the arteries. For example, when a blood pressure reading is given as 120/80, 80 represents the diastolic value.

Diathermy: A classification of therapeutic modality that uses high-frequency electrical energy to heat subcutaneous tissues.

Dipole: A pair of equal and opposite charges separated by a distance.

Direct access: Health-care services can be provided without physician referral. Note that a physician referral is often required for third-party reimbursement.

Direct current: The uninterrupted, one-directional flow of electrons.

Disposition: The patient's current physical status and projected course of recovery.

Divergence: The spreading of a beam or wave.

DNA: See Deoxyribonucleic acid.

Doctrine: A statement of fundamental government policy.

Dorsal columns: The large bundle of fibers in the dorsal spinal cord formed by ascending primary afferent fibers that carry touch and proprioceptive sensation.

Dorsal columns/medial lemniscal system: The ascending fiber system that conveys fine touch and proprioception from spinal cord to the thalamus.

Dorsolateral fasciculus: The small bundle of fibers in the dorsolateral spinal cord formed by ascending primary afferent fibers that carry pain and temperature sensation.

Due care: An established responsibility for an individual to respond to a given situation in a certain manner.

Duty cycle: The ration between the pulse duration and the pulse interval: Duty cycle = Pulse duration/(Pulse duration + Pulse interval) × 100.

Dynamometer: A device used for measuring muscular strength.

Dyskinesia: A defect in the ability to perform voluntary joint movement.

Ecchymosis: A blue-black discoloration of the skin caused by movement of blood into the tissues. In the later stages, the color may appear as a greenish-brown or yellow.

Ectopic: Outside or away from its normal position; in an abnormal position or sequence.

Eddy: A circular current of fluid, often moving against the main flow.

Edema: An excessive accumulation of serous fluids.

Effective radiating area (ERA): The portion of an ultrasonic transducer's (sound head) surface that emits ultrasonic energy.

Efferent: Carrying impulses away from a central structure. Nerves leaving the central nervous system are efferent nerves.

Efficacy: The ability of a modality or treatment regimen to produce the intended effects.

Effleurage: Massage using long, deep strokes.

Electromagnetic field: The lines of force created by positive and negative poles.

Electromagnetic radiation: Energy found on the electromagnetic spectrum capable of traveling near the speed of light and exhibiting both electrical and magnetic properties.

Electromagnetic spectrum: A continuum ordered by the wavelength or frequency of the energy produced.

Electromyogram: A recording of the electrical charges associated with the contraction of a muscle.

Electron: A negatively charged atomic particle.

Electro-osmotic: Pertaining to the movement of ions as a result of electrical charges. Positive ions move away from the positive pole toward the negative pole; negative ions move away from the negative pole toward the positive pole.

Electropiezo: The vibration caused by an alternating current being passed through a crystal.

Electrostatic field: A field created by static electricity.

Embolism: Blockage of a blood vessel by a blood clot or other foreign substance.

Emigration: Passage of white blood corpuscles through the walls of capillaries and veins during inflammation.

Encapsulated receptor: A sensory receptor formed by a nerve fiber and surrounding connective tissue cells.

Endogenous opiates: Pain-inhibiting substances produced in the brain. These include endorphins and enkephalins.

Endorphin: A morphine-like neurohormone produced from b-lipotropin in the pituitary. Endorphins are thought to increase the pain threshold by binding to receptor sites.

Endothelial cells: Flat cells lining the blood and lymphatic vessels and the heart.

Enkephalin: A substance released by the body that reduces the perception of pain by bonding to pain receptor sites.

Enthesopathy: Pathology of the bony attachment of tendon, ligament, or joint capsule.

Epicritic pain: Pain that is well localized.

Epidemiology: The study of the distribution, rates, and causes of injuries and illness within a specified population. This information may then be used to prevent future occurrence.

Epiphyseal plates: Growth plates of bones.

Epithelial tissue: Tissue that forms the outer skin and lines the body's cavities. This type of tissue has a high potential to regenerate.

Ergometer: A device used to measure the amount of work performed by the legs or arms.

Evaporation: The change from a liquid to a gas state.

Exhaustion stage: The third and final stage in the general adaptation syndrome; the stage when cell death occurs.

External fixation: A fracture-setting technique incorporating the use of metal rods that extend through the skin and are attached to a device outside the body.

Extracellular: Outside the cell membrane.

Extravasation: To exude from or pass out of a vessel into the tissues, said of blood, lymph, or urine.

Exudate: Fluid that collects in a cavity and has a high concentration of cells, protein, and other solid matter.

Far infrared: The portion of the light spectrum located between 1500 and 12,500 nm.

Far ultraviolet: The portion of the light spectrum located between 180 and 290 nm.

Farad: A measure of the storage capability of capacitors. One farad stores a charge of 1 coulomb when 1 V is applied.

Fascia: Fibrous connective tissue found in muscle, beneath the skin, and in the viscera.

Fascia, deep: Found within muscle, this type of fascia is high in collagen content. The fascial fibers are arranged parallel to the line of stress.

Fascia, superficial: Found between the skin and underlying muscle. Superficial fascia has a random, loose fibrous arrangement.

Fibrin: A filamentous protein formed by the action of thrombin on fibrinogen.

Fibrinogen: A protein present in the blood plasma, essential for the clotting of blood.

Fibrinolysis: Pathological breaking up of fibrin.

Fibromyalgia: Chronic inflammation of a muscle or connective tissue.

Fibrosis: An abnormally large formation of inelastic fibrous tissue.

First-order neurons: Sensory nerves that course outside the central nervous system and have their bodies in a dorsal root ganglion.

Flavoprotein: A protein involved in oxidation within a cell.

Flux: A residual electromagnetic field created by two unlike charges.

Focal compression: Applying direct pressure to soft tissue surrounded by prominent structures.

Footcandle: A measure of light equal to 1 lumen per square foot. One lumen is the amount of light emitted by one international candle.

Foramen: An opening (e.g., in a bone) to allow the passage of blood vessels or nerves.

Free nerve endings: The unencapsulated receptor of pain and thermal primary afferent fibers. Unlike the encapsulated receptor organs, free nerve endings have no connective tissue capsule and appear to be bare nerve fibers. Within their membranes, however, are thermal, mechanical, and chemical receptor molecules.

Free radical: A highly reactive molecule having an odd number of electrons. Free radical production plays an important role in the progression of an ischemic injury.

Frequency: The number of times an event occurs in 1 second; measured in hertz (cycles per second) or pulses per second.

Fresnel zone: See Near field.

Functional scoliosis: Lateral curvature of the spinal column in the frontal plane caused as the spinal column attempts to compensate for postural deficits such as leg length discrepancy. Functional scoliosis is also known as protective scoliosis.

GaAs laser: Laser produced by the excitation of gallium arsenide.

Gallium arsenide lasers: See GaAs laser.

Galvanic current: A low-voltage direct current.

Galvanic effect: The migration of ions as the result of the application of a galvanic current.

Gamma globulin: An infection-fighting blood protein.

Gamma-motoneurons: Efferent motor nerves that innervate the intrafusal fibers of a muscle spindle.

Ganglia: A cluster of neurons in the peripheral nervous system.

Gauss: A unit of magnetic strength.

General adaptation syndrome: A theory stating that the body has a common mechanism for adapting to stress. The three stages of this response are alarm, resistance, and exhaustion.

Glycolytic pathway: A complex chemical reaction that yields adenosine triphosphate (ATP) from glucose.

Golgi tendon organ: A sensory nerve ending found in tendons and aponeuroses that detects tension within the muscle. When the tension reaches a threshold, muscle activity of the contracting muscle is inhibited and the antagonistic muscle is facilitated.

Granulation tissue: Delicate tissue composed of fibroblasts, collagen, and capillaries formed during the revascularization phase of wound healing.

Granuloma: A hard mass of fibrous tissue.

Gross negligence: Total failure to provide what would normally be deemed proper in a given situation.

Grotthus-Draper, law of: A law stating that there is an inverse relationship between the amount of penetration and absorption. The more energy that is absorbed by the superficial tissues, the less that remains to be transmitted to underlying tissues.

Ground: An electrical connection that provides a path for leaked current to return safely to the earth.

Ground fault: A disruption in the electrical circuitry where the current exits from the normal path.

Ground-fault interrupter: An interrupter that discontinues the current flow when a ground fault is detected.

Ground substance: Material occupying the intercellular spaces in bone, fibrous connective tissue, cartilage, or bone (also known as matrix).

Growth factors: Substances that stimulate the production of specific types of cells.

Habituation: A function of the central nervous system that filters out nonmeaningful information.

Half-layer value: The depth, measured in cm, at which 50% of the ultrasonic energy has been absorbed by the tissues.

Heat capacity: See Thermal capacity.

Health Insurance Portability and Accountability Act: Federal legislation that ensures patient confidentiality during the electronic transfer of medical records.

Helium neon laser: See HeNe laser.

Hemarthrosis: Blood in a joint.

Hematoma: A mass of blood confined to a limited area, resulting from the subcutaneous leakage of blood.

Hemodynamic: The systemic and local characteristics of blood flow.

Hemoglobinemia: An excessive proportion of hemoglobin in plasma as the result of the separation of hemoglobin from red blood cells.

Hemorrhage: Bleeding from veins, arteries, or capillaries.

HeNe laser: Laser produced by the excitation of helium and neon atoms.

Henry: A measure of inductance (H). One henry induces an electromagnetic force of 1 V when the current changes at a rate of 1 A per second.

Heparin: An inflammatory mediator produced by the mast cells of the liver. It inhibits the clotting process by preventing the transformation of prothrombin into thrombin.

Hertz (Hz): The number of cycles per second.

High frequency (electrical stimulation): An electrical current having a frequency greater than 100,000 cps.

High TENS: The application of transcutaneous electrical nerve stimulation possessing high-frequency, short-duration pulses and applied at the sensory level.

HIPAA: See Health Insurance Portability and Accountability Act.

Histamine: A blood-thinning chemical released from damaged tissue during the inflammatory process. Its primary function is vasodilation of arterioles and increased vascular permeability in venules.

Hives: See Urticaria.

Homeostasis: State of equilibrium in the body and its systems that provides a stable internal environment.

Homunculus: A map of the body's surface across a brain region, usually a gyrus of the cerebral cortex.

Hunting response: A vascular response to cold application marked by a series of vasoconstrictions and vasodilations. This response has been shown to occur only in limited body areas.

Hydrocortisone: An anti-inflammatory drug that closely resembles cortisol.

Hydropic: Relating to edema; an excessive amount of fluid.

Hydrostatic: Relating to the pressure of liquids in equilibrium or to the pressure they exert.

Hydrostatic pressure: The pressure of blood within the capillary.

Hyperalgesia, primary: Pain resulting from a lowering of the nerve's threshold.

Hyperalgesia, secondary: The spreading of pain caused by chemical mediators being released into the painful tissues.

Hyperemia: A red discoloration of the skin caused by increased blood flow. The skin turns white when pressure is applied.

Hypermobile: An abnormally large amount of motion.

Hypersensitive: Abnormally increased sensitivity; a condition in which there is an exaggerated response by the body to a stimulus.

Hypertension: High blood pressure.

Hyperthermia: Increased core temperature.

Hyperthyroidism: Metabolic disorder characterized by the overproduction of endocrine hormones and includes conditions such as Graves' disease and gonad tumors.

Hypertrophic: Increased size.

Hypertrophy: To develop an increase in bulk, for example, in the cross-sectional area of muscle.

Hypomobile: An abnormal limitation of normal motion.

Hyporeflexia: Diminished function of the reflexes.

Hypotension: Low blood pressure.

Hypothalamus: The body's thermoregulatory center.

Hypothermia: Decreased core temperature.

Hypoxia: Lack of an adequate supply of oxygen.

ICD codes: See International Classification of Disease codes.

Immediate treatment: Used in the initial management of orthopedic injuries. Immediate treatment is composed of four components: rest, ice, compression, and elevation.

Impedance: The resistance to flow of an alternating current resulting from inductance and capacitance.

Impedance plethysmography: A determination of blood flow based on the amount of electrical resistance in the area.

Inductance: The degree to which a varying current can induce voltage, expressed in henries (H).

Induration: The hardening of tissue often caused by the deposition of fibroconnective cells.

Infection: A disease state produced by the invasion of a contaminating organism.

Inflammation: Tissue reaction to injury.

Inflammatory response, acute: The stage of the body's response to injury that attempts to isolate and localize the trauma.

Inflammatory response, maturation phase: The stage of injury response during which the body attempts to restore the orientation and function of the injured tissues.

Inflammatory response, proliferation phase: The stage of injury response during which the body prepares to rebuild the damaged tissues.

Infrapatellar: The distal portion of the patella including the patellar tendon.

Infrared light: Electromagnetic energy possessing a wavelength between 780 and 12,500 nm. Infrared light is invisible to the human eye.

Injury potential: Disruption of a tissue's normal electrical balance as a result of injury.

Innervated: Normal and sufficient nerve supply to a muscle, body area, and so on.

Institutional Review Board (IRB): An institutional agency that oversees medical investigations involving humans or animals by assuring compliance with federal regulations. In research involving humans, the IRB functions to protect the rights and health of the subjects.

Interferon gamma: A group of proteins released by white blood cells and fibroblasts when devouring the unwanted tissues. The gamma classification is also referred to as "angry macrophages" because of their heightened phagocytic activity.

Interleukin-8 (IL-8): Primarily produced by endothelial cells and macrophages, IL-8 enables immune cells into the tissues and acts as a chemotaxic for neutrophils.

Internal capsule: A massive band of ascending and descending fibers in the forebrain that connect the cerebral cortex to thalamus, brain stem, and spinal cord.

Internal fixation devices: Wires, screws, plates, or pins used to repair fractures.

International Classification of Disease codes (ICD): Standard nomenclature used to code injury and disease. ICD codes are used for research and reimbursement purposes.

Interneuron: A neuron connecting two nerves.

Interpulse interval: The elapsed time between the conclusion of one pulse and the start of the next.

Interstitial: Between the tissues.

Intra-articular: Within a joint.

Intracellular: Within the membrane of a cell.

Intramedullary rod: An internal fixation device placed with the marrow of fractured bone.

Intrapulse interval: The period within a discrete pulse when the current is not flowing. The duration of the intrapulse interval cannot exceed the duration of the interpulse interval.

Intrauterine device (IUD): A plastic or metal coil inserted within the uterus to prevent pregnancy.

Inverse square law: A law stating that the intensity of the energy striking the tissues is proportional to the square of the distance between the source of the energy and the tissues: Energy received = Energy at the source ÷ Distance from the source squared.

Ion: An atom, or group of atoms, with a net charge other than zero.

Iontophoresis: Introduction of ions into the body through the use of an electrical current.

Ipsilateral: On the same side of the body.

Ischemia: Local and temporary deficiency of blood supply caused by obstruction of circulation to a part.

Isoelectric point: The point at which positive and negative electrical points are equal. The electrical baseline of zero.

Isokinetic (contractions): A muscle contraction against a variable resistance where a limb moves through the range of motion at a constant speed.

Isometric: Muscle contraction without appreciable joint motion.

Isotonic (contractions): Muscle contraction through a range of motion against a constant resistance.

Joule: Basic unit of work in the International System of Units. One joule equals 0.74 foot-pounds of work. Joules = Coulombs × Volts.

Keloid: A nodular, firm, movable, and tender mass of dense, irregularly distributed collagen scar tissue in the dermis and subcutaneous tissue. Common in the African-American population, keloid scarring tends to occur after trauma or surgery.

Keratin: A dry, fibrous protein that replaces cytoplasm in the cells of the stratum corneum.

Kilohertz (kHz): One thousand cycles per second.

Kinetic energy: The energy possessed by an object by virtue of its motion.

Kinins: A group of polypeptides that dilate arterioles, serve as strong chemotactics, and produce pain. They are primarily involved in the inflammatory process in the early stages of vascular response.

Labile cells: Cells located in the skin, intestinal tract, and blood possessing good regenerative abilities.

Lactic acid: A cellular waste product produced by muscular contraction or cell metabolism. A fatiguing carbohydrate.

Laminectomy: Surgical removal of the lamina from a vertebra.

Laser: Acronym for *Light Amplification by Stimulated Emission of Radiation*. A highly organized beam of light.

Latent: Delayed period between the stimulus and the response.

Legal guardian: An individual who is legally responsible for the care of an infant or minor.

Leukocytes: White blood cells that serve as scavengers.

Leukotrienes: Fatty acids that cause smooth muscle contraction, increase vascular permeability, and attract neutrophils.

Libel: Defamation of character by the written word.

Limbic system: System in the brain that controls emotion.

Lipid: A broad category of fat-like substances.

Lissauer's tract: See Dorsolateral fasciculus.

Lordosis: The forward curvature of the cervical and lumbar spine.

Low frequency (electrical stimulation): An electrical current having a frequency of less than 1000 cps.

Low TENS: The application of transcutaneous electrical nerve stimulation using low-frequency, long-duration pulses, applied at a motor-level intensity.

Lucid: Of clear and rational mind.

Luminous infrared: See Near infrared.

Lupus: A chronic disorder of the body's immune system that affects the skin, joints, internal organs, and neurological system.

Lymphangitis: Inflammation of the lymphatic vessels draining an extremity. This condition is most often associated with inflammation or infection.

Lymphatic return: A return process similar to that of the venous network but specializing in the removal of interstitial fluids.

Lymphedema: Swelling of the lymph nodes caused by blockage of the vessels by protein-rich substances.

Macerated: Skin that has been softened by soaking in water.

Macrophage: A cell having the ability to devour particles; a phagocyte.

Magnetic resonance image (MRI): A view of the body's internal structures obtained through the use of magnetic and radio fields.

Malaise: Discomfort, mental fogginess, or disorientation. Often associated with infection or fever.

Malfeasance: The performance of an unlawful or improper act.

Malpractice: Negligence on the part of a professional person serving in the line of duty.

Malunion fracture: The faulty or incorrect healing of bone.

Margination: A state in which platelets and leukocytes, normally flowing in the bloodstream, begin to tumble along the walls of the vessel.

Master points: Points that, according to the theory of acupuncture, connect skin areas to deeper energy channels. Stimulating master points results in systemic changes.

McGill Pain Questionnaire: One of many pain rating scales, a method using pictures, scales, and words to describe the location, type, and magnitude of pain.

Mechanoreceptors: See Mechanosensitive receptors.

Mechanosensitive receptors: Nerve endings that are sensitive to mechanical pressure.

Medial lemniscus: The large bundle of fibers in the dorsal spinal cord formed by ascending second-order axons that carry touch and proprioceptive sensation.

Mediators: Chemicals that act through indirect means.

Medium: A material used to promote the transfer of energy. An object or substance that permits the transmission of energy through it.

Medium frequency (electrical stimulation): An electrical current having a frequency of 1000 to 100,000 cps.

Megahertz (MHz): One million cycles per second.

Melanin: Pigmentation of the hair, skin, and eye produced by melanocytes.

Meningitis: Inflammation of the membranes of the brain or spinal cord.

Meridians: In acupuncture, primary pathways through which the body's energy flows.

Messenger RNA (mRNA): Serves as the blueprint for protein synthesis.

Metabolism: The sum of physical and chemical reactions taking place within the body.

Metabolite: A by-product of metabolism.

Mho: The measure of a material's electrical conductance; the mathematical reciprocal of electrical resistance.

Microcoulomb: The charge produced by 10^{-6} electrons.

Micrometer (μm): 1/1,000,000 of a meter.

Microstreaming: During ultrasound application, the localized flow of fluids resulting from cavitation.

μm: Micrometer, 1/1,000,000 of a meter.

Microvolt (μV): One microvolt equals 1/1,000,000 of a volt.

Midline and intralaminar nuclei: Several medially placed thalamic nuclei that receive ascending pain information from the anterior lateral fasciculus and reticular nuclei.

Millivolt (mV): One millivolt equals 1/1000 of a volt.

Misfeasance: The improper performance of an otherwise lawful act.

Mitochondria: The portion of the cell—the "power plant"—that generates a cell's energy in the form of adenosine triphosphate (ATP).

Modality: The application of a form of energy to the body that elicits an involuntary response.

Modulate: To regulate or adjust.

Modulation: Regulation or adjustment.

Monochromatic: Light that consists of only one color.

Monocyte: A white blood cell that matures to become a macrophage.

Monophasic current: The unidirectional flow of electrons that is interrupted by discrete periods of noncurrent flow.

Monopolar stimulation: The application of electrical stimulation in which the current density under one set of electrodes (the active electrodes) is much greater than that under the other electrode (the dispersive electrode). All of the effects of the treatment should be experienced only under the active electrodes.

Motor-level stimulation: Electrical stimulation applied at an output intensity that produces a visible muscle contraction without activating pain fibers.

Motor nerve: A nerve that provides impulses to muscles.

Motor point: An area on the skin used to stimulate motor nerves.

Motor unit: A group of skeletal muscle fibers that are innervated by a single motor nerve.

Mottling: A blotchy discoloration of the skin.

Muscle, cardiac: Muscle associated with the heart and responsible for the pumping of blood.

Muscle guarding: A voluntary or subconscious contraction of a muscle to protect an injured area.

Muscle, skeletal: Responsible for the movement of the body's joints.

Muscle, smooth: Contractile tissue that is associated with the body's hollow organs. Smooth muscle is not under voluntary control.

Muscle spindle: An organ located within the muscular tissue that detects the rate and magnitude of a muscle contraction.

Muscular tissue: Tissue composed of smooth (found in the internal organs) cardiac and skeletal muscle; has the ability to actively shorten and passively lengthen.

Myelin: A fatty layer around nerves.

Myelinated: Having a fat-like outer coating (myelin) that serves as insulation for nerves.

Myocardial: Pertaining to the middle layer of the heart walls.

Myofibroblasts: Fibroblasts that have contractile properties.

Myoglobin: A blood-based protein that stores oxygen in the tissues.

Myonecrosis: Death of muscle tissue.

Myosin: Noncontractile muscle protein.

Myositis: Inflammation of muscular tissue.

Myositis ossificans: Ossification or deposition of bone in muscle fascia, resulting in pain and swelling.

Nanometer: One-billionth (10^{-9}) of a meter.

Nanosecond: One-billionth (10^{-9}) of a second.

Near field: The portion of an ultrasonic beam that is close to the sound head.

Near infrared: The range of infrared light that is closest to visible light, with wavelengths ranging between 770 and 1500 nm on the electromagnetic spectrum. Also known as luminous infrared.

Near ultraviolet: The range of light having wavelengths between 290 and 390 nm on the electromagnetic spectrum. This is the portion of the ultraviolet spectrum that is located the closest to visible light.

Necrosin: Increases the permeability of a cell membrane.

Necrosis: Cell death.

Negligence, gross: Intentional and conscious act or omission committed by an individual, with reckless disregard for the consequences.

Negligence, ordinary: Departure from the standard of care or duty. See also Omission and Commission.

Neoplasm: Abnormal tissue such as a tumor that grows at the expense of healthy organisms.

Neoprene: A synthetic rubber material.

Nervous tissue: Tissue possessing the ability to conduct electrochemical impulses.

Neuralgia: Pain following the path of a nerve; a hypersensitive nerve.

Neurapraxia: A temporary loss of function in a peripheral nerve.

Neurological: Pertaining to the nervous system.

Neuroma: Swelling or other mass formation around a nerve (Neuro = nerve; oma = tumor).

Neuropathy: Destruction, trauma, or inhibition of a nerve.

Neutron: An electrically neutral particle found in the center of an atom.

Nociceptive stimulus: Impulse giving rise to the sensation of pain.

Nociceptors: Specialized receptors on nerves that transmit pain impulses.

Nonfeasance: Failure to act when there is a duty to act.

Nonunion fracture: Fracture that fails to heal spontaneously within a normal time frame.

Norepinephrine: A hormone that causes vasoconstriction.

Normative data: Information that can be used to describe a specific population.

Noxious: Harmful, injurious, or painful. Capable of producing pain.

Noxious-level stimulation: Application of electrical stimulation that produces pain; caused by activation of C fibers.

Noxious-level TENS: Brief, intense electrical stimulation (above the threshold of pain) that is thought to activate the release of endogenous opiates.

Nucleus (Nuclei): A cluster of neurons in the CNS.

Nucleus cuneatus: A nucleus in the caudal medulla that relays fine touch and proprioceptive information from the upper body to the thalamus.

Nucleus gracilis: A nucleus in the caudal medulla that relays fine touch and proprioceptive information from the lower body to the thalamus.

Nucleus pulposus: The gelatinous middle of an intervertebral disk.

Numbness: Lack of sensation in a body part.

Occiput: The posterior base of the skull.

Occupational Safety and Health Administration (OSHA): A federal agency responsible for ensuring safe working conditions. This agency has enforcement powers and is capable of levying fines against employers.

Ohm: Unit of electrical resistance required to develop 0.24 calorie of heat when 1 A of current is applied for 1 second.

Ohm's law: A law stating that current is directly proportional to resistance: Amperage = Voltage/Resistance (I = V/R).

Omission: Failure to respond to a situation in which actions are necessary to limit or reduce harm.

Ordinary negligence: Failure to act as a reasonable and prudent person would act under similar circumstances.

Organelle: A specialized portion of a cell that performs a specific function, such as the mitochondria and the Golgi apparatus.

Orthotics: The use of orthopedic devices for correcting deformity or malalignment.

Osteoarthritis: Degeneration of a joint's articular surface.

Osteoblast: A cell involved in the formation of new bone.

Osteoclast: A cell that absorbs and removes unwanted bone.

Osteogenesis: Healing of fracture sites through the formation of callus, followed by the deposition of collagen and bone salts.

Osteomyelitis: Inflammation of the bone marrow and adjacent bone.

Osteophyte: A branching bony outgrowth.

Osteoporosis: A porous condition resulting in thinning of bone. Most commonly seen (but not exclusively) in postmenopausal women.

Outcome measures: Data that are used to evaluate the efficacy of a treatment program or protocol.

Overload principle: A principle stating that for strength gains to occur, the body must be subjected to more stress than it is accustomed to. This is accomplished by increasing the load, frequency, or duration of exercise.

Oxyhemoglobin: Hemoglobin that is carrying oxygen found in the arterial system.

Ozone: Formed by the grouping of three oxygen atoms (O_3). Ozone is present in the atmosphere, where it filters out ultraviolet light (especially in the C band), helping to prevent certain forms of cancer.

Pacinian corpuscles (pacinian receptors): Large encapsulated receptor organs found in the skin and deeper tissues. These rapid adapting receptors are best activated by an alternating stimulus, for example, a tuning fork. Within the joints, they assist in relaying proprioceptive information.

Pain threshold: The level of noxious stimulus required to alert the individual to possible tissue damage.

Pain tolerance: The amount of time an individual can endure pain.

Palliative: Pain relief without addressing the cause of the pain. Treatment only of the symptoms.

Pallor: Lack of color in the skin.

Paradoxical (Paradox): Two seemingly contradictory statements that are nonetheless true.

Parallel circuit: An electrical circuit in which electrons have more than one route to follow.

Pathology: Changes in structure or function caused by disease or trauma.

Pavementing: Adherence of platelets to the vessel walls in multiple layers to form a patch over the injury site.

Peak-to-peak value: The sum of a pulse's maximum deviation above and below the baseline.

Penetration: Depth at which energy absorption takes place.

Perfusion: Local blood flow that supplies tissues and organs with oxygen and nutrients.

Periaqueductal gray nucleus: A midbrain nucleus that lies around the cerebral aqueduct. This nucleus regulates pain sensation through descending multisynaptic projections to the dorsal horn.

Periosteal pain: A deep-seated ache resulting from overly intense application of ultrasonic energy that irritates the bone's periosteum.

Peripatellar: Around the patella.

Peripheral vascular disease: A syndrome describing an insufficiency of arteries and/or veins for maintaining proper circulation (also known as PVD).

pH (potential of hydrogen): A measure of acidity or alkalinity (bases). A neutral solution has a pH of 7. Acids have a pH of less than 7; bases have a pH greater than 7.

Phagocyte: A classification of scavenger cells that ingest and destroy unwanted substances in the body.

Phagocytosis: The ingestion and digestion of bacteria and particles by phagocytes.

Phase: Individual sections of a single pulse that remain on one side of the baseline for a period.

Phase duration: The amount of time for a single phase to complete its route. During monopolar application, the terms "phase duration" and "pulse duration" are equivalent. The phase duration must be sufficient to cause depolarization.

Phonophoresis: The introduction of medication into the body through the use of ultrasonic energy.

Phosphocreatine: A compound that is important in muscle metabolism.

Photon: A unit of light energy that has zero mass, no electrical charge, and an indefinite life span.

Physical medicine codes: Billing codes used to describe rehabilitation and treatment services rendered.

Physis: The growth plate of bone.

Piezoelectric crystal: A crystal that produces positive and negative electrical charges when it is compressed or expanded.

Pitting edema: An exudate-rich form of edema characterized by being easily indented by pressure (hence, "pitting").

Placebo: A substance of no objective curative value given to a patient to satisfy a need for treatment or used as a control treatment in an experimental study. Interestingly, this word means "I shall please" in Latin.

Platelet: A free-flowing cell fragment in the bloodstream.

Pneumothorax: The collection of air in the pleural cavity (a void between the lungs and rib cage) that inhibits the lung's ability to expand.

Policies and procedures manual: An administrative manual that describes the operation of a department or agency.

Polymodal: Capable of being depolarized by different types of stimuli.

Polymorph: A type of white blood cell; a granulocyte.

Porphyria: Inherited disorder of hemoglobin, myoglobin, or cytochromes that results in light sensitivity and other complaints.

Postpolio syndrome: Musculoskeletal symptoms, including pain and atrophy, that affect patients 25 to 30 years after the original polio symptoms occurred.

Potential of hydrogen: See pH.

Power (electrical): See Watt.

Precedent: A previous ruling that serves as a guide in future legal action.

Precursor: A substance that is formed before changing into its final state or substance.

Prepatellar: Around the patella.

Primary afferent fiber: The complete nerve fiber—both peripheral and central process—of a first-order neuron.

Primary hyperalgesia: Increased pain sensation near the site of injury.

Pronation: An inward flattening and tilting of the foot, resulting in the lowering of the medial longitudinal arch.

Propagation (Propagate): Transmission through a medium.

Prothrombin: A chemical found in the blood that reacts with an enzyme to produce thrombin.

Proton: A positively charged atomic particle.

Protopathic pain: Poorly localized pain sensation.

Psoralen: A group of substances that produce inflammation of the skin when exposed to sunlight or ultraviolet light.

Psychogenic: Pain of mental rather than physical origin.

Pulsatile current: See Pulsed current.

Pulse charge: The number of coulombs contained in one electrical pulse.

Pulse duration: The amount of time from the initial nonzero charge to the return to a zero charge, including the intrapulse interval.

Pulse frequency: The number of electrical pulses that occur in a 1-second period.

Pulse interval: (ultrasound): The amount of time between ultrasonic pulses.

Pulse period: The period of time between the initiation of a pulse and the initiation of the subsequent pulse, including the phase duration(s), intrapulse interval, and interpulse interval.

Pulse width: See Pulse duration.

Pulsed current: A flow of electrons marked by discrete periods of nonelectron flow.

Q10 effect: Describes the relationship between tissue temperature and cell metabolism. For each 10°C increase in temperature, the cell's metabolism increases by a factor of 2 to 3.

Quadripolar stimulation: Electrical stimulation applied with two channels.

Radiant energy: Heat that is gained or lost through radiation.

Radiation: The transfer of electromagnetic energy that does not require the presence of a medium.

Radicular: Distally radiating pain caused by spinal nerve root involvement.

Range of motion: The distance, measured in degrees, that a limb moves in one plane (e.g., flexion-extension, adduction-abduction).

Raynaud's phenomenon: A vascular reaction to cold application or stress that results in a white, red, or blue discoloration of the extremities. The fingers and toes are the first to be affected.

Rebound vasoconstriction: A reflex constriction of blood vessels caused by prolonged exposure to extreme temperatures.

Reflection: The return of waves from an object.

Refraction: The bending of a wave as it passes through an object.

Regeneration (tissue): Restoration of damaged tissues with cells of the same type and function as the damaged cells.

Reimbursement: Payment for services rendered.

Replacement (tissue): Replacement of damaged tissues by cells of a different type from the original.

Resistance stage: The second stage in the general adaptation syndrome. During this stage, the body adapts to the stresses placed on it.

Resistor (electrical): A material that has few free electrons and opposes the flow of electricity. Within the body, tissues having a low water content are considered resistors.

Resonating: Vibrating.

Respondeat superior: See Vicarious liability.

Reticular nuclei (reticular formation): A diffuse network of cells and fibers located in the brain stem. The reticular formation influences alertness, waking, sleeping, and certain reflexes.

Retinaculum: A fibrous membrane that holds an organ or body part in place.

Retinoid: Topical medication consisting of retinoic acid. Used to treat psoriasis and severe acne.

Rheobase: The minimum amount of voltage under the negative pole that is required for depolarization when a direct current is applied to living tissues.

Ribonucleic acid: Controls protein synthesis.

Rickets: Common in children, a vitamin D deficiency that results in inadequate deposition of lime salts, altering the shape, structure, and function of bone.

RNA: See Ribonucleic acid.

Root-mean-square (RMS) value: A conversion of the electrical power delivered by an alternating current into the equivalent direct current power, calculated by multiplying the peak value by 0.707.

Salicylates: A family of analgesic compounds that includes aspirin.

Satellite cell: Spindle-shaped cell that assists in the repair of skeletal muscle.

Sclerotome: A portion of bone that is supplied by a spinal nerve root.

Scoliosis: Lateral curvature of the spinal column in the frontal plane. See also Functional scoliosis and Structural scoliosis.

Secondary hypoxic injury: Cell death resulting from a lack of oxygen.

Second-order neuron: A nerve having its body located in the spinal cord. It connects second- and third-order neurons (nerves having their bodies in the thalamus and extending into the cerebral cortex).

Sedation: The result of calming nerve endings.

Sedative: An agent that causes sedation.

Self-treatment: Treatment or rehabilitation performed by the patient without direct supervision, including home treatment programs.

Sensitization: The process of being made sensitive to a specific substance.

Sensory-level stimulation: Electrical stimulation applied at an intensity at which sensory nerves are stimulated without also producing a muscle contraction.

Sequential compression: Compression of an extremity characterized by a distal to proximal flow.

Series circuit: A circuit in which the current has only one path to follow.

Serotonin: A substance that causes local vasodilation and increases permeability of the capillaries.

Sham: A device that has no physiological effect on the body (e.g., an ultrasound unit with the output intensity set to zero). Sham devices are often used during research to determine the actual biophysical effects of a treatment by comparing the results of an actual treatment to a patient who is receiving no treatment.

Silica: A finely ground form of sand capable of holding water.

Singlet oxygen: An uncharged form of oxygen that can selectively destroy cells.

Slander: Defamation of character by the spoken word.

Somatic: Pertaining to the body.

Somatic receptive field: Area to which a stimulus is applied to obtain the optimum response.

Somatosensory cortex: An area in the cerebral cortex, located in the postcentral gyrus of the parietal lobe, that is important in the perception of touch and proprioception and in the localization of pain sensation.

Specific gravity: The ratio of the density of a substance to the density of pure water taken as a standard when both densities are obtained by weighing in air.

Specific heat: The ratio of a substance's thermal capacity to that of water, which has a thermal capacity of 1. The specific heats of the three states of water are: ice 0.50, water 1, and steam 0.48.

Spherocytosis: An anemic condition in which red blood cells assume a spheroid shape.

Spondylolisthesis: Forward slippage of the lower lumbar vertebrae on the vertebrae above.

Spondylolysis: The breaking down of a vertebral structure.

Sprain: A stretching or tearing of ligaments.

Stable cavitation: The gentle expansion and contraction of bubbles formed during ultrasound application.

Stabile cells: Cells possessing some ability to regenerate.

Standard precautions: See Universal precautions.

Standards of practice: The criteria against which an individual's performance is measured.

Standing orders: A "blanket prescription" from a physician describing how injuries are to be managed when the physician is not present.

Standing wave: A single-frequency wave formed by the collision of two waves of equal frequency and speed traveling in opposite directions. The energy with a standing wave cannot be transmitted from one area to another and is focused in a confined area.

States of matter: The three forms of physical matter: solid, liquid, and gas. Using water as an example, we see the three states of matter as ice, water, and steam.

Statute of limitations: A legal time limit allowed for the filing of a lawsuit.

Strain: A stretching or tearing of tendons or muscles.

Stratum basale: The deepest layer of the lining of the uterus.

Stratum corneum: The outermost, nonliving portion of the epidermis.

Stress: A force that disrupts the normal homeostasis of a system.

Structural scoliosis: Lateral curvature of the spinal column caused by malformed vertebrae and/or intervertebral discs.

Subacute: Between the acute and chronic stages of the inflammatory stages.

Subcutaneous: Beneath the skin.

Subjective: Symptoms stated by the patient that are not externally apparent, such as pain. Personal beliefs and attitudes may alter subjective symptoms.

Substance P: A neurotransmitter thought to be responsible for the transmission of pain-producing impulses.

Summation: An overlap of muscle contractions that is caused by electrical stimulation.

Synapse: The junction at which two nerves communicate.

Synapse, chemical: The junction between two nerves that is characterized by a synaptic cleft. Chemical neurotransmitters carry the impulse from one nerve to the next.

Synapse, electrical: The junction between two nerves that is characterized by a gap junction. The nervous impulse is transferred directly to the subsequent nerve.

Synapse, excitatory: The release of the neurotransmitter tends to activate the postsynaptic nerve.

Synapse, inhibitory: The release of the neurotransmitter increases the nerve's resting potential, decreasing the probability that the nervous impulse will be propagated.

Synovitis: Inflammation of the synovial membrane.

Synovium: Membrane lining the capsule of a joint.

Systemic: Affecting the body as a whole.

T cell: A transmission cell that connects sensory nerves to the central nervous system. Not to be confused with T cells found in the immune system. See Tract cell.

Temporal average intensity: The average amount of power delivered to the body during pulsed ultrasound.

Tendinitis: Inflammation of the tendon.

Tendinopathy: Any disease or trauma involving a muscle's tendon, tissues surrounding the tendon, or the tendon's insertion into the bone.

Tendinosis: Degeneration of a tendon from repetitive microtrauma or collagen degeneration within a tendon.

Tensile strength: The ability of a structure to withstand a pulling force along its length. Resistance to tear.

Tesla: A unit of magnetic strength. 1 tesla = 1000 gauss.

Tetany: Total contraction of a muscle achieved through the recruitment and contraction of all motor units.

Thalamus: Gray matter located at the base of the brain.

Therapeutic: Having healing properties.

Thermal capacity: The number of heat units required to raise a unit of mass by 1°C.

Thermal conductivity: The quantity of heat (in calories per second) passing through a 1-cm-thick by 1-cm-wide substance having a temperature gradient of 1°C.

Thermolysis: Chemical decomposition caused by heating.

Thermoreceptors: Sensory receptors that detect temperature.

Thermotherapy: The application of therapeutic heat to living tissues.

Third-order neuron: A nerve having its body located in the thalamus and extending into the cerebral cortex.

Thoracic duct: A central collection point for the lymphatic system. The contents of the thoracic duct are routed into the left subclavian vein, where it returns to the blood system.

Thrombin: An enzyme formed in the blood of a damaged area.

Thrombophlebitis: Inflammation of the veins.

Thrombosis: The formation or presence of a blood clot within the vascular system.

Tissue hydrostatic pressure: The pressure that moves fluids from the tissues into the capillaries.

Tonic contraction: Prolonged contraction of a muscle.

Tract cell: Second-order neuron of the pain and temperature pathways. The axons of these cells cross the midline of the spinal cord and ascend in the anterior lateral fasciculus. Tract cells are sometimes called T cells, but this should not be confused with the T cells of the immune system. See T cell.

Transcutaneous: Through the skin.

Transdermally (transdermal): Introduction of medication to the subcutaneous tissues through unbroken skin.

Transducer: A device that converts one form of energy to another.

Transduction: The process of converting a stimulus into action potentials.

Transfer: Assisted patient mobility, such as when moving from a wheelchair to a bed.

Transient cavitation: See Unstable cavitation.

Translation: Sliding or gliding of opposing articular surfaces.

Trigger point: A localized area of spasm within a muscle.

Turf burn: A deep abrasion caused by friction between the skin and artificial playing surfaces.

Twitch contraction: Repeated muscle contraction characterized by the fibers returning to their original length subsequent to the next contraction. Twitch contractions are distinguishable from each other.

Tympanic membrane: The eardrum.

Type I muscle fibers: Muscle fibers that generate a relatively low level of force but can sustain contractions for a long period. Geared to aerobic activity, these muscle fibers are also referred to as tonic or slow-twitch fibers.

Type II muscle fibers: Muscle fibers that generate a large amount of force in a short time. Geared to anaerobic activity, they are also referred to as phasic or fast-twitch fibers.

Ultraviolet light: Energy on the electromagnetic spectrum having a wavelength between 180 and 390 nm. Ultraviolet light is invisible to the human eye.

Universal precautions: A series of steps, established by OSHA, that individuals should take to avoid accidental exposure to blood-borne pathogens.

Unstable cavitation: The violent oscillation and subsequent rupture of bubbles during ultrasound application at too high an intensity.

Upper motor neuron lesion: A spinal cord lesion resulting in paralysis, loss of voluntary movement, spasticity, sensory loss, and pathological reflexes.

Uremic pruritus: Itching caused by increased blood content in urine.

Urticaria: Skin vascular reaction to an irritant characterized by red, itchy areas, wheals, or papules. Commonly referred to as hives.

Valence shell: An imaginary shell in which the electrons responsible for chemical reactivity orbit around the nucleus of an atom.

Vascular endothelial growth factor (VEGF): Encourages capillary formation that precedes bone healing.

Vasoconstriction: Reduction in a blood vessel's diameter, resulting in a decrease in blood flow.

Vasodilation: Increase in a blood vessel's diameter, resulting in an increase in blood flow.

Vasomotor: Muscles and their associated nerves acting on arteries and veins that cause constriction and/or dilation.

Venous stasis ulcer: Ischemic necrosis and ulceration of tissue, especially that overlying bony prominences, caused by prolonged pressure. Also referred to as decubitus ulcers or bedsores.

Ventral posterior lateral nucleus: A nucleus in the posterior thalamus that receives fibers from the anterior lateral fasciculus and medial lemniscus.

Ventral white commissure: The bundle of fibers in the spinal cord through which second-order pain fibers cross the midline before entering the anterior lateral fasciculus.

Venule: A small vein exiting from a capillary.

Vicarious liability: Liability of employers for the acts of their employees.

Visceral: Pertaining to organs of the body.

Viscosity: The resistance of a fluid to flow.

Visible light: Electromagnetic energy possessing a wavelength between 390 and 760 nm. Visible light is a combination of violet, indigo, blue, green, yellow, orange, and red.

Vitamin D: Needed for bone formation and normal endocrine, intestine, and brain function.

Voltage: A measure of the potential for electrons to flow.

Volumetric measurement: Determination of the size of a body part by measuring the amount of water it displaces.

Wallerian degeneration: Gradual physiological breakdown of a nerve axon that has been severed from its body.

Watt: A unit of electrical power. For an electrical current: Watts = Voltage × Amperage.

Weaning: Decreasing dependence on a substance or device by gradually reducing its use.

White light: See Visible light.

Wide dynamic range cells (neurons): Neurons in the spinal cord and thalamus that respond to a broad range of mechanical pressures. They respond to both touch and pain.

Withdrawal reflex: A multisynaptic spinal reflex that is normally elicited by a noxious stimulus. Muscle groups are activated so that the body is moved away from the damaging stimulus.

Work hardening: Job-specific exercises used to prevent work-related injuries or to rehabilitate injured workers.

X-ray: An electromagnetic wave 0.05 to 100 Å in length that is able to penetrate most solid matter.

Index

Page numbers followed by "f" denote figures, "t" denote tables, and "b" denote boxes